Textbook of Hematology

Textbook of Hematology

Edited by **Brian Jenkins**

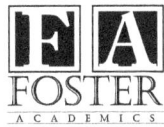

FA

FOSTER
ACADEMICS

New Jersey

Published by Foster Academics,
61 Van Reypen Street,
Jersey City, NJ 07306, USA
www.fosteracademics.com

Textbook of Hematology
Edited by Brian Jenkins

International Standard Book Number: 978-1-63242-450-1 (Hardback)

The publisher's policy is to use permanent paper from mills that operate a sustainable forestry policy. Furthermore, the publisher ensures that the text paper and cover boards used have met acceptable environmental accreditation standards.

Trademark Notice: Registered trademark of products or corporate names are used only for explanation and identification without intent to infringe.

Printed in the United States of America.

Contents

Preface

Blood is the carrier of oxygen and oxygen in turn is responsible for all the biological activities inside the body. Hematology is the study of blood and deals with the treatment and diagnosis of problems related to it such as anemia, myeloma, leukemia, lymphoma, blood clots, etc. This book provides comprehensive insights into this field. It studies in detail the various components of blood such as hemoglobin, platelets, blood cells, etc. This book is a collective contribution of a renowned group of international experts. It is a complete source of knowledge on the present status of this important field. Students, researchers, experts and all associated with this discipline will be benefitted from this book.

Various studies have approached the subject by analyzing it with a single perspective, but the present book provides diverse methodologies and techniques to address this field. This book contains theories and applications needed for understanding the subject from different perspectives. The aim is to keep the readers informed about the progress in the field; therefore, the contributions were carefully examined to compile novel researches by specialists from across the globe.

Indeed, the job of the editor is the most crucial and challenging in compiling all chapters into a single book. In the end, I would extend my sincere thanks to the chapter authors for their profound work. I am also thankful for the support provided by my family and colleagues during the compilation of this book.

Editor

Achievement of Therapeutic Goals with Low-Dose Imiglucerase in Gaucher Disease: A Single-Center Experience

Irina Tukan,[1] Irith Hadas-Halpern,[1] Gheona Altarescu,[2] Ayala Abrahamov,[1] Deborah Elstein,[1] and Ari Zimran[1]

[1] *Shaare Zedek Medical Center, Affiliated to the Hadassah-Hebrew University School of Medicine, Ein Karem 91031, Israel*
[2] *Gaucher Clinic and Preimplantation Genetics Unit, Shaare Zedek Medical Center, Affiliated to the Hadassah-Hebrew University School of Medicine, Ein Karem 91031, Israel*

Correspondence should be addressed to Deborah Elstein; elstein@szmc.org.il

Academic Editor: David Varon

Gaucher disease, a lysosomal storage disorder, is a multisystem disorder with variable and unpredictable onset and severity. Disease-specific enzyme replacement therapy (ERT) has been shown to reverse or ameliorate disease-specific hepatosplenomegaly and anemia and thrombocytopenia. ERT also impacts bone manifestations, including bone crises, bone pain, and appearance of new osteonecrosis, and improves bone mineral density to varying degrees. The objective of this study was to assess achievement of predefined therapeutic goals based on international registry outcomes for Israeli patients with Gaucher disease receiving imiglucerase for four consecutive years on a low-dose regimen followed in a single center. All data were taken from patient files. The therapeutic goals were taken from standards published in the literature for disease-specific clinical parameters. Among 164 patients at baseline, values for spleen and liver volumes, hemoglobin and platelet counts, and Z-scores for lumbar spine and femoral were significantly different from the goal. After four years ERT, there was a significant improvement ($P = 0.000$) in each of the therapeutic goal parameters from baseline. 15.2% of these patients achieved all hematology-visceral goals. In children, there was achievement of linear growth and puberty. This survey highlights the good overall response in symptomatic patients receiving low-dose ERT with imiglucerase in Israel.

1. Introduction

Gaucher disease, a prevalent lysosomal storage disorder, is a multisystem disorder with variable and unpredictable onset and severity especially in the common nonneuronopathic form [1]. Patients with nonneuronopathic (type 1) Gaucher disease may suffer from varying degrees of splenomegaly, hepatomegaly, thrombocytopenia, bleeding tendencies, anemia, hypermetabolism, skeletal pathology, growth retardation in children, and/or pulmonary disease; invariably, health-related quality of life is affected. Age of onset may be in any decade of life, and there are no apparent triggers to onset; yet there are also periods of quiescence even in patients with severe manifestations such as debilitating and irreversible skeletal complications. Disease characteristics, including genotype, provide only a statistical estimation of the expected trajectory of the signs and symptoms of the disease for any particular patient.

Disease-specific enzyme replacement therapy (ERT) with mannose-terminated glucocerebrosidase (alglucerase, Ceredase, Genzyme Corporation, Cambridge, MA, USA) was introduced in 1991 [2]. Subsequently, a recombinant enzyme (imiglucerase, Cerezyme, Genzyme Corporation, Cambridge, MA) superseded the placental product [3, 4] and has been shown to reverse or ameliorate many of the visceral and hematological manifestations of Gaucher disease. ERT also impacts bone manifestations, including bone crises, bone pain, and appearance of new osteonecrosis in the joints and pathological fractures, and improves bone mineral density (BMD) to varying degrees [5]. However, due to the variable patterns of onset, progression, and severity, the initiation of treatment and the evaluation of the therapeutic response have often been controversial [6].

In 2004, a group of international experts in Gaucher disease [7] defined a set of therapeutic goals for the primary parameters of Gaucher disease that would benchmark successful interventions. These "goals" reflected the experience recorded for ERT with imiglucerase and as such also provided a means to assess alternative therapies and modalities as they enter the clinical arena. The goals as described at that time were derived from a decade of experience and data from more than 3000 patients treated with imiglucerase as reported to the International Collaborative Gaucher Group (ICGG); the registry is supported by the Genzyme Corporation (now a Sanofi company). Specifically, the achieved therapeutic response, respectively, in the realms of anemia, thrombocytopenia, hepatomegaly, splenomegaly, (four features of) skeletal pathology, and health-related quality of life (HRQoL) following a minimum of four years of imiglucerase exposure was equal to the therapeutic goal for that feature. However, monitoring these therapeutic goal achievements has proved difficult even among registry cohorts because more than half the patients evaluated had incomplete/partial clinical responses relative to these therapeutic goals [8]. Nonetheless, among the findings [8] garnered from these studies is that the higher-dose regimen (60 units/kg body weight/every-other-week) achieves a more rapid response relative to that achieved with lower doses (15 units/kg body weight/every-other-week) in the key disease-specific parameters of anemia, thrombocytopenia, and spleen and liver sizes; also see [3].

The purpose of the current study was to assess achievement of the therapeutic goals for patients receiving imiglucerase for four consecutive years on a constant low-dose regimen which is the standard in Israel for symptomatic Gaucher disease [9].

2. Methods

Our local institutional review board (Helsinki Committee) deemed that patient consent was not required for this retrospective analysis.

Beginning in 1992 [4], all patients who initiated ERT with imiglucerase were included if there was a complete data set from advent of ERT and after approximately 4 years of uninterrupted exposure to imiglucerase and at a constant dosage of 15 units/kg body weight/every-other-week for most of the adults and 30/kg body weight/every-other-week for most of the children (<14 years at start of ERT and <18 years at end of study). These dosing regimens are those that are standard for all patients who have been approved for ERT by the Gaucher Committee of the Israeli National Ministry of Health.

All data were taken from patient files. Laboratory tests were performed in the central hematology laboratory of the Shaare Zedek Medical Center. Spleen and liver volumes were performed by ultrasonography by a single senior radiologist (IH-H) using the three long axes with the organ volume considered a multiplicand of these [10].

Complaints of bone pain at any site were culled from the patient files.

Evidence of new osteonecrosis was based on radiological evidence in comparison to the full plain X-ray set taken at presentation in all patients; new complaints and/or functional changes were indications for complaint-specific radiological work-up in any patient at any time.

Bone mineral density (BMD) and Z-scores were performed using dual energy X-ray absorptiometry (DXA; Hologic, Bedford, MA, USA) at the lumbar spine (LS) and femoral neck (FN) according to the manufacturer's instructions.

The therapeutic goals were taken from Pastores et al. [7] for the clinical parameters. For pediatric patients who entered the study at age <14 years, achievement of puberty and (pediatric) height was also included.

Since our clinic does not provide tools of health-related quality of life as part of the annual follow-up protocol, this feature of the therapeutic goals is not included.

2.1. Statistical Analysis. Descriptive statistics were used and one-sample (two-tailed) Student's t-test was applied to ascertain whether goals were achieved after four years of ERT. A significance level of 5% was predetermined. Logistic regressions with start and end measures as independent and/or predictors were employed when controlling for the possible confounders and/or proposed predictors of gender, age, and splenic status to control for these factors that might impact attainment of the therapeutic goal.

3. Results

There were 164 patients who met the criteria for inclusion; that is, they had been receiving a constant dose for approximately four years from advent of ERT.

There were 42 patients for whom there was documentation about puberty and/or pediatric height while on ERT (ages 4–14 years at start of study).

Of all patients, 65 patients (39.6%) were male; the mean age was 39.7 years, range 8–78 years, at end of the four years. There were 59 patients (36%) who were homozygous for the N370S mutations, and the rest had various compound heterozygous genotypes but not all with one N370S allele. There were 35 patients (21.3%) who were splenectomized.

Table 1 presents the mean values at baseline and after four years of ERT with imiglucerase and the percent achieving respective therapeutic goals. Table 2 provides the therapeutic goals as per Pastores et al. [7] for comparison as to the expectations regarding values that are "at goal" at presentation or at any point thereafter. According to these criteria, not all disease-specific parameters are expected to normalize within four years, and hence comparison to local normal values was not employed. Importantly, <10% were at goal for anemia at baseline, and in addition, despite the fact that 21% of patients were splenectomized, the mean platelet counts at baseline was below the lower limit of the normal range. The mean BMD Z-scores for LS and FN were both in the negative range with the mean LS Z-score in the osteopenic range; despite the fact that children and splenectomized patients were included, only 70% were at goal at baseline for BMD Z-scores.

TABLE 1: Baseline values for surveyed parameters and after 4 years ($n = 164$), P value between value of difference at four years from baseline, and percent of patients achieving goal for that parameter at four years (Student's t-test and logistic regression with significance level of 5% were predetermined.). Therapeutic goals are as described by Pastores et al. (2004) [7] and as presented in Table 2.

	Hemoglobin (gm/dL)	Platelet counts (×10/mm^3)	Spleen (US) index volume ($n = 129$)	Liver (US) index volume	Bone pain	New bone crises	New osteonecrosis	LS BMD	LS Z-score ($n = 114$)	FN BMD	FN Z-score ($n = 112$)	Pediatric height	Puberty
Mean ± SD baseline	10.95 ± 1.77	125.61 ± 85.00	2595.18 ± 2423.57	5259.95 ± 3048.00	0.57 ± 0.50	0.09 ± 0.28	0.22 ± 0.41	1.00 ± 0.13	[−1.48]±1.43	1.02 ± 0.19	[−0.92]±1.88	101.57±24.15	0.00
Mean ± SD 4 years	12.72 ± 1.74	177.01 ± 100.86	1645.43 ± 1356.71	4119.49 ± 1571.65	0.38 ± 0.49	0.02 ± 0.16	0.06 ± 0.24	1.06 ± 0.07	[−1.13]±1.18	0.98 ± 0.19	[−0.80]±1.61	145.74±22.33	0.51 ± 0.51
P value	0.000	0.000	0.000	0.000	0.000	0.000	0.000	0.000	0.000	0.000	0.000	0.000	0.000
% at goal at 4 years	81.7%	68.9%	60.0%	53.1%	59.9%	93.8%	92.6%	NA	69.9%	NA	70.6%	100%	48.8%

US: ultrasound; NA: not applicable.

TABLE 2: Long-term goals (2–5 years) for adults (Pastores et al., 2004 [7]).

Anemia	Women: increasing hemoglobin concentration to ≥11 g/dL; Men: increasing hemoglobin concentration to ≥12 g/dL; Maintaining improved hemoglobin value achieved in first 1-2 years
Thrombocytopenia	Moderate thrombocytopenia at baseline $(60-120 \times 10^9/\text{L})$: Increase platelet count 1.5 to 2 times by 1 Year, and approach low normal platelet count values by 2 Year. Severe thrombocytopenia at baseline $(<60 \times 10^9/\text{L})$: increasing platelet count 1.5 times by 1 Year and continuing to improve platelet counts slightly (2 times by 2 Year)
Splenomegaly	Decreasing spleen volume by 30–50% within 1 Year; reducing and maintaining spleen volume to ≤2–8 times normal or decreasing volume by 50–60% by 2–5 Years
Hepatomegaly	Decreasing liver volume by 20–30% within 1-2 Years; reducing and maintaining liver volume to 1.0 to 1.5 times normal or reducing liver volume by 30–40% by 3–5 Years
Bone pain	Lessening or eliminating bone pain in 1-2 years
Bone crises	Preventing bone crises
Osteonecrosis	Preventing osteonecrosis and joint collapse
Skeletal pathology	Improving trabecular BMD by 3–5 years

TABLE 3: Percent of patients achieving therapeutic goals in 4 years.

Therapeutic goal	Current study ($n = 164$)	Change in 4 years
Anemia	9.1% to 81.7%	72.6%
Thrombocytopenia	20.7% to 68.9%	48.2%
Splenomegaly	60.0% at 4 years	ND
Hepatomegaly	53.1% at 4 years	ND
No bone pain	42.1% to 59.9%	17.8%
No bone crises	91.5% to 93.8%	2.3%
No osteonecrosis	78.7% to 92.6%	13.9%
LS Z-score	69.9% at 4 years	ND
FN Z-score	70.6% at 4 years	ND

*ND: not done.

At baseline, values for the four hematology-visceral parameters and BMD Z-scores for LS and FN were significantly different than the goal as per Table 2. At the end of four years, there was a significant improvement ($P = 0.000$) in each of the parameters from baseline; between 60% and 94% of patients achieved the respective goals at four years. 15.2% of all the patients achieved therapeutic goals in both hematological and visceral parameters within 4 years.

For the pediatric patients, because not all the children had achieved the age of sexual maturation at the end of the study, then, as to be expected, only some of them achieved the goal (albeit statistically significant for the group). Similarly, for these children, but also for the young adults who had not achieved the age of peak bone density (25–30 years), the goal was improvement in the absolute value of BMD (as versus improvement in T-scores which were not used in this study for this reason), and this was statistically significant after four years for the cohort.

Table 3 shows achievement of therapeutic goals after four years in the current cohort on low-dose (mean = 34.2 units/kg/4 weeks) imiglucerase. Table 3 also shows the differences in percentages from baseline to four years where possible. The current cohort had 35 patients (21.3%) who were splenectomized at baseline and would be expected to have high-normal platelet counts: but only 37 patients (22.6%) had platelet counts >150,000/mm^3 at baseline, and not all of these were the splenectomized patients.

For the goal of BMD (at both LS and FN), only an improvement in absolute values was considered as achieving the therapeutic goal (see above); however, for the respective Z-scores, achieving a normal value of 0 or better (non-negative score) was considered as achieving the therapeutic goal.

When logistic regression was applied to ascertain the effect of gender, age, or spleen status on each of the hematological (hemoglobin and platelet counts) and visceral (spleen and liver size), the only significant effect was on liver size by gender ($P = 0.013$) and age ($P = 0.008$) where achievement of the goal of decreasing liver size was less in males and in younger patients, respectively. However, when applying analysis of variance (ANOVA) post hoc with the therapeutic goal of each of the above four parameters, respectively, as a dependent variable and the other variables constant (gender, genotype, age, and parameter values at start and end), all were significant ($P = 0.000$).

4. Discussion

With more than two decades of experience with imiglucerase, there is abundant evidence of its effectiveness in amelioration of the disease-specific parameters of Gaucher disease. Nonetheless, the issue of dosage has never been resolved in a practical sense. In 1995, the seminal papers on safety and efficacy of imiglucerase in the context of two clinical trials were published, which, respectively, showed approximately equivalent efficacy of the recombinant enzyme imiglucerase relative to placenta-derived alglucerase at 60 units/kg/infusion [3] and equivalent efficacy at low-frequency (every-other-week) relative to high frequency (three times a week) in a low-dose (15 units/kg/infusion) regimen [4]. While the manufacturer (Genzyme Corporation, Cambridge, MA, USA) originally recommended the high-dose regimen, countries with limited health budgets were not uncomfortable to adopt the low-dose regimen. Nonetheless, it was also obvious that higher dosing regimens were able to achieve better numerical values than those achieved at lower doses. Indeed, by cognizance of these findings and despite the fact that the starting regimens for ERT in Israel are 15 units/kg and 30 units/kg biweekly for adults and children, respectively, in the past there had always been recourse to the Israeli National Gaucher Committee to request doubling of the dose for those patients whose response was deemed inadequate by the treating physician. Nonetheless, with regard to the responses to imiglucerase based on a recent analysis of ICGG data [11] that demonstrated differences in response in favor of higher dosages, the actual clinical significance of those differences in patients who may have responded well to lower doses (albeit more slowly) is debatable [12].

However, along with acknowledging the importance of inducing a rapid response in patients with life-threatening symptoms and signs, there is an appreciation of the actual symptoms and signs of most patients with type 1 Gaucher disease at presentation which are not life-threatening. It is the case in many of the wealthier countries that all identified patients with Gaucher disease are treated, and mostly at the high-dose regimen. This is dramatically different in less wealthy countries such as Israel where only symptomatic patients who meet the disease-specific severity criteria of a national Gaucher Committee are eligible for governmental reimbursement/support of this expensive therapy. This is clearly evident in the baseline characteristics of the current cohort versus that of Weinreb et al. [8] (which also includes some patients from our clinic). The overall implication from the current data as a stand-alone report about the effect of low-dose regimen in achieving the standard therapeutic goals is that even in very symptomatic patients there will be a beneficial response within four years. The percent of patients achieving those goals is not greatly different than those benchmarked by Weinreb et al. [8]. Although some may contend that the quality of these comparisons (of achievement of goals for disease-specific parameters and also for the nonparametric markers) is imperfect, making interpretation difficult, in that the Gaucher community has come to accept the Pastores et al. criteria as a benchmark of therapeutic response, we are comfortable with these outcomes using low-dose regimens.

The means for all parameters including pediatric height and achievement of puberty were significantly lower than expected at baseline based on goals to achieve improved status and/or normalization. This underscores the fact that the patients in this cohort were approved for ERT by virtue of comparable objective criteria; that is, they presented with these same criteria in order to be eligible for ERT. In all parameters, there was a significant increase in mean values from baseline to four years. It is also noteworthy that the mean platelet counts were below the normal range at baseline despite a large percentage of splenectomized patients. This reflects the fact that for some patients who initiated ERT many years after splenectomy (most often in childhood in the era before ERT), platelet counts did not remain in the upper normal range, and the progressive decrease in counts was a continuing marker of disease severity.

Regarding achievement of age-specific goals in the pediatric patients, it is important to note that, in a report from the ICGG of the effect of imiglucerase on children [13], median height Z-score was −1.4 at baseline but required eight years of ERT to approximate the median value for the normal population. In the current cohort, virtually all the children,

who were at least 18 years at the end of the 4-year study period, had achieved midparental height within four years.

Drilling down to the outcomes presented here for the entire cohort, one notes that genotype was not predictive of achieving any of the goals, despite the fact that there was a majority of patients who were compound heterozygotes (and not necessarily with even one N370S allele). Age and gender impacted achieving goals only for liver size for which this may be an idiosyncratic finding and for which we have no clinical comparator.

Limitations of this study are that it is both retrospective and dependent on patients for whom there were all the parameters at nearly exactly four years from the advent of ERT. This paradigm disallowed those who do not come for annual followups, are not in Israel at the fourth annual followup, and those who either did or did not achieve the goals at a point earlier than four years but were recruited to clinical trials for switchover to a different ERT.

Another limitation is the issue of compliance with the ERT regimen because it was based on patients' claim of compliance.

The most important limitation of the study is that the evaluation of the therapeutic goals was at four years when the Pastores et al. [7] timeline for some of the goals is within one or two years. However, this limitation can be explained as derivative from the objectives of the study because the results in the current cohort were intended to also be compared to those of Weinreb et al. [8] who also used an approximately four-year interval.

5. Conclusions

In conclusion, this retrospective look at the achievement of therapeutic goals in a single Israeli center using low-dose imiglucerase in a real-life setting relative to what has heretofore been reported vis a vis the achievement of these goals at a mean of higher doses highlights the good overall response to imiglucerase in symptomatic patients. The issue of the clinical relevance of achieving goals has been raised with regard to the goal of improving hemoglobin because in Gaucher disease it has been shown to be correlated with the risk of avascular necrosis [14]. The goal for hemoglobin was achieved within four years in this cohort. It is also assumed that the remaining goals were achieved at a comparable timeline to the cohort at a higher mean ERT doses and that most patients approached improvement if not having actually achieved normalization of all parameters. The differential in responses among patients with Gaucher disease may be due to several reasons including (1) signs that are considered disease-specific but are actually multi-factorial such as bone pain; (2) differences in target organs/tissues before advent of ERT such as infarcted spleens and/or nodular livers that are poorly responsive to ERT [15]; (3) idiosyncratic events such as pregnancies or viral infections that impact hematological parameters and/or splenomegaly at the time of analysis; (4) associated diseases, being related or unrelated to Gaucher disease; and (5) adverse reactions to ERT whether as a hypersensitivity reaction or antibody formation that in some cases reduce efficacy and/or timeliness of response. Nonetheless, ERT with imiglucerase at a low-dose regimen benefits patients with respect to the predetermined therapeutic goals.

Acknowledgment

The help of Dr. Aviad (Emeritus, Open University, Jerusalem, Israel) in performing all the statistical analyses is gratefully acknowledged.

References

[1] A. Zimran and D. Elstein, "Lipid storage diseases," in *Williams Hematology*, M. A. Lichtman, T. Kipps, U. Seligsohn, K. Kaushansky, and J. T. Prchal, Eds., pp. 1065–1071, McGraw-Hill, New York, NY, USA, 8th edition, 2010.

[2] N. W. Barton, R. O. Brady, J. M. Dambrosia et al., "Replacement therapy for inherited enzyme deficiency: macrophage-targeted glucocerebrosidase for Gaucher's disease," *The New England Journal of Medicine*, vol. 324, no. 21, pp. 1464–1470, 1991.

[3] G. A. Grabowski, N. W. Barton, G. Pastores et al., "Enzyme therapy in type 1 Gaucher disease: comparative efficacy of mannose-terminated glucocerebrosidase from natural and recombinant sources," *Annals of Internal Medicine*, vol. 122, no. 1, pp. 33–39, 1995.

[4] A. Zimran, D. Elstein, E. Levy-Lahad et al., "Replacement therapy with imiglucerase for type 1 Gaucher's disease," *The Lancet*, vol. 345, no. 8963, pp. 1479–1480, 1995.

[5] N. J. Weinreb, J. Charrow, H. C. Andersson et al., "Effectiveness of enzyme replacement therapy in 1028 patients with type 1 Gaucher disease after 2 to 5 years of treatment: a report from the Gaucher registry," *The American Journal of Medicine*, vol. 113, no. 2, pp. 112–119, 2002.

[6] N. J. Weinreb, "Advances in Gaucher disease: therapeutic goals and evaluation and monitoring guidelines," *Seminars in Hematology*, vol. 41, no. 4, supplement 5, pp. 1–3, 2004.

[7] G. M. Pastores, N. J. Weinreb, H. Aerts et al., "Therapeutic goals in the treatment of Gaucher disease," *Seminars in Hematology*, vol. 41, no. 5, supplement 5, pp. 4–14, 2004.

[8] N. Weinreb, J. Taylor, T. Cox, J. Yee, and S. vom Dahl, "A benchmark analysis of the achievement of therapeutic goals for type 1 Gaucher disease patients treated with imiglucerase," *The American Journal of Hematology*, vol. 83, no. 12, pp. 890–895, 2008.

[9] D. Elstein, A. Abrahamov, I. Hadas-Halpern, A. Meyer, and A. Zimran, "Low-dose low-frequency imiglucerase as a starting regimen of enzyme replacement therapy for patients with type I Gaucher disease," *Quarterly Journal of Medicine*, vol. 91, no. 7, pp. 483–488, 1998.

[10] D. Elstein, I. Hadas-Halpern, Y. Azuri, A. Abrahamov, Y. Bar-Ziv, and A. Zimran, "Accuracy of ultrasonography in assessing spleen and liver size in patients with Gaucher disease: comparison to computed tomographic measurements," *Journal of Ultrasound in Medicine*, vol. 16, no. 3, pp. 209–211, 1997.

[11] G. A. Grabowski, K. Kacena, J. A. Cole et al., "Dose-response relationships for enzyme replacement therapy with imiglucerase/alglucerase in patients with Gaucher disease type 1," *Genetics in Medicine*, vol. 11, no. 2, pp. 92–100, 2009.

[12] E. Sidransky, G. M. Pastores, and M. Mori, "Dosing enzyme replacement therapy for Gaucher disease: older, but are we wiser?" *Genetics in Medicine*, vol. 11, no. 2, pp. 90–91, 2009.

[13] H. Andersson, P. Kaplan, K. Kacena, and J. Yee, "Eight-year clinical outcomes of long-term enzyme replacement therapy for 884 children with Gaucher disease type 1," *Pediatrics*, vol. 122, no. 6, pp. 1182–1190, 2008.

[14] A. Khan, T. Hangartner, N. J. Weinreb, J. S. Taylor, and P. K. Mistry, "Risk factors for fractures and avascular osteonecrosis in type 1 Gaucher disease—a study from the international collaborative Gaucher group (ICGG) Gaucher registry," *Journal of Bone and Mineral Research*, vol. 27, no. 8, pp. 1839–1848, 2012.

[15] P. Stein, A. Malhotra, A. Haims, G. M. Pastores, and P. K. Mistry, "Focal splenic lesions in type I Gaucher disease are associated with poor platelet and splenic response to macrophage-targeted enzyme replacement therapy," *Journal of Inherited Metabolic Disease*, vol. 33, no. 6, pp. 769–774, 2010.

Characterization of Zebrafish von Willebrand Factor Reveals Conservation of Domain Structure, Multimerization, and Intracellular Storage

Arunima Ghosh,[1] **Andy Vo,**[2] **Beverly K. Twiss,**[2] **Colin A. Kretz,**[1] **Mary A. Jozwiak,**[3] **Robert R. Montgomery,**[3] **and Jordan A. Shavit**[2]

[1] *Life Sciences Institute, University of Michigan, Ann Arbor, MI 48109, USA*
[2] *Department of Pediatrics, University of Michigan, Room 8301 Medical Science Research Building III, 1150 W. Medical Center Drive, Ann Arbor, MI 48109-5646, USA*
[3] *Blood Research Institute, Medical College of Wisconsin, Milwaukee, WI 53226, USA*

Correspondence should be addressed to Jordan A. Shavit, jshavit@umich.edu

Academic Editor: Elspeth Payne

von Willebrand disease (VWD) is the most common inherited human bleeding disorder and is caused by quantitative or qualitative defects in von Willebrand factor (VWF). VWF is a secreted glycoprotein that circulates as large multimers. While reduced VWF is associated with bleeding, elevations in overall level or multimer size are implicated in thrombosis. The zebrafish is a powerful genetic model in which the hemostatic system is well conserved with mammals. The ability of this organism to generate thousands of offspring and its optical transparency make it unique and complementary to mammalian models of hemostasis. Previously, partial clones of zebrafish *vwf* have been identified, and some functional conservation has been demonstrated. In this paper we clone the complete zebrafish *vwf* cDNA and show that there is conservation of domain structure. Recombinant zebrafish Vwf forms large multimers and pseudo-Weibel-Palade bodies (WPBs) in cell culture. Larval expression is in the pharyngeal arches, yolk sac, and intestinal epithelium. These results provide a foundation for continued study of zebrafish Vwf that may further our understanding of the mechanisms of VWD.

1. Introduction

Vertebrates possess a complex closed circulatory system that requires balanced coordination of various factors that serve to maintain blood flow as well as prevent exsanguination when the system is breached. This is known as hemostasis and consists of a complex array of cellular elements, as well as a network of proteins known as the coagulation cascade. The latter have been highly conserved at the genomic level throughout vertebrate evolution, including mammals, birds, reptiles, and fish [1–3].

One of the central components of coagulation is von Willebrand factor (VWF), deficiencies of which are the basis for the bleeding disorder von Willebrand disease (VWD). The mammalian *VWF* gene consists of 52 exons, and the largest, exon 28, contains several functional domains that are frequently mutated in VWD [4]. VWF is a 260 kDa (kilodalton) secreted glycoprotein that assembles into multimers of over 10,000 kDa [5]. At sites of injury, high molecular weight VWF multimers bind to receptors in the vascular subendothelium and tether platelets to form the primary hemostatic plug [6]. Much of our knowledge of VWF function is derived from characterization of mutations in humans and various mammalian model organisms, including mouse, dog, horse, cat, pig, and rabbit [7, 8]. However, relatively little information is available in other vertebrate models, such as the teleost *Danio rerio* (zebrafish). Teleost fish possess highly conserved orthologs of nearly all blood coagulation factors [1, 3] and have been shown to develop thrombosis in response to a laser-induced injury

[9]. Zebrafish embryonic development is external, rapid, and transparent, greatly simplifying phenotypic screening. Circulation begins approximately 24 hours after fertilization, and vascular development has been well characterized [10]. Forward genetic screens with chemical mutagenesis have been performed to study cardiogenesis, vasculogenesis, and angiogenesis [11–14].

Recently exon 28 was cloned from zebrafish, and conservation of several VWF functions was demonstrated [15], and *in silico* assembly of full length zebrafish *vwf* has also been described [16]. We now report cloning and characterization of the full length zebrafish *vwf* cDNA. Zebrafish Vwf demonstrates conservation of primary human VWF domain structure, as well as the ability to form pseudo-Weibel-Palade bodies (WPBs) and large multimers in cell culture. Unlike mammalian species, at the stages examined it does not appear to be expressed widely in developing endothelium.

2. Material and Methods

2.1. Cloning of Full Length Zebrafish vwf cDNA. Total mRNA was prepared from a single adult zebrafish using TRIzol (Invitrogen, Carlsbad, California). Total cDNA was synthesized with Superscript III reverse transcriptase after priming with random hexamers (Invitrogen). The *vwf* cDNA was assembled in four overlapping PCR amplified fragments using genomic sequence from Zv6 as a template to design primers (Table 1). Unique restriction sites contained in the overlapping sequences were used to sequentially assemble each of the four PCR products into the vector pCR4-TOPO (Invitrogen). The 5′ and 3′ UTRs (untranslated regions) were amplified by RACE (rapid amplification of cDNA ends, Ambion) with ends that overlapped unique restriction sites in the assembled clone. The external RACE primers were designed with restriction sites for the unique 5′ and 3′ vector sites, NotI and SpeI, respectively.

2.2. Multispecies Alignments. Non-zebrafish VWF amino acid sequences were downloaded from the UCSC Genome Browser, http://genome.ucsc.edu/ [17], aligned using ClustalW2, http://www.ebi.ac.uk/Tools/msa/clustalw2/ [18, 19], with output display through BOXSHADE 3.21, http://www.ch.embnet.org/software/BOX_form.html. Domain comparisons were performed using two sequence protein BLAST (Basic Local Alignment Search Tool) with the default settings through the National Center for Biotechnology Information, http://blast.ncbi.nlm.nih.gov/.

2.3. Plasmid Cloning of vwf cDNA. The assembled *vwf* cDNA was cloned into pcDNA3.1/V5-HISA (Invitrogen), which has an 8 amino acid linker, producing pzVwf/V5-HISA. Since expression of tagged human VWF has been shown to be more robust with an 18–20 amino acid linker (R. Montgomery and S. Haberichter, unpublished observations), we amplified this linker from a human VWF/Myc-HIS construct (pVWF/Myc-HIS, linker sequence in Table 1) and cloned it into the 3′ XhoI-PmeI sites (derived from pcDNA3.1/V5-HISA) of pzVwf/V5-HISA, producing pzVwf/Myc-HIS. The human pVWF-EGFP plasmid contains the same linker sequence.

p*fli*-zVwf-EGFP was constructed by inserting the *vwf* cDNA into Tol2-*fli*-EGFP [20] in frame with *egfp*.

2.4. Immunofluorescence Analysis. HEK293T cells were maintained in DMEM (Sigma; St Louis, MO) supplemented with 10% fetal bovine serum, 100 U/mL penicillin, and 100 μg/mL streptomycin (Sigma). Cells were grown on cover slips until they reached 50–80% confluence, followed by transfection using FuGENE (Roche, Penzberg, Germany) as per manufacturer's instructions. The transfected cover slips were washed in phosphate buffered saline (PBS) and fixed in 10% formalin at room temperature for 25 minutes, followed by fixation/permeabilization at 4°C for 10 minutes in 100% ice cold methanol. After rehydration in PBS for 5 minutes, the cells were incubated with mouse anti-Myc (Santa Cruz Biotechnology, Santa Cruz, California) and rabbit anti-calnexin (Novus Biologicals, Littleton, Colorado) antibodies at dilutions of 1 : 100 and 1 : 500, respectively, at 4°C overnight. Cells were then washed three times in PBS (5 minutes each) and incubated with goat anti-mouse antibody coupled to Alexa Fluor 488 and goat anti-rabbit antibody coupled to Alexa Fluor 594, both at 1 : 200 dilutions for 60 minutes at room temperature. After an additional three washes in PBS, the cover slips were mounted with Prolong Antifade Gold (Invitrogen) and viewed on an inverted Olympus (Melville, New York) confocal microscope. Processing was completed with Olympus FluoView version 5.0.

2.5. Vwf Multimer Analysis. HEK293T (human embryonic kidney) cells were cultured and transfected with pzVwf/V5-HISA or an untagged full length human VWF expressing plasmid (pCineoVWF), as previously described [21]. Conditioned medium from pzVwf/V5-HISA transfected cells was purified over nickel columns per manufacturer's instructions (GE Healthcare Life Sciences, Uppsala, Sweden). Supernatants were analyzed by electrophoresis through a 0.8% (w/v) HGT(P) agarose (FMC Bioproducts, Rockland, Maine) stacking gel and a 1.5% (w/v) HGT(P) agarose running gel containing 0.1% sodium dodecyl sulfate for 16 hours at 40 volts using the Laemmli buffer system and western blotting as previously described [21]. Primary antibodies were a 1 : 5 mixture of anti-V5 antibody (Invitrogen) and anti-HIS antibody (AbD Serotec, Oxford, United Kingdom) or a mixture of monoclonal anti-human VWF antibodies Avw1, 5, and 15 [22].

2.6. Maintenance of Zebrafish Lines and Production of Embryos. Adult zebrafish (AB, TL, EK) were maintained and bred according to standard methods [23]. Embryos collected immediately after fertilization were maintained at 28.5°C and treated with 1-phenyl-2-thiourea (PTU) at 6–8 hpf (hours post fertilization) until fixation in order to prevent pigment formation. At specific time points, embryos were dechorionated or euthanized with tricaine, fixed using 4% paraformaldehyde in PBS overnight at 4°C, and stored at −20°C in methanol up to one month [24].

2.7. RNA Isolation and cDNA Synthesis for RT-PCR of Embryos and Larvae. Total RNA was extracted from at least three

TABLE 1: List of primers and sequences.

Reference number	Sequence	Description
92	AGTCGGCAGCACATACACAC	vwf cloning, assembly of fragment 1 (EcoRI-BstBI)
93	ATCCGACAGGTCAGTTCAC	vwf cloning, assembly of fragment 1 (EcoRI-BstBI)
94	CCTGCAGCTTAAACCCAAAG	vwf cloning, assembly of fragment 2 (BstBI-AvaI)
95	AAAGCTTCATCGTCCAGCTC	vwf cloning, assembly of fragment 2 (BstBI-AvaI)
96	CTGTTGACGGCAAGTGCTAA	vwf cloning, assembly of fragment 3 (AvaI-SbfI)
97	TCTCCTGATGCTGGACACAC	vwf cloning, assembly of fragment 3 (AvaI-SbfI)
98	GACGGCAGTGTAACGACAGA	vwf cloning, assembly of fragment 4 (SbfI-ApaLI)
99	CCTGCAAGAGAGCCGATAAC	vwf cloning, assembly of fragment 4 (SbfI-ApaLI)
116	TGCGTGCTGAATCAAACTGT	vwf cloning, 3′ RACE (ApaLI-SpeI), SpeI vector derived
128	AGTCGCCAGGGAATTCATAA	vwf cloning, 5′ RACE (NotI-EcoRI), NotI vector derived
130	TTTGATTGACATTTTTATTTATTTGTAGTTTA	vwf cloning, amplification of 3′ UTR
543	gatttaggtgacactatagCGACATGCAAGTGCAGAAGT	424 bp vwf riboprobe (exon 28) with SP6 promoter overhang
544	taatacgactcactataggGCTGGGTTTTGCTGTAGGAG	424 bp vwf riboprobe (exon 28) with T7 promoter overhang
545	gatttaggtgacactagGGAGTTATCGGCTCTCTTGC	441 bp vwf riboprobe (exons 47–52) with SP6 promoter overhang
546	taatacgactcactataggACACAGACTTGCTGCCACAC	441 bp vwf riboprobe (exons 47–52) with T7 promoter overhang
	CTCGAGAGAATTCCACCACACTGGACTAGTGGATC	
	CGAGCTCGGTACCAAGCTTGGGCCCGAACAAAAAC	
	TCATCTCAGAAGAGGATCTGAATAGCGCCGTCGAC	XhoI-PmeI human VWF linker sequence (includes Myc/HIS tag)
	CATCATCATCATCATCATTGAGTTTAAAC	

biological replicates per experimental condition using TRIzol RNA isolation reagent (Invitrogen) according to the manufacturer's instructions. RNA (1 μg) was reverse-transcribed using random hexamers and SuperScript III reverse transcriptase (Invitrogen). First-strand cDNA aliquots from each sample served as templates in PCR reactions using primers for *vwf*.

2.8. In Situ Hybridization. In situ hybridization was performed essentially as described with a few modifications [24]. Full length *vwf* cDNA in pCR4-TOPO was linearized with NotI and SpeI (antisense and sense transcripts, respectively) and transcribed *in vitro* using T3 and T7 (Ambion, Austin, Texas), respectively, with digoxigenin labeled nucleotides followed by alkaline hydrolysis per manufacturer's instructions (Roche). Alternatively, 424 and 441 bp fragments were amplified from full length cDNA using primers with SP6 or T7 overhangs (Table 1) and transcribed *in vitro* with digoxigenin labeled nucleotides. Prior to hybridization, riboprobes were heated to 80°C for 3–5 minutes and chilled immediately on ice for at least 5 minutes. Stained embryos were photographed using a Leica MXFLIII stereofluorescent microscope with an Olympus DP-70 digital camera. Embedding was in JB-4 resin as described [25], followed by sectioning at 4–6 μm using a Leica RM2265 ultramicrotome. Imaging of sections was with an Olympus BX-51 upright light microscope and Olympus DP-70 high-resolution digital camera.

3. Results

3.1. Cloning and Characterization of Zebrafish vwf cDNA. According to genomic sequence, the zebrafish *vwf* locus is located on chromosome 18 just downstream of *cd9*, maintaining conservation of synteny with mammalian species [15]. The full length *vwf* cDNA was assembled by RT-PCR of four overlapping fragments from total adult zebrafish cDNA, followed by RACE to complete the 5′ and 3′ UTRs (Section 2). The full length sequence is one amino acid shorter than human VWF with 46% overall identity (Table 2). Alignment of zebrafish Vwf to human VWF using BLAST shows clear delineation of all known domains (Figure 1(a)) with varying degrees of conservation (Table 2). The least conserved are the A1 and A2 domains, which encompass the entirety of exon 28 (Table 2). As in mammals, the *vwf* locus consists of 52 exons, but only spans 81 kb (kilobases), as opposed to 176 kb and 134 kb in the human and murine genomes, respectively. Previous iterations of the zebrafish genome (prior to Zv7) predicted that exon 28 was split into two exons [17]. Both sequence data from this report and previous work [15, 16] demonstrate clearly that the intervening sequence is actually exonic.

Other key features of human VWF are identifiable with varying degrees of conservation. The propeptide cleavage site, Arg-Ser, is highly conserved across all species examined except for medaka, and is a part of the extended RX(R/K)R motif (Figure 1(b)) [26]. The putative ADAMTS13 cleavage site in the A2 domain, Phe-Leu, is discernible due to mammalian orthology of flanking residues and is conserved across

TABLE 2: Human/zebrafish Vwf domain conservation.

Domain	Identities (%)	Positives (%)	Human length	zebrafish length
D1	51	70	352	351
D2	64	79	360	359
D′	51	71	90	88
D3	56	69	376	370
A1	36	57	220	233
A2	28	56	193	193
A3	42	58	202	207
D4	39	54	372	382
B1	58	73	35	34
B2	52	64	26	30
B3	67	83	25	25
C1	50	58	116	107
C2	48	63	119	117
CK	42	64	90	91
Total	46	62	2813	2812

Alignment of human and zebrafish amino acid sequences using BLAST (http://blast.ncbi.nlm.nih.gov/). Percentage identity represents exact amino acid matches, while positives indicate conserved substitutions. Domain length is in amino acids.

all fish species (Figure 1(c)). However, the presumed Phe-Leu cleavage site is only somewhat similar to the highly conserved mammalian and avian Tyr-Met cleavage sequence (Figure 1(c)). More importantly, there is conservation of a leucine orthologous to human Leu^{1603} (Figure 1(c)), which has been shown to be critical for ADAMTS13-mediated proteolysis of VWF [27].

A number of disulfide bonds are required for dimerization and multimerization of human VWF [6]. These are mediated by cysteines at positions 1099, 1142, and several in the C-terminal cystine knot (CK), at 2771, 2773, and 2811, all of which are conserved in zebrafish Vwf. In fact, nearly all cysteine residues are completely conserved, with the exception of Cys^{1669} and Cys^{1670}, located at the C-terminus of the A2 domain [16] and absent in all fish species examined. There was one cysteine present solely in medaka, four residues N-terminal to the propeptide cleavage site, but its absence in other species makes its significance unclear. There is a cysteine in zebrafish Vwf at position 4, which is not conserved in mammalian species, although genomic sequence information for the other teleost species is absent in this region.

3.2. Expression of Vwf in Mammalian Cell Culture. In order to determine if zebrafish Vwf can multimerize, we expressed V5/HIS tagged *vwf* cDNA in HEK293T cells. A ladder of high molecular weight multimers was detected using a mixture of anti-V5 and anti-HIS antibodies (Figure 2). This included high molecular weight multimers similar in size to human VWF (Figure 2).

The zebrafish *vwf* cDNA was cloned into an expression vector in frame with a Myc-HIS tag using the same linker as a human *VWF* cDNA construct. The latter, when transfected into HEK293T cells, is known to form pseudo-WPBs

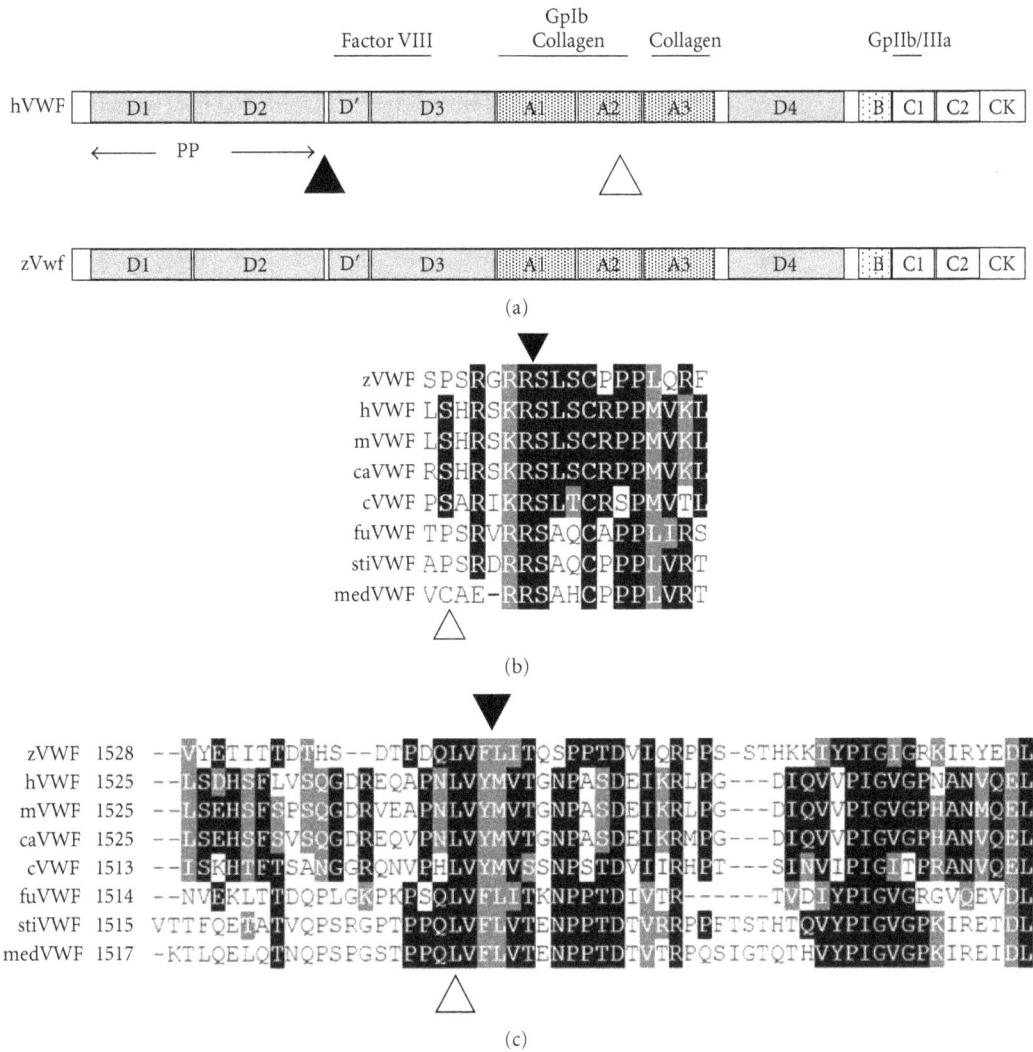

FIGURE 1: Domain organization of human VWF and multispecies alignment of the VWF propeptide and ADAMTS13 cleavage sites and flanking sequences. Sequence alignment was performed using ClustalW2 followed by output using BOXSHADE (Section 2). (a) Domain organization of human VWF. Upper notations indicate known protein-protein interaction domains (Gp: glycoprotein). The solid triangle indicates the propeptide (PP) cleavage site, and the open triangle indicates the ADAMTS13 cleavage site. "B" indicates domains B1–B3. (b) Alignment of sequences surrounding the Arg-Ser (RS, indicated by the solid triangle) human propeptide cleavage site demonstrates a high degree of conservation. Note the extended RX(R/K)R motif present in all species except for medaka. The open triangle indicates the presence of an unconserved cysteine in medaka Vwf. (c) Alignment at the human ADAMTS13 cleavage site (YM, indicated by the solid triangle) and flanking sequences demonstrates conservation of the Tyr-Met residues in mammalian and avian species, but a Phe-Leu putative site in teleost fish. The invariant Leu (human residue 1603) is indicated by a white triangle. z: zebrafish; h: human; m: mouse; ca: canine; c: chicken; fu: fugu; st: stickleback; med: medaka.

[28, 29]. These structures are produced after VWF has been processed into high molecular weight multimers in the Golgi apparatus. Using an anti-Myc antibody we were able to identify elongated structures consistent with pseudo-WPBs in zebrafish *vwf* transfected cells (Figures 3(d) and 3(g)). These were morphologically similar to those found in human *VWF* transfected cells (Figure 3(a)). Staining with an anti-calnexin antibody to localize endoplasmic reticulum (ER, Figures 3(b), 3(e), and 3(h)) demonstrated no overlap between the structures (Figures 3(c), 3(f), and 3(i)), as expected for WPBs and pseudo-WPBs [28, 29].

3.3. Developmental Patterns of vwf Expression. RT-PCR of whole embryos up to 96 hpf demonstrated increasing levels of *vwf* expression, with the most intense expression at 96 hpf (Figure 4(f)). Whole-mount *in situ* hybridization was used to localize expression from the middle of gastrulation (8 hpf) to 120 hpf. Expression of *vwf* is weakly detectable throughout the embryo at 8 hpf (Figure 4(a)). Stronger expression is observed in 12-hour embryos as a more diffuse pattern throughout the embryo (Figure 4(b)). At 48 hours there is diffuse expression cranially, which extends caudally (Figure 4(c)). At 96–120 hours, strong expression is present

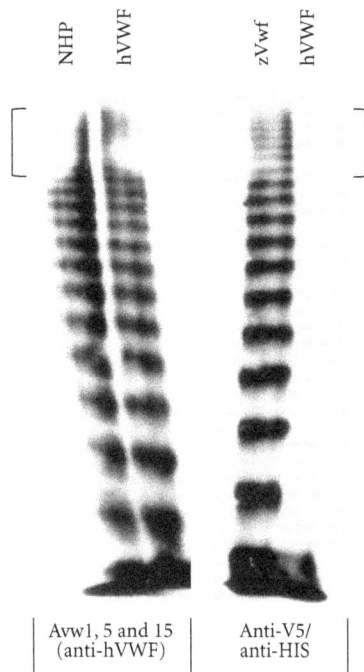

FIGURE 2: Multimerization of zebrafish Vwf in mammalian cell culture demonstrates high molecular weight multimers similar to human VWF. HEK293T cells were transfected with pzVwf/V5-HISA, expressing V5-HIS tagged zebrafish Vwf (zVwf), or pCineoVWF, expressing untagged human VWF (hVWF). Normal human plasma (NHP) and zebrafish and human supernatants were separated by agarose gel electrophoresis, transferred by western blotting, and detected with either a pool of monoclonal anti-hVWF antibodies (Avw1, 5, 15, left panel) or a mixture of anti-V5 and anti-HIS antibodies (for tagged zVwf, right panel). The anti-V5/HIS combination detects zVwf with a multimer pattern, including high molecular weight multimers, indistinguishable from that typically observed for human VWF (brackets indicate high molecular weight multimers for both zebrafish and human VWF).

in the pharyngeal arches, intestinal epithelium, and inner layer of the yolk sac (Figures 4(e), 4(g), and 4(h)).

4. Discussion

VWD is due to quantitative or qualitative deficiency of VWF and has been described in several mammals, including human, horse, cat, pig, rabbit, and dog [7, 8]. Identification and characterization of the human *VWF* cDNA [30–33] enabled the eventual identification of many of these pathogenic mutations as well as partial or full length sequence information in numerous mammalian species [34]. The zebrafish genome project [35] assisted in the identification of much of the *vwf* cDNA [15, 16], but this did not include the complete 5′ and 3′ UTRS. We have now completed cloning and characterization of the full length zebrafish *vwf* cDNA.

We found that *vwf* displays widespread expression in early embryonic development and then becomes more restricted at the larval stage. Mammalian *VWF* is widely expressed in vascular endothelial cell beds of the adult mouse [36], and VWF protein is an established clinical pathologic

marker of human vasculature [37]. However, it has not been examined in the developing vertebrate. We hypothesized that there would be widespread expression of zebrafish *vwf* in developing vasculature, but instead found an early broad and then later restricted pattern. A previous study in zebrafish identified Vwf protein expression within the vasculature at the larval stage, although the source was not determined [15]. Therefore one possible explanation for the discrepancy with our results is that larval intravascular Vwf is not produced in endothelial cells but rather comes from the yolk sac or pharyngeal arches. Alternatively, endothelial *vwf* mRNA expression might not be present until later in development.

The expression seen in early embryonic development may possibly reflect maternally derived transcripts [38], while later expression is clearly of embryonic/larval origin. There is no prior evidence for a role of VWF in gastrulation, although the expression in the pharyngeal arches is intriguing. These structures develop into gills [39], the organs responsible for oxygen exchange in fish. The highest levels of mammalian *Vwf* mRNA expression have been identified in the lung [36], suggesting the possibility of an evolutionary conserved role of VWF in these structures.

In order to produce functional VWF activity, high molecular weight multimers are assembled in the trans-Golgi, packaged into WPBs, and secreted. This is followed by circulation in the blood and tethering of platelets to sites of vessel injury, forming the primary platelet plug [6]. It has been previously shown that zebrafish thrombocytes will aggregate in a Vwf-dependent fashion and that morpholino-mediated knockdown results in increased bleeding times and hemorrhage [15]. In this paper we have demonstrated that zebrafish Vwf has the ability to multimerize and form pseudo-WPBs in mammalian cell culture. Taken together, these data suggest that the basic mechanisms of zebrafish Vwf function appear to be conserved.

Previous studies have shown evidence for the presence of the Vwf receptor, GpIb, on thrombocytes in zebrafish and chicken [40, 41]. If thrombocytes bind Vwf as platelets do in mammals, one might expect a high degree of conservation of the Vwf A1 domain, which encodes the GpIb-binding site. The A2 domain, which encodes the Adamts13 cleavage site, is required for the production of properly sized Vwf multimers. When cleavage is reduced, vascular occlusion can occur, while when enhanced, bleeding results [42]. However, there are notable differences between mammalian and non-mammalian vertebrate systems. Despite the overall amino acid similarity and conservation of synteny of Vwf, the A1 and A2 domains display the largest degree of divergence when compared to humans. It is tempting to speculate that the A1 domain has evolved a relatively increased or decreased ability to bind thrombocytes in compensation for the latter's lesser or greater role in the initiation of primary hemostasis. Shear forces required to expose the A1 and A2 domains are likely to be different in zebrafish compared to mammals. Despite their functional similarities, nucleated thrombocytes are clearly different from anucleate platelets, suggesting the possibility that the two function quite differently. Studies of avian thrombocytes, which are also nucleated, have led to the

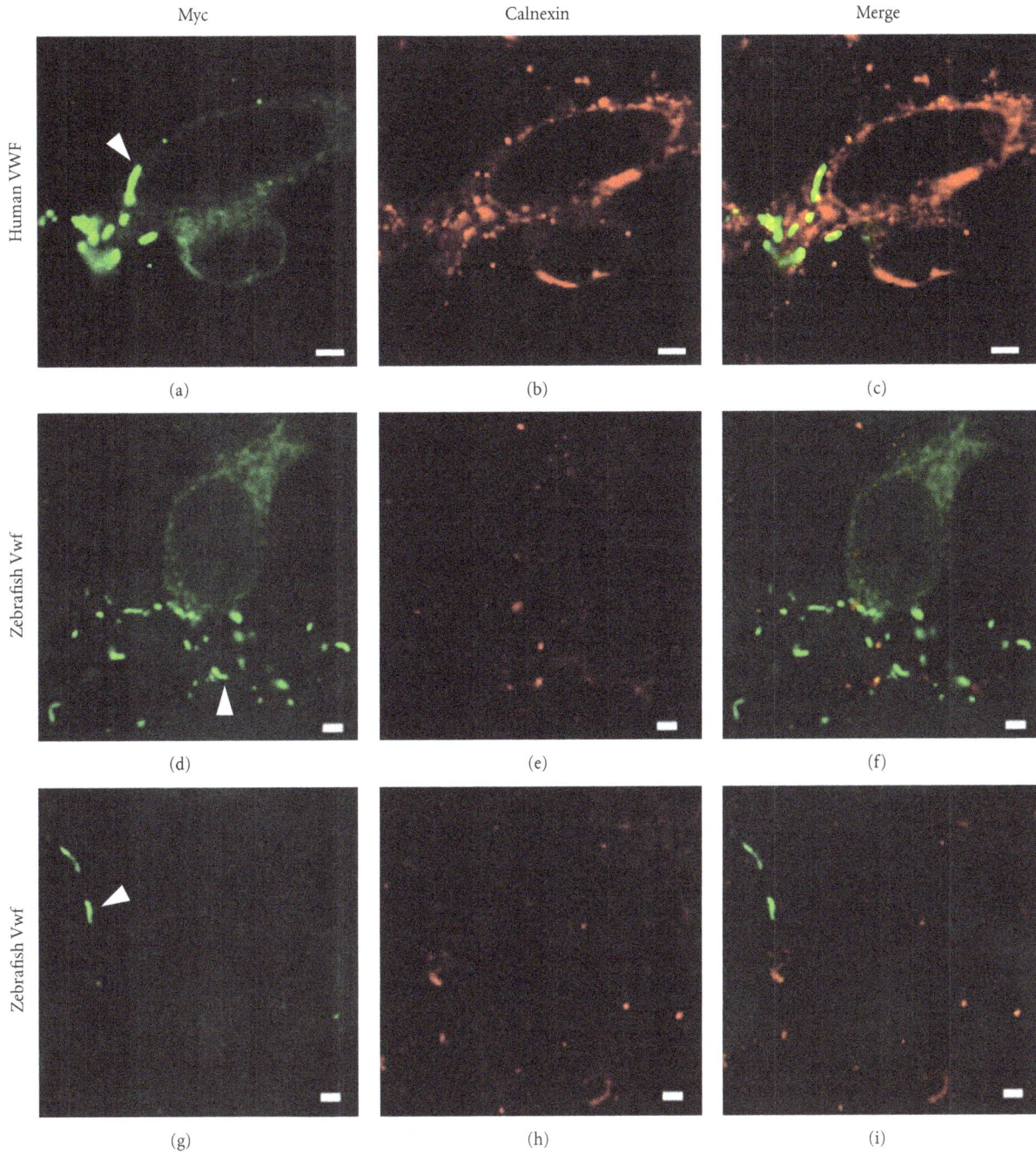

FIGURE 3: Zebrafish Vwf forms pseudo-Weibel-Palade bodies (pseudo-WPBs) in mammalian cell culture. pVWF/Myc-HIS (human VWF, (a–c)) or pzVwf/Myc-HIS (zebrafish Vwf, (d–i)) plasmids were transfected into HEK293T cells. Anti-Myc antibody conjugated to Alexa Fluor 488 (green channel, (a, d, g)) was used for detection and anti-calnexin antibody conjugated to Alexa Fluor 594 (red channel, (b, e, h)) labeled endoplasmic reticulum (ER). Both constructs demonstrate formation of elongated Myc positive and ER negative structures (absence of yellow signal in the merged panels, (c, f, i)) characteristic of pseudo-WPBs (examples are indicated in (a, d), and (g) by arrowheads). Scale bars, 2.5 μm.

hypothesis that human cardiovascular disease may be related to the existence of platelet rather than thrombocyte-initiated primary hemostasis [41]. Further understanding of the role of thrombocytes and Vwf in zebrafish and avian hemostasis may have potential implications for the treatment of bleeding and thrombotic disorders.

Acknowledgments

The authors thank the University of Michigan Sequencing and Genotyping Core, and Dave Siemieniak, Susan Spaulding, Kristen Lessl, and Toby Hurd for technical assistance, and Evan Sadler for helpful suggestions. The authors would

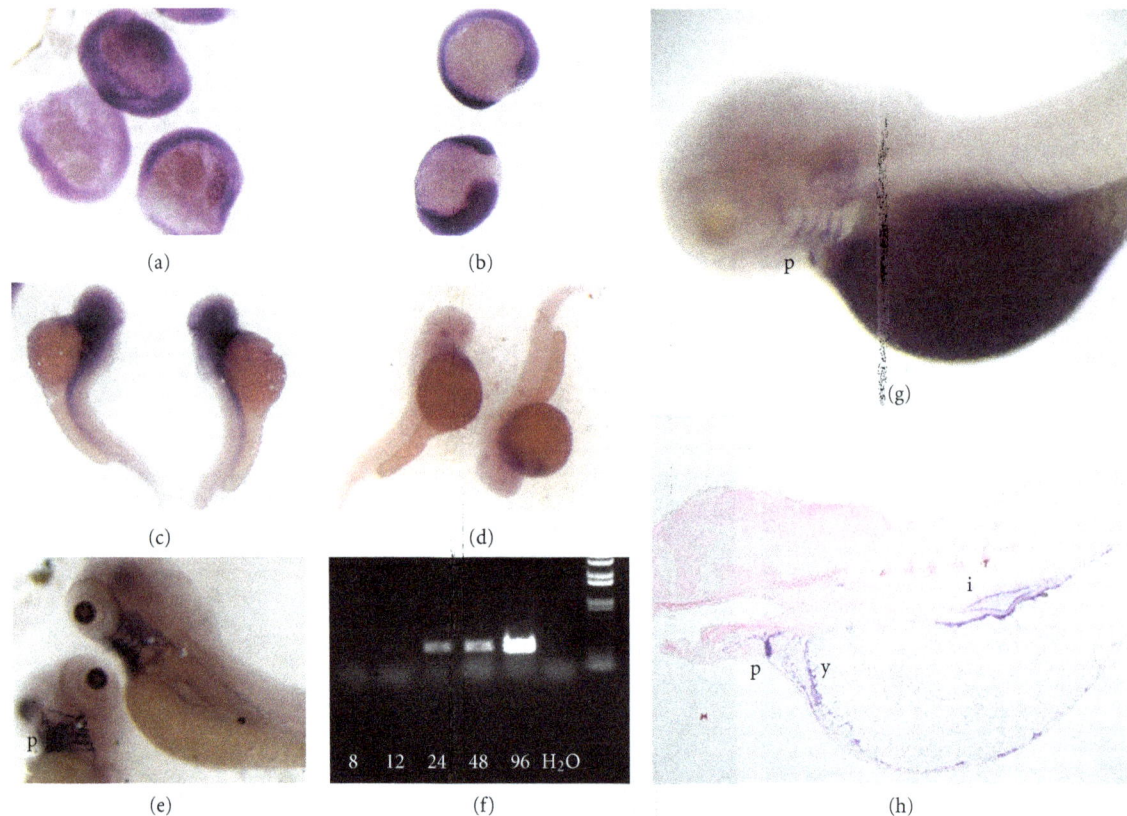

FIGURE 4: Developmental expression of *vwf* mRNA. Wild type zebrafish offspring were isolated from 8 to 120 hpf, fixed, and *in situ* hybridization was performed (Section 2). (a) Examination at 8 hpf demonstrates weak expression throughout the entire embryo, and staining was completely absent from a sense control. (b) Diffuse expression continues at 12 hpf (staining was completely absent from a sense control), followed by more restricted expression cranially with a stripe that extends caudally at 48 hpf (c). Figure 4(d) is a sense probe as negative control at 48 hpf. (e) 96 hpf shows strong expression in the pharyngeal arches. (f) RT-PCR of cDNA isolated from whole zebrafish embryos and larvae from 8–96 hpf. (g, h) Analysis at 120 hpf shows continued expression in the pharyngeal arches, as well as inner yolk sac layer and intestinal epithelium. Experiments in (a–e) used full length *vwf* riboprobes. Results in (g, h) are representative of hybridization with exon 28 and exon 47–52 riboprobes (Section 2, Table 1). Abbreviations: p: pharyngeal arches; y: inner layer of yolk sac; i: intestinal epithelium.

especially like to thank David Ginsburg for support and critical reading of the paper. This work was supported by American Heart Association no. 0675025N, the Bayer Hemophilia Awards Program, and the Diane and Larry Johnson Family Scholar Award (J.A.S.), as well as National Institutes of Health P01-HL081588 and R01-HL033721 (R.R.M.).

References

[1] C. J. Davidson, R. P. Hirt, K. Lal et al., "Molecular evolution of the vertebrate blood coagulation network," *Thrombosis and Haemostasis*, vol. 89, no. 3, pp. 420–428, 2003.

[2] C. J. Davidson, E. G. Tuddenham, and J. H. McVey, "450 million years of hemostasis," *Journal of Thrombosis and Haemostasis*, vol. 1, no. 7, pp. 1487–1494, 2003.

[3] Y. Jiang and R. F. Doolittle, "The evolution of vertebrate blood coagulation as viewed from a comparison of puffer fish and sea squirt genomes," *Proceedings of the National Academy of Sciences of the United States of America*, vol. 100, no. 13, pp. 7527–7532, 2003.

[4] W. C. Nichols and D. Ginsburg, "Von Willebrand disease," *Medicine*, vol. 76, no. 1, pp. 1–20, 1997.

[5] R. Schneppenheim and U. Budde, "Von Willebrand factor: the complex molecular genetics of a multidomain and multifunctional protein," *Journal of Thrombosis and Haemostasis*, vol. 9, no. 1, pp. 209–215, 2011.

[6] J. E. Sadler, "Von Willebrand factor assembly and secretion," *Journal of Thrombosis and Haemostasis*, vol. 7, supplement s1, pp. 24–27, 2009.

[7] D. Ginsburg and E. J. W. Bowie, "Molecular genetics of von Willebrand disease," *Blood*, vol. 79, no. 10, pp. 2507–2519, 1992.

[8] G. Levy and D. Ginsburg, "Getting at the variable expressivity of von Willebrand disease," *Thrombosis and Haemostasis*, vol. 86, no. 1, pp. 144–148, 2001.

[9] P. Jagadeeswaran, R. Paris, and P. Rao, "Laser-induced thrombosis in zebrafish larvae: a novel genetic screening method for thrombosis," *Methods in Molecular Medicine*, vol. 129, pp. 187–195, 2006.

[10] K. R. Kidd and B. M. Weinstein, "Fishing for novel angiogenic therapies," *British Journal of Pharmacology*, vol. 140, no. 4, pp. 585–594, 2003.

[11] J. N. Chen, P. Haffter, J. Odenthal et al., "Mutations affecting the cardiovascular system and other internal organs in zebrafish," *Development*, vol. 123, pp. 293–302, 1996.

[12] D. Y. Stainier, B. Fouquet, J. N. Chen et al., "Mutations affecting the formation and function of the cardiovascular system in the zebrafish embryo," *Development*, vol. 123, pp. 285–292, 1996.

[13] S. W. Jin, W. Herzog, M. M. Santoro et al., "A transgene-assisted genetic screen identifies essential regulators of vascular development in vertebrate embryos," *Developmental Biology*, vol. 307, no. 1, pp. 29–42, 2007.

[14] E. E. Patton and L. I. Zon, "The art and design of genetic screens: zebrafish," *Nature Reviews Genetics*, vol. 2, no. 12, pp. 956–966, 2001.

[15] M. Carrillo, S. Kim, S. K. Rajpurohit, V. Kulkarni, and P. Jagadeeswaran, "Zebrafish von Willebrand factor," *Blood Cells, Molecules, and Diseases*, vol. 45, no. 4, pp. 326–333, 2010.

[16] L. T. Dang, A. R. Purvis, R. H. Huang, L. A. Westfield, and J. E. Sadler, "Phylogenetic and functional analysis of histidine residues essential for pH-dependent multimerization of von willebrand factor," *Journal of Biological Chemistry*, vol. 286, no. 29, pp. 25763–25769, 2011.

[17] P. A. Fujita, B. Rhead, A. S. Zweig et al., "The UCSC genome browser database: update 2011," *Nucleic Acids Research*, vol. 39, no. 1, pp. D876–D882, 2011.

[18] M. Goujon, H. McWilliam, W. Li et al., "A new bioinformatics analysis tools framework at EMBL-EBI," *Nucleic Acids Research*, vol. 38, supplement 2, pp. W695–W699, 2010.

[19] M. A. Larkin, G. Blackshields, N. P. Brown et al., "Clustal W and clustal X version 2.0," *Bioinformatics*, vol. 23, no. 21, pp. 2947–2948, 2007.

[20] D. A. Buchner, F. Su, J. S. Yamaoka et al., "Pak2a mutations cause cerebral hemorrhage in redhead zebrafish," *Proceedings of the National Academy of Sciences of the United States of America*, vol. 104, no. 35, pp. 13996–14001, 2007.

[21] S. L. Haberichter, S. A. Fahs, and R. R. Montgomery, "Von Willebrand factor storage and multimerization: 2 independent intracellular processes," *Blood*, vol. 96, no. 5, pp. 1808–1815, 2000.

[22] J. Schullek, J. Jordan, and R. R. Montgomery, "Interaction of von Willebrand factor with human platelets in the plasma milieu," *Journal of Clinical Investigation*, vol. 73, no. 2, pp. 421–428, 1984.

[23] M. Westerfield, *The Zebrafish Book. A Guide For the Laboratory Use of Zebrafish (Danio Rerio)*, University of Oregon Press, Eugene, Ore, USA, 4th edition, 2000.

[24] C. Thisse and B. Thisse, "High-resolution in situ hybridization to whole-mount zebrafish embryos," *Nature Protocols*, vol. 3, no. 1, pp. 59–69, 2008.

[25] J. Sullivan-Brown, M. E. Bisher, and R. D. Burdine, "Embedding, serial sectioning and staining of zebrafish embryos using JB-4 resin," *Nature Protocols*, vol. 6, no. 1, pp. 46–55, 2011.

[26] A. Rehemtulla and R. J. Kaufman, "Preferred sequence requirements for cleavage of pro-von Willebrand factor by propeptide-processing enzymes," *Blood*, vol. 79, no. 9, pp. 2349–2355, 1992.

[27] Y. Xiang, R. de Groot, J. T. B. Crawley, and D. A. Lane, "Mechanism of von Willebrand factor scissile bond cleavage by a disintegrin and metalloproteinase with a thrombospondin type 1 motif, member 13 (ADAMTS13)," *Proceedings of the National Academy of Sciences of the United States of America*, vol. 108, no. 28, pp. 11602–11607, 2011.

[28] G. Michaux, L. J. Hewlett, S. L. Messenger et al., "Analysis of intracellular storage and regulated secretion of 3 von Willebrand disease-causing variants of von Willebrand factor," *Blood*, vol. 102, no. 7, pp. 2452–2458, 2003.

[29] J. W. Wang, K. M. Valentijn, H. C. de Boer et al., "Intracellular storage and regulated secretion of von Willebrand factor in quantitative von Willebrand disease," *Journal of Biological Chemistry*, vol. 286, no. 27, pp. 24180–24188, 2011.

[30] D. Ginsburg, R. I. Handin, and D. T. Bonthron, "Human von Willebrand Factor (vWF): isolation of complementary DNA (cDNA) clones and chromosomal localization," *Science*, vol. 228, no. 4706, pp. 1401–1406, 1985.

[31] D. C. Lynch, T. S. Zimmerman, and C. J. Collins, "Molecular cloning of cDNA for human von Willebrand factor: authentication by a new method," *Cell*, vol. 41, no. 1, pp. 49–56, 1985.

[32] J. E. Sadler, B. B. Shelton-Inloes, and J. M. Sorace, "Cloning and characterization of two cDNAs coding for human von Willebrand factor," *Proceedings of the National Academy of Sciences of the United States of America*, vol. 82, no. 19, pp. 6394–6398, 1985.

[33] C. L. Verweij, C. J. M. de Vries, B. Distel et al., "Construction of cDNA coding for human von willebrand factor using antibody probes for colony-screening and mapping of the chromosomal gene," *Nucleic Acids Research*, vol. 13, no. 13, pp. 4699–4717, 1985.

[34] ISTH SSC VWF Database, http://www.vwf.group.shef.ac.uk/index.html.

[35] S. C. Ekker, D. L. Stemple, M. Clark, C. B. Chien, R. S. Rasooly, and L. C. Javois, "Zebrafish genome project: bringing new biology to the vertebrate genome field," *Zebrafish*, vol. 4, no. 4, pp. 239–251, 2007.

[36] K. Yamamoto, V. de Waard, C. Fearns, and D. J. Loskutoff, "Tissue distribution and regulation of murine von Willebrand factor gene expression in vivo," *Blood*, vol. 92, no. 8, pp. 2791–2801, 1998.

[37] M. R. Wick and J. L. Hornick, "Immunohistology of soft tissue and osseous neoplasms," in *Diagnostic Immunohistochemistry*, D. J. Dabbs, Ed., pp. 83–136, Saunders, 3rd edition, 2010.

[38] A. F. Schier, "The maternal-zygotic transition: death and birth of RNAs," *Science*, vol. 316, no. 5823, pp. 406–407, 2007.

[39] C. B. Kimmel, W. W. Ballard, S. R. Kimmel, B. Ullmann, and T. F. Schilling, "Stages of embryonic development of the zebrafish," *Developmental Dynamics*, vol. 203, no. 3, pp. 253–310, 1995.

[40] P. Jagadeeswaran, J. P. Sheehan, F. E. Craig, and D. Troyer, "Identification and characterization of zebrafish thrombocytes," *British Journal of Haematology*, vol. 107, no. 4, pp. 731–738, 1999.

[41] A. A. Schmaier, T. J. Stalker, J. J. Runge et al. et al., "Occlusive thrombi arise in mammals but not birds in response to arterial injury: evolutionary insight into human cardiovascular disease," *Blood*, vol. 118, no. 13, pp. 3661–3669, 2011.

[42] J. E. Sadler, "Von Willebrand factor: two sides of a coin," *Journal of Thrombosis and Haemostasis*, vol. 3, no. 8, pp. 1702–1709, 2005.

3

Sonoclot Signature Analysis in Patients with Liver Disease and Its Correlation with Conventional Coagulation Studies

Priyanka Saxena,[1] Chhagan Bihari,[1] Archana Rastogi,[2] Savita Agarwal,[2] Lovkesh Anand,[3] and Shiv Kumar Sarin[3]

[1] Department of Hematology, Institute of Liver and Biliary Sciences, D-1, Vasant Kunj, New Delhi 110070, India
[2] Department of Pathology, Institute of Liver and Biliary Sciences, D-1, Vasant Kunj, New Delhi 110070, India
[3] Department of Hepatology, Institute of Liver and Biliary Sciences, D-1, Vasant Kunj, New Delhi 110070, India

Correspondence should be addressed to Chhagan Bihari; drcbsharma@gmail.com

Academic Editor: John Roback

Introduction. Liver disease patients have complex hemostatic defects leading to a delicate, unstable balance between bleeding and thrombosis. Conventional tests such as PT and APTT are unable to depict these defects completely. *Aims.* This study aimed at analyzing the abnormal effects of liver disease on sonoclot signature by using sonoclot analyzer (which depicts the entire hemostatic pathway) and assessing the correlations between sonoclot variables and conventional coagulation tests. *Material and Methods.* Clinical and laboratory data from fifty inpatients of four subgroups of liver disease, including decompensated cirrhosis, chronic hepatitis, cirrhosis with HCC and acute-on-chronic liver failure were analyzed. All patients and controls were subjected to sonoclot analysis and correlated with routine coagulation parameters including platelet count, PT, APTT, fibrinogen, and D-dimer. *Results.* The sonoclot signatures demonstrated statistically significant abnormalities in patients with liver disease as compared to healthy controls. PT and APTT correlated positively with SONACT ($P < 0.008$ and <0.0015, resp.) while platelet count and fibrinogen levels depicted significant positive and negative correlations with clot rate and SONACT respectively. *Conclusion.* Sonoclot analysis may prove to be an efficient tool to assess coagulopathies in liver disease patients. Clot rate could emerge as a potential predictor of hypercoagulability in these patients.

1. Introduction

Patients with liver disease show significant changes in the hemostatic system. Consequently, routine diagnostic tests such as platelet count, prothrombin time (PT), and activated partial thromboplastin time (APTT) are frequently abnormal. However, interpretation of these tests is much less accurate in patients with complex hemostatic disorders as can be found in patients with liver disease [1]. It is now established that patients with liver disease not only have bleeding tendencies but may develop thrombotic complications as well [2].

The inability of PT-INR and APTT to predict the bleeding risk can be explained by the fact that they incompletely reflect the coagulation process. The parallel decline in the level of natural anticoagulants leading to a prothrombotic tendency is not depicted by these tests. Additionally, significant variations in the INR values have been reported in liver disease patients

when tested in different laboratories. Due to this poor reproducibility of INR values, models for end stage liver disease (MELD) score variations up to 12 points have been noted [3]. This could lead to significant discrepancies in the management of these patients.

Standard coagulation tests such as PT and APTT do not incorporate cellular elements. They tend to provide data on isolated aspects of coagulation cascade and overlook factors such as rate of clot formation, time taken for maximal clot retraction, and maximal clot strength. Instead, viscoelastic devices such as sonoclot provide *in vitro* assessment of global coagulation. Sonoclot may also be useful in diagnosing systemic fibrinolysis, though it may not reflect localized clot breakdown by plasmin. Most conventional coagulation tests end when the first fibrin strands are developing, whereas viscoelastic coagulation tests begin at this point and continue throughout clot development, retraction, and lysis [4].

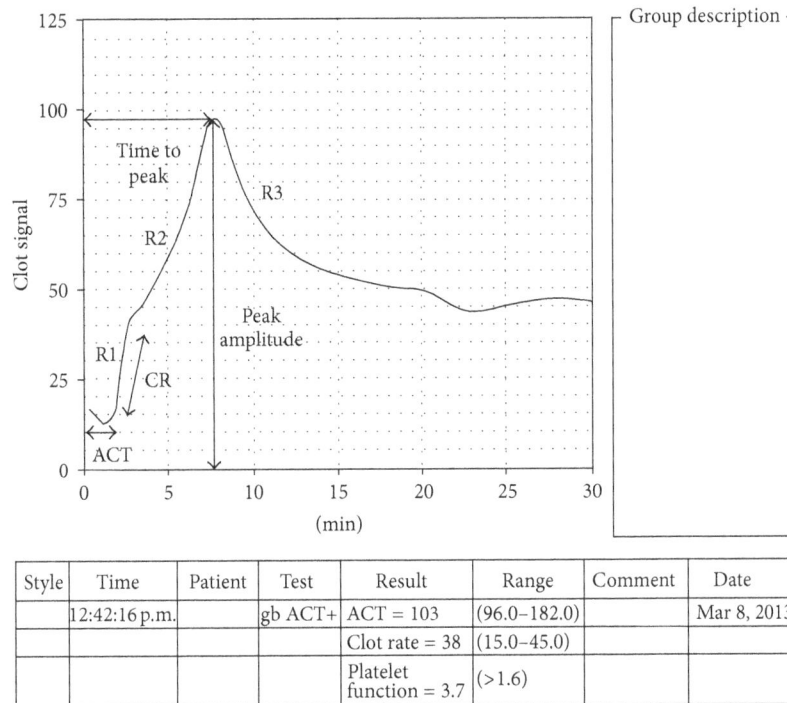

Style	Time	Patient	Test	Result	Range	Comment	Date
	12:42:16 p.m.		gb ACT+	ACT = 103	(96.0–182.0)		Mar 8, 2013
				Clot rate = 38	(15.0–45.0)		
				Platelet function = 3.7	(>1.6)		

FIGURE 1: Normal sonoclot signature ACT (SONACT: activated clotting time), CR: clot rate.

This study was carried out to analyze the abnormalities of sonoclot signature in patients with liver diseases including chronic hepatitis, decompensated cirrhosis, compensated cirrhosis with hepatocellular carcinoma, and acute-on-chronic liver failure. The sonoclot signature parameters studied included sonoclot activated clotting time (SONACT), clot rate (CR), platelet function (PF), time to peak (TP), peak amplitude (PA), and R2 peak character. We also aimed to establish a correlation between the above mentioned sonoclot parameters and conventional coagulation tests like PT, international normalized ratio (INR), APTT, fibrinogen levels, platelet count, and D-dimer levels in these patients.

2. Sonoclot Coagulation and Platelet Function Analyzer, Sienco Inc., Arvada, CO, USA

The sonoclot analyser was introduced by von Kaulla et al. in 1975. Sonoclot measurements are based on detection of viscoelastic changes in the whole blood sample. The instrument provides information on the entire hemostatic process in the form of a qualitative graph known as sonoclot signature along with several quantitative measurements [5].

The quantitative measurements include sonoclot activated clotting time (SONACT) which is the onset time in seconds till the beginning of fibrin formation. The rate of fibrin formation from fibrinogen is depicted by the gradient of primary slope (R1) and is known as clot rate (CR). It is expressed in units per minute. The secondary slope (R2) reflects fibrin polymerization and platelet-fibrin interaction. The R2 peak indicates completion of fibrin formation and has two variables, the time to peak (in minutes), which is

an index of the rate of conversion of fibrinogen to fibrin, and peak amplitude (expressed in units), which is an index of fibrinogen concentration. The downward slope (R3) after the peak is produced as platelets induce contraction of the completed clot. In cases of low platelet counts and/or poor platelet function, a shallow R3 slope is obtained. Hence, the R3 slope gradient determines the number of available platelets and the level of platelet function and is recorded as platelet function (PF) by the analyzer (Figure 1). In patients with accelerated fibrinolysis, the decrease in signal after the R3 slope can be clinically used as a measure of fibrinolysis [6].

3. Material and Methods

3.1. Patients and Control. An observational study was carried out over a period of three months wherein data of 50 adult inpatients without any anticoagulation therapy with liver disease in a superspeciality liver institute were analyzed. The study also included 10 healthy controls from voluntary donors at the blood bank. None of the candidates in the control group had any other apparently known disease. Exclusion criteria for controls were presence of any chronic medical condition (especially coagulopathies), patients on anticoagulation, and individuals on long term medications.

Patients were classified into four groups:

(1) Group 1 (G1) or decompensated cirrhosis (D. cirrhosis) included 16 (32%) patients with decompensated cirrhosis which was defined by histological presence of regenerative nodules surrounded by fibrosis with clinical stage 3 or 4 [7] along with presence of ascites,

TABLE 1: Demographic and clinical data.

Demographic data	Patient groups ($N = 50$)			Control group ($N = 10$)
Male : female	34 : 16			6 : 4
Age mean ± SD	50.7 ± 10.68			34.2 ± 9.4
Clinical data	Patient groups			
	G1 ($N = 16$)	G2 ($N = 14$)	G3 ($N = 11$)	G4 ($N = 09$)
History of bleed	4 (25%)	1 (7%)	1 (9%)	—
Hepatic encephalopathy	8 (50%)	3 (21%)	—	4 (44%)
Sepsis	6 (37.5%)	3 (21%)	1 (9%)	3 (33%)

G1: group 1 (decompensated cirrhosis), G2: group 2 (noncirrhotic liver disease), G3: group 3 (cirrhotic HCC), G4: group 4 (ACLF).

variceal haemorrhage, encephalopathy, or jaundice [8]. This group comprised eight patients with alcoholic cirrhosis, one patient with hepatitis C-related cirrhosis, five patients with cryptogenic cirrhosis, and two patients with nonalcoholic steatohepatitis (NASH) induced cirrhosis.

(2) Group 2 (G2) or chronic hepatitis (CH) included 14 (28%) patients with chronic liver disease (CLD) other than cirrhosis (chronic hepatitis group). This group comprised four patients with chronic alcoholic hepatitis, seven patients with chronic viral hepatitis, and three patients with chronic cholestatic hepatitis.

(3) Group 3 (G3) or cirrhosis included 11 (22%) patients with compensated cirrhosis who had an additional finding of hepatocellular carcinoma (HCC).

(4) Group 4 (G4) or acute-on-chronic liver failure (ACLF) included nine (18%) patients with acute on chronic liver failure (ACLF) as defined by the Asia Pacific Association for the Study of the Liver (APASL). The APASL's definition of ACLF is "acute hepatic insult manifesting as jaundice and coagulopathy, complicated within 4 weeks by ascites and/or encephalopathy in a patient with previously diagnosed or undiagnosed chronic liver disease" [9].

(5) A fifth group (control group) was created which comprised 10 voluntary healthy controls.

Patients in G3 (cirrhosis) were segregated from G1 (D. cirrhosis) (though both groups consisted of patients with cirrhosis) because there is sufficient recent evidence to indicate that compensated and decompensated cirrhosis are two separate entities and should be analyzed separately [8, 10]. In our study, the patient group of compensated cirrhosis had an additional finding of HCC.

3.2. Demographic Data and Clinical Presentation. The clinical profile of the patients including age, sex, clinical presentation, underlying liver disease, and bleeding history was recorded and summarized in Table 1.

There were 34 male (68%) and 16 female (32%) patients. The minimum age was 29 years while the maximum age was 70 years with a mean age of 50.7 years (SD ± 10.68). The control group consisted of 6 male (60%) and 4 female (40%) patients. The minimum age was 20 years and the maximum was 52 years with a mean age of 34.2 years (SD ± 9.4).

The most common cause in G1 (D. cirrhosis) was alcoholic liver disease. Eight patients (50%) in the group were clinically reported to have hepatic encephalopathy. Additionally, four patients (44.4%) in G4 (ACLF) also had hepatic encephalopathy. A total of 13 patients out of 50 (26%) developed features of sepsis, six of which belonged to G1 (D. cirrhosis) (37.5%), three belonged to G2 (CH) (21%), one belonged to G3 (cirrhosis) (9%), and three belonged to G4 (ACLF) (33%). History of bleeding was present in six patients (12%) who included four patients from G1 (D. cirrhosis), one patient from G2 (CH), and one patient from G3 (cirrhosis) (Table 1). Bleeding from varices was the commonest with four patients (66.7%) having history of variceal bleed (multiple emesis and/or melena), one patient with history of intra-abdominal bleed, and one patient having mucosal bleeds.

3.3. Laboratory Tests. The platelet count of all the patients as well as control group was carried out on a hematology autoanalyzer (Coulter Hmx Hematology Analyser; Beckman Coulter Inc., Brea, California, USA).

For coagulation parameters, blood from patients and controls was collected in two citrated tubes containing buffered sodium citrate (0.109 M, 3.2%) in the ratio blood : anticoagulant 9 : 1. The citrated samples were processed within half an hour of collection. One of the tubes containing citrated blood was centrifuged and plasma was obtained. The plasma was run on fully automated coagulometer (Sysmex CA 1500; Sysmex Corporation, Kobe, Japan) and values of PT, INR, APTT, and fibrinogen were recorded. The remainder of the plasma was used for determination of D-dimer levels by a semiquantitative rapid latex agglutination slide test (D-Di test, Diagnostica Stago S.A.S., France).

The other tube containing citrated whole blood was used for sonoclot analysis. 340 μL of citrated whole blood was added to gb ACT+ (glass bead activated ACT) cuvette prewarmed to 37°C along with 20 μL of CaCl$_2$. Sonoclot signature was obtained and recorded for a period of 30 minutes on sonoclot analyzer (Sonoclot Coagulation and Platelet Function Analyzer, Sienco Inc., Arvada, CO, USA).

SONACT, CR, and PF were calculated by the instrument and recorded accordingly. TP and PA were calculated manually from the signature. The R2 peak character was recorded as a qualitative parameter according to the type of peak obtained on the R2 slope of the signature. R2 peaks were classified as sharp (well-defined peaks, Figure 1), dull (poorly defined peaks, Figure 2(a)), and flat signature (Figure 2(b)).

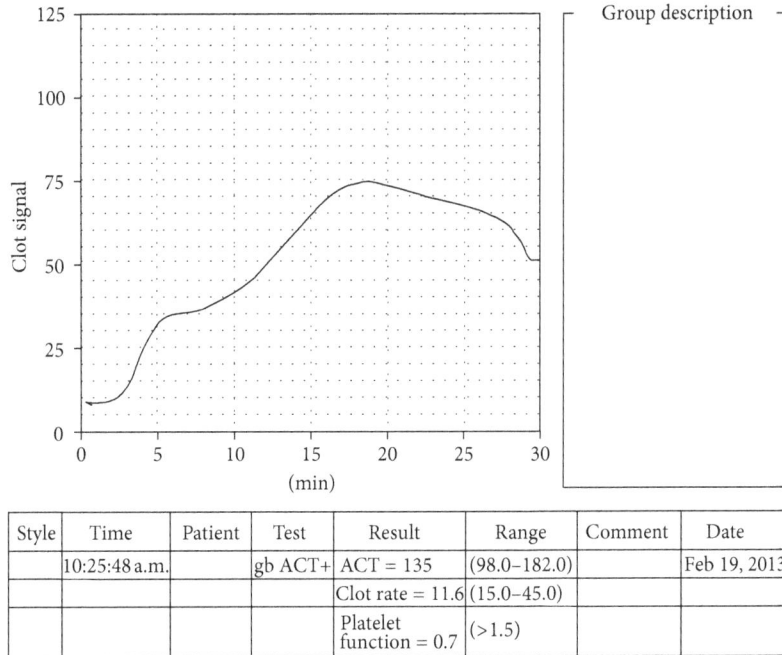

Style	Time	Patient	Test	Result	Range	Comment	Date
	10:25:48 a.m.		gb ACT+	ACT = 135	(98.0–182.0)		Feb 19, 2013
				Clot rate = 11.6	(15.0–45.0)		
				Platelet function = 0.7	(>1.5)		

(a)

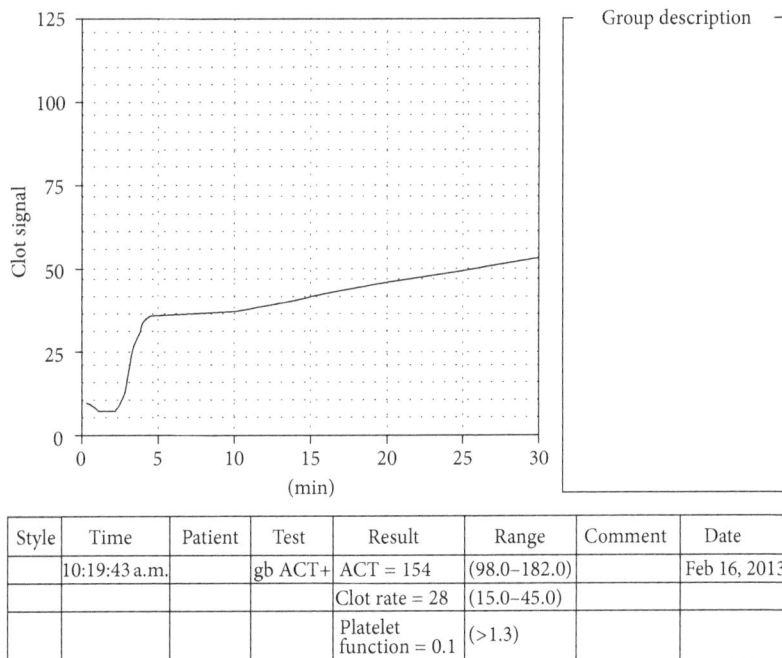

Style	Time	Patient	Test	Result	Range	Comment	Date
	10:19:43 a.m.		gb ACT+	ACT = 154	(98.0–182.0)		Feb 16, 2013
				Clot rate = 28	(15.0–45.0)		
				Platelet function = 0.1	(>1.3)		

(b)

FIGURE 2: (a) Dull rounded peak on sonoclot signature. (b) Flat sonoclot signature.

3.4. *Statistical Methods.* The coagulation profiles of the patients as well as controls were groupwise tabulated. Quantitative data in different groups were expressed by median, mean, and standard deviation. Qualitative data was expressed as percentages. The sonoclot parameters obtained for different groups were compared with controls using the Wilcoxon signed rank test. The statistically significant difference between the patient groups and controls was reported using the Wilcoxon critical values table (at alpha = 0.05 level).

Correlations between sonoclot parameters and conventional coagulation tests were calculated using Spearman's rank correlation and calculated P value. P value was considered significant if less than 0.05.

4. Results

Sonoclot signature parameters in different groups of liver disease as well as control group were studied.

TABLE 2: Comparison between sonoclot parameters in different groups.

Group		G1	G2	G3	G4	Control
SONACT	Mean ± SD (s)	176.31 ± 51.41	146.14 ± 41.76	130.09 ± 31.23	152.44 ± 13.22	137 ± 24.46
	Median (s)	164	147	140	148	143.5
	W_C	88*	27*	22*	23*	—
CR	Mean ± SD (u/min)	29.41 ± 11.31	42.5 ± 17.64	44.54 ± 10.44	34.88 ± 11.54	31.6 ± 7.63
	Median (u/min)	30	44.5	48	30	44
	W_C	50*	59*	56*	11*	—
PF	Mean ± SD	1.54 ± 1.08	2.29 ± 1.31	2.97 ± 0.84	1.36 ± 1.13	2.53 ± 0.76
	Median	1.5	2.7	3.0	1.4	2.45
	W_C	98*	07⸸	45*	31*	—
TP	Mean ± SD (min)	20.5 ± 10.2	11.5 ± 7.6	9.5 ± 10.4	15.3 ± 11.9	11.8 ± 2.8
	Median	17	9.5	6	10	11.5
	W_C	116*	18⸸	44*	11*	—
PA	Mean ± SD (units)	75.31 ± 25.13	91.07 ± 21.94	97.91 ± 8.61	71.94 ± 24.99	95.7 ± 7.48
	Median	80	95	100	75	93.5
	W_C	88*	05⸸	32*	33*	—
	W_T	29	21	10	05	—

G1: group 1 (decompensated cirrhosis), G2: group 2 (noncirrhotic liver disease), G3: group 3 (cirrhotic HCC), G4: group 4 (ACLF).
SONACT: sonoclot activated clotting time, CR: clot rate, PF: platelet function, TP: time to peak, PA: peak amplitude.
SD: standard deviation.
W_C: calculated Wilcoxon test statistic (patient groups versus controls), W_T: tabulated Wilcoxon critical value of alpha = 0.05 ($W_c > W_T$ is considered to be statistically significant).
* Significantly different values as compared to control group.
⸸ Values are not significantly different as compared to controls.

SONACT. SONACT prolongation was seen maximally in G1 (D. cirrhosis) followed by the G4 (ACLF). The variations in SONACT values were also most pronounced in G1 (D. cirrhosis) as compared to other groups. A statistically significant difference was obtained between the SONACT values in patient groups as compared to controls (Table 2).

CR. Mean value of CR was highest in G3 (cirrhosis) and lowest in G1 (D. cirrhosis). The control group was most consistent showing minimal variations in CR. The CR values in patient groups demonstrated a statistically significant difference as compared to the control group (Table 2).

PF. Mean value of PF was lowest in G4 (ACLF) followed by G1 (D. cirrhosis). The difference in PF values between control group and G2 (CH) did not reach levels of statistical significance while the other groups depicted a statistically significant difference as compared to controls (Table 2).

TP. Mean value of TP was the highest in G1 (D. cirrhosis) followed by G4 (ACLF). Deviations from the mean value were much less in the control group. Again, the difference in values between control group and G2 (CH) did not reach levels of statistical significance (Table 2).

PA. Mean value of PA was lowest in G4 (ACLF) closely followed by G1 (D. cirrhosis). All the patient groups except for G2 (CH) demonstrated a statistically significant difference as compared to the control group (Table 2).

TABLE 3: Comparison between R2 peak characters in different groups.

R2 peak in	G1	G2	G3	G4	Control group
Sharp peak (%)	18.75	71.43	90.9	11.11	100
Dull peak (%)	50	7.14	9.1	66.67	00
Flat (%)	31.25	21.43	0	22.22	00

G1: group 1 (decompensated cirrhosis), G2: group 2 (noncirrhotic liver disease), G3: group 3 (cirrhotic HCC), G4: group 4 (ACLF).

4.1. R2 Peak Character. All the R2 peaks in the control group were sharp, well-defined peaks. In contrast, G1 (D. cirrhosis) and G4 (ACLF) showed grossly abnormal R2 peaks with G1 (D. cirrhosis) having around half of the patient population with dull peaks and maximum numbers of flat sonoclot signatures and G4 (ACLF) having around two-thirds of the patients with dull, poorly defined R2 peaks and few flat signatures as well (Table 3). One patient in G1 (D. cirrhosis) (NASH induced cirrhosis) depicted hyperfibrinolysis on sonoclot signature (Figure 3).

Sonoclot parameters and conventional coagulation tests were correlated and studied in patients with liver disease. A significant positive correlation was found between PT-INR, APTT and SONACT ($r = 0.36$, $P < 0.008$ (PT) and $r = 0.43$, $P < 0.0015$ (APTT)) and TP ($r = 0.49$, $P < 0.0002$ (PT) and $r = 0.34$, $P < 0.01$ (APTT)). PT and APTT were found to weakly correlate with CR and PA ($r = -0.46$, $P < 0.0006$ and

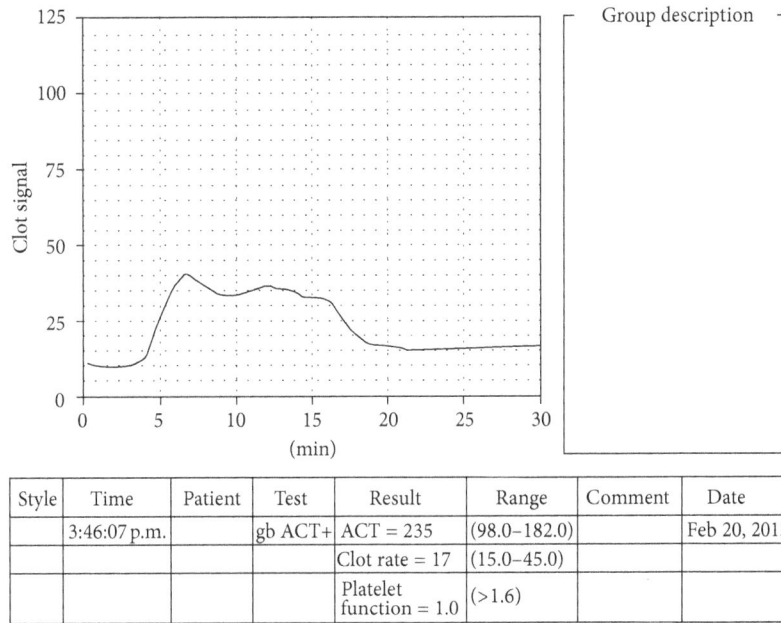

FIGURE 3: Hyperfibrinolysis as detected on sonoclot signature. The characteristic rise of the signature as depicted by R2 peak (suggestive of fibrin gel tightening by platelets) is not seen. Platelet function is subnormal (as calculated from the R3 gradient by the analyser). The hyperfibrinolysis in this case was confirmed by inspecting the sample in the cuvette immediately after the test procedure and was found to be in liquid state.

TABLE 4: Correlation obtained between sonoclot parameters and conventional coagulation variables in patients with liver disease.

Conventional tests		PT-INR	APTT	Fibrinogen	D-dimer	Platelet count
		P value (r: correlation coefficient)				
Sonoclot parameters	SonACT	<0.008 ($r = 0.36$)	<0.0015 ($r = 0.43$)	<0.037 ($r = -0.29$)	0.39 ($r = 0.12$)	<0.01 ($r = -0.34$)
	CR	<0.0025 ($r = -0.41$)	<0.0025 ($r = -0.41$)	<0.004 ($r = 0.39$)	0.96 ($r = -0.005$)	<0.03 ($r = 0.3$)
	PF	0.07 ($r = -0.25$)	0.2 ($r = -0.16$)	<0.001 ($r = 0.44$)	0.89 ($r = 0.02$)	<0.0001 ($r = 0.62$)
	TP	<0.0002 ($r = 0.49$)	<0.01 ($r = 0.34$)	<0.0001 ($r = -0.56$)	0.12 ($r = 0.22$)	<0.0001 ($r = -0.61$)
	PA	<0.0006 ($r = -0.46$)	<0.008 ($r = -0.36$)	<0.0001 ($r = 0.56$)	0.6 ($r = -0.08$)	<0.0002 ($r = 0.5$)

PT: prothrombin time, INR: international normalized ratio, APTT: activated partial thromboplastin time.
SONACT: sonoclot activated clotting time, CR: clot rate, PF: platelet function, TP: time to peak, PA: peak amplitude.
r: Spearmans rank correlation coefficient.
P value is significant if <0.05.

$r = -0.36$, $P < 0.008$, resp.). As the coagulation was activated by glass beads in the sonoclot analyser, these parameters may not accurately correlate with PT and APTT. We also found a significant positive correlation between fibrinogen levels, platelet counts and CR, PF, PA and a significant negative correlation between these two conventional parameters and SONACT and TP. Regarding the D-dimer levels, statistically significant levels were not obtained with any of the sonoclot parameters (Table 4).

Similar correlations were also obtained between the coagulation variables (both sonoclot and conventional) and history of bleed without reaching levels of statistical significance.

5. Discussion

The coagulopathy of liver disease is complex and often unpredictable. While coagulopathy is the hallmark of ACLF group,

the diagnostic tests of coagulation are frequently abnormal in patients with decompensated cirrhosis too [11]. Most of the sonoclot parameters in our study also demonstrate statistically significant abnormalities in decompensated cirrhotics and ACLF group while the noncirrhotic category shows comparatively fewer abnormalities. Prolonged SONACT and shortened CR in these cases can be attributed to decreased synthesis of Vitamin K dependent factors (II, VII, IX, and X). Additionally, prolonged TP and decreased PF could be a result of thrombocytopenia caused by splenic sequestration. Also, impaired platelet aggregation responses to adenosine diphosphate, arachidonic acid, collagen, and thrombin lead to low PF values on sonoclot analysis in chronic liver disease [12].

Despite clear evidence of an increased tendency for bleeding in patients with liver disease, many circumstances also promote local and systemic hypercoagulable states [11, 13].

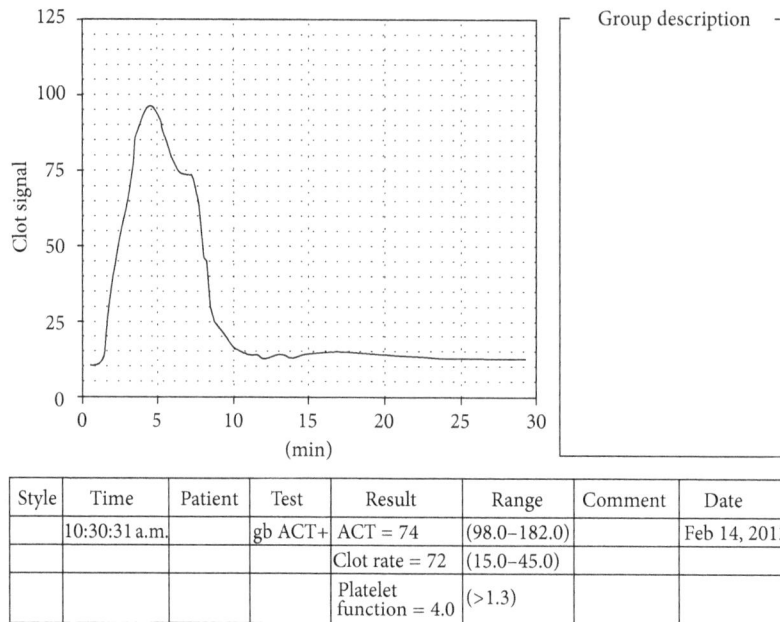

Style	Time	Patient	Test	Result	Range	Comment	Date
	10:30:31 a.m.		gb ACT+	ACT = 74	(98.0–182.0)		Feb 14, 2013
				Clot rate = 72	(15.0–45.0)		
				Platelet function = 4.0	(>1.3)		

FIGURE 4: Hypercoagulability (ACT of sample < ACT normal range, CR of sample ≫ CR normal range). The steep slope of the signature is depicted by increased clot rate (72 units/min). The characteristic rise of the graph (as seen by increased peak amplitude) and sharp peak depict strong clot retraction by platelets. Note also the time to peak which is very short (<5 minutes). The platelet function is very good (as calculated by the R3 gradient).

The routine coagulation tests give no insight regarding the hypercoagulable tendency in patients with liver disease. Due to lack of proper measurement tools to identify those patients who are prone to develop clots, there is reliance on clinical endpoints like deep vein thrombosis, portal vein thrombosis, and so forth to detect the presence of hypercoagulability in these patients [14].

Assessment of prothrombotic states has been carried out in cancer patients, using sonoclot analyser, by studying significantly increased CRs. This study used powdered celite as contact activator instead of glass beads [15]. In our study, the highest mean CR was observed in the cirrhotic HCC group followed by the chronic hepatitis group (Table 2). Some of the CRs of the patients in these groups were quite high as compared to the control group (reaching as high as 72 units/min in one of the patients (Figure 4) (biological reference range: 15–45 units/min)). These abnormal values could help to define the underlying state of hypercoagulability in these patients. As our study did not include the subsequent followup of these cases, the predictive value of CR regarding the prothrombotic tendency cannot be demonstrated with certainty in these patients. Nevertheless, this sonoclot parameter has ample potential to be explored as a predictor of hypercoagulable state in liver diseases.

Hypercoagulable states in cirrhosis have been attributed to decrease in the levels of natural anticoagulant proteins (protein C, protein S, and antithrombin III) and increase in factor VIII and von Willebrand factor levels [1]. Additionally, it is suggested that prothrombotic tendencies are common in HCC patients due to the ability of tumor cells to secrete procoagulants/fibrinolytic inhibitor factors and inflammatory cytokines [16]. Also, elevated homocysteine levels in

patients with HCC have been implicated in thromboembolic tendencies [16]. (Whether the coagulation abnormalities detected in cirrhotic-HCC group in our study were purely because of cirrhosis or influenced by an additional finding of HCC or due to both could not be assessed as the number of cases in this group was not sufficient for such analysis).

The correlation between conventional coagulation tests and sonoclot parameters is rather limited [17, 18]. In this study we have tried to compare the sonoclot parameters with conventional tests so as to be able to replace the need for several coagulation tests in these patients with sonoclot. SONACT and TP have shown a statistically significant positive correlation with PT-INR and APTT and a statistically significant negative correlation with platelet count and fibrinogen levels, whereas CR and PA have demonstrated a statistically significant negative correlation with PT-INR and APTT and a highly significant positive correlation with fibrinogen levels and platelet count. These findings are in agreement with other studies aiming to establish similar correlations [19, 20]. These sonoclot variables once obtained, may subsequently be used to predict the PT-INR and APTT values as well as fibrinogen levels in liver disease patients.

The D-dimer levels in this study have not shown any statistically significant correlation with the sonoclot parameters. D-dimer levels may act as marker for enhanced fibrinolytic activity and disseminated intravascular coagulation (DIC) [21]. However, the increased levels do not always indicate hyperfibrinolysis. In our study, eight patients had very high levels of plasma D-dimers out of which only one patient had hyperfibrinolytic tracing on sonoclot signature. This finding may be related to some studies which show that, in spite of increased levels of D-dimer, actual incidence of hyperfibrinolysis in patients of cirrhosis is quite less and elevated levels of D-dimers may merely be because of coagulation activation cascade [22, 23]. Certain studies have pointed out that the indicators of fibrinolysis such as D-dimer, are breakdown products which have a relatively short half-life. It is likely that the clearance of these molecules is delayed in patients of liver disease resulting in falsely elevated D-dimer levels [24].

As sonoclot effectively measures global hemostasis by monitoring the viscosity changes in blood during initiation of coagulation and development of clot [25], it is immune to the levels of by-products of fibrin breakdown in plasma and may prove to be a better method for detection of hyperfibrinolysis.

Hyperfibrinolysis can be accurately assessed by TEG [26, 27]. As both TEG and sonoclot are based on similar principles, fibrinolysis as detected by sonoclot may be comparable to TEG fibrinolysis. However, it is important to note that fibrinolysis might not always be apparent on sonoclot and localized clot breakdown by plasmin may not be depicted by this method. Hence, the sensitivity of sonoclot to detect the process of fibrinolysis needs to be studied further especially in conjunction with other markers of fibrinolysis before substantiating the importance of this test in cases of hyperfibrinolysis.

As it has already been described in several studies [28, 29], none of the standard tests of coagulation in this study depicted any significant correlation with history of bleed in patients with liver disease. Unfortunately, none of the sonoclot parameters also had any statistically significant correlation with bleeding history in these patients.

Alternative tests such as thromboelastography (TEG), thrombin generation test (TGT), and clotting factor assays should be explored to predict bleeding and hypercoagulability in liver disease. TEG has been applied in liver disease patients to assess global coagulation. Stravitz et al. have noted normal TEG parameters in spite of prolonged PT-INR values in liver injury patients [30].

TEG has certain disadvantages like increased failure rates of the test procedure. In our experience, sonoclot has proved to be more durable than TEG requiring fewer repetitions. Also, SONACT is considered more specific as it represents the initial clot formation and reflects clotting factor defects whereas TEG reaction time (R) gives information about a more mature and developed fibrin clot [31].

Individual factor assays have also been used to define hemostatic disorders in liver disease but their main disadvantage is that they do not give information on the entire coagulation process. Also, they are more time-consuming and expensive and may show significant interlaboratory variations [32]. In contrast, sonoclot provides overall picture of coagulation profile in a single test procedure.

Hemostatic defects in liver disease have been assessed by several coagulation measures including individual factor assays, TEG and sonoclot. Not only is the assessment of factor levels cumbersome, but it also fails to give complete information on the coagulation system. TEG, like sonoclot, is a global assay of coagulation but the reaction time obtained does not accurately define the initial clotting process. Hence,

sonoclot assay is quite an accurate tool, comparable to TEG for assessing global coagulopathic disorders in liver disease.

TGT has also shown utility in assessing bleeding or thrombotic risks and may be used to predict the coagulopathy of liver disease [33]. Studies have shown that the balance of procoagulants and anticoagulants in patients with cirrhosis was normal when thrombin generation was measured in presence of thrombomodulin even though PT and APTT were prolonged [34]. Hence, this test should be developed in appropriate clinical trials as a predictor of bleeding as well as thrombosis in liver disease [35].

6. Conclusion

Sonoclot analyzer can be used as an effective tool to assess coagulation defects in liver disease patients as statistically significant differences are obtained on sonoclot signatures especially in the ACLF and decompensated cirrhotic groups as compared to normal healthy individuals.

The statistically significant correlations between routine tests and sonoclot parameters prove that this global test of coagulation should be used in conjunction with the standard tests to define the hemostatic profile in liver disease as conventional tests alone have shown poor reproducibility with bleeding and thrombotic risks. CR on sonoclot signature may prove to be an effective guide for predicting thrombosis in patients of liver disease in the future. Similarly, the detection of hyperfibrinolysis on sonoclot needs to be explored further in relation with TEG and plasma D-dimer levels.

Acknowledgments

The authors gratefully acknowledge Mrs. Deepti Srivastava for her statistical inputs and Mrs. Rekha and Mr. Alok for laboratory data entry.

References

[1] T. Lisman, S. H. Caldwell, A. K. Burroughs et al., "Hemostasis and thrombosis in patients with liver disease: the ups and downs," *Journal of Hepatology*, vol. 53, no. 2, pp. 362–371, 2010.

[2] P. G. Northup, V. Sundaram, M. B. Fallon et al., "Hypercoagulation and thrombophilia in liver disease," *Journal of Thrombosis and Haemostasis*, vol. 6, no. 1, pp. 2–9, 2008.

[3] T. Lisman, Y. van Leeuwen, J. Adelmeijer et al., "Interlaboratory variability in assessment of the model of end-stage liver disease score," *Liver International*, vol. 28, no. 10, pp. 1344–1345, 2008.

[4] M. A. Mcmichael and S. A. Smith, "Viscoelastic coagulation testing: technology, applications, and limitations," *Veterinary Clinical Pathology*, vol. 40, no. 2, pp. 140–153, 2011.

[5] M. T. Ganter and C. K. Hofer, "Coagulation monitoring: current techniques and clinical use of viscoelastic point-of-care coagulation devices," *Anesthesia and Analgesia*, vol. 106, no. 5, pp. 1366–1375, 2008.

[6] D. A. Hett, D. Walker, S. N. Pilkington, and D. C. Smith, "Sonoclot analysis," *British Journal of Anaesthesia*, vol. 75, no. 6, pp. 771–776, 1995.

[7] R. de Franchis, "Evolving consensus in portal hypertension. Report of the Baveno IV consensus workshop on methodology

of diagnosis and therapy in portal hypertension," *Journal of Hepatology*, vol. 43, no. 1, pp. 167–176, 2005.

[8] G. Garcia-Tsao, J. Bosch, and R. J. Groszmann, "Portal hypertension and variceal bleeding—unresolved issues. Summary of an American Association for the study of liver diseases and European Association for the study of the liver single-topic conference," *Hepatology*, vol. 47, no. 5, pp. 1764–1772, 2008.

[9] S. K. Sarin, A. Kumar, J. Almeida et al., "Acute on chronic liver failure (ACLF): consensus recommendations of the Asia Pacific Association for the Study of the Liver (APASL)," *Hepatology International*, vol. 3, pp. 269–282, 2009.

[10] A. Zipprich, G. Garcia-Tsao, S. Rogowski, W. E. Fleig, T. Seufferlein, and M. M. Dollinger, "Prognostic indicators of survival in patients with compensated and decompensated cirrhosis," *Liver International*, vol. 39, pp. 1407–1414, 2012.

[11] R. Jalan, P. Gines, J. C. Olson et al., "Acute on chronic liver failure," *Journal of Hepatology*, vol. 57, pp. 1336–1348, 2012.

[12] M. Senzolo, P. Burra, E. Cholongitas, and A. K. Burroughs, "New insights into the coagulopathy of liver disease and liver transplantation," *World Journal of Gastroenterology*, vol. 12, no. 48, pp. 7725–7736, 2006.

[13] P. G. Northup, "Hypercoagulation in liver disease," *Clinics in Liver Disease*, vol. 13, no. 1, pp. 109–116, 2009.

[14] P. G. Northup, M. M. McMahon, A. P. Ruhl et al., "Coagulopathy does not fully protect hospitalized cirrhosis patients from peripheral venous thromboembolism," *American Journal of Gastroenterology*, vol. 101, no. 7, pp. 1524–1528, 2006.

[15] J. L. Francis, D. A. Francis, and G. J. Gunathilagan, "Assessment of hypercoagulability in patients with cancer using the Sonoclot analyzer(TM) and thromboelastography," *Thrombosis Research*, vol. 74, no. 4, pp. 335–346, 1994.

[16] D. N. Samonakis, I. E. Koutroubakis, A. Sfiridaki et al., "Hypercoagulable states in patients with hepatocellular carcinoma," *Digestive Diseases and Sciences*, vol. 49, no. 5, pp. 854–858, 2004.

[17] B. L. D. Schaer, A. I. Bentz, R. C. Boston, J. E. Palmer, and P. A. Wilkins, "Comparison of viscoelastic coagulation analysis and standard coagulation profiles in critically ill neonatal foals to outcome," *Journal of Veterinary Emergency and Critical Care*, vol. 19, no. 1, pp. 88–95, 2009.

[18] M. Furuhashi, N. Ura, K. Hasegawa et al., "Sonoclot coagulation analysis: new bedside monitoring for determination of the appropriate heparin dose during haemodialysis," *Nephrology Dialysis Transplantation*, vol. 17, no. 8, pp. 1457–1462, 2002.

[19] T. Miyashita and M. Kuro, "Evaluation of platelet function by Sonoclot analysis compared with other hemostatic variables in cardiac surgery," *Anesthesia and Analgesia*, vol. 87, no. 6, pp. 1228–1233, 1998.

[20] J. J. Liszka-Hackzell and G. Ekback, "Analysis of the information content in sonoclot data and reconstruction of coagulation test variables," *Journal of Medical Systems*, vol. 26, no. 1, pp. 1–8, 2002.

[21] S. S. Adam, N. S. Key, and C. S. Greenberg, "D-dimer antigen: current concepts and future prospects," *Blood*, vol. 113, no. 13, pp. 2878–2887, 2009.

[22] N. Bennani-Baiti and H. A. Daw, "Primary hyperfibrinolysis in liver disease: a critical review," *Clinical Advances in Hematology & Oncology*, vol. 9, no. 3, pp. 250–252, 2011.

[23] D. Prisco and E. Grifoni, "The role of D-dimer testing in patients with suspected venous thromboembolism," *Seminars in Thrombosis and Hemostasis*, vol. 35, no. 1, pp. 50–59, 2009.

[24] F. Violi, D. Ferro, S. Basili et al., "Hyperfibrinolysis resulting from clotting activation in patients with different degrees of cirrhosis," *Hepatology*, vol. 17, no. 1, pp. 78–83, 1993.

[25] M. A. Lyew and W. C. Spaulding, "Template for rapid analysis of the Sonoclot signature," *Journal of Clinical Monitoring*, vol. 13, no. 4, pp. 273–277, 1997.

[26] A. Chen and J. Teruya, "Global hemostasis testing thromboelastography: old technology, new applications," *Clinics in Laboratory Medicine*, vol. 29, no. 2, pp. 391–407, 2009.

[27] R. Kaku, M. Matsumi, M. Ichiyama et al., "Massive bleeding due to hyperfibrinolysis during living-related liver transplantation for terminal liver cirrhosis, report of two cases," *Masui*, vol. 52, no. 11, pp. 1195–1199, 2003.

[28] J. B. Segal and W. H. Dzik, "Paucity of studies to support that abnormal coagulation test results predict bleeding in the setting of invasive procedures: an evidence-based review," *Transfusion*, vol. 45, no. 9, pp. 1413–1425, 2005.

[29] K. Ewe, "Bleeding after liver biopsy does not correlate with indices of peripheral coagulation," *Digestive Diseases and Sciences*, vol. 26, no. 5, pp. 388–393, 1981.

[30] R. T. Stravitz, T. Lisman, V. A. Luketic et al., "Minimal effects of acute liver injury/acute liver failure on hemostasis as assessed by thromboelastography," *Journal of Hepatology*, vol. 56, no. 1, pp. 129–136, 2012.

[31] K. A. Tanaka, F. Szlam, H. Y. Sun, T. Taketomi, and J. H. Levy, "Thrombin generation assay and viscoelastic coagulation monitors demonstrate differences in the mode of thrombin inhibition between unfractionated heparin and bivalirudin," *Anesthesia and Analgesia*, vol. 105, no. 4, pp. 933–939, 2007.

[32] P. G. Northup and S. H. Caldwell, "Coagulation in liver disease: a guide for the clinician," *Clinical Gastroenterology and Hepatology*, vol. 11, pp. 1064–1074, 2013.

[33] H. C. Hemker, R. Al Dieri, E. de Smedt, and S. Béguin, "Thrombin generation, a function test of the haemostatic-thrombotic system," *Thrombosis and Haemostasis*, vol. 96, no. 5, pp. 553–561, 2006.

[34] A. Tripodi, F. Salerno, V. Chantarangkul et al., "Evidence of normal thrombin generation in cirrhosis despite abnormal conventional coagulation tests," *Hepatology*, vol. 41, no. 3, pp. 553–558, 2005.

[35] R. Kar, S. S. Kar, and S. K. Sarin, "Hepatic coagulopathy-intricacies and challenges, a cross sectional descriptive study of 110 patients from a superspeciality institute of North India with review of literature," *Blood Coagulation and Fibrinolysis*, vol. 24, pp. 175–180, 2013.

4

Approach to Management of Thrombotic Thrombocytopenic Purpura at University of Cincinnati

N. Abdel Karim,[1,2] **S. Haider,**[1] **C. Siegrist,**[1,2] **N. Ahmad,**[1]
A. Zarzour,[2] **J. Ying,**[3] **Z. Yasin,**[4] **and R. Sacher**[1,2,5]

[1] Department of Internal Medicine, University of Cincinnati College of Medicine, Cincinnati, OH 45267, USA
[2] Division of Hematology and Oncology, University of Cincinnati College of Medicine, 231 Albert Sabin Way, Cincinnati, OH 45267, USA
[3] Department of Environmental Health, University of Cincinnati College of Medicine, Cincinnati, OH 45267, USA
[4] Department of Hematology and Oncology, Baylor College of Medicine, Houston, TX 76706, USA
[5] Hoxworth Blood Center, University of Cincinnati College of Medicine, Cincinnati, OH 45267, USA

Correspondence should be addressed to N. Abdel Karim; nagla.karim@uc.edu

Academic Editor: Estella M. Matutes

Thrombotic Thrombocytopenic Purpura (TTP) is a rare hematologic emergency, congenital or acquired, characterized by ischemic damage of various organs because of platelet aggregation. It is the common name for adults with microangiopathic hemolytic anemia, thrombocytopenia, with or without neurologic or renal abnormalities, and without another etiology; children without renal failure are also described as TTP. Plasma exchange (PE) is the main stay of treatment in combination with steroids and immunosuppressive therapies. The monoclonal antibody against CD20 Rituximab decreases the production of antibodies from B lymphocytes and it is used for antibodies-mediated diseases including TTP. We present our data on retrospective analysis of rituximab in treatment of TTP at University of Cincinnati in a series of 22 patients from 1997 to 2009. Our results showed that PE with immunosuppressive therapy resulted in decreased duration of PE, relapse rate, and increased duration of remission in patients with TTP.

1. Introduction

TTP is a rare hematologic emergency in which various organs, mainly the brain and kidneys, are affected by ischemic damage due to platelets aggregations. It is characterized by thrombocytopenia, MAHA, fever, and neurological and renal abnormalities; however, this pentad is not necessary for diagnosis. TTP may be congenital or acquired as a result of HIV, connective tissue disorder, cancers, drugs like quinine, mitomycin C, cyclosporine, oral contraceptives, and ticlopidine or it may be idiopathic. Only thrombocytopenia and MAHA without another clinically apparent etiology (e.g., disseminated intravascular coagulation, malignant hypertension, severe preeclampsia, sepsis, and systemic malignancy) are required to suspect the diagnosis of TTP and to initiate PE.

MAHA is defined as nonimmune hemolysis (i.e., negative direct antiglobulin test) with prominent red cell fragmentation (schistocytes) observed on the peripheral blood smear.

The pathogenesis may be autoimmune in nature since autoantibodies against ADAMTS13 (acronym for a Disintegrin and a Metalloproteinase with Thrombospondin-1 Motifs, 13th member of the family), which cleaves von Willebrand Factor (vWF), are typically present in most cases of idiopathic TTP. These antibodies cause the absence of ADAMTS 13 protease activity and the persistence of vWF. Subsequently the procoagulation tendency dominates and causes the systemic abnormalities. The mainstay of treatment for patients with TTP is PE in conjunction with steroids. The mortality rate of TTP prior to the use of PE was approximately 90 percent [1–3] and is currently 20 percent or less in patients

TABLE 1: Characteristics of patients in PE and PE + R/C arm.

Variable	Category	All (N = 22)	PE (13)	PE + R/C (9)	P value
Age		41.5	46	38	0.3771
Gender	Female	19 (86.4%)	10 (76.9)	9 (100)	0.2403
Race	African-American	16 (72.7%)	8 (61.5%)	8 (88.9%)	0.3330
New/Relapsed	Relapsed	5 (22.7%)	1 (7.7%)	4 (44.4%)	0.1159
Pregnancy	Yes	3 (13.6%)	3 (23.1%)	0 (0%)	0.2403
Schistocytes	Present	21 (95.5%)	12 (92.3%)	9 (100%)	1.000
Proteinuria	Yes	9 (40.9%)	4 (30.8%)	5 (55.6%)	0.3842
Died		6 (27.3%)	6 (46.2%)	0 (0%)	0.0461
Platelets (×1000)		15.5 (0.03, 60)	21 (4, 60)	8 (0.03, 27)	0.0839
WBC		10.4 (3.7, 16.4)	10.8 (4.1, 10.8)	8.9 (3.7, 16.4)	0.6706
Hb		8.5 (4.4, 10.7)	8.8 (6.4, 10.2)	7.4 (4.4, 10.7)	0.3602
Reticulocytes		4.9 (3.0, 12.3)	4.0 (3.0, 12.3)	7.1 (4.2, 11.5)	0.3624
Creatinine		1.0 (0.04, 9.8)	1.4 (0.4, 9.8)	1.0 (0.5, 1.9)	0.2018
LDH		827.5 (225, 2437)	1000 (225, 2302)	698 (226, 2437)	0.7283
Duration of PE		252 (53, 2624)	284 (53, 2337)	220 (69, 2624)	0.7418
Time between 1st PE and 1st Ritual		—	—	69 (0, 2375)	

treated with PE [3–5]. PE reverses the platelet consumption responsible for the thrombus formation and symptoms in TTP.

Although the majority of patients with TTP achieve remission with PE + steroids therapy [6], more than one-third of the patients survive the acute phase relapse within 10 years [7]. Different immunosuppressive therapies (such as intravenous immunoglobulins, vincristine, cyclophosphamide) [8–11] and splenectomy [12] have been suggested with no definitive benefit.

Rituximab is a monoclonal antibody directed against CD20 which is specific to B lymphocytes. It depletes the production of antibodies from these lymphocytes and thus has been used for antibodies-mediated diseases including TTP. Here we report our experience at the University of Cincinnati for over a decade of using Rituximab in the treatment of TTP patients.

2. Aims and Methodology

The objective of this study was to review the medical records of patients diagnosed with TTP at the University of Cincinnati between the period of 1997 and 2009 and compare the outcome of patients who received PE alone to those who were treated with PE in combination with Rituximab-based chemotherapy (PE + R/RC). The variables reviewed were patient's demographics, types of treatment received (i.e., PE alone versus PE + R/RC), duration of PE, remission rate, and duration of remission. IRB approval was obtained and patient's outcome was followed during this period of time. Rituximab was added to the treatment if there is no response after 4 weeks of PE or there is brief response with relapse in 4 weeks. It was given at 375 mg/sq. meter every week for four doses.

3. Statistical Analysis

Numerical and categorical variables were summarized using median (range) and frequency (in %), respectively.

Nonparametric Wilcoxon rank sum tests were used to compare medians between groups while frequencies were compared using Fisher's exact test. For patients in the PE + R/RC group, their duration time using PE only was compared to that of PE and R/RC combined using a Wilcoxon signed-rank test. All patients were followed up to their last visit or death after treatment. Survival curves were estimated and plotted using a Kaplan-Meier survival method and compared between PE and PE + R/RC groups using a log rank test. All statistical analyses were performed using a SAS 9.2 (SAS, Cary, NC) package. P values <0.05 were considered statistically significant.

4. Results

A total of 22 patients were studied. The median (range) of age was 41.5 (17 to 61) and the female : male ratio was 19 : 3. Thirteen patients (59%) were treated with PE only while the rest of 9 patients (41%) were treated with PE + R/RC. Please see Table 1. All patients in the PE + R/RC group were female. Among the rest of 10 female patients in the PE group, 3 were found pregnant. All patients started the treatment at the time of diagnosis, only one patient started the next day because of issues with the functioning of line. Patient's baseline clinical characteristics (presence of proteinuria, presence of schistocytes on blood smear, white blood cells count, hemoglobin levels, reticulocytes count, creatinine levels, and LDH levels) showed no difference between the two groups.

The median (range) of duration of PE was 284 (53, 337) days in the PE group. In the PE + R/RC group, the median (range) of duration using Rituximab only (R/RC only) was 151 (30, 291) days, shorter than that of the PE group (P = 0.0912). However, the entire duration of PE in the PE + R/RC group was 220 (69, 624) days, which showed no difference to the duration in the PE group (P = 0.742).

It is important to underline this point because the decrease in duration of PE reflects a faster achievement of remission of the disease. Although PE is known to decrease the mortality rate of TTP from 90 percent (prior to the use of PE) to 20 percent, the procedure itself may have adverse reactions, such as pneumothorax, hemorrhage, local and systemic infection at catheter site, venous thrombosis, catheter obstruction, citrate anticoagulant-induced symptoms of hypocalcemia, (paresthesias, muscle cramps, nausea and vomiting, hypotension, and tetany), allergic symptoms including anaphylactoid reactions, or transfusion-related acute lung injury (TRALI) [13].

All patients in the PE + R/RC were followed by a median (range) of 41 (7, 88) months and all survived. Patients in the PE group were followed by 20 (8, 77) months and 6 (46.2%) died after treatment. From the review of charts, we were able to identify the cause of death as intracranial hemorrhage in 1 patient and five deaths were attributed to catheter-related sepsis. Thus the death rate was higher in the PE group ($P = 0.046$) and underlines the importance of immunosuppression using rituximab in the treatment of TTP. Nevertheless, the 3 pregnant women in the PE group were all alive. Figure 1 shows survival curves in the two groups. The PE group showed a lower survival curve than that of the PE + R/RC group, which was a flat line at 100% given that all survived up to the last visit ($P = 0.011$).

5. Discussion

There is rationale for the use of rituximab in patients with TTP who do not respond promptly to PE and steroids or who have a relapse. Such patients almost always have severe ADAMTS13 deficiency and a demonstrable inhibitor. We were not able to find ADAMTS 13 values from retrospective analysis of the charts. However, this rationale is not often present during their first episode, as information concerning ADAMTS13 activity is generally not available at the time PE is instituted. Patients with a more severe course and more neurologic abnormalities, who either do not respond to PE, develop worsening disease in spite of continuing PE plus glucocorticoids, or have relapsing disease, may benefit from more intensive immunosuppressive treatment.

Rituximab can be administered during a course of PE. The dose of rituximab should be given immediately after the apheresis procedure to avoid unnecessary removal of the antibody. Although plasmapheresis removes much of the rituximab, PE on the day following rituximab treatment does not appear to impair rituximab's effectiveness [14]. This may be because the standard rituximab dose used ($375 \, \mathrm{mg/m}^2$) may exceed the dose required to deplete autoantibody-producing B cells. No increase in infections was documented during the first year of follow-up in the rituximab-treated group.

On review of the literature, Goyal et al. showed that 4 out of 12 patients (33%) who received PE and rituximab relapsed after 62 ± 8.5 months achieving remission [15].

There are no randomized trials evaluating the benefit of combining rituximab with PE. However, observational studies have suggested good outcomes in some settings. Rituximab should be considered in the management of TTP along with PE and well-designed prospective studies are needed to evaluate its role in TTP.

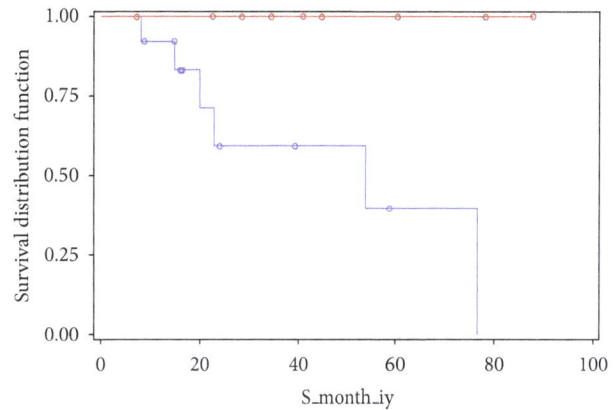

FIGURE 1: Survival curves of PE + R/C (red) versus PE (blue) alone arm.

6. Conclusion

TTP is adequately treated with PE in the acute setting; however, PE with immunosuppressive therapy trending towards a decreased duration of PE, relapse rate, and increased duration of remission. Prospective studies with immunosuppressive therapy upfront are needed to substantiate this.

References

[1] E. L. Amorosi and J. E. Ultmann, "Thrombotic thrombocytopenic purpura: report of 16 cases and review of the literature," *Medicine*, vol. 45, no. 2, pp. 139–160, 1966.

[2] G. Remuzzi and S. Garella, "HUS and TTP: variable expression of a single entity," *Kidney International*, vol. 32, no. 2, pp. 292–308, 1987.

[3] H. von Baeyer, "Plasmapheresis in thrombotic microangiopathy-associated syndromes: review of outcome data derived from clinical trials and open studies," *Therapeutic Apheresis*, vol. 6, no. 4, pp. 320–328, 2002.

[4] J. A. Kremer Hovinga, S. K. Vesely, D. R. Terrell, B. Lämmle, and J. N. George, "Survival and relapse in patients with thrombotic thrombocytopenic purpura," *Blood*, vol. 115, no. 8, pp. 1500–1511, 2010.

[5] G. A. Rock, K. H. Shumak, N. A. Buskard et al., "Comparison of plasma exchange with plasma infusion in the treatment of thrombotic thrombocytopenic purpura," *The New England Journal of Medicine*, vol. 325, no. 6, pp. 393–397, 1991.

[6] C. L. Balduini, L. Gugliotta, M. Luppi et al., "High versus standard dose methylprednisolone in the acute phase of idiopathic thrombotic thrombocytopenic purpura: a randomized study," *Annals of Hematology*, vol. 89, no. 6, pp. 591–596, 2010.

[7] K. H. Shumak, G. A. Rock, and R. C. Nair, "Late relapses in patients successfully treated for thrombotic thrombocytopenic purpura," *Annals of Internal Medicine*, vol. 122, no. 8, pp. 569–572, 1995.

[8] J. M. Durand, P. Lefevre, G. Kaplanski, and J. Soubeyrand, "Ineffectiveness of high-dose intravenous gammaglobulin infusion in thrombotic thrombocytopenic purpura," *American Journal of Hematology*, vol. 42, no. 2, article 234, 1993.

[9] J. M. Durand, P. Lefevre, G. Kaplanski, H. Telle, and J. Soubeyrand, "Vincristine for thrombotic thrombocytopenia purpura," *The Lancet*, vol. 340, no. 8825, pp. 977–978, 1992.

[10] N. T. J. O'Connor, M. J. O'Shea, and L. F. Hill, "Vincristine for thrombotic thrombocytopenic purpura," *The Lancet*, vol. 340, no. 8817, p. 490, 1992.

[11] M. Udvardy and K. Rak, "Cyclophosphamide for chronic relapsing thrombotic thrombocytopenic purpura," *The Lancet*, vol. 336, no. 8729, pp. 1508–1509, 1990.

[12] M. A. Crowther, N. Heddle, C. P. M. Hayward, T. Warkentin, and J. G. Kelton, "Splenectomy done during hematologic remission to prevent relapse in patients with thrombotic thrombocytopenic purpura," *Annals of Internal Medicine*, vol. 125, no. 4, pp. 294–296, 1996.

[13] M. A. Rizvi, S. K. Vesely, J. N. George et al., "Complications of plasma exchange in 71 consecutive patients treated for clinically suspected thrombotic thrombocytopenic purpura-hemolytic-uremic syndrome," *Transfusion*, vol. 40, no. 8, pp. 896–901, 2000.

[14] V. McDonald, K. Manns, I. J. Mackie, S. J. Machin, and M. A. Scully, "Rituximab pharmacokinetics during the management of acute idiopathic thrombotic thrombocytopenic purpura," *Journal of Thrombosis and Haemostasis*, vol. 8, no. 6, pp. 1201–1208, 2010.

[15] J. Goyal, J. Adamski, J. L. Lima, and M. B. Marques, "Relapses of thrombotic thrombocytopenic purpura after treatment with rituximab," *Journal of Clinical Apheresis*, 2013.

5

Post-Autologous (ASCT) Stem Cell Transplant Therapy in Multiple Myeloma

Zeina Al-Mansour and Muthalagu Ramanathan

Division of Hematology/Oncology, School of Medicine, University of Massachusetts, 55 Lake Avenue North, Worcester, MA 01655, USA

Correspondence should be addressed to Muthalagu Ramanathan; muthalagu.ramanathan@umassmemorial.org

Academic Editor: Shaji Kumar

Autologous stem cell transplant (ASCT) is the standard of care in transplant-eligible multiple myeloma patients and is associated with significant improvement in progression-free survival (PFS), complete remission rates (CR), and overall survival (OS). However, majority of patients eventually relapse, with a median PFS of around 36 months. Relapses are harder to treat and prognosis declines with each relapse. Achieving and maintaining "best response" to initial therapy is the ultimate goal of first-line treatment and sustained CR is a powerful surrogate for extended survival especially in high-risk multiple myeloma. ASCT is often followed by consolidation/maintenance phase to deepen and/or maintain the response achieved by induction and ASCT. Novel agents like thalidomide, lenalidomide, and bortezomib have been used as single agents or in combination. Thalidomide use has been associated with a meaningful improvement in PFS and EFS, however, with substantial side effects. Data with lenalidomide maintenance after-ASCT is favorable, but the optimal duration of lenalidomide maintenance is still unclear. Bortezomib use has been associated with superior outcomes, predominantly in high-risk myeloma patients. Combination regimens utilizing a proteasome inhibitor (i.e., bortezomib) with an immunomodulatory drug (thalidomide or lenalidomide) have provided the best outcomes. This review article serves as a review of the best available evidence in post-ASCT approaches in multiple myeloma.

1. Introduction

Autologous stem cell transplant (ASCT) is the standard of care in transplant-eligible patients, based on several phase III trials and meta-analyses in the mid-1990s showing significant improvement in progression-free survival (PFS) and complete remission rates (CR) as well as overall survival (OS) [1–3]. In their IFM-90 trial, Attal et al. reported superior outcomes of high-dose chemotherapy (HDC) followed by ASCT compared to conventional chemotherapy alone, with improvement noted in OS (57%), complete remission rate CR (22%) and event-free survival EFS (16%), as well as median OS improvement to 57 months versus 44 months [1]. However, majority of patients eventually relapsed with a median PFS of around 36 months. Unfortunately, relapses are harder to treat and prognosis declines with each relapse. Therefore, achieving and maintaining "best response" to initial therapy is the ultimate goal of first-line treatment.

Several studies have shown that sustained CR for 3 years or more from treatment initiation is a powerful surrogate for extended survival especially in high-risk multiple myeloma [4].

The treatment algorithm for newly diagnosed multiple myeloma (MM) has evolved over the last two decades with the incorporation of novel agents in myeloma induction regimens prior to ASCT [5, 6]. Improved outcomes when used before ASCT were the basis for the use of these agents in the post-ASCT setting as a means to *deepen* and *maintain* the response achieved by HDC-ASCT in myeloma patients. The benefit of maintenance therapy is thought to be due to suppression of clonal proliferation of myeloma cancer cells thereby delaying or preventing relapse.

In this review article, we will briefly review the significance of the depth of response to induction chemotherapy and will focus on how to deepen or maintain response by means of a consolidation approach, maintenance, or both.

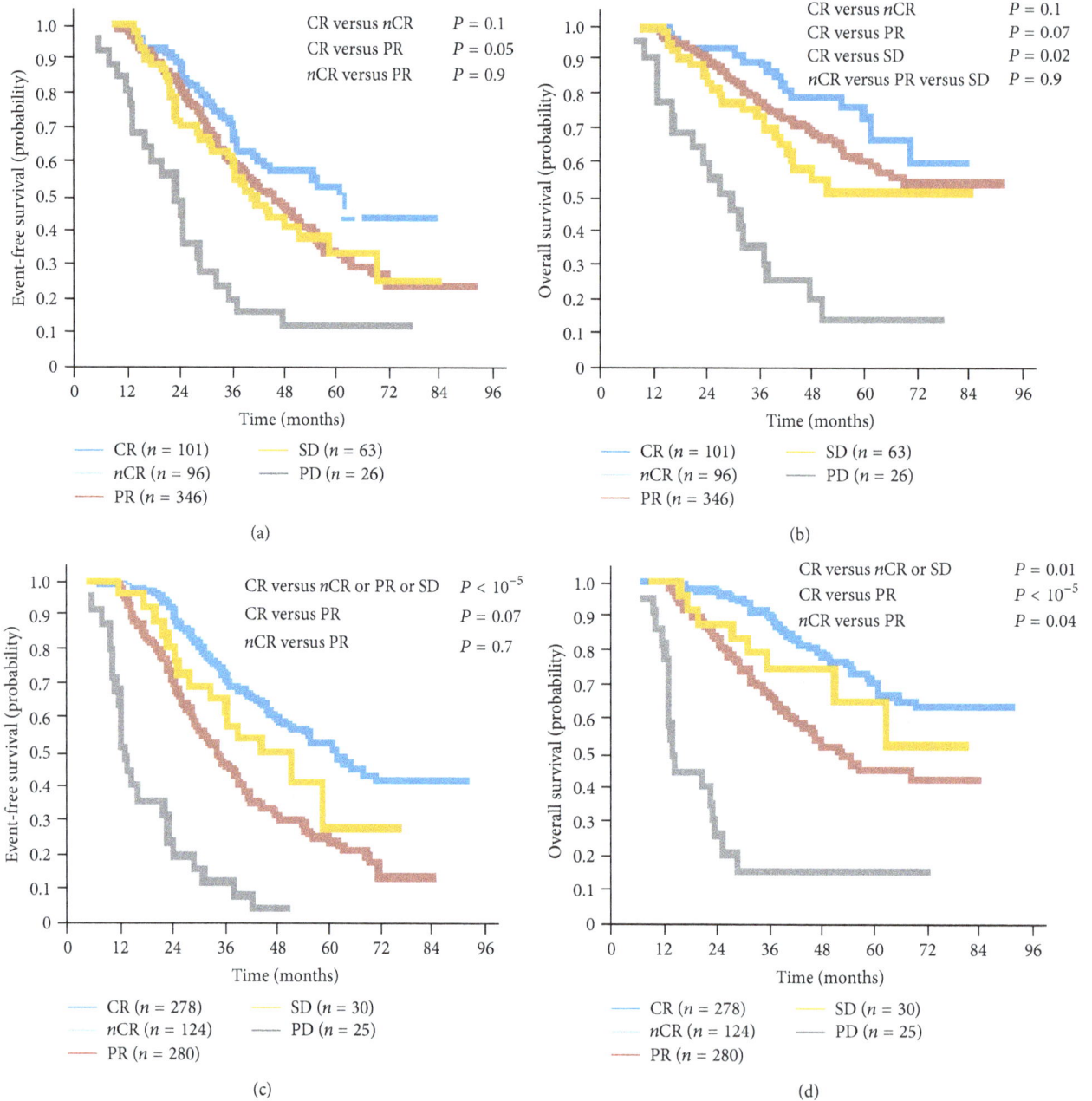

FIGURE 1: Achievement of CR is associated with improvement in survival outcomes after induction as well as after ASCT (adapted with permission from [10]).

2. Significance of Depth of Response to Chemotherapy

Multiple studies have suggested a survival advantage from attaining a deeper response to induction chemotherapy and HDC-ASCT, and sustained CR was shown to be a surrogate for OS in myeloma population [7–14] (see Figure 1). In a meta-analysis of 21 studies including 4,990 patients in 10 prospective and 11 retrospective studies, highly significant associations between maximal response and survival outcomes were demonstrated [7]. However, it remains uncertain whether this just reflects underlying disease biology (i.e., prognostic marker) versus a specific treatment effect, especially since the definition of CR was historically ununified until the development of the IMWG treatment response criteria [8, 9].

Furthermore, achieving stringent CR (sCR), as defined by IMWG criteria, is associated with even better outcomes compared to CR, with median time-to-progression of 50 months with sCR versus 20 months with CR [11, 12]. The benefit is more pronounced when comparing OS outcomes (see Figure 2).

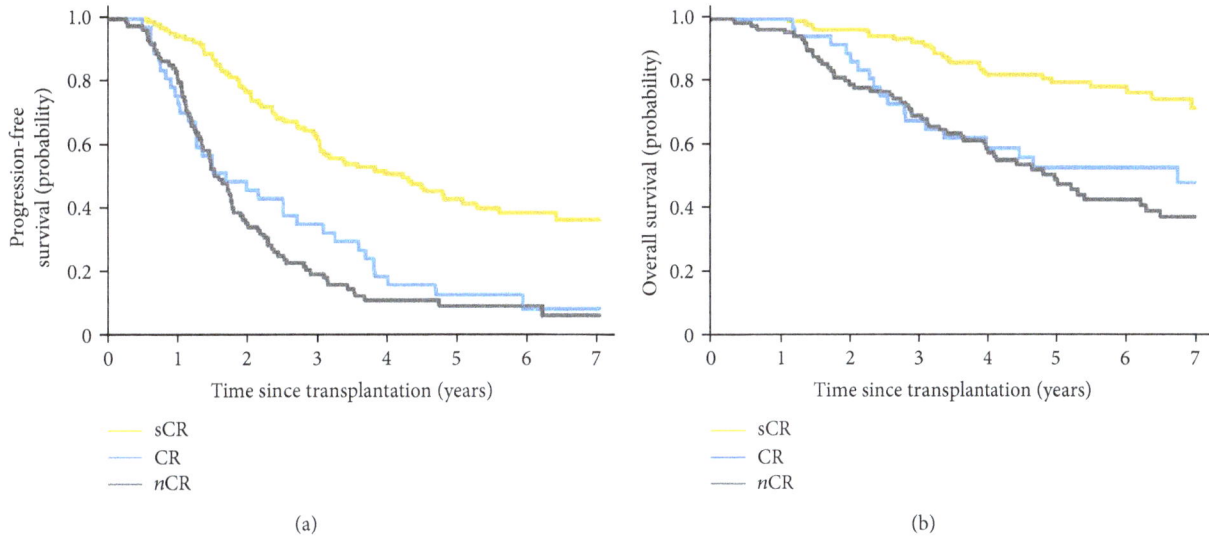

FIGURE 2: sCR is associated with superior PFS and OS compared to CR (adapted from [11]).

2.1. Evaluation of Minimal Residual Disease (MRD). The techniques for assessing disease burden in MM have evolved over time. Sensitive methods to detect MRD have been used to evaluate either immunophenotypic response or molecular response [13, 14, 18, 19]. In their recent article about *Controversies in the Assessment of Minimal Residual Disease in MM*, Corradini et al. reviewed the clinical significance of MRD negativity using highly sensitive techniques and concluded that, at the present time, the goal of assessing MRD is for risk stratification and to evaluate response to novel agents particularly in the context of clinical trials [20].

Immunophenotypic response assessment by multiparameter flow cytometry (MFC) was evaluated after ASCT in a subset of patients enrolled in Myeloma Research Council (MRC) IX, the Spanish GEM 2000, and GEM 2005 trials. Absence of MRD at D + 100 was associated with statistically significant improvement in both PFS and OS in patients with favorable and adverse cytogenetics [13, 21, 22]. Additionally, persistent MRD by MFC at D + 100 (HR 8.0, $P = 0.005$) and high-risk cytogenetics by FISH (HR 17.3, $P = 0.002$) were the only independent factors that predicted unsustained CR and shortened OS [22].

Molecular response can be assessed by either PCR-based techniques (either fluorescent or allele-specific oligonucleotide PCR) or next generation sequencing (NGS). MRD assessment by PCR was evaluated in several trials and homogenously showed that lower levels of MRD were associated with markedly better survival and longer disease-free periods [14, 23–25].

It should be noted, though, that these results were based on subsets of patients enrolled in the cited trials where MRD assessment was done only in those who had a bone marrow sample at D + 100 (in those assessed by MFC), thus raising concern for selection bias. Additionally, variety of technical factors can affect the sensitivity, specificity, and applicability of MFC such as time of sampling with respect to treatment, number of markers, number of cells counted,

and marrow cellularity. On the other hand, PCR and NGS, despite being very sensitive for MRD detection, are limited by the technical complexity and the lack of validated threshold to separate high from low MRD to better allow establishment of prognostic variables [21–26].

In conclusion, all methods reliably differentiated between MRD-positive versus -negative cases and successfully correlated MRD negativity with improved outcomes. MFC appears to have the greatest applicability, whereas PCR and NGS demonstrated higher sensitivity. Other techniques for MRD assessment such as detection of circulating tumor cells and whole-body PET-CT/MRI seem to have potential to add sensitivity for MRD detection, especially in extramedullary disease and/or oligo- or nonsecretory MM [26]. However, these approaches are still investigational and need further validation in the context of clinical trials.

3. Consolidation and Maintenance Strategies in MM

Despite the remarkable improvement in the outcome of MM treatment over the last two decades with the use of immunomodulatory and novel agents, MM remains an incurable disease. Multiple studies over the last few years have examined the role of maintenance, consolidation, or both to eliminate residual disease after HDC-ASCT in MM. Consolidation is typically a short course, more intensive, with the main goal of deepening the response achieved by induction chemotherapy and HDC-ASCT. Maintenance is given for a prolonged period of time with the goal of preventing/delaying disease progression. Both approaches showed favorable outcomes in terms of delaying relapse and need for second line intensive therapy. However, it remains unclear whether there is a significant survival advantage to justify the cost and toxicity of continued treatment. The ideal regimen should be easy to deliver, convenient to use, cost-effective, have modest toxicity and lead to improved PFS and ideally OS over retreatment at relapse [27, 28].

Historically, interferons (IFN) and glucocorticoids were the first agents studied in the maintenance setting after induction. Berenson et al. compared alternate-day oral prednisone at 2-dose levels (10 mg versus 50 mg) in a subset of patients achieving at least 25% tumor reduction following induction therapy during their enrollment in SWOG 9210 trial ($n = 125$). Significant improvements were noted in both PFS (14 versus 5 months, $P = 0.003$) and OS (37 versus 26 months, $P = 0.05$) favoring those receiving the 50 mg dose [29].

4. Post-ASCT Strategies in MM

Multiple studies have examined the role of consolidation and/or maintenance following HDC-ASCT to eliminate residual disease in MM. IFN-α was evaluated in 2 major studies and showed improved PFS, however, with substantial side effects and no survival benefit [30, 31]. Glucocorticoids were compared to IFNs and produced similar remission rates, but reinduction at relapse was more successful in those who received post-ASCT IFN [32].

4.1. Thalidomide Use after ASCT. Several randomized trials evaluated the use of thalidomide after ASCT [15, 16, 33–38] (see Table 1). Thalidomide's use has been associated with a meaningful improvement in PFS (by approximately 10 months) and EFS. However, the efficacy of thalidomide maintenance was counterbalanced by the significant rate of both acute and long-term side effects leading to discontinuation of the drug in a substantial number of patients ranging between 30–80% by 2 years in different studies [15, 16, 33–35, 37–45].

Due to increased toxicity of maintenance thalidomide, significant improvement in overall survival outcomes was not observed.

In their 2012 meta-analysis, IMWG reviewed 6 randomized trials with a total of 2786 patients evaluating thalidomide use after HDC-ASCT in myeloma [46]. Thalidomide maintenance was associated with significant improvement in PFS (HR 0.65; 95% CI 0.59–0.72) and OS (HR 0.84; 95% CI 0.73–0.97); however, there was considerable heterogeneity among individual trials, likely due to variability in inclusion criteria and salvage treatment of choice at disease progression/relapse (see Figures 3 and 4).

In conclusion, thalidomide use after ASCT appeared to have appeared to be most beneficial in MM with standard-risk disease. It may be more efficacious when combined with a proteasome inhibitor or glucocorticoids, as discussed below [9]. However, in considering such an approach, one should be vigilant about the risk/benefit ratio in individual patients taking into account their comorbidities and residual toxicities from previous treatment, given the considerable discontinuation rate secondary to toxicity noted in different studies.

4.2. Lenalidomide Use after ASCT. Two major phase III trials evaluated the role of lenalidomide use after HDC-ASCT in MM and showed improvement in PFS and TTP [47–49]. In the IFM 2005-02 trial, Attal et al. evaluated lenalidomide after ASCT in 614 patients where all study subjects received 2 cycles of lenalidomide consolidation and then got randomized to either lenalidomide maintenance arm (10 mg/day for 3 months and then 15 mg/day) or placebo until disease progression, intolerable side effects, or death [47]. However, at a median of 32 months, maintenance was discontinued when an interim analysis showed increased risk of second primary malignancies (SPMs) with lenalidomide maintenance. At a median follow-up of 45 months, lenalidomide maintenance was associated with improvement in median PFS (41 months versus 23 months in the placebo arm, HR 0.50, $P < 0.001$). However, OS rate at 5 years from diagnosis was similar in both arms.

In comparison, CALGB-100104 trial that evaluated lenalidomide maintenance after ASCT did not include a consolidation phase and it permitted crossover [48]. 460 patients were randomized, after achieving at least stable disease after ASCT, to either lenalidomide maintenance (10 mg/day for 3 months and then 15 mg/day) or placebo until disease progression, intolerance, or death. Interim analysis at 4 years showed significant improvement in TTP (42 months in lenalidomide arm versus 27 months in the placebo arm; $P < 0.001$).

A subgroup analysis showed that patients treated with lenalidomide induction therapy had significantly longer survival if they received lenalidomide maintenance, compared to those who received a placebo. The same analysis also showed that lenalidomide maintenance did not provide a survival advantage for patients who were treated with thalidomide induction therapy, patients who had elevated β-2 microglobulin levels, or patients who achieved a CR prior to the start of maintenance therapy or placebo.

Based on these results, the study was unblinded and 82 out of 128 patients in the placebo arm crossed over to the lenalidomide maintenance arm. Dr. McCarthy updated the results of CALGB-100104 trial in 2013 at the International Myeloma Workshop in Japan. Intention-to-treat analysis conducted at a median follow-up of 48 months after crossover showed median TTP of 50 months in the lenalidomide maintenance arm versus 27 months in the placebo arm. OS benefit was maintained at 48 months (median OS not reached in the lenalidomide maintenance arm versus 73 months in the placebo group, $P = 0.008$). Interestingly, OS analysis of patients crossing over from placebo to lenalidomide within 6–12 months of randomization showed significant benefit from lenalidomide maintenance [49].

The difference in survival results between the CALGB and IFM trials may be due to differences in induction consolidation and maintenance therapies.

In the IFM trial, one half got VAD and one quarter got augmented with DICEP, 20% of patients got two transplants, and maintenance was discontinued at a median of 32 months from the start. Longer follow-up and additional studies might clarify the differences in results.

Most recently, Palumbo et al. reported results of the open-label, randomized, phase III study comparing melphalan 200 mg/m^2 followed by ASCT versus melphalan-prednisone-lenalidomide (MPR). This study also compared lenalidomide

TABLE 1: Thalidomide trials in the post-ASCT setting.

Study (authors)	N	Maintenance phase study arms	EFS	PFS	OS
IFM 99-02 (Attal et al.) AM [33]	597	A: no maintenance B: pamidronate C: pamidronate/thalidomide (400 mg/d)	A: 36% B: 37% C: 52% ($P < 0.009$)		A: 77% B: 74% C: 87% ($P < 0.04$)
TT-2* (Barlogie et al.) AM [34]	668	A: thalidomide 100 mg/d × 1 year → 50 mg/d until PD B: no maintenance	A: 6 years B: 4.1 years ($P = 0.001$)		A: 57% B: 44% ($P = 0.09$)
HOVON-50 (Lokhorst et al.) AM [35]	556	A: VAD induction → IFN-α maintenance B: TAD induction → thalidomide maintenance	A: 22 months B: 34 months ($P < 0.001$)	A: 25 months B: 35 months ($P < 0.001$)	A: 60 months B: 73 months ($P = 0.77$)
MRC myeloma IX intensive group (Morgan et al.) AM [15]	493	A: thalidomide (50–100 mg/d) B: no maintenance	A: 30 months B: 27 months ($P = 0.003$)		A: 75 months B: 80 months ($P = 0.26$)
BMT CTN-0102 (Krishnan et al.) AM [16]	436	A: dexamethasone/thalidomide (200 mg/d) B: no maintenance		A: 49% B: 43% ($P = 0.08$)	A: 80% B: 81% ($P = 0.82$)
(Maiolino et al.) AM [36]	108	A: dexamethasone/thalidomide (200 mg/d) B: dexamethasone		A: 64% B: 30% ($P = 0.002$)	A: 85% B: 70% ($P = 0.27$)
ALLG MM-6 (Spencer et al.) AM [37]	269	A: prednisolone/thalidomide 100–200 mg/d × 12 months B: prednisolone		A: 42% B: 23% ($P < 0.001$)	A: 86% B: 75% ($P = 0.004$)
NCIC CTG MY10 (Stewart et al.) AM [38]	332	A: prednisone/thalidomide (200 mg/d) B: no maintenance		A: 28 months B: 17 months ($P < 0.0001$)	A: 68% B: 60% ($P = 0.21$)

*Both arms in TT-2 received the same 4 induction cycles followed by double ASCT and 4 cycles of consolidation (Figure 6). Thalidomide was given in arm A at a dose of 400 mg/d during induction, 100 mg/d during ASCT, and 200 mg/d during consolidation.

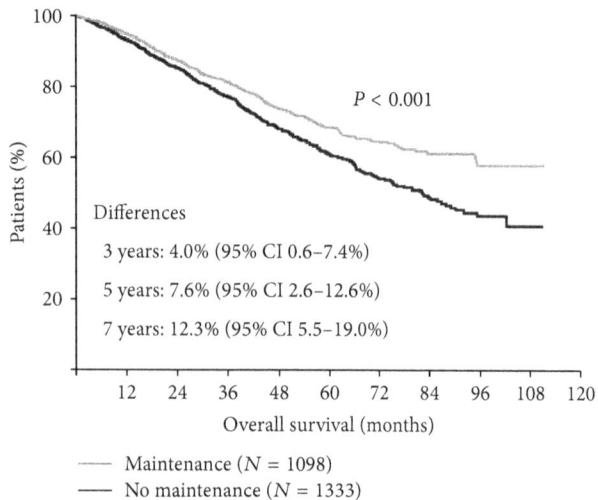

FIGURE 3: Meta-analysis of thalidomide maintenance showing OS benefit (adapted from [15]).

maintenance to no maintenance after high-dose melphalan or MPR consolidation. In comparison to no maintenance, lenalidomide maintenance significantly reduced the risk of progression independently of previous induction/consolidation regimen (PFS 41.9 versus 21.6 months, $P < 0.001$) with a trend towards improved 3-year OS rates in the lenalidomide maintenance arm (88% versus 79.2%, $P = 0.14$). Response rates improved during maintenance therapy in both high-dose melphalan and MPR arms. Interestingly, despite a similar CR rate, PFS improved in those who received high-dose melphalan in comparison to MPR chemotherapy. One possible explanation stated by authors is that response was assessed with standard laboratory tests rather than MRD detection by immunophenotypic or molecular techniques which may have revealed subtle differences in response between the two groups [50]. The concept of PFS2, defined as the time from initial randomization to time of objective disease progression after next-line therapy or death from any cause, was recently proposed as a surrogate to OS, particularly in trials evaluating maintenance in MM. This is due to the fact that effective salvage therapies are likely to be available at relapse which is thought to be the main reason for the lack of any statistically significant survival advantage noted across the trials addressing this topic [51].

4.2.1. Second Primary Malignancies (SPMs) after Lenalidomide Maintenance.

Enthusiasm for lenalidomide maintenance after HDC-ASCT in MM was subdued by the concern for increased risk of SPMs reported in both IFM and CALGB trials. Interim analysis of IFM trial showed increased risk of SPMs (3.1 versus 1.2 per 100 patients per year) in the lenalidomide maintenance arm [47]. Based on this, lenalidomide maintenance was halted. CALGB trial reported risk of SPMs of 12% in the maintenance versus 6% in the placebo arm ($P = 0.034$) [29]. However, in the CALGB trial maintenance was continued and, of notice, no new cases of SPMs were reported with longer follow-up [49].

The incidence of SPMs following lenalidomide exposure was reviewed in a recently published meta-analysis of 7 randomized trials including 2620 patients treated with lenalidomide versus 598 patients treated with no lenalidomide exposure [52]. Risk of SPMs at 5 years was 6.9% versus 4.8% (HR 1.1; 95% CI 1.03–2.34) which was statistically significant for second primary hematologic malignancies only. This increased risk is thought to be driven by treatment strategies combining lenalidomide with oral melphalan, suggesting that alkylator-free alternatives might be a better combination when using lenalidomide for myeloma patients.

On the other hand, acute myeloid leukemia (AML) and myelodysplasia (MDS) were reported in high frequency in untreated patients with monoclonal gammopathy of undetermined significance (MGUS) [53]. This suggests that hematopoietic stem cell or microenvironmental defect may be leading to the increased risk of hematological malignancies rather than the effect of chemotherapy exposure alone.

In conclusion, data with lenalidomide maintenance after ASCT is favorable. However, the optimal duration of lenalidomide maintenance is still unclear. Lenalidomide provides the most benefit in those who fail to achieve CR or very good partial response (VGPR), by IMWG criteria, after ASCT.

4.3. Bortezomib Use after ASCT.

The use of bortezomib in the post-ASCT setting in myeloma was evaluated in multiple randomized trials as consolidation, maintenance and in combination with other agents [39, 54, 55]. In the Nordic Myeloma Study Group trial, single-agent bortezomib consolidation given as 20 doses after ASCT resulted in 7-month improvement in PFS compared to placebo ($P = 0.007$); however, no OS benefit was seen. This approach seemed to be most beneficial for patients achieving less than a VGPR after induction and ASCT [54].

HOVON-65 trial evaluated bortezomib given during induction and during maintenance in 827 newly diagnosed myeloma patients [39]. Patients receiving bortezomib had improved PFS compared to those who received nonbortezomib induction regimens ($P = 0.006$). There was a trend towards improvement in 5-year OS survival rates (61% with bortezomib regimens versus 55% in nonbortezomib arm) but this did not reach statistical significance ($P = 0.07$). Bortezomib maintenance significantly improved nCR/CR rate from 31% to 49%, which was found, in a landmark analysis, to be associated with better PFS and OS at 12 months. However, in this trial, no random assignment for maintenance therapy was performed; and, therefore, the effect of that cannot be independently assessed. Furthermore, the major part of the difference in nCR/CR rates between the two groups was observed after induction and ASCT favoring the bortezomib arm. Equivalent upgrade of response was noted with either bortezomib or thalidomide maintenance. Nonetheless, maintenance treatment with bortezomib was much better tolerated than thalidomide maintenance, with fewer patients stopping treatment prematurely. Subgroup analysis showed that the superior outcomes with bortezomib were predominantly accomplished in patients with high-risk disease and myeloma-related renal failure or those with

Study	Number of patients		Odds ratio (95% CI)	P value for interaction
IFM-9902	597		0.61 (0.33–1.13)	0.040
Spencer et al.	243		0.43 (0.21–0.91)	0.004
Total therapy 2	668		0.82 (0.60–1.12)	0.090
Ludwig et al.	128		0.93 (0.53–1.66)	0.810
Myeloma IX Assuming effective Salvage therapy	820		0.77 (0.55–1.07)	0.040
All studies	2456		0.75 (0.64–0.87)	<0.001

0   0.25   0.5   0.75   1   1.25   1.5   1.75   2

Favors
maintenance

Favors
no maintenance

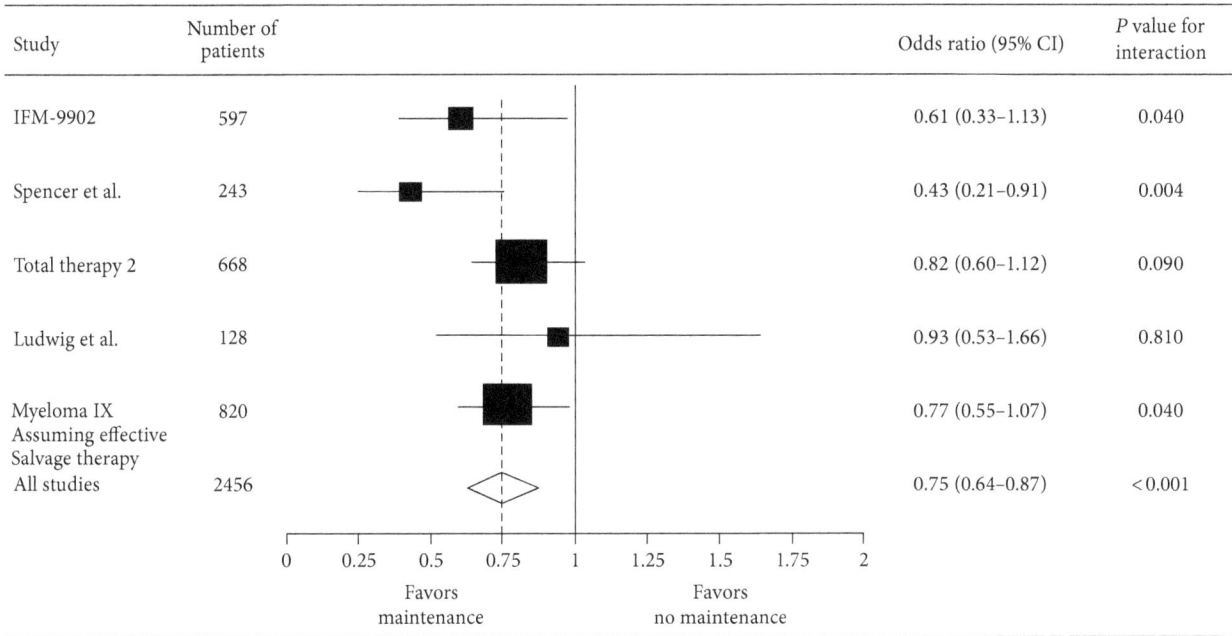

FIGURE 4: Collective data from thalidomide trials favoring maintenance (adapted from [16]).

del(17p) and del(13q) [39]. In patients with increased serum creatinine, both median PFS (30 versus 13 months, $P = 0.004$) and OS (54 versus 21 months, $P < 0.001$) were significantly improved in the bortezomib-containing arm compared to those who did not receive bortezomib. In patients with normal serum creatinine, PFS remained superior in the bortezomib arm, whereas OS was similar in both groups. Patients with abnormal FISH results for del(13q14), t(4; 14), and del(17p13) were compared with patients without the abnormality. PFS was worse in all patients with del(13q14) regardless of the treatment arm whereas OS in patient with del(13q14) was similar to those who did not carry the deletion. Of note, OS in patients with the deletion was significantly better in the bortezomib arm in comparison to the nonbortezomib arm. In patients with del(17p13), both PFS (median 22 versus 12 months, $P = 0.01$) and OS (median > 54 months versus 24 months, $P = 0.003$) were significantly better in the bortezomib arm. The presence of t(4; 14) was associated with worse outcomes compared to patients without this translocation. There was a trend towards better outcomes in patients with t(4; 14) who received bortezomib-containing regimen; however, this did not reach statistical significance. This leads us to the conclusion that the use of bortezomib in the post-ASCT setting can potentially overcome the adverse effects of abnormal cytogenetics, a subgroup that has always been associated with inferior outcomes.

4.4. Combination Regimens after ASCT. Trials in the recent years focused on combination regimens for consolidation/maintenance after ASCT. The Spanish PETHEMA study was a 3-arm randomized trial that evaluated bortezomib/thalidomide maintenance after ASCT versus single-agent IFN or single-agent thalidomide for a period of 3 years [55]. After a median follow-up of 24 months from

maintenance initiation, PFS was significantly longer in bortezomib/thalidomide arm (78%) compared with thalidomide arm (63%) or IFN arm (49%), with no relevant difference in side effects except for higher incidence of neuropathy in the combination arm. Interestingly, the improvement in PFS was primarily seen in patients with low-risk cytogenetics, contrary to what was reported by HOVON-65 trial. This discrepancy might be in part due to different bortezomib dosing and duration (52 doses over 2 years in HOVON-65 versus 48 doses over 3 years in PETHEMA trial).

Cavo et al. evaluated the combination bortezomib/thalidomide/dexamethasone (VTD) versus thalidomide/dexamethasone (TD) as consolidation therapy after ASCT in 474 newly diagnosed myeloma patients [17]. After consolidation, CR (60.6% versus 46.6%) and nCR (73.1% versus 60.9%) rates were significantly higher for VTD arm versus TD arm. Notably, VTD consolidation significantly increased CR/nCR rates compared to pretransplant rates, whereas TD did not. With a median follow-up of 30.4 months from initiation of consolidation, 3-year PFS was significantly longer for the VTD group versus TD group (60% versus 48%). Furthermore, PFS curves in the VTD arm were almost superimposable regardless of the presence or absence of cytogenetic abnormality, whereas patients who received TD consolidation and carried abnormal cytogenetics had significantly worse outcomes (Figure 5).

Total therapy (TT) trials are series of studies conducted by the Arkansas Myeloma Group utilizing all active antimyeloma agents upfront to achieve a maximal tumor cytoreduction and thereby increase the frequency and duration of CR, with the goal of extending PFS and OS (see Figure 6).

The introduction of bortezomib in the post-ASCT setting started with TT-3A (VTD-PACE for 2 cycles as consolidation

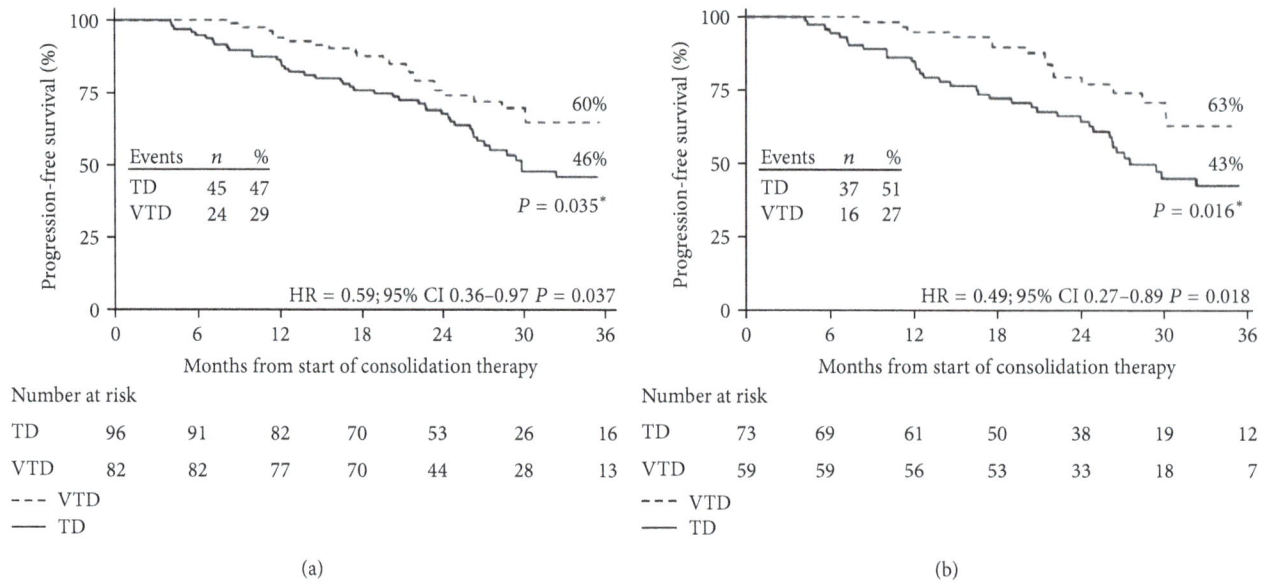

FIGURE 5: Kaplan-Meier curves for PFS from the landmark of starting consolidation therapy according to the presence or absence of cytogenetic abnormalities. The figure shows PFS for patients with no cytogenetic abnormality or with del(13q) positivity but lack of t(4; 14) and del(17p) or t(4; 14) and/or del(17p) positivity which received VTD consolidation therapy (a) or TD consolidation therapy (b). *P value according to log-rank test (adapted from [17]).

FIGURE 6: It summarizes the series of Total therapy trials. VAD: vincristine, doxorubicin, and dexamethasone; HD-Cyt: high-dose cyclophosphamide; EDAP: etoposide, dexamethasone, cytarabine, and cisplatin; TD-PACE: thalidomide, dexamethasone, cisplatin, doxorubicin, cyclophosphamide, and etoposide; VTD: bortezomib, thalidomide, and dexamethasone; VRD: bortezomib, lenalidomide, and dexamethasone.

followed by either VTD for 1 year or TD for 2 years). The upfront addition of bortezomib resulted in improved outcomes, compared with TT-2 trials that randomized patients upfront to receive/not receive thalidomide as part of induction, consolidation, and maintenance. To validate these findings along with bortezomib pharmacogenomic data, a successor trial TT-3B enrolled another 177 patients. TT-3A and TT-3B were identical in design, except for the fact that the maintenance phase of TT-3B included VRD (using lenalidomide instead of thalidomide) and was continued for 3 years

rather than 1 year in TT-3A (Figure 6). Comparing results of TT-3A and TT-3B, the difference between OS (87% in TT-3B versus 85% in TT-3A) and EFS (83% in TT-3B versus 80% in TT-3A) at 2 years was not statistically significant [56, 57]. When examined in the context of GEP-defined risk, TT-3A and TT-3B result curves were superimposable for both low-risk and high-risk groups. However, more patients with GEP-defined high risk were included in TT-3B versus TT-3A (22% versus 15%, $P = 0.038$). Despite more adverse features in TT-3B and overall higher-risk population, all outcomes (OS, EFS, and CR duration) were similar in the 2 protocols suggesting that 3-year maintenance with a bortezomib-containing regimen is superior to shorter maintenance, along with the reportedly more effective immunomodulatory effect of lenalidomide compared to thalidomide used in TT-3A [56–58]. Furthermore, according to multivariate analysis, deletion TP53 conferred inferior OS and EFS in TT-2 but not in TT-3. The major difference between TT-2 and TT-3 is the addition of bortezomib in induction, consolidation, and maintenance phases. This provides further evidence that the use of proteasome inhibitors in all treatment phases can potentially negate the adverse consequences of deletion TP53, likely through a synergistic mechanism [59].

Most recently, Nooka et al. reported results of a single-arm trial evaluating consolidation and maintenance therapy with lenalidomide, bortezomib, and dexamethasone (RVD) in patients with high-risk cytogenetics, defined as del TP53, del(1p), t(4; 14), or t(14; 16). Patients received different induction regimens followed by ASCT and subsequently RVD maintenance for 3 years followed by lenalidomide until disease progression. Following initiation of RVD maintenance, 51% of patients achieved sCR with 96% achieving at least VGPR as best response. Median PFS for all patients was 32 months and 3-year OS of 93% was reported [60].

Furthermore, in their recent phase II IFM study, Roussel et al. reported high-quality response and favorable tolerability. This phase II trial included 31 newly diagnosed MM patients who were eligible for ASCT. Overall, 27% of patients were classified as having high-risk chromosomal abnormalities based on either having a del(17p) or t(4; 14) abnormality, determined by FISH. Patients received three cycles of RVD and then proceeded to ASCT. Two months after recovery of blood counts, patients who had not progressed received consolidation therapy consisting of two cycles of RVD. Patient subsequently received maintenance therapy with continuous lenalidomide (Revlimid) for one year. Responses deepened significantly after ASCT and consolidation therapy in comparison to responses at the end of induction: 40% reaching sCR versus 10%; 58% of patients were MRD-negative versus 16%. Responses also improved further for some patients during maintenance therapy. After all treatment sequences, 68% of patients had achieved MRD negativity. At a median follow-up of 39 months, the estimated 3-year PFS and OS were 77% and 100%, respectively [61]. None of the patients who had achieved MRD negativity relapsed within three years of diagnosis. Of note, PFS was significantly lower at 23% in patients who had never reached MRD negativity. The most common side effect during lenalidomide maintenance therapy was low blood cell counts.

4.5. Maintenance Using Immunotherapeutics and Future Modalities. Dendritic cell vaccination, an example of this approach, works by induction of idiotype-specific T- and B-cell response that can stimulate the body's own immune system to fight and eradicate myeloma cells following administration of idiotype-protein pulsed dendritic cells. Although this seems to be a safe strategy, it has not shown any effects on survival and, to date, remains experimental [62–64].

Other forms of immunotherapy include the monoclonal antibody Elotuzumab (anti-CS1) and Daratumumab (anti-CD38) that have activity both as single agents and in combination with other novel therapeutics. Novel proteasome inhibitors such as Carfilzomib, Marizomib, Ixazomib, and Oprozomib may provide better outcomes in the future. Antibodies to various myeloma cell markers, such as CD40, CD56, CD74, IL-6, TRAIL, and RANKL, combined with proteasome inhibitors, conventional chemotherapy, and/or immunomodulatory agents, may serve as maintenance targets for future research with an ultimate goal of significantly improving OS or potentially curing multiple myeloma [27, 65].

5. Summary and Recommendations

Over the last decade, the trials mentioned above have led to markedly improved outcomes in myeloma and answered multiple questions regarding optimal induction regimens as well as highlighting the importance of consolidation/maintenance after ASCT in the era of novel agents. While considering consolidation/maintenance strategies after HDC-ASCT,

one needs to take into careful consideration the cost and toxicity involved with the different strategies in order to improve outcomes. The use of sensitive techniques to detect MRD provides a stratification tool to guide further treatment following ASCT.

Patients with low-risk disease and normal cytogenetics, who achieve CR or sCR (per IMWG criteria) after ASCT, especially if this excellent response can be confirmed by MRD negativity, may forgo further therapy after ASCT. These patients will need to be closely followed for evidence of relapse. Patients with high-risk cytogenetics and those with low-/standard-risk cytogenetics who achieve less than a CR should be considered for maintenance treatment. Average time to start consolidation/maintenance is typically 60–100 days after ASCT.

Nooka et al. have reported excellent outcomes for patients with high-risk cytogenetics using combination RVD followed by lenalidomide maintenance. However, this needs further validation in a phase II/III trial design to confirm these superior results. Roussel regimen (2 cycles of RVD followed by lenalidomide maintenance) is promising particularly in the setting of less than a CR with HDC-ASCT.

Our institutional approach for high-risk cytogenetics and low-/standard-risk cytogenetic patients who are still MRD positive after HDC-ASCT is an approach similar to Roussel regimen's with continuation of RVD beyond 2 cycles until achievement of MRD negativity followed by lenalidomide maintenance as long as tolerated or until progression.

Conflict of Interests

The authors declare that there is no conflict of interests regarding the publication of this paper.

References

[1] M. Attal, J.-L. Harousseau, A.-M. Stoppa et al., "A prospective, randomized trial of autologous bone marrow transplantation and chemotherapy in multiple myeloma," *The New England Journal of Medicine*, vol. 335, no. 2, pp. 91–97, 1996.

[2] J. A. Child, G. J. Morgan, F. E. Davies et al., "High-dose chemotherapy with hematopoietic stem-cell rescue for multiple myeloma," *The New England Journal of Medicine*, vol. 348, no. 19, pp. 1875–1883, 2003.

[3] J. Koreth, C. S. Cutler, B. Djulbegovic et al., "High-dose therapy with single autologous transplantation versus chemotherapy for newly diagnosed multiple myeloma: a systematic review and meta-analysis of randomized controlled trials," *Biology of Blood and Marrow Transplantation*, vol. 13, no. 2, pp. 183–196, 2007.

[4] B. Barlogie, E. Anaissie, J. Haessler et al., "Complete remission sustained 3 years from treatment initiation is a powerful surrogate for extended survival in multiple myeloma," *Cancer*, vol. 113, no. 2, pp. 355–359, 2008.

[5] M. Cavo and M. Baccarani, "The changing landscape of myeloma therapy," *The New England Journal of Medicine*, vol. 354, no. 10, pp. 1076–1078, 2006.

[6] M. Cavo, S. V. Rajkumar, A. Palumbo et al., "International myeloma working group consensus approach to the treatment of multiple myeloma patients who are candidates for autologous

stem cell transplantation," *Blood*, vol. 117, no. 23, pp. 6063–6073, 2011.

[7] H. J. K. van de Velde, X. Liu, G. Chen, A. Cakana, W. Deraedt, and M. Bayssas, "Complete response correlates with long-term survival and progression-free survival in high-dose therapy in multiple myeloma," *Haematologica*, vol. 92, no. 10, pp. 1399–1406, 2007.

[8] B. G. M. Durie, J.-L. Harousseau, J. S. Miguel et al., "International uniform response criteria for multiple myeloma," *Leukemia*, vol. 20, no. 9, pp. 1467–1473, 2006.

[9] R. A. Kyle and S. V. Rajkumar, "Criteria for diagnosis, staging, risk stratification and response assessment of multiple myeloma," *Leukemia*, vol. 23, no. 1, pp. 3–9, 2009.

[10] J. J. Lahuerta, M. V. Mateos, J. Martínez-López et al., "Influence of pre- and post-transplantation responses on outcome of patients with multiple myeloma: sequential improvement of response and achievement of complete response are associated with longer survival," *Journal of Clinical Oncology*, vol. 26, no. 35, pp. 5775–5782, 2008.

[11] P. Kapoor, S. K. Kumar, A. Dispenzieri et al., "Importance of achieving stringent complete response after autologous stem-cell transplantation in multiple myeloma," *Journal of Clinical Oncology*, vol. 31, no. 36, pp. 4529–4535, 2013.

[12] A. A. Chanan-Khan and S. Giralt, "Importance of achieving a complete response in multiple myeloma, and the impact of novel agents," *Journal of Clinical Oncology*, vol. 28, no. 15, pp. 2612–2624, 2010.

[13] B. Paiva, M.-B. Vidriales, J. Cerveró et al., "Multiparameter flow cytometric remission is the most relevant prognostic factor for multiple myeloma patients who undergo autologous stem cell transplantation," *Blood*, vol. 112, no. 10, pp. 4017–4023, 2008.

[14] J. Martinez-Lopez, J. J. Lahuerta, F. Pepin et al., "Prognostic value of deep sequencing method for minimal residual disease detection in multiple myeloma," *Blood*, vol. 123, no. 20, pp. 3073–3079, 2014.

[15] G. J. Morgan, W. M. Gregory, F. E. Davies et al., "The role of maintenance thalidomide therapy in multiple myeloma: MRC Myeloma IX results and meta-analysis," *Blood*, vol. 119, no. 1, pp. 7–15, 2012.

[16] A. Krishnan, M. C. Pasquini, B. Logan et al., "Autologous haemopoietic stem-cell transplantation followed by allogeneic or autologous haemopoietic stem-cell transplantation in patients with multiple myeloma (BMT CTN 0102): a phase 3 biological assignment trial," *The Lancet Oncology*, vol. 12, no. 13, pp. 1195–1203, 2011.

[17] M. Cavo, L. Pantani, M. T. Petrucci et al., "Bortezomib-thalidomide-dexamethasone is superior to thalidomide-dexamethasone as consolidation therapy after autologous hematopoietic stem cell transplantation in patients with newly diagnosed multiple myeloma," *Blood*, vol. 120, no. 1, pp. 9–19, 2012.

[18] M. Ladetto, M. Brüggemann, L. Monitillo et al., "Next-generation sequencing and real-time quantitative PCR for minimal residual disease detection in B-cell disorders," *Leukemia*, vol. 28, no. 6, pp. 1299–1307, 2014.

[19] M. Cavo, C. Terragna, G. Martinelli et al., "Molecular monitoring of minimal residual disease in patients in long-term complete remission after allogeneic stem cell transplantation for multiple myeloma," *Blood*, vol. 96, no. 1, pp. 355–357, 2000.

[20] P. Corradini, M. Cavo, H. Lokhorst et al., "Molecular remission after myeloablative allogeneic stem cell transplantation

predicts a better relapse-free survival in patients with multiple myeloma," *Blood*, vol. 102, no. 5, pp. 1927–1929, 2003.

[21] A. C. Rawstron, J. A. Child, R. M. de Tute et al., "Minimal residual disease assessed by multiparameter flow cytometry in multiple myeloma: impact on outcome in the Medical Research Council Myeloma IX Study," *Journal of Clinical Oncology*, vol. 31, no. 20, pp. 2540–2547, 2013.

[22] B. Paiva, N. C. Gutiérrez, L. Rosiñol et al., "High-risk cytogenetics and persistent minimal residual disease by multiparameter flow cytometry predict unsustained complete response after autologous stem cell transplantation in multiple myeloma," *Blood*, vol. 119, no. 3, pp. 687–691, 2012.

[23] J. Martinez-Lopez, E. Fernández-Redondo, R. García-Sánz et al., "Clinical applicability and prognostic significance of molecular response assessed by fluorescent-PCR of immunoglobulin genes in multiple myeloma: results from a GEM/PETHEMA study," *British Journal of Haematology*, vol. 163, no. 5, pp. 581–589, 2013.

[24] M. H. C. Bakkus, Y. Bouko, D. Samson et al., "Post-transplantation tumour load in bone marrow, as assessed by quantitative ASO-PCR, is a prognostic parameter in multiple myeloma," *British Journal of Haematology*, vol. 126, no. 5, pp. 665–674, 2004.

[25] M. E. Sarasquete, R. García-Sanz, D. González et al., "Minimal residual disease monitoring in multiple myeloma: a comparison between allelic-specific oligonucleotide real-time quantitative polymerase chain reaction and flow cytometry," *Haematologica*, vol. 90, no. 10, pp. 1365–1372, 2005.

[26] N. Biran, S. Ely, and A. Chari, "Controversies in the assessment of minimal residual disease in multiple myeloma: clinical significance of minimal residual disease negativity using highly sensitive techniques," *Current Hematologic Malignancy Reports*, 2014.

[27] P. L. McCarthy and T. Hahn, "Strategies for induction, autologous hematopoietic stem cell transplantation, consolidation, and maintenance for transplantation-eligible multiple myeloma patients," *Hematology/The Education Program of the American Society of Hematology*, vol. 2013, no. 1, pp. 496–503, 2013.

[28] R. Mihelic, J. L. Kaufman, and S. Lonial, "Maintenance therapy in multiple myeloma," *Leukemia*, vol. 21, no. 6, pp. 1150–1157, 2007.

[29] J. R. Berenson, J. J. Crowley, T. M. Grogan et al., "Maintenance therapy with alternate-day prednisone improves survival in multiple myeloma patients," *Blood*, vol. 99, no. 9, pp. 3163–3168, 2002.

[30] D. Cunningham, R. Powles, J. Malpas et al., "A randomized trial of maintenance interferon following high-dose chemotherapy in multiple myeloma: long-term follow-up results," *British Journal of Haematology*, vol. 102, no. 2, pp. 495–502, 1998.

[31] B. Barlogie, R. A. Kyle, K. C. Anderson et al., "Standard chemotherapy compared with high-dose chemoradiotherapy for multiple myeloma: final results of phase III US intergroup trial S9321," *Journal of Clinical Oncology*, vol. 24, no. 6, pp. 929–936, 2006.

[32] R. Alexanian, D. Weber, M. Dimopoulos, K. Delasalle, and T. L. Smith, "Randomized trial of alpha-interferon or dexamethasone as maintenance treatment for multiple myeloma," *The American Journal of Hematology*, vol. 65, no. 3, pp. 204–209, 2000.

[33] M. Attal, J. L. Harousseau, S. Leyvraz et al., "Maintenance therapy with thalidomide improves survival in patients with multiple myeloma," *Blood*, vol. 108, no. 10, pp. 3289–3294, 2006.

[34] B. Barlogie, M. Pineda-Roman, F. van Rhee et al., "Thalidomide arm of total therapy 2 improves complete remission duration and survival in myeloma patients with metaphase cytogenetic abnormalities," *Blood*, vol. 112, no. 8, pp. 3115–3121, 2008.

[35] H. M. Lokhorst, B. Van Der Holt, S. Zweegman et al., "A randomized phase 3 study on the effect of thalidomide combined with adriamycin, dexamethasone, and high-dose melphalan, followed by thalidomide maintenance in patients with multiple myeloma," *Blood*, vol. 115, no. 6, pp. 1113–1120, 2010.

[36] A. Maiolino, V. T. M. Hungria, M. Garnica et al., "Thalidomide plus dexamethasone as a maintenance therapy after autologous hematopoietic stem cell transplantation improves progression-free survival in multiple myeloma," *American Journal of Hematology*, vol. 87, no. 10, pp. 948–952, 2012.

[37] A. Spencer, H. M. Prince, A. W. Roberts et al., "Consolidation therapy with low-dose thalidomide and prednisolone prolongs the survival of multiple myeloma patients undergoing a single autologous stem-cell transplantation procedure," *Journal of Clinical Oncology*, vol. 27, no. 11, pp. 1788–1793, 2009.

[38] A. K. Stewart, S. Trudel, N. J. Bahlis et al., "Arandomized phase 3 trial of thalidomide and prednisone as maintenance therapy afterASCT in patients withMMwith a quality-of-life assessment: the national cancer Institute of Canada clinicals trials group myeloma 10 trial," *Blood*, vol. 121, no. 9, pp. 1517–1523, 2013.

[39] P. Sonneveld, I. G. H. Schmidt-Wolf, B. Van Der Holt et al., "Bortezomib induction and maintenance treatment in patients with newly diagnosed multiple myeloma: results of the randomized phase III HOVON-65/ GMMG-HD4 trial," *Journal of Clinical Oncology*, vol. 30, no. 24, pp. 2946–2955, 2012.

[40] S. Feyler, A. Rawstron, G. Jackson, J. A. Snowden, K. Cocks, and R. J. Johnson, "Thalidomide maintenance following high-dose therapy in multiple myeloma: a UK myeloma forum phase 2 study," *British Journal of Haematology*, vol. 139, no. 3, pp. 429–433, 2007.

[41] B. Barlogie, G. Tricot, E. Anaissie et al., "Thalidomide and hematopoietic-cell transplantation for multiple myeloma," *The New England Journal of Medicine*, vol. 354, no. 10, pp. 1021–1030, 2006.

[42] M. Zangari, F. Van Rhee, E. Anaissie et al., "Eight-year median survival in multiple myeloma after total therapy 2: roles of thalidomide and consolidation chemotherapy in the context of total therapy 1," *British Journal of Haematology*, vol. 141, no. 4, pp. 433–444, 2008.

[43] B. Barlogie, G. Tricot, E. Rasmussen et al., "Total therapy 2 without thalidomide in comparison with total therapy 1: role of intensified induction and posttransplantation consolidation therapies," *Blood*, vol. 107, no. 7, pp. 2633–2638, 2006.

[44] B. Barlogie, M. Attal, J. Crowley et al., "Long-term follow-up of autotransplantation trials for multiple myeloma: update of protocols conducted by the intergroupe francophone du myeloma, southwest oncology group, and university of arkansas for medical sciences," *Journal of Clinical Oncology*, vol. 28, no. 7, pp. 1209–1214, 2010.

[45] S. Z. Usmani, R. Sexton, A. Hoering et al., "Second malignancies in total therapy 2 and 3 for newly diagnosed multiple myeloma: influence of thalidomide and lenalidomide during maintenance," *Blood*, vol. 120, no. 8, pp. 1597–1600, 2012.

[46] H. Ludwig, B. G. M. Durie, P. McCarthy et al., "IMWG consensus on maintenance therapy in multiple myeloma," *Blood*, vol. 119, no. 13, pp. 3003–3015, 2012.

[47] M. Attal, V. Lauwers-Cances, G. Marit et al., "Lenalidomide maintenance after stem-cell transplantation for multiple myeloma," *The New England Journal of Medicine*, vol. 366, no. 19, pp. 1782–1791, 2012.

[48] P. L. McCarthy, K. Owzar, C. C. Hofmeister et al., "Lenalidomide after stem-cell transplantation for multiple myeloma," *The New England Journal of Medicine*, vol. 366, no. 19, pp. 1770–1781, 2012.

[49] H. Ludwig, J. S. Miguel, M. A. Dimopoulos et al., "International Myeloma Working Group recommendations for global myeloma care," *Leukemia*, vol. 28, no. 5, pp. 981–992, 2014.

[50] A. Palumbo, F. Cavallo, F. Gay et al., "Autologous transplantation and maintenance therapy in multiple myeloma," *The New England Journal of Medicine*, vol. 371, no. 10, pp. 895–905, 2014.

[51] M. A. Dimopoulos, M. T. Petrucci, R. Foà et al., "PFS2 in elderly patients with newly diagnosed multiple myeloma (NDMM): results from the MM-015 study," *Blood*, vol. 122, no. 21, p. 405, 2013.

[52] A. Palumbo, S. Bringhen, S. K. Kumar et al., "Second primary malignancies with lenalidomide therapy for newly diagnosed myeloma: a meta-analysis of individual patient data," *The Lancet Oncology*, vol. 15, no. 3, pp. 333–342, 2014.

[53] S. Mailankody, R. M. Pfeiffer, S. Y. Kristinsson et al., "Risk of acute myeloid leukemia and myelodysplastic syndromes after multiple myeloma and its precursor disease (MGUS)," *Blood*, vol. 118, no. 15, pp. 4086–4092, 2011.

[54] U.-H. Mellqvist, P. Gimsing, O. Hjertner et al., "Bortezomib consolidation after autologous stem cell transplantation in multiple myeloma: a Nordic Myeloma Study Group randomized phase 3 trial.," *Blood*, vol. 121, no. 23, pp. 4647–4654, 2013.

[55] L. Rosiñol, A. Oriol, A. I. Teruel et al., "Superiority of bortezomib, thalidomide, and dexamethasone (VTD) as induction pretransplantation therapy in multiple myeloma: a randomized phase 3 PETHEMA/GEM study," *Blood*, vol. 120, no. 8, pp. 1589–1596, 2012.

[56] B. Nair, F. Van Rhee, J. D. Shaughnessy Jr. et al., "Superior results of total therapy 3 (2003-33) in gene expression profiling-defined low-risk multiple myeloma confirmed in subsequent trial 2006-66 with VRD maintenance," *Blood*, vol. 115, no. 21, pp. 4168–4173, 2010.

[57] F. Van Rhee, J. Szymonifka, E. Anaissie et al., "Total Therapy 3 for multiple myeloma: prognostic implications of cumulative dosing and premature discontinuation of VTD maintenance components, bortezomib, thalidomide, and dexamethasone, relevant to all phases of therapy," *Blood*, vol. 116, no. 8, pp. 1220–1227, 2010.

[58] S. Z. Usmani, J. Crowley, A. Hoering et al., "Improvement in long-term outcomes with successive total therapy trials for multiple myeloma: are patients now being cured?" *Leukemia*, vol. 27, no. 1, pp. 226–232, 2013.

[59] J. D. Shaughnessy, Y. Zhou, J. Haessler et al., "TP53 deletion is not an adverse feature in multiple myeloma treated with total therapy 3," *British Journal of Haematology*, vol. 147, no. 3, pp. 347–351, 2009.

[60] A. K. Nooka, J. L. Kaufman, S. Muppidi et al., "Consolidation and maintenance therapy with lenalidomide, bortezomib and dexamethasone (RVD) in high-risk myeloma patients," *Leukemia*, vol. 28, no. 3, pp. 690–693, 2014.

[61] M. Roussel, V. Lauwers-Cances, N. Robillard et al., "Front-line transplantation program with lenalidomide, bortezomib, and dexamethasone combination as induction and consolidation followed by lenalidomide maintenance in patients with multiple

myeloma: a phase II study by the intergroupe francophone du myélome," *Journal of Clinical Oncology*, vol. 32, no. 25, pp. 2712–2717, 2014.

[62] Q. Yi, R. Desikan, B. Barlogie, and N. Munshi, "Optimizing dendritic cell-based immunotherapy in multiple myeloma," *British Journal of Haematology*, vol. 117, no. 2, pp. 297–305, 2002.

[63] S. J. Harrison and G. Cook, "Immunotherapy in multiple myeloma—possibility or probability?" *British Journal of Haematology*, vol. 130, no. 3, pp. 344–362, 2005.

[64] L. Hansson, A. O. Abdalla, A. Moshfegh et al., "Long-term idiotype vaccination combined with interleukin-12 (IL-12), or IL-12 and granulocyte macrophage colony-stimulating factor, in early-stage multiple myeloma patients," *Clinical Cancer Research*, vol. 13, no. 5, pp. 1503–1510, 2007.

[65] N. C. Munshi and K. C. Anderson, "New strategies in the treatment of multiple myeloma," *Clinical Cancer Research*, vol. 19, no. 13, pp. 3337–3344, 2013.

6

Characteristics and Results of the Treatment of Multiple Myeloma in the Subject under the Age of 65 at the University Hospital of Yopougon in Abidjan, Côte d'Ivoire

Diebkilé Aïssata Tolo, Duni Sawadogo, Danho Clotaire Nanho, Boidy Kouakou, N'Dogomo Méité, Roméo Ayémou, Paul Kouéhion, Mozart Konan, Yassongui Mamadou Sékongo, Emeraude N'Dhatz, Ismaël Kamara, Alexis Silué, Kouassi Gustave Koffi, and Ibrahima Sanogo

Department of Clinical Hematology, Yopougon Teaching Hospital, P.O. Box 632, Abidjan 21, Cote d'Ivoire

Correspondence should be addressed to Diebkilé Aïssata Tolo; aissata_tolo@yahoo.fr

Academic Editor: Aldo Roccaro

We retrospectively studied 30 cases of multiple myeloma in patients under the age of 65, diagnosed from 1991 to 2005 in the clinical hematology department of the University Hospital of Yopougon that is a hospital incidence of 2.9 cases/year. The age of patients ranged from 34 to 64 years, with a mean age of 49 years and a sex ratio of 1.73. The professional activity was variable with 3% of radiographers and 10% of farmers. Clinically, the dominant sign was bone pain in 83% of cases. Myeloma was secretory in 93% of cases. It was Ig G-type in 86%, kappa-type in 66% of cases. 86% of patients were anemic, 20% had creatinine >20 mg/L, and 10% had serum calcium >120 mg/L. Geodes were found in 80% of cases. 53% were at stage III of DURIE and SALMON. Complications were infectious (33%), renal (20%), and hemorrhagic (7%). Chemotherapy regimens were VAD (10%), VMCP (30%), and VMCP/VBAP (60%) with 47% of partial responses, 33% of stable disease, and 7% of very good quality partial responses. The outcome developed towards death in 37% and causes of death were renal in 46% of cases. The median survival was only 5.1 months.

1. Introduction

Multiple myeloma or Kahler disease is a malignant proliferation of an abnormal plasma cell clone secreting a complete or incomplete immunoglobulin. It, respectively, accounts for 10% and 20% of malignant hemopathies in the Caucasian and Black American. It is a condition of the subject of more than 50 years of age. Its incidence increases with age: 5 per 100,000 individuals at the age of 60 and 20 per 100,000 individuals at the age of 80. The average age at diagnosis is 64 years. It is slightly more common in men than in women [1].

Positive diagnosis of multiple myeloma is not always easy. It requires a combination of clinical arguments (general condition, bone syndrome), biological arguments (study of marrow, study of protein in the blood and urine, hemoglobin level, serum calcium, and creatinine), and radiological arguments (X-ray of the skeleton) [2].

The outcome is punctuated by multiple complications such as bone, renal, infectious, metabolic, neurological, hemorrhagic complications, and cachexia.

Initially the prognostic classification was based on that of DURIE and SALMON but currently it is the ISS (International Staging System) with two parameters albumin and $\beta2$ microglobulin, which is used. In addition, some cytogenetic abnormalities such as del (13q), t(11; 14), t(4; 14), t(14; 16), and del (17p) have a major prognostic value. They have poor prognosis [3–6]. Mortality is 4.1/100,000 inhabitants/year in Europe [3].

Therapeutically, the treatment is not recommended for patients at stage I of DURIE and SALMON; on the other hand for stages II and III, treatment will be established taking into account the patient's age [3]. If, in developed countries, patients under the age of 65 receive intensive treatment with bone marrow graft particularly, this is not the case in

Côte d'Ivoire. What were the results of treatment in these patients in our context of exercise and what were the features of their myeloma?

2. Patients and Methods

Our study was carried out in the Clinical Hematology Department of the University Hospital of Yopougon in Côte d'Ivoire. It was retrospective and descriptive and focused on the records of patients hospitalized for symptomatic multiple myeloma, diagnosed in the period from January 1991 to August 2005 by myelogram, the study of protein in the blood and urine, hemoglobin level, serum calcium, creatinine, skeletal X-ray according to SWOG criteria (Southern Western Oncology Group) and ROTI (multiple myeloma-related organ or tissue impairment: elevation of serum calcium, anemia, kidney failure, and bone lesions) [6, 7], and who had received chemotherapy. Thirty patients were included in the study. The patients with asymptomatic multiple myeloma and monoclonal gammopathies of undetermined significance were not selected. Each medical record was operated using an individual survey form with collection of epidemiological parameters (age, sex, occupation, and socioeconomic status), clinical parameters (performance status, bone pain), biological parameters (bone marrow plasma cells, type of monoclonal immunoglobulin, type of light chain, Bence Jones proteinuria, hemoglobin level, serum calcium, and creatinine), radiological parameters (geodes, demineralization, bone tumors, and bone fractures), evolutionary parameters (classification of DURIE and SALMON, progressive complications, and death), and therapeutic parameters according to the index of standardized generalized response (complete remission or CR, very good partial response or VGPR, partial response or PR, stable disease, progression, and relapse) (Table 2).

The socioeconomic status was assessed using indirect criteria: habitat type, occupation, ability to meet the cost of prescriptions, and number of dependent children.

CR corresponds to the negativity of monoclonal immunoglobulin in the blood and urine and to bone marrow plasma cells <5%.

VGPR corresponds to serum monoclonal immunoglobulin decreased by 90% and to urinary immunoglobulin <100 mg/24 H.

PR corresponds to serum monoclonal immunoglobulin decreased by 50%, urinary monoclonal immunoglobulin decreased by 90%, and free light chains decreased by 50%.

Stable disease corresponds to the lack of criteria for CR, VGPR, and PR.

Progression criteria are 25% increase of serum or urine monoclonal immunoglobulin or free light chains assay, an increase of 10% of the bone marrow plasma cells, appearance of new bone or extra bone lesions, and a level of calcium greater than 2.65 mmol/L.

The criteria for relapse are appearance of new bone or extra bone lesions, a level of serum calcium greater than 2.65 mmol/L, hemoglobin level lowering to 2 g/dL, and a level of creatinine greater than 20 mg/L (177 μmol/L); the

Kaplan Meier plot of cumulative survival for column 1. Variable censure: censured variable.

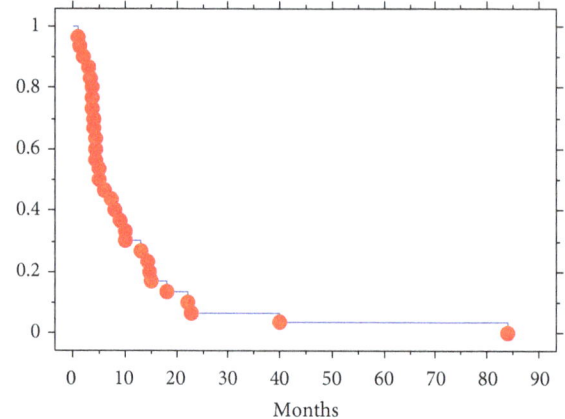

FIGURE 1: Overall survival curve.

monoclonal component alone is not taken into account for relapse [7].

Therapeutically, three chemotherapy regimens were used in our patients (VAD: vincristine, adriamycin, dexamethasone protocol, VMCP: vincristine, melphalan, cyclophosphamide, prednisone protocol, VMCP/VBAP: VMCP/vincristine, carmustine, adriamycin, prednisone alternate protocol) in spaced treatments of 4 to 6 weeks associated with adjuvant therapies (bisphosphonates, antiemetics, and potassium).

Data were analyzed using Epi-Info software version 6.04b, Statview. The calculation of overall survival was performed according to the Kaplan Meier method with the existence in the record of an inclusion date (admission date) and a date of final assessment (date of death or the latest information mentioned in day, month, and year (dd-mm-yyyy)) (Figure 1).

3. Results

From January 1991 to August 2005, the diagnosis of symptomatic multiple myeloma was made in 30 patients under the age of 65, out of a total number of 44 cases of myeloma. The epidemiological, clinical, and biological features of these patients are summarized in Table 1.

4. Discussion

This study of multiple myeloma was carried out because very few data exist on the international level concerning the myeloma of the Ivorian.

The Clinical Hematology Department of the University Hospital of Yopougon is the only center of therapeutic management of hematological malignancies.

Out of a total of 44 cases of symptomatic multiple myeloma diagnosed from 1991 to 2005, in 15 years, we had a hospital incidence of 2.9 cases/year. The prevalence increased steadily with age: 10% among patients under the age of 40, 33% among 40–51-year-old patients, and 57% among 52–64-year-old patients. In addition, patients under the age of

TABLE 1: Epidemiological, clinical, and biological features of patients.

Variables	Numbers (%)
Age (years): average and extremes: 49 (34–64)	
<40	3 (10)
40–51	10 (33)
52–64	17 (57)
Sex: sex ratio: 1.73	
Male	19 (63)
Female	11 (37)
Professional occupations	
Executives	8 (27)
Housewives	4 (13)
Informal sector	4 (13)
Others	14 (47)
Socioeconomic status	
Low	8 (27)
Average	17 (57)
High	5 (16)
Performance status	
0 and 1	3 (10)
2 and 3	24 (80)
4	3 (10)
Bone syndrome	
Bone pains	25 (83)
Bone tumors	1 (3)
Fractures	10 (33)
Bone marrow plasma cells	
10 to 30%	18 (60)
>30	12 (40)
Whether secretory or not	
Secretory	28 (93)
Nonsecretory	2 (7)
Type of monoclonal immunoglobulin	
Ig G	26 (86)
Ig A	2 (7)
Light chains myeloma	2 (7)
Type of light chain	
Kappa	20 (86)
Lambda	2 (7)
Undetermined	2 (7)
Hemoglobin level (g/dL)	
<8	13 (43)
8–12	13 (43)
>12	4 (14)
Serum creatinine (mg/L)	
<20	24 (80)
>20	6 (20)
Calcium (mg/L)	
<120	27 (90)
>120	3 (10)
Bence Jones proteinuria (mg/24 H)	
<12	24 (80)
>12	6 (20)

Other professional activities: radiographer, farmers, policeman, traders, and teachers.

TABLE 2: Radiological, evolutional, and therapeutic features.

Variables	Numbers (%)
Radiological signs	
Geodes	24 (80)
Demineralization	12 (40)
Bone tumors	1 (3)
Fractures	10 (33)
Seats of fractures	
Femur	6 (20)
Humerus	2 (7)
Rib	1 (3)
Tibia	1 (3)
Stage of DURIE and SALMON	
Stage I	0 (0)
Stage II	14 (47)
Stage III	16 (53)
Complications	
Acute renal failure	2 (7)
Chronic renal failure	2 (7)
Infectious	10 (33)
Hemorrhagic	2 (7)
Therapeutic protocols	
VAD	3 (10)
VMCP	9 (30)
VMCP/VBAP	18 (60)
Therapeutic responses	
CR	0 (0)
VGPR	2 (7)
PR	14 (47)
Stable disease	10 (33)
Progression	4 (13)
Relapse	0 (0)
Outcome	
Living and on treatment	6 (20)
Lost to followup	13 (43)
Dead	11 (37)
Causes of death	
Progression	3 (27)
Renal complication	5 (46)
Infectious complication	3 (27)
Survival (median and extreme values in months)	5.1 (0–84)

65 accounted for 68.2% of all of our myelomas. Thus, the predominance of young patients under the age of 65 is one of the epidemiological features of our myelomas, whereas, in Europe, 40% of patients are under the age of 65 and less than 2% are under the age of 40 [8]. The average age of onset in Europe is typically around 65 to 70 years [6, 8]. The average age of our study population was 49 years, with extremes of 34 and 64. Our low average age is due to our type of sampling (study population aged under 65), and also due to the age pyramid of the African populations. However, all authors agree that myeloma is rare before the age of 40 and that it is

predominant among the male subject, as shown in our study [4, 6, 9].

In our study population, the occupation was very variable, ranging from executives to the informal sector and housewives. Exposure to ionizing radiation is the only established risk factor. This risk was found in one patient who was a radiographer. No case of family myeloma was noted. Some authors mentioned environmental factors (pesticides, herbicides, and fertilizers), especially among farmers who accounted for 10% of our study population [1].

Clinically, a bone syndrome was found in 83% of cases. It was characterized by bone pains associated or not with a bone tumor (3%) or a fracture (33%). Thus, bone pain was the dominant clinical sign in our patients, not relieved by conventional analgesics. The performance status was 2 or 3 in 80% of cases, most often associated with asthenia due to anemia or other evolutionary complications particularly recurrent infections (33%), renal failure (20%), and bleeding (7%). Infections were urogenital in 5 cases, pulmonary in 2 cases, ENT in 1 case, mucocutaneous in 1 case, and musculoskeletal in 1 case [1, 6].

Paraclinically, anemia was found in 86% of cases. This anemia was severe <8 g/dL in 43% of cases in our study population. In the literature we have, anemia is observed in 40–73% of cases [6, 9]. Bone marrow plasma cells were between 10 and 30% in 60%, the monoclonal immunoglobulin of type G in 86%, the kappa light chains in 66%, and secretory myeloma in 93%. Creatinine was <20 mg/L in 80% and serum calcium <120 mg/L in 90%. Radiological signs were dominated by geodes (80%) [10, 11]. No patient received magnetic resonance imaging (MRI) or serum determination of free light chains or cytogenetic examination for the detection of chromosomal abnormalities.

In terms of outcome, myeloma was at stage II of DURIE and SALMON in 47% of cases and at stage III in 53% of cases. The ISS (International Staging System) could not be assessed because the determination of $\beta2$ microglobulin could not be performed in the majority of patients.

Therapeutically, we only resorted to chemotherapy associated with bisphosphonates in our patients because we did not have bone marrow graft. Three chemotherapy regimens were used: VAD protocol (10%), VMCP protocol (30%), and VMCP/VBAP alternate protocol (60%). These treatments resulted in 47% of partial responses, 7% of very good partial responses, 33% of stable disease, and 13% of progression. No case of complete remission or relapse was recorded [7]. The absence of complete remission is due to the lack of intensification and the poor compliance by the fact that most patients do not complete their treatment plan, mostly for financial problems, given that 84% of our patients were of low socioeconomic conditions.

Four parameters have influenced our responses to treatment:

   (i) the absence of bone marrow transplant and new drugs for multiple myeloma (Bortezomib, IMiDs),

   (ii) the large number of patients lost to followup (43%),

   (iii) the fact that the Black has a mortality rate higher than the Caucasian [12],

   (iv) the problems of access to antimitotics: patients who are mostly of low socioeconomic status are obliged to buy medicines at exorbitant prices for their treatment.

Despite this, our results can be considered acceptable since our complete remission rate was 47%. This rate is close to that of Alexanian et al. in the US and Wan in China who have obtained, respectively, 55% and 59.09% with a protocol including vincristine, VAD [13, 14].

Our challenge that is to improve our response rate will probably be taken up because the service has new treatments for multiple myeloma.

Concerning the outcome of patients, 13 were lost to followup, that is, 43%, 11 had died, that is, 37%, and 6 were still alive and on treatment, that is, 20%. We have no data concerning the monitoring of the cohort of 6 patients alive from 2005 to 2013. This is the reason why the maximum survival time was 84 months in our Kaplan Meier curve. So there is no median followup of this cohort. The causes of death were renal in 47% and infectious in 27%, related to the progression of the disease in 27%. The median overall survival was 5.1 months with extremes ranging from 0 to 84 months. The probability of survival at 6 months was 51% and at 3 years 6.7%. But it should be noted that currently the gold standard in subjects under the age of 65 is the VTD (velcade, thalidomide, dexamethasone) protocol, and we have this protocol at our disposal since October 2010. But only well-off patients have access to it, given its relatively high cost. But in our regions, there is no international clinical trial for multiple myeloma at the moment.

References

[1] A. B. Chaubert, F. Delacretaz, and P. M. Schmidt, "Myélome multiple," *Schweizerische Medical Forum*, vol. 5, pp. 309–316, 2005.

[2] R. Bataille, "Myélome multiple: traitements symptomatiques et antitumoraux," in *Encycl Méd Chir*, Hématologie, p. 17, Elsevier, Paris, France, 1996.

[3] J.-L. Harousseau and M. Dreyling, "Multiple myeloma: ESMO clinical practice guidelines for diagnosis, treatment and followup," *Annals of Oncology*, vol. 21, no. 5, pp. v155–v157, 2010.

[4] W. J.-Dong, M. Chang-Ki, and H. Kyungja, "Impact of genetic abnormalities on the prognoses and clinical parameters of patients with multiple myeloma," *Annals of Laboratory Medicine*, vol. 33, no. 4, pp. 248–254, 2013.

[5] D. E. Reece, "Recent trends in the management of newly diagnosed multiple myeloma," *Current Opinion in Hematology*, vol. 16, no. 4, pp. 306–312, 2009.

[6] A. Palumbo and C. Cerrato, "Diagnosis and therapy of multiple myeloma," *The Korean Journal of Internal Medicine*, vol. 28, no. 3, pp. 263–273, 2013.

[7] J. M. Bird, R. G. Owen, S. D'Sa et al., "Guidelines for the diagnosis and management of multiple myeloma 2011," *British Journal of Haematology*, vol. 154, no. 1, pp. 32–75, 2011.

[8] A. Oranger, C. Carbone, and M. Grano, "Cellular mechanisms of multiple myeloma bone disease," *Clinical and Developmental Immunology*, vol. 2013, Article ID 289458, 14 pages, 2013.

[9] A. Dispenzieri and R. A. Kyle, "Multiple myeloma: clinical features and indications for therapy," *Best Practice and Research*, vol. 18, no. 4, pp. 553–568, 2005.

[10] R. A. Kyle, M. A. Gertz, T. E. Witzig et al., "Review of 1027 patients with newly diagnosed multiple myeloma," *Mayo Clinic Proceedings*, vol. 78, no. 1, pp. 21–33, 2003.

[11] G. R. Shaw, "Nonsecretory plasma cell myeloma—becoming even more rare with serum free light-chain assay: a brief review," *Archives of Pathology and Laboratory Medicine*, vol. 130, no. 8, pp. 1212–1215, 2006.

[12] D. Pulte, M. T. Redaniel, H. Brenner, L. Jansen, and M. Jeffreys, "Recent improvement in survival of patients with multiple myeloma: variation byethnicity," *Leukemia Lymphoma*. In press.

[13] R. Alexanian, B. Barlogie, and S. Tucker, "VAD-based regimens as primary treatment for multiple myeloma," *American Journal of Hematology*, vol. 33, no. 2, pp. 86–89, 1990.

[14] J. Wan, "Therapeutic efficacy analysis of VD regimen and VAD regimen for multiple myeloma," *Zhongguo Shi Yan Xue Ye Xue Za Zhi*, vol. 21, no. 3, pp. 647–649, 2013.

7

Prognostic Significance of Serum Free Light Chains in Chronic Lymphocytic Leukemia

Katerina Sarris,[1] Dimitrios Maltezas,[1] Efstathios Koulieris,[1] Vassiliki Bartzis,[1]
Tatiana Tzenou,[1] Sotirios Sachanas,[1] Eftychia Nikolaou,[1] Anna Efthymiou,[1]
Katerina Bitsani,[1] Maria Dimou,[1] Theodoros P. Vassilakopoulos,[1] Marina Siakantaris,[1]
Maria K. Angelopoulou,[1] Flora Kontopidou,[1] Panagiotis Tsaftaridis,[1] Nikolitsa Kafasi,[2]
Gerasimos A. Pangalis,[1] Panayiotis P. Panayiotidis,[1] Stephen Harding,[3]
and Marie-Christine Kyrtsonis[1]

[1] Hematology Section of the First Department of Propedeutic Internal Medicine, Laikon University Hospital, Agiou Thoma 17, 11527 Athens, Greece
[2] Immunology Department, Laikon General Hospital, Agiou Thoma 17, 11527 Athens, Greece
[3] The Binding Site Ltd, B15 1QT, Birmingham, UK

Correspondence should be addressed to Marie-Christine Kyrtsonis; mck@ath.forthnet.gr

Academic Editor: Shaji Kumar

Background. Serum free light chains (sFLC), the most commonly detected paraprotein in CLL, were recently proposed as useful tools for the prognostication of CLL patients. *Objective.* To investigate the prognostic implication of sFLC and the summated FLC-kappa plus FLC-lambda in a CLL patients' series. *Patients and Methods.* We studied 143 CLL patients of which 18 were symptomatic and needed treatment, while 37 became symptomatic during follow-up. Seventy-two percent, 18%, and 10% were in Binet stage A, B and C, respectively. Median patients' followup was 32 months (range 4–228). *Results.* Increased involved (restricted) sFLC (iFLC) was found in 42% of patients, while the summated FLC-kappa plus FLC-lambda was above 60 mg/dL in 14%. Increased sFLC values as well as those of summated FLC above 60 were related to shorter time to treatment ($P = 0.0005$ and $P = 0.000003$, resp.) and overall survival ($P = 0.05$ and $P = 0.003$, resp.). They also correlated with β2-microglobulin ($P = 0.009$ and $P = 0.03$, resp.), serum albumin ($P = 0.009$ for summated sFLC), hemoglobin ($P < 0.001$), abnormal LDH ($P = 0.037$ and $P = 0.001$, resp.), Binet stage ($P < 0.05$) and with the presence of beta symptoms ($P = 0.004$ for summated sFLC). *Conclusion.* We confirmed the prognostic significance of sFLC in CLL regarding both time to treatment and survival and showed their relationship with other parameters.

1. Introduction

Chronic lymphocytic leukemia is the most common type of leukemia in the Western world accounting for 40% of all leukemias. It affects mainly elderly patients as the median age of diagnosis is about 72 years and the male to female ratio is 2 : 1. So far, Rai and Binet staging systems are used for predicting CLL patients' outcome. Other prognostic markers, which have been established but mainly concern symptomatic CLL patients, are lymphocyte CD38 expression, presence of ZAP-70, immunoglobulin (Ig) heavy gene mutation status, and cytogenetic profile [1–6]. In symptomatic

patients the presence of unmutated Ig heavy chain variable region, the presence of ZAP-70, and CD-38 expression predict worse clinical outcome. Chromosomal abnormalities with importance for disease prognosis are deletion of long arm of chromosome 13, deletion of petit arm of chromosome 17 (del p17), and deletion of the long arm of chromosome 11 (del q11) with the first indicating a better prognosis than the last ones. Nevertheless the presence of these factors in patients does not signify that they should start treatment in the absence of symptomatic disease.

Immunoglobulins (Igs) are produced by terminally differentiated B cells (either plasma cells or long lived memory cells), with the capacity to produce antibodies with high affinity for the immunizing antigen which are composed by 2 heavy and 2 light chains [7]. During this procedure a small excess amount of light chains are produced and released in the plasma/serum in the form of serum immunoglobulin free light chains (sFLC). It has recently been found that 38% of patients eventually developing CLL displayed abnormal sFLC ratio (FLCR) up to 10 years before CLL diagnosis and another 16% had polyclonal sFLC elevation in the same time frame preceding diagnosis [8].

Recent data have shown that serum free light chains and their ratio may constitute prognostic factors in CLL [9–15]. Serum free light assays have already been shown to improve detection, management, and prognostication in plasma cell dyscrasias [16–18]. In diffuse large B-cell lymphomas, increased levels of sFLC were shown to be an independent, adverse prognostic factor for overall survival (OS). Also abnormal sFLC ratio can help in CNS lymphomas diagnosis [19]. Recently abnormal sFLC ratio was found to play an important prognostic role in multiple myeloma [16], AL Amyloidosis [20], and Waldestrom's macroglobulinemia [17]. Moreover, abnormal FLCR is considered a risk factor for the progression of MGUS [21], solitary plasmacytoma [22], and smoldering myeloma [23] into multiple myeloma.

It is of great importance to identify simple prognostic markers that could be widely applied in clinical practice and with low cost, in order to predict the group of asymptomatic patients that will shortly require therapy [24]. We therefore tested the eventual prognostic implication of sFLC in a cohort of CLL patients at diagnosis.

2. Patients and Methods

2.1. Patients. Frozen sera from patients that fulfilled the 1996 CLL criteria [25] were drawn at diagnosis in 143 consecutive CLL patients with available sera. At presentation 18 (13%) of them needed immediate treatment, while all the others were asymptomatic and were only regularly followed. During followup 37 (26%) developed symptoms and required treatment administration. Seventy-two percent, 18%, and 10% of patients were in Binet stage A, B, and C respectively.

Patients' standard workup at diagnosis included physical examination and whole body CT scanning for the evaluation of eventual lymph node swelling and organomegaly, complete blood counts and cell morphology evaluation on blood smears, bone marrow aspiration and biopsy, blood or marrow lymphocyte immunophenotype, and biochemical background including serum lactate dehydrogenase (LDH) and serum protein electrophoresis, while serum beta-2-microglobulin and fluorescent *in situ* hybridization (FISH) studies for del p17 and del q11, were tested in a subset of patients only (48% and 24%, resp.).

Light chain restriction was established by flow cytometry or bone marrow biopsy immunohistochemistry. The patients' characteristics can be seen in Table 1; median patients' followup was 32 months (range 4–228).

TABLE 1: Patients' characteristics.

Number of patients	143
Median age	63 years (range 37–87)
Sex male/female	64/79 (45%/55%)
Rai stage	
0	64 (45%)
I	46 (32%)
II	14 (10%)
III	14 (10%)
IV	5 (3%)
Binet stage	
A	89 (62%)
B	31 (22%)
C	23 (16%)
Lymphadenopathy	79 (55%)
Splenomegaly	23 (16%)
LDH (>normal upper limit)	20 (14%)
Hemoglobin, g/dL, median (range)	13,5 (4–17,8)
White blood cell counts, $\times 10^9$/L, median (range)	21,600 (7–600)
Lymphocytes absolute value, $\times 10^9$/L, median (range)	14 (5–580)
Beta-2-microglobulin, mg/L median (range)*	2,5 (1,18–8,8)
CD38 expression > 20%	14 (10%)
FISH and IGVH status**	34 (24%)
Symptomatic	18 (12,5%)
Median followup	32 months (range 4–228)

*Evaluated in 69 patients.
**The percentage of patients that were positive is too small to be evaluated.

2.2. Methods. Serum free light chain values were retrospectively determined by nephelometry (Freelite™, the Binding Site Birmingham, UK) in frozen sera drawn at diagnosis.

Abnormal sFLC and FLCR values were defined as any values out of the 95th percent percentile normal ranges reported by the manufacturer [26, 27], meaning 3.3 to 19.4 mg/L for kappa free light chain, 5.7 to 26.3 mg/L for lambda free light chain, and 0.31 to 1.2 for FLCR. In this series, all patients but one had normal serum creatinine, so abnormal FLC values were assessed without adjustment for renal failure.

We evaluated the prognostic significance of the summated sFLC, using as cut off values (1) their median level, (2) the value of 60 mg/L proposed by Morabito et al. [15] that performed a receiver operating characteristics analysis in order to establish the most suitable sFLC ($\kappa + \lambda$) cutoff value and showed it was 60.6 mg/mL (area under the curve = 0.62; $P < 0.0001$), (3) we additionally tested arbitrarily a cutoff of 50 mg/L, because few early stage CLL patients had a summated FLC above 60 mg/L.

Statistical analysis was performed using SPSS v15.0. Correlations between disease variables derived from patients' standard workout at diagnosis and sFLC values were evaluated by the chi square test when assessed as categorical variables and by the Kendall's test if one of them was categorical.

With regard to survival and time to first treatment (TFT), the prognostic significance of abnormal sFLC and ratios were determined by univariate Cox regression analysis. Kaplan Meier method was used for pictorial representation of survival and TFT.

3. Results

3.1. sFLC Values in Patients. Sixty-nine percent of patients presented with kappa light chain restriction and 31% with lambda monoclonality.

Kappa sFLC ranged from 2.54 to 196 mg/L (median 19.2 mg/L) and lambda from 9.19 to 121 mg/L (median 20 mg/L) in kappa-and lambda-restricted patients, respectively. Increased involved (restricted) sFLC (iFLC), either kappa or lambda, were found in 42% of patients.

sFLC ratio (FLCR) ranged from 0.02 to 496 (median 0.95). Abnormal FLCR values, suggesting light chain paraprotein presence, were present in 30% of patients.

The summated FLC-kappa plus FLC-lambda ranged from 9.4 to 217.4 mg/L (median 33,1 mg/L); it was higher than 60 mg/L in 14%.

3.2. Correlations between sFLC Values and Disease Markers. iFLC and summated sFLC kappa + lambda > 60 significantly correlated with Binet stage (P = 0.039 and P = 0.02, resp.), the presence of lymphadenopathy (P = 0.02 and 0.05, resp.), hemoglobin level (negatively), (P = 0.000003 and P = 0.0002, resp.), white blood cells counts (P < 0.01 both), lymphocyte absolute number (P < 0.01 both), serum immunoglobulin IgG level (P = 0.025 and 0.01, resp.), abnormal LDH (P = 0.037 and 0.001 resp.), beta-2-microglobulin (P = 0.009 and 0.03, resp.), serum albumin (P = 0.009 only for FLC kappa + lambda > 60), and with the presence of beta-symptoms (P = 0.004 only for summated sFLC > 60) (Figure 1).

No correlations were found with the presence of spleen enlargement and CD38 expression while the number of cases tested for del p17, del q11, and IGVH status are too small to reach conclusions.

FLCR did not show any significant correlation with disease variables.

3.3. Correlations between sFLC, FLCR, Summated sFLC Values and, Survival

3.3.1. Time to First Treatment (TFT). Increased involvment sFLC (iFLC) values as well as values of summated sFLC kappa + lambda > 60 were related to shorter TFT (P = 0.0005 and P = 0.000003, resp.) as shown in Figure 2, while neither values of summated FLC were above median nor was FLCR.

3.3.2. Overall Survival (OS). Increased iFLC and summated sFLC above 60 correlated with shorter OS (P = 0.05 and P = 0.003, resp.) as shown in Figure 3, while neither values of summated FLC above were median nor was FLCR.

3.4. Other Variables with Prognostic Importance on OS and TFT. We also evaluated the prognostic value of some other routine laboratory variable tested during diagnostic workup, namely, Binet stage, beta-2-microglobulin, serum albumin, and LDH. Hemoglobin levels, platelet counts, and lymphocyte doubling time were not assessed as they constitute, by definition, criteria to start treatment. IGVH status and FISH results for adverse genetic markers were not assessed, as they were available in only a minority of patients.

Binet stage correlated with both TFT and OS (P < 0.001 for both). Abnormal (above normal upper limit) LDH correlated with OS (P = 0.001) but not with TFT.

Beta-2-microglobulin above 3.5 mg/L correlated with TFT (P < 0.001) but not with OS. Serum albumin correlated neither with TFT nor with OS.

However, because the number of patients is too small for a comprehensive modeling, prognostic models combining iFLC or summated FLC with other variables of adverse outcome were not assessed.

4. Discussion

Although CLL is usually an indolent disease and may not require treatment for years, some patients can experience a much more aggressive disease and a shorter survival. The general rule is that symptomatic CLL patients need treatment immediately while the others should be regularly followed. Existing established clinical and genetic prognostic markers and staging systems apply very well to symptomatic patients but not always to asymptomatic ones that represent about 2/3 of all CLL patients. For these patients overall survival (OS) highly depends on the time to first treatment (TFT).

The most frequent paraprotein produced in CLL is serum free light chain in almost up to 50% of the patients. Accordingly, we also found increased involved FLC in more than 40% of patients and an abnormal FLCR, thus, confirming the monoclonal nature of sFLC in 30% of cases.

It has recently been shown that sFLC and their sum above 60.6 mg/L may contribute usefully to prognosis [15], mainly with regard to TFT. The first group that studied sFLC prognostic contribution in CLL was the one of Pratt et al. [10]. Using a Cox regression analysis, they identified 4 independent prognostic variables for overall survival, namely, Zap-70, β2-microglobulin, M-IgVH, and abnormal sFLC ratio. Patients with CLL with an abnormal sFLC ratio were significantly more likely to have U-IgVH, a Zap-70 positivity, a lymphocyte doubling time less than 12 months, and a high β2-microglobulin. In a similar way, in a study involving 84 patients with CLL, Perdigao et al. [13] showed a correlation among abnormal sFLCr, TFT, IgVH mutational status, and survival. In their study of 34 patients with CLL in various stages (median age, 66 years; male-female ratio of 1.9 : 1; median time from diagnosis, 41.5 months), Ruchlemer et al. found [28] an abnormal sFLCr in 53% of cases, which mostly correlated with advanced disease stage and increased κ chain. In a separate group of 120 patients with CLL (serum samples collected before initiation or 6 months after

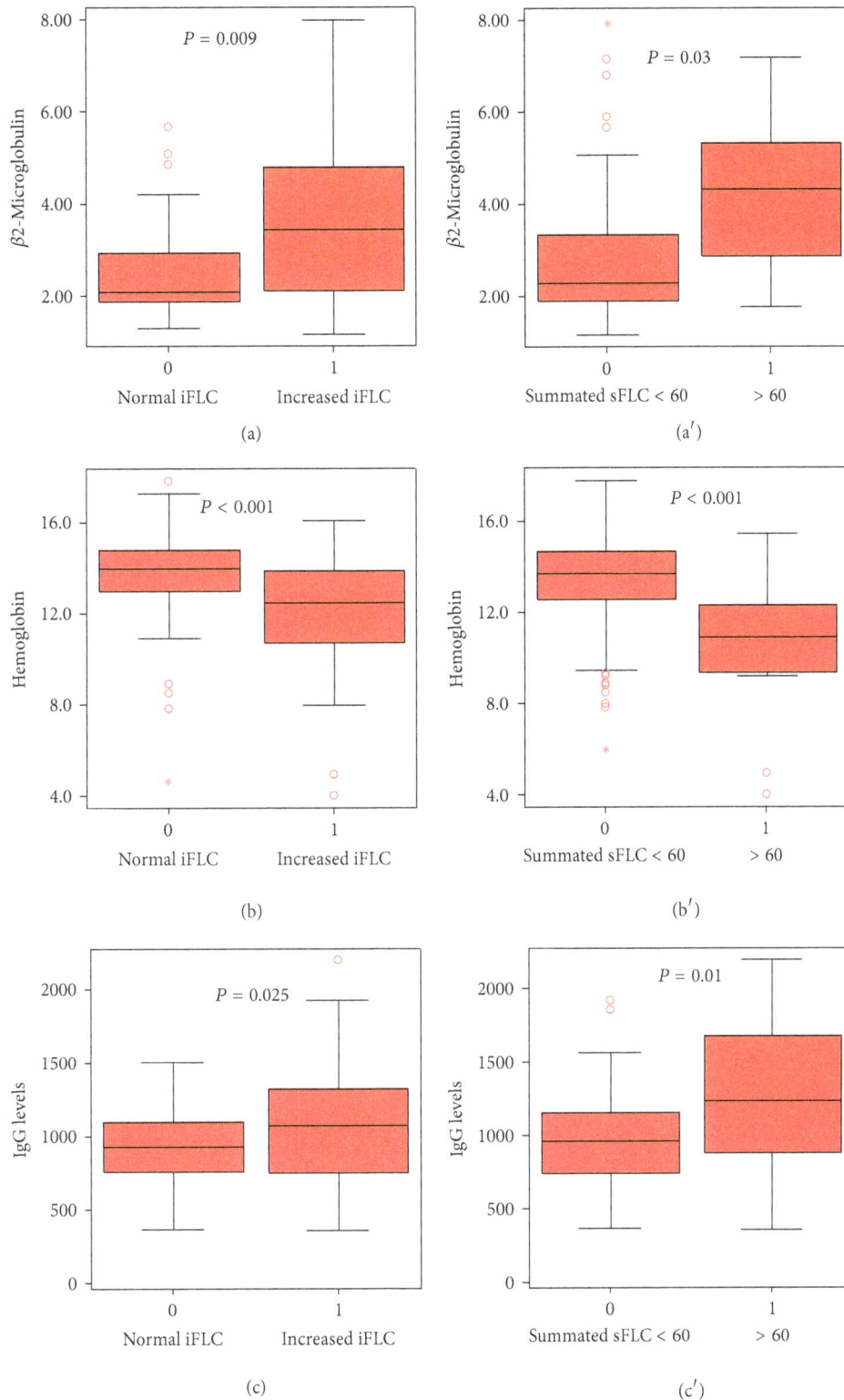

FIGURE 1

cessation of treatment), 71 patients (59%) had abnormal FLCR. In addition to improving M-protein detection in CLL, it was shown that abnormal low FLCR (indicating lambda FLC involvement) was associated with worse outcome. In addition, no correlation was found between sFLC and other prognostic factors (ZAP-70, CD38, cytogenetic markers, and Binet stage) implying, according to the authors, that sFLC is an independent prognostic factor in patients with CLL [9].

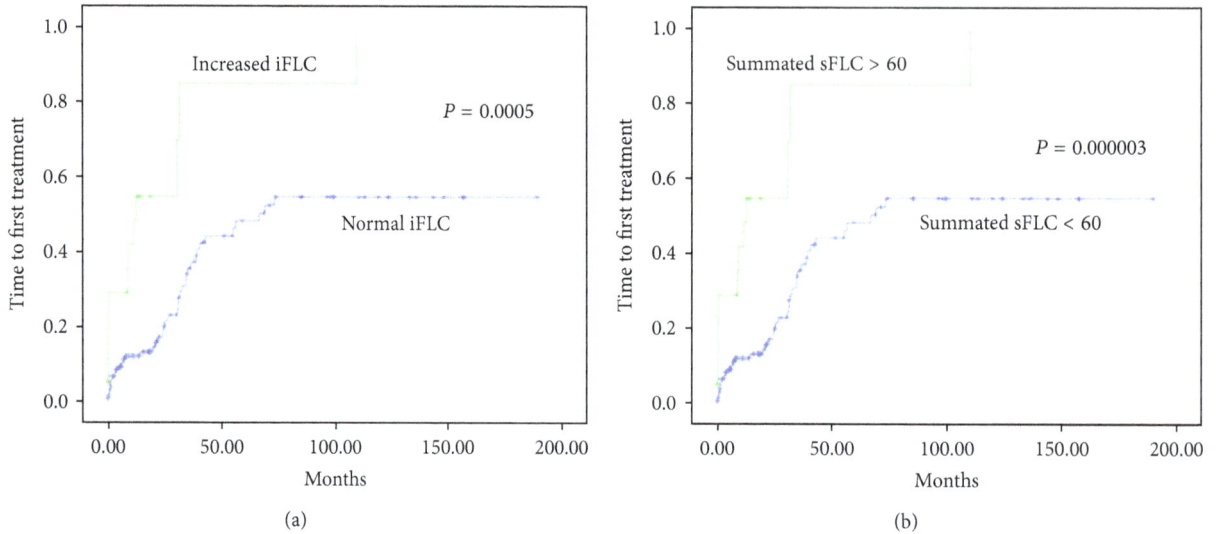

(a)   (b)

FIGURE 2

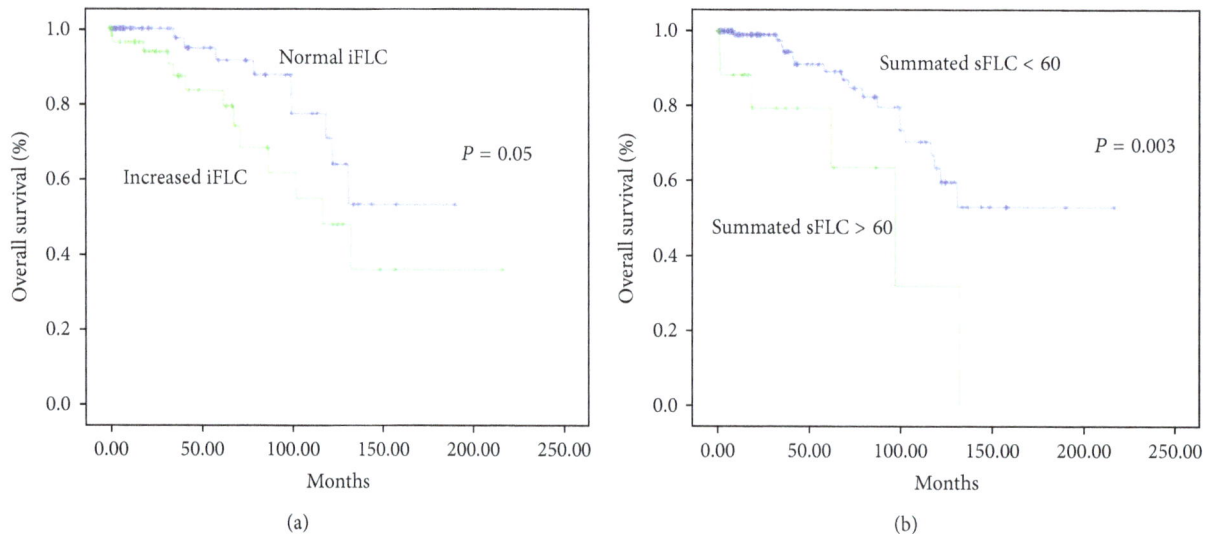

(a)   (b)

FIGURE 3

Unlike these results, we found a correlation between iFLC or the summated sFLC and Binet stage.

In their recent study, Maurer et al. [14] classified 339 newly diagnosed patients with CLL into 3 types: type 1 with elevated κ or λ FLC and abnormal sFLCr (monoclonal, $n = 57$ patients), type 2 with elevated kappa or lambda FLC and normal sFLCr (polyclonal, $n = 52$ patients), and type 3 with normal range kappa and lambda FLC and abnormal FLCR (monoclonal, $n = 54$ patients). Patients were followedup for a median of 47 months. Forty-nine percent of patients with sFLC abnormalities had a worse TFT and overall survival than those with normal sFLC. The authors concluded that sFLC is an important prognostic factor and is maintained after adjustment for Rai staging, with different types of sFLC abnormality affecting prognosis to various degrees.

In 2010, Yegin et al. [11] in their retrospective study assessed the prognostic value of sFLC levels and FLCR in

a cohort of 101 patients with CLL (median age, 62 years; male-female ratio, 68 : 33) followedup for a median of 29 (range, 1.1–234) months. sFLC levels were found to be high in 55 patients (54.5%), with 30 patients (29.7%) having abnormal FLCR, in agreement with our results. Median TFT was shorter in patients with high sFLC levels but not in low-risk patients with CLL. In addition, median TFT was not statistically different between patients with normal and abnormal FLCR. The median overall survival was shorter in patients with both high sFLC levels and abnormal FLCR, but this did not remain valid in the multivariate analysis, probably because of the small sample. Furthermore, patients with high sFLC levels and abnormal FLCR expressed higher CD38 levels and positivity, thus, indicating that these biomarkers are involved in stimulation of B-cell receptor on CLL proliferating cells. However, we did not find any correlation with CD38 expression.

The finding that increased polyclonal sFLC also constituted an adverse marker for time to first treatment (TFT) in CLL was firstly reported by Maurer et al. [14] and almost immediately confirmed by Morabito et al. [15] that evaluated the sum of absolute kappa and lambda sFLC and found that the prognostic impact of the summated sFLC (kappa + lambda) value above 60.6 mg/L was a superior prognosticator of TFT than FLCR [15].

In our study, increased sFLC were found in 42% of the patients, while the summated FLC-kappa plus FLC-lambda was higher than 60 mg/dL in 14%. Increased involvement of sFLC (iFLC) values and values of summated sFLC above 60 were related to shorter TFT and OS, in agreement with the aforementioned publications; we additionally tested the prognostic potential of the summated FLC using as cutoff the median value and confirmed that the value of 60 mg/L was a better cutoff. We also found significant correlations with disease variables. Likewise, iFLC and/or summated sFLC above 60 correlated with β2-microglobulin, serum albumin, negatively with hemoglobin, white blood cell and lymphocyte counts, abnormal LDH, Rai and Binet stage, and with the presence of lymphadenopathy and beta-symptoms. The relationship with IgG is very interesting and its significance remains to be fully evaluated. The observed correlations of sFLC with β2-microglobulin, albumin, and IgG are reported here for the first time and their interpretation remains to be further studied.

In the present study, Binet stage was, as expected, of prognostic relevance with regard to TFT and OS, while abnormal serum LDH was predictive of a worse outcome and increased beta-2-microglobulin of a shorter TFT. However, the number of patients is too small to build prognostic models associating iFLC or summated FLC with other variables of adverse outcome. This should be done in larger series.

5. Conclusion

The results of our study confirmed the significance of sFLC in CLL with regard to TFT and OS, showed their relationship with adverse prognostic clinical and laboratory parameters and suggested, in accordance with others, that these tests should be included in CLL patients' initial workout, as they offer additional prognostic information.

Abbreviations

sFLC: Serum free light chains
iFLC: Involved serum free light chains
FLCR: Free light chain ratio
TFT: Time to first treatment
OS: Overall survival
CLL: Chronic lymphocytic leukemia
IGVH Ig: Heavy chain variable region.

Acknowledgments

The authors would like to thank the Binding Site Ltd, for graciously providing then with the kits used in the study.

References

[1] T. J. Hamblin, Z. Davis, A. Gardiner, D. G. Oscier, and F. K. Stevenson, "Unmutated Ig V(H) genes are associated with a more aggressive form of chronic lymphocytic leukemia," *Blood*, vol. 94, no. 6, pp. 1848–1854, 1999.

[2] R. N. Damle, T. Wasil, F. Fais et al., "Ig V gene mutation status and CD38 expression as novel prognostic indicators in chronic lymphocytic leukemia," *Blood*, vol. 94, no. 6, pp. 1840–1847, 1999.

[3] T. J. Hamblin, J. A. Orchard, R. E. Ibbotson et al., "CD38 expression and immunoglobulin variable region mutations are independent prognostic variables in chronic lymphocytic leukemia, but CD38 expression may vary during the course of the disease," *Blood*, vol. 99, no. 3, pp. 1023–1029, 2002.

[4] Z. Matral, K. Lin, M. Dennis et al., "CD38 expression and Ig VH gene mutation in B-cell chronic lymphocytic leukemia," *Blood*, vol. 97, no. 6, pp. 1902–1903, 2001.

[5] M. Crespo, F. Bosch, and N. Villamor, "Zap-70 expression as a surrogate for IgV-region mutations in CLL," *New England Journal of Medicine*, vol. 348, pp. 1764–1775, 2003.

[6] H. Döhner, S. Silgenbauer, A. Benner et al., "Genomic aberrations and survival in CLL," *New England Journal of Medicine*, vol. 343, pp. 1910–1916, 2000.

[7] M. C. Kyrtsonis, E. Koulieris, V. Bartzis et al., "Monoclonal immunoglobulin," in *Multiple Myeloma—A Quick Reflection on the Fast Progress*, R. Hajek, Ed., 2013.

[8] H.-T. Tsai, N. E. Caporaso, R. A. Kyle et al., "Evidence of serum immunoglobulin abnormalities up to 9.8 years before diagnosis of chronic lymphocytic leukemia: a prospective study," *Blood*, vol. 114, no. 24, pp. 4928–4932, 2009.

[9] J. Matschke, L. Eisele, L. Sellman et al., "Abnormal free light chain ratio in chronic lymphocytic leukemia: a new prognostic factor?" *Blood*, vol. 114, article 1237, 2009.

[10] G. Pratt, S. Harding, R. Holder et al., "Abnormal serum free light chain ratios are associated with poor survival and may reflect biological subgroups in patients with chronic lymphocytic leukaemia," *British Journal of Haematology*, vol. 144, no. 2, pp. 217–222, 2009.

[11] Z. A. Yegin, Z. N. Özkurt, and M. Yàci, "Free light chain: a novel predictor of adverse outcome in chronic lymphocytic leukemia," *European Journal of Haematology*, vol. 84, no. 5, pp. 406–411, 2010.

[12] K. M. Charafeddine, M. N. Jabbour, R. H. Kadi, and R. T. Daher, "Extended use of serum free light chain as biomarker in lymphoproliferative disorders," *American Journal of Clinical Pathology*, vol. 137, pp. 890–897, 2012.

[13] J. Perdigao, M. J. Cabrai, N. Costa et al., "Prognostic factors in CLL: is serum free light chain ratio a new biological marker?" *Annals of Oncology*, vol. 19, article 204, 2008.

[14] M. J. Maurer, J. R. Cerhan, J. A. Katzmann et al., "Monoclonal and polyclonal serum free light chains and clinical outcome in chronic lymphocytic leukemia," *Blood*, vol. 118, no. 10, pp. 2821–2826, 2011.

[15] F. Morabito, R. De Filippi, L. Laurenti et al., "The cumulative amount of serum-free light chain is a strong prognosticator in chronic lymphocytic leukemia," *Blood*, vol. 118, no. 24, pp. 6353–6361, 2011.

[16] M.-C. Kyrtsonis, T. P. Vassilakopoulos, N. Kafasi et al., "Prognostic value of serum free light chain ratio at diagnosis in multiple myeloma," *British Journal of Haematology*, vol. 137, no. 3, pp. 240–243, 2007.

[17] A. Moreau, X. Leleu, R. Manning et al., "Serum free light chains in Waldestroms macroglobulinemia," *Blood*, vol. 108, article 2420a, 2006.

[18] F. van Rhee, V. Bolejack, K. Hollmig et al., "High serum-free light chain levels and their rapid reduction in response to therapy define an aggressive multiple myeloma subtype with poor prognosis," *Blood*, vol. 110, no. 3, pp. 827–832, 2007.

[19] R. Schroers, A. Baraniskin, C. Heute et al., "Detection of free immunoglobulin light chains in cerebrospinal fluids of patients with central nervous system lymphomas," *European Journal of Haematology*, vol. 85, no. 3, pp. 236–242, 2010.

[20] S. Kumar, A. Dispenzieri, J. A. Katzmann et al., "Serum immunoglobulin free light-chain measurement in primary amyloidosis: prognostic value and correlations with clinical features," *Blood*, vol. 116, no. 24, pp. 5126–5129, 2010.

[21] S. V. Rajkumar, R. A. Kyle, T. M. Therneau et al., "Serum free light chain ratio is an independent risk factor for progression in MGUS," *Blood*, vol. 106, pp. 812–817, 2005.

[22] D. Dingli, R. A. Kyle, S. V. Rajkumar et al., "Immunoglobulin free light chains and solitary plasmacytoma of bone," *Blood*, vol. 108, no. 6, pp. 1979–1983, 2006.

[23] A. Dispenzieri, R. A. Kyle, J. A. Katzmann et al., "Immunoglobulin free light chain ratio is an independent risk factor for progression of smoldering (asymptomatic) multiple myeloma," *Blood*, vol. 111, no. 2, pp. 785–789, 2008.

[24] T. Zeniz, S. Frohling, D. Mertens et al., "Moving from prognostic to predictive factors in CLL," *Best Practice and Research Clinical Haematology*, vol. 23, pp. 1171–1184, 2010.

[25] M. Hallek, B. D. Cheson, D. Catovsky et al., "Guidelines for the diagnosis and treatment of chronic lymphocytic leukemia: a report from the International Workshop on Chronic Lymphocytic Leukemia updating the National Cancer Institute-Working Group 1996 guidelines," *Blood*, vol. 111, no. 12, pp. 5446–5456, 2008.

[26] A. R. Bradwell, "Chapter 5. Normal ranges and reference intervals," in *Serum Free Light Chain Analysis (Plus Hevylite)*, pp. 36–44, 6th edition, 2010.

[27] A. R. Bradwell, H. D. Carr-Smith, G. P. Mead et al., "Highly sensitive, automated immunoassay for immunoglobulin free light chains in serum and urine," *Clinical Chemistry*, vol. 47, no. 4, pp. 673–680, 2001.

[28] R. Ruchlemer, C. Reinus, E. Paz et al., "Free light chains, monoclonal proteins and chronic lymphocytic leukaemia," *Blood*, vol. 110, article 4697a, 2007.

8

Acquired Myelodysplasia or Myelodysplastic Syndrome: Clearing the Fog

Ethan A. Natelson[1] and David Pyatt[2,3]

[1] Professor of Clinical Medicine, Weill-Cornell Medical School and Director, Transitional Residency Program, Houston Methodist Hospital, 6550 Fannin Street, Suite 1001, Houston, TX 77030, USA
[2] Summit Toxicology, LLP, 1944 Cedaridge Circle, Superior, CO 80026, USA
[3] Schools of Pharmacy and Public Health, The University of Colorado, Denver, CO 80026, USA

Correspondence should be addressed to Ethan A. Natelson; enatelson@tmhs.org

Academic Editor: Giuseppe G. Saglio

Myelodysplastic syndromes (MDS) are clonal myeloid disorders characterized by progressive peripheral blood cytopenias associated with ineffective myelopoiesis. They are typically considered neoplasms because of frequent genetic aberrations and patient-limited survival with progression to acute myeloid leukemia (AML) or death related to the consequences of bone marrow failure including infection, hemorrhage, and iron overload. A progression to AML has always been recognized among the myeloproliferative disorders (MPD) but occurs only rarely among those with essential thrombocythemia (ET). Yet, the World Health Organization (WHO) has chosen to apply the designation myeloproliferative neoplasms (MPN), for all MPD but has not similarly recommended that all MDS become the myelodysplastic neoplasms (MDN). This apparent dichotomy may reflect the extremely diverse nature of MDS. Moreover, the term MDS is occasionally inappropriately applied to hematologic disorders associated with acquired morphologic myelodysplastic features which may rather represent potentially reversible hematological responses to immune-mediated factors, nutritional deficiency states, and disordered myelopoietic responses to various pharmaceutical, herbal, or other potentially myelotoxic compounds. We emphasize the clinical settings, and the histopathologic features, of such AMD that should trigger a search for a reversible underlying condition that may be nonneoplastic and not MDS.

1. Introduction

Despite advances in cytogenetic and flow cytometric analyses, aberrant cellular morphology, as identified in the peripheral blood and bone marrow, remains the defining feature leading to a clinical diagnosis of myelodysplastic syndrome (MDS). Certain laboratory values such as blood cell count and cell volume measurements are accurate and reproducible, and the results are not open to dispute, as is the presence of particular unique and obvious morphologic findings such as the presence of acquired Pelger-Huët granulocytes and tear-drop erythrocytes in the peripheral blood or large numbers of ringed sideroblasts or increased numbers of myeloblasts in the bone marrow. Other observations such as reduced mature myeloid cell cytoplasmic granulation

and the presence of dimorphic erythrocyte or dysmorphic megakaryocytic populations are more subtle. However, what constitutes a significant variation from normal in each of the three major cell lines in the bone marrow remains very observer dependent. Unfortunately, we are only occasionally but usefully reminded that not all clear-cut examples of acquired and persistent myelodysplasia represent MDS or neoplasia [1, 2].

The difficulty with morphology, alone, in establishing a diagnosis of MDS is evident in the evolution of the current World Health Organization [WHO] classification system for MDS with respect to the acquired refractory sideroblastic disorders. Germing and associates suggested that careful morphological review allowed some separation within the initial MDS classification system of those individuals with acquired idiopathic sideroblastic anemia (AISA) who were more likely to have an illness that would terminate in AML from those who might not have a neoplastic or preleukemic condition. They separated 232 individuals with MDS associated with ringed sideroblasts into two groups, one without significant myelodysplastic features among nonerythroid bone marrow cells and the other exhibiting such dyspoiesis among multiple cell lines. The 38% with selective erythroid aberrations and the 62% with a more multilineage dysplasia, respectively, exhibited different clinical courses, frequency of cytogenetic defects, and survival patterns [3]. Earlier, other authors had also proposed that AISA was not a uniform illness and that some affected individuals actually had a "benign" form of the disorder [4].

Such an arbitrary distinction among those with a sideroblastic MDS was subsequently adopted in the WHO MDS classification as refractory anemia with ringed sideroblasts (RARS) and refractory cytopenia with multi-lineage dysplasia and ringed sideroblasts (RCMD-RS). However, a uniform concordance with this dual classification among experts in the field seemed hopelessly lacking. In Pavia, Italy, experienced hematopathologists classified only 28% of 60 such MDS cases with ringed sideroblasts as RCMD-RS while their colleagues in Dusseldorf, Germany, opined that 76% of their 119 patients with MDS and ringed sideroblasts fell into this category [5]. To solve this dilemma of lack of agreement in classification, the WHO simply eliminated the category of RCMD-RS with the publication of their 2008 fascicle. The result was that the diagnosis of RARS seems to be disappearing as fewer hematopathologists seem to be willing to commit to a unilineage myelodysplasia in their interpretation of bone marrow morphology. Thus, RARS, which once amounted to more than 10% of all MDS, despite the original inclusion of the myeloproliferative disease, chronic myelomonocytic leukemia [CMML] as MDS now only accounted for 1.1% of all MDS in a recently analyzed group of 611 cases [6]. Nevertheless, many clinical hematologists still recognize RARS as a specific entity and wonder why the morphology-based separation between the two ends of a bell-shaped curve, which may represent perhaps the single most distinctive form of MDS, was even attempted [7].

Current and suggested future MDS classifications seem to focus primarily on survival statistics or risk for evolution into AML to complement prognostic scoring systems [8]. Such data are not useful for epidemiological studies searching for the etiology of the initial process or necessarily dictating the therapy of specific types of MDS as advocated and applicable for other complex hematologic disorders such as the non-Hodgkin lymphomas [NHL]. Figure 1 indicates the age-related incidence and an estimated frequency distribution of subsets of MDS that relate with etiologic circumstances or associations rather than survival risk.

The ability to "see" and report myelodysplasia where none is likely to exist was emphasized in a recent blinded study involving inspection of the bone marrow aspirate slides of 120 healthy prospective bone marrow donors with normal blood counts by four allegedly experienced morphologists [9]. Here, more than 10% of the bone marrow cells were found to exhibit myelodysplasia involving one cell line in 37% of this cohort,

among two cell lines in 31%, and among all three cell lines in 6.5% of these individuals, none of whom would be reasonably expected to have either myelodysplasia or MDS. Such observations speak to the inherent weakness of morphologic interpretation in current WHO MDS classification systems despite attempts at clarification [10].

When a clinical hematologist is confronted by a bone marrow study interpreted as MDS, typically, that diagnosis has been made with a little difficulty and is thought likely to be correct [10]. However, both the presence and the absence of certain supportive clinical observations and laboratory findings and the disease setting should give a pause for thought and avoid tacit acceptance of the diagnosis without consideration and exclusion of other potential entities. As a prominent medical educator, and Master of the American College of Physicians (MACP), cautions us, *"From time to time almost all of us practice what I call elephant medicine. Like elephants in the circus ring—the trunk of one holding on to the tail of the other—we plod mindlessly along, following without question the diagnoses and decisions of our colleagues"* [11]. Some of these cautionary circumstances and histological observations in relation to a diagnosis of MDS are outlined in the list below, and several combined features may be present in any particular example. Some of these caveats deserve a specific comment, and we include brief, illustrative summaries of three cases that represent AMD but not MDS, in which one of the authors (Ethan A. Natelson) was a consultant.

Clinical and laboratory features where AMD may not represent MDS.

(1) Young age (<40).

(2) Lack of erythrocyte macrocytosis.

(3) Lack of cytogenetic aberrations.

(4) Presence of ringed sideroblasts.

(5) Amegakaryocytic thrombocytopenia.

(6) Multiple vacuoles in erythroid and/or myeloid precursor cells.

(7) Absence of increased numbers of myeloid blast forms.

(8) Prior use of prolonged antibiotic therapy.

(9) A history of herbal and/or unregulated alternative medication use.

(10) Evidence of systemic or cutaneous autoimmune conditions preceding myelodysplasia.

(11) Human immunodeficiency virus (HIV) infection.

2. Results

2.1. Patient Age. The incidence of MDS increases dramatically with advancing age, and MDS is uncommon among individuals younger than 50 years, where it accounts for only 6-7% of all MDS and much less when the diagnosis is restricted to a *de novo* presentation [12–14]. In a recent MDS cohort without such restriction, only 3 of 70 patients were younger than 40 years [15]. The overall incidence of MDS in the United States per 100,000 individuals aged 70–79 is

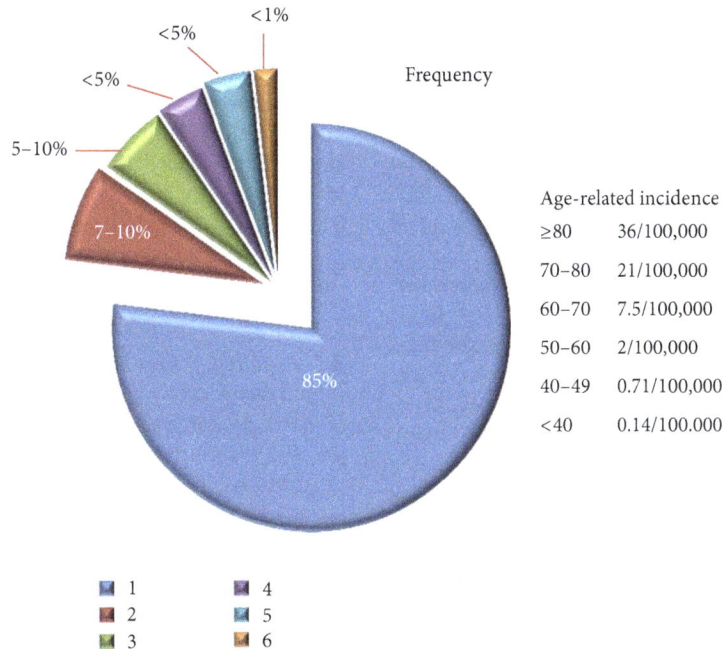

FIGURE 1: Age-related incidence of MDS and frequency estimates of MDS subsets. (1) *De novo* MDS (primary): estimates are 85% of all MDS. About 45–50% manifest cytogenetic abnormalities evident by standard analysis with recurring examples being del (5q), del (7q), del (20q), and trisomy 8. (2) Secondary MDS: estimates are 7–12% of all MDS with >80% relating to prior therapy with mutagenic chemicals and/or radiation (therapy-related, t-MDS). Chromosome aberrations are present in >90%, particularly involving chromosomes 5 and 7, and often associated with complex cytogenetics and poor prognosis. (3) Cigarette smoking is strongly associated with MDS/AML and directly relates with the total amount smoked and current smoking at diagnosis. (4) Subsets of MDS characterized by ringed sideroblasts may have different causation from other MDS syndromes. (5) Perhaps 5–10% of individuals with MDS as defined only by morphologic aberrations and cytopenias and with clinical features suggesting autoimmune disease may respond favorably to immunosuppressive therapy. (6) Occupational/environmental chemical exposures are thought to cause <1% of all MDS with benzene-related disease some fraction of this amount.

20.94 and in those less than 40 years only 0.14 [16]. Other consistently noted specific features of this younger group with MDS include the infrequency of a hypocellular bone marrow and the infrequency of RARS morphology, the latter observation particularly striking among children [13, 17]. Thus, when evaluating a young adult with a presumptive diagnosis of MDS associated with large numbers of ringed sideroblasts, normal cytogenetics, and no increase in blast forms, one should always seek to identify an alternative diagnosis.

2.2. Absence of Erythrocyte Macrocytosis. Mean corpuscular red blood cell volume (MCV) measurements above 100 fl occur in less than 2% of the general population but are nearly a universal finding among patients with MDS, where the MCV is often above 106 fl and may be as high as 140 fl, particularly among those individuals with RARS. Thus, to be referred an individual with suspected MDS featuring a sideroblastic anemia associated with a normal MCV, and in the absence of chromosomal aberrations, and where vitamin B-12 and folic acid deficiency have been excluded, certain alternate maladies should immediately come to mind. For example, despite the impressive numbers of ringed sideroblasts, both lead and arsenic poisoning typically are associated with an MCV in the normal range [18, 19]. Copper deficiency, which may be a consequence of bariatric surgery, and excessive use of zinc, also causes an anemia with a refractory sideroblastic

bone marrow appearance but usually with a normal or even reduced MCV, unless other vitamin deficiencies are present [20–23]. Copper deficiency may also result in multiple cytoplasmic vacuoles among the bone marrow erythroid and myeloid precursors, which is not a feature of MDS [21, 23]. Additionally, copper deficiency has been associated with the presence of multiple clumps of hematogones (clusters of lymphoid precursors) in the bone marrow which should not, but may be, confused with increased numbers of blast cells suggesting MDS/AML [21].

2.3. Sideroblastic Anemia. As discussed in the previous section, reversible sideroblastic anemias may occur in a number of circumstances including prolonged use of certain antibiotics such as chloramphenicol, linezolid, pyrazinamide, isoniazid, rifampin, and some tetracyclines [24, 25]. In this group the myelodysplasia that results may from time to time also be associated with the acquired or pseudo Pelger-Huët anomaly of abnormal granulocyte nuclear segmentation. The presence of such atypical mature but bilobed granulocytes in the peripheral blood is often sought as a diagnostic marker of MDS [26–29]. Perhaps not well appreciated, a number of drugs may also cause the pseudo-Pelger-Huët nuclear anomaly. It is increasingly noted in organ transplant patients receiving immunosuppressive medications and, in particular, tacrolimus and mycophenolate mofetil [28, 29]. Thus, it is not surprising that the combined aberrant morphology of drug-induced sideroblastic anemia with pseudo Pelger-Huët cells might well be misinterpreted as clear-cut evidence of MDS [30]. For example, in a large cohort of patients with MDS, a statistically significant increased incidence of MDS was reported to be associated both with tuberculosis and with the use of herbal or traditional medications [31]. However, large and well-controlled epidemiological studies show no association of MDS with tuberculosis or other infectious diseases [32]. Moreover, lead, arsenic, and mercury poisoning as described in the previous section have been reported as contaminants of unregulated traditional medications and may cause refractory sideroblastic anemias. Thus, the observed, statistically significant association of MDS with tuberculosis and herbal medications in this study likely represents inclusion of AMD cases in the analysis [31]. Later commented on further, one of the first examples of effective treatment of apparent MDS with immunosuppressive therapy was described in a patient with RARS [33].

2.4. Absence of Cytogenetic Aberrations. Certainly, examples of MDS without numerical or molecular cytogenetic aberrations occur but are uncommon, particularly in secondary or therapy-related MDS. As cytogenetic analysis has become more sophisticated and accompanied by specific and comprehensive fluorescent *in situ* hybridization (FISH) probe panels and the developing nucleotide polymorphism array technology, the frequency of a normal cytogenetic result in MDS with a cellular bone marrow has been greatly reduced [34]. Particularly in the proper setting, the lack of a demonstrable cytogenetic abnormality should always increase suspicion that MDS may not be the correct diagnosis despite persistent morphologically evident myelodysplasia. Conversely, 14 recurring cytogenetic aberrations that allow a presumptive diagnosis of MDS to be established despite inconclusive cellular morphology are outlined in a recent review of MDS classification [35].

2.5. Absence of an Increase in Myeloid Blast Forms. Whether a bone marrow demonstrating 10% or more myeloblasts should still be considered a form of MDS, rather than AML, has always been a very controversial issue [2]. Certainly, major cancer centers have often advocated treating such patients with acute myeloid leukemia [AML] chemotherapy protocols, and the associated hematological illness is clearly a neoplasm and would not be confused with AMD. Currently, diagnostic blast cell percentages in MDS/AML continue to be enumerated by morphology, but advances in flow cytometry are likely to ultimately prove a more accurate measure and to define other cellular features which may improve specificity in the diagnosis of MDS [34, 36].

2.6. An Associated or Preceding Autoimmune Disorder. Many have commented on the association of autoimmune disease preceding or coincident to the development of hematological abnormalities consistent with MDS, and this association has also been well documented by epidemiological studies [32, 33,

37–43] Some suggest that as many as 10% of all MDS represent an immune-related illness [37]. Particularly, profound myelodysplasia consistent with MDS may occur following the onset of certain cutaneous disorders such as Sweet syndrome, bullous pemphagoid, several forms of vasculitis, with certain rheumatoid disorders including relapsing polychondritis, polyneuropathy, and inflammatory bowel disease [37, 40–43]. Remission from both the skin disease and the associated MDS may occur simultaneously with effective immune-mediated therapy, as in our Case 2.

2.7. Acquired Amegakaryocytic Thrombocytopenia with Cellular Bone Marrow. While thrombocytopenia in the setting of MDS is common and may be associated with reduced numbers and dysmyelopoietic-appearing megakaryocytes, acquired amegakaryocytic thrombocytopenia with a cellular bone marrow is unusual in MDS but has been described in association with lupus erythematosis and thymoma and as an immune consequence of several disorders [44]. It may also respond favorably to immunosuppressive therapy as in our Case 1. Again, in concert with other clinical and laboratory manifestations of what appears to be MDS, amegakaryocytic thrombocytopenia may be a clue to search for an alternate diagnosis.

2.8. Vacuolization of Bone Marrow Erythroid and Myeloid Precursor Cells. Years ago, extensive vacuole formation, particularly in the cytoplasm and even the nucleus of bone marrow erythroid precursors, was a hallmark of chloramphenicol toxicity. Today, a similar process has been noted with toxicity to the antibiotics linozolid and certain tetracyclines. This finding has been also described with arsenic poisoning and copper deficiency where it may affect both myeloid and erythroid cells and is well known as a consequence of alcohol-induced hematological toxicity along with ringed sideroblasts [21, 23, 24, 45]. Importantly, it is highly unlikely to be the primary or sole feature of MDS, as in our Case 3, and its presence should immediately suggest a medication review and a search for a possible recent bone marrow toxic exposure.

Case 1. A 29-year-old white woman who worked in the home as a computer specialist had been scheduled for her initial visit at a bone marrow transplant center in order to discuss, and then undergo, allogeneic stem cell transplantation for progressive cytopenias consequent to MDS. Features of two prior bone marrow studies allowed multiple hematopathologists and her hematologist to concur with the diagnosis of MDS. However, fearful of the complications of bone marrow transplantation, she had been referred to yet another hematologic consultation by her primary physicians not for a review of the diagnosis but simply to convince her of the need for urgent transplantation. Several months earlier she first began to experience easy bruising and was found to have a hemoglobin concentration of 11.0 gm/dL with a platelet count of 63,000/cu mm. She was thought to have idiopathic thrombocytopenic purpura [ITP], but, despite therapy with corticosteroids and Win-Rho SD immune globulin, she became progressively pancytopenic and had required blood transfusions. Numerous laboratory studies including antinuclear antibody, Coombs' tests, serum vitamin B-12, folate, serum copper and blood lead levels, parvovirus, hepatitis A, B, and C panels, and HIV titres gave normal results as did CT scans of the chest and abdomen. Her CBC now showed a hemoglobin concentration of 6.6 gm/dL with an MCV of 107 fl. Her total leukocyte count was 2,100/cu mm with a neutropenia, and she had a platelet count of 8,000/cu mm.

Her peripheral blood film showed macrocytosis, teardrop, and other abnormally shaped erythrocytes. The two bone marrow specimens were similar, with about 70% cellularity and with only rare megakaryocytes. Erythropoiesis was increased in activity and extremely dyspoietic. Iron stains showed numerous ringed sideroblasts. Granulocytopoiesis was reduced in activity with mild dysplastic changes. Blast cells were not increased. Routine cytogenetic studies had twice given normal (diploid) results. For the first time, in evaluating the cause for her myelodysplasia and cytopenias, the history was elicited that she had suffered a spontaneous miscarriage shortly before she began to experience excessive bruising. The event was known to her primary care physician, who attributed no significance to it, and her referring hematologist was unaware of it. Now, suspecting a diagnosis of pregnancy-induced pancytopenia based upon the unusual spectrum of peripheral blood and bone marrow findings and prior clinical experience, she was treated with a course of anti-thymocyte globulin and oral danazol, as described in a previous publication [46]. Within a few months she fully recovered a normal blood count and was advised not to again become pregnant.

However, a year later, asymptomatic and with a normal CBC, she again became pregnant. Her pancytopenia and macrocytosis soon reappeared within the first trimester, and the cytopenias were more profound than on her first presentation. The platelet count was now 2,000/cu mm with a total leukocyte count of 2,200/cu mm with a neutropenia, and she again required blood transfusions. She declined the suggestion by her high-risk obstetrician of a therapeutic termination of pregnancy. She received low-dose prednisone and cyclosporine and required frequent platelet and red blood cell transfusions throughout the pregnancy but uneventfully came to term with only continuous severe bruising. A healthy female infant with a normal blood count was delivered by C-section. She then received oral mycophenolate mofetil and prednisone and within 4 months achieved a normal blood count, and all medications were discontinued. She later underwent bilateral tubal ligation and remained well with a normal CBC, five years later.

Pregnancy-induced pancytopenia is a rare disorder that may occur with the first pregnancy where it may be mild and spontaneously remit to reappear with subsequent pregnancies, often with increasing severity. In this regard, it is similar to the rare syndrome of circulating inhibitor of factor VIII induced by pregnancy, and the infant is not affected by the process. While the peripheral blood and bone marrow, at first glance, seem typical of MDS, the constellation of teardrop erythrocytes in the peripheral blood, increased bone marrow cellularity with erythroid hyperplasia, amegakaryocytic thrombocytopenia, and ringed sideroblasts in a young woman in the proper clinical setting should suggest the correct diagnosis and not MDS.

In a recent publication calling for all MDS to be renamed as the myelodysplastic neoplasms (MDN), the authors' comment was "··· *The risk of non-MDS patients being treated erroneously as having MDS is relatively low*" [47]. Certainly, this patient might argue that point, particularly if she were required to convince her insurance company that she did not have a malignancy and underwent an unnecessary allogeneic stem cell transplant procedure!

Case 2. A 52-year-old white attorney with type II diabetes mellitus developed a macular pruritic rash on his upper arms typical of Sweet syndrome that, over several months, became generalized and excoriated. Various topical preparations, antihistamines, and pulse steroid doses were not helpful. He experienced a 20-pound weight loss and developed intermittent fever. He became anemic and thrombocytopenic. He underwent upper and lower endoscopies which gave normal results as did CT scans of the chest and abdomen. His hemoglobin concentration was 10 gm/dL with an MCV of 105 fl. The total leukocyte count was 7,000/cu mm with a monocytosis and the platelet count 102,000/cu mm. A bone marrow study revealed an 80% cellular marrow with an increase in megakaryocytes and trilineage dysplasia, particularly evident in erythroid elements. Iron stores were normal without ringed sideroblasts. Blast forms were not increased. His bone marrow was interpreted by the hematopathology department as consistent with MDS. Cytogenetic studies gave normal results.

Considering an immune-related AMD, he received a trial of oral prednisone and 6-mercaptopurine, and his hemoglobin improved to 14.0 gm/dL with a normal MCV and a platelet count of 232,000/cu mm. His skin rash faded but reappeared when the immunosuppressive drugs were tapered and discontinued. His platelet count then fell to 44,000/cu mm and his hemoglobin concentration to 8.6 gm/dL. Prednisone was resumed, and mycophenolate mofetil substituted for the 6-mercaptopurine. Now, 3 years later and receiving only 500 mg of mycophenolate mofetil daily, aside from his usual diabetic medications, his skin rash is well controlled, his CBC is normal with a normal MCV, and he is asymptomatic.

Sweet syndrome has been described in MDS, AML, and NHL but often abruptly affects younger individuals with no evident underlying neoplasm and typically responds well to immunosuppressive therapy [41, 42]. Its presence preceding the presumptive cytopathological diagnosis of MDS without cytogenetic aberrations or an increase in myeloblasts and a cellular bone marrow should suggest that MDS may not be the correct diagnosis of AMD and prompt a trial of immunosuppressive therapy.

Case 3. A 56-year-old white man, who was employed as mechanic, and was a heavy smoker, developed severe, generalized, and disabling arthritis, thought by his rheumatologists to represent seronegative rheumatoid arthritis. His blood counts and chemistries initially gave normal results. Over a period of 2 years he received courses of at least five different nonsteroidal anti-inflammatory agents. When this therapy proved ineffective, he received oral methotrexate for several months, along with continued anti-inflammatory medications. He then underwent a bone marrow study because over this two-year period his hemoglobin concentration had declined from 14.3 gm/dL to 12.6 gm/dL and his total leukocyte count from 7,000/cu mm to 3,300/cu mm, with a neutropenia. His platelet count remained in the normal range. The striking morphological abnormality in the bone marrow was extensive vacuolization, particularly among the myeloid cell precursors. There was no increase in blast forms, and cytogenetic studies gave normal (*diploid*) results. He was thought to have MDS but required no specific therapy for this illness. Over time, his anemia spontaneously improved, but he remained with mild neutropenia and with a normal platelet count until he died 5 years later from complications of pulmonary fibrosis, a well-known association with the rheumatoid diseases [48]. It was alleged in a legal action, later dropped, that on the basis of his bone marrow study he had MDS, caused by his exposure, years earlier, to benzene, as it was contained in diesel and other fuels he worked with. As discussed, vacuolization of bone marrow precursors is not a primary feature of MDS, and his mild and nonprogressive cytopenias were likely treatment-related.

3. Discussion

Despite our current knowledge and growing laboratory expertise, whether a prolonged hematopoietic myelodysplastic reaction associated with cytopenias but without a distinct pattern of clonal cytogenetic aberration or increase in blast forms is actually MDS, as we currently employ this term for risk assessment, may remain uncertain. Such an unusual circumstance is presented by the work of Irons and associates in China, involving individuals with alleged major exposures to pure benzene and who manifest unusual and complex bone marrow histology frequently associated with bone marrow hypoplasia, multilineage dysplasia, atypical eosinophilia, and phagocytic histiocytes, among other features [6, 49, 50]. A similar type of general hypocellular bone marrow histology with eosinophilia was described among a large Brazilian cohort with chronic benzene poisoning, but a long-term followup to determine recovery or progression to MDS, AML, aplastic anemia, or other illness was never described, and cytogenetic studies apparently were not done [51]. This cohort was not described as having MDS and, one would assume, rather thought to have a form of chronic myelosuppression, capable of recovery, but possibly with later risk for onset of AML, as described in Aksoy's work in Turkey [52].

In Irons and associates two initial reports, this distinctive hematological toxicity to benzene was described simply with morphologic descriptive terms such as dysplasia and dyserythropoiesis [49, 50]. In their most recent publication, these cases are classified as MDS. However, more than twice as many subjects were placed in the MDS-U (*unclassifiable*) category as their control subjects with MDS [6]. MDS-U is a seldom-employed subset of MDS, and, with such few cases, a separate survival risk assessment is not available [36]. Nevertheless, 80% of Irons and associates' cases were alive at

60 months, with a continuing flat survival analysis at the time of publication compared with the nonbenzene exposed MDS group with a steadily declining survival, circa 25%, at that follow-up interval. The latter observation would be consistent with the usual survival statistics in MDS and far superior to survival characteristics in typical chemical-induced MDS [53]. Moreover, Irons and associates' cohort, overall, had a lesser frequency of chromosome aberrations than routinely seen in *de novo* MDS and far less frequently than described in chemical-induced or secondary MDS, even among other individuals with their hematological illness claimed to be related to solvent and petrochemical exposures and exhibiting high frequencies of aberrations in chromosomes 5 and 7 and the 5 q-syndrome.

Other medical groups in China, where major and prolonged benzene exposures are still possible, have classified their alleged examples of benzene-induced hematotoxicity in a different manner than Irons and associates. In one report the authors separate 41 such patients as representing either aplastic anemia, pancytopenia (*presumably signifying chronic myelosuppression*), or MDS, with the latter diagnosis only accounting for 4 members of this cohort [54]. They emphasize that many of these subjects responded favorably to removal from continuing benzene exposure along with the use of androgens and immunosuppressive medications. As Irons and associates observed, their few cases with MDS also had excellent long-term survival [6, 54].

A caveat is that cytogenetic studies in China for MDS/ AML have shown a differing frequency of particular aberrations than among Western patients, with an increased frequency of trisomy 8 and a very reduced incidence of the 5q-syndrome as well as a marked increase in t (15; 17) acute promyelocytic leukemia [55, 56]. Another confounding factor might be the frequent use of traditional or herbal preparations among this population [31]. We would not suggest arbitrarily classifying this seemingly unique AMD as something other than MDS, but we prefer to await a longer followup on the index patients and to see if others observe this unique type of hematologic toxicity and outcome among different ethnic populations with exposures to similar levels of benzene.

Olnes and Sloan have demonstrated that, in selected patients with MDS, a significant number may respond favorably to immunosuppressive therapy and observed a complete remission in 18% of 31 evaluable patients, including one manifesting a small clone with trisomy 13 [40]. This patient received treatment with alemtuzumab, a monoclonal antibody directed against the T cell marker, CD 52, which has also produced favorable responses in nonneoplastic associated autoimmune hemolytic anemia as well as in B cell neoplasms such as chronic lymphocytic anemia [57]. They also suggest that the ideal candidates for a trial of immunosuppressive therapy are younger individuals with low risk forms of MDS but did not feel that the degree of marrow cellularity was a predictor of favorable response. The trisomy 13 was a concern but, by analogy, small clones of trisomy 15 associated with pancytopenia may spontaneously regress associated with improvement in the pancytopenia, and a small aberrant clone does not always imply preleukemic syndromes [43, 58]. Thus, the presence of small clones of certain cytogenetic aberrations should not eliminate consideration of a trial of immunosuppressive therapy, although the ideal drug combination to employ is not established. Patients with trisomy 8, even with hypocellular bone marrows, may respond favorably to immunosuppressive therapy possibly for reasons apart from classical mechanisms in autoimmune disorders [59]. Many other agents and drug combinations have been effective in immune-related therapy of MDS and include tissue necrosis factor-α (TNF-α) inhibitors and compounds that may bind with T-lymphocyte CD receptors and modify the expression of interleukin-2 and other cytokine production [34, 60].

In MDS with hypocellular bone marrow, this circumstance may be difficult to clearly separate from aplastic anemia where favorable responses to drugs such as antithymocyte globulin [ATG] are often seen. Nevertheless, we believe that a young individual with MDS, regardless of bone marrow cellularity and normal cytogenetics, particularly when associated with morphologic features such as sideroblastic anemia or amegakaryocytic thrombocytopenia occurring in the clinical setting of autoimmune illness, are with high likelihood of achieving a favorable response to immunosuppressive medications. As emphasized, it seems critical to initiate therapy with immunosuppressive regimens early in the course of MDS in order to favorably impact the long-term result [60]. This may seem difficult to recommend in a patient with low-risk MDS who is not particularly symptomatic. Nevertheless, delaying such therapy may contribute to the adverse immune response by facilitating the continuing presentation of apoptotic cell-generated autoantigens to T-lymphocytes.

Bone marrow flow cytometry (FC) analysis may be useful in an attempt to separate MDS from other causes of persistent cytopenias, including forms of hypoplastic anemia. Its application can identify specific aberrations in both immature and maturing cell compartments among the hematopoietic cell lineages but, as yet, it is not reliable as a single parameter to segregate MDS as a specific diagnosis [61]. There may be no universal FC marker pattern to prove MDS in all cases because of the heterogenous nature of the disorder. The information obtained by FC is most useful with analysis of lineage fidelity or infidelity among the immature myeloid progenitor cells and least useful with disorders of megakaryocyte lineage. It is particularly difficult to use FC to isolate MDS from nonneoplastic conditions characterized by cytopenias and a normal basic cytogenetic pattern. Nevertheless, guidelines are being established to describe a FC panel as normal, suggestive of MDS, or consistent with MDS [61]. Repeated FC assessments are recommended, particularly in low-risk and/or inconclusive MDS patients, to document changes and monitor the course of the disease.

The WHO MDS classification seems to favor a parallel association with risk stratification [62]. Since the usual survival risk of MDS-U is claimed to be similar to that in the RCMD subset, and, since only 6% of 2032 patients with MDS were classified as MDS-U, a recent recommendation is that the MDS-U category simply be eliminated from the WHO MDS classification scheme and combined with RCMD [63]. This approach would recapitulate the fate of the former RARS-MD MDS subset. Since the category of MDS-U requires <10% cellular dysplasia, it would then be difficult to find a suitable home in this proposed WHO MDS system for many of these subjects classified as MDS by Irons and associates [6].

Whether or not all MDS should be considered neoplasms and whether or not Irons and associates' experience with persistent cytopenias among heavily benzene-exposed individuals should be classified as MDS and as neoplasms are just some of the unanswered questions in this field. There is considerable information that immune dysregulation plays an important role in the onset and progression of MDS both confounding a certain confirmation of the diagnosis and its uniform classification as a malignancy. The most straight-forward evidence of this influence is the favorable therapeutic response seen among certain patients with MDS, as defined by current diagnostic criteria, who are treated with medications with immunosuppressive activity. The frequency of long-term control of the illness with this form of therapy is uncertain, but as many as 30% of all MDS cases exhibit some hematologic improvement when treated with a variety of immunosuppressive agents [60]. What remains unclear are the underlying mechanisms by which the immune system may regulate myeloid cell development and either promote the disease or modulate progressive failure of normal hematopoiesis.

In low-risk forms of MDS, based upon current stratification schemes, among those with bone marrow hypocellularity, increased apoptosis of bone marrow cells is an established pathogenic mechanism resulting in ineffective hematopoiesis. Several compelling lines of evidence suggest that disruption of the differentiation of hematopoietic progenitor cells and their increased apoptosis is immunologically mediated [64–70]. Moreover, in many examples of low-risk MDS, inflammatory cytokines appear to be driving the disordered immune response, including the observed increase in apoptosis. Many investigators have reported aberrations in the TNF-α pathway in immunosuppressive-responsive examples of MDS [66, 69, 71–77]. TNF-α plays a fundamental role in mediating apoptotic pathways among multiple cell types, and an increased production or deregulated role could result in the observed bone marrow pathology. At least in low-risk MDS, there is also support for the involvement of various components of the innate immunity pathway such as natural killer [NK] cells and macrophages [76, 78–80]. The increased frequency of NK and activated macrophages in the MDS bone marrow may increase the elaboration of cytokines such as gamma interferon and TNF-α and other proapoptotic cytokines, which, in turn, results in the observed increase in apoptosis and peripheral blood cytopenias [76, 81, 82]. NK-cell mediated cytotoxicity toward aberrant cell precursors occurs in many low-risk examples of MDS [78]. Macrophages are believed to play important roles in bone marrow regulation and hematopoiesis via contact with adhesion molecules [80, 83]. Apoptosis occurs in low-risk MDS cases among both clonal and nonclonal progenitor cells, but this feature begins to decrease as the MDS evolves toward a more malignant phenotype [84].

The increase in apoptosis observed in low-risk MDS is thought to be a key step in the pathology of this disorder. However, there may be additional modifying immunological events in play that collectively result in the observed morphological dyspoiesis. Dysplasia-associated antigens released by degenerating cells that are processed by antigen-presenting cells may initiate an adaptive immune response that may influence the course of the illness [76]. Evidence in support of active involvement of the immune system includes an increase in the number and activation of various effector cells, promoting an autoimmune environment. There is a clear relationship between autoimmunity and some forms of bone marrow failure and dysplasia [76, 85]. The autoimmune-promoting environment in example of low-risk MDS includes increased levels of proapoptotic cytokines, increased numbers of helper T cells, altered humeral immunity, and reduced levels of regulatory T cells [Treg]. Treg cells are CD-4 and Fox-P3 positive and are known to play an important role in immune surveillance and self-tolerance and in suppressing autoimmunity [76, 86]. It has been suggested that reduced numbers of Treg cells and other immunological changes may result in T cell-mediated inhibition of normal hematopoiesis [76, 78–80].

TNF-α mediated apoptosis may be a highly relevant mechanism to promoting bone marrow dysplasia reported following excessive benzene exposure [48–50, 86]. Previous reports indicate that benzene metabolites and TNF-α act synergistically to induce apoptosis in CD-34+, bone marrow progenitor cells [87–89]. Further, epidemiologic evidence suggests that polymorphisms in TNF-α, resulting in deregulated TNF-α production, increase susceptibility to benzene-induced hematopoietic toxicity [49, 87, 90]. There is also limited evidence that immunosuppressive therapy provides therapeutic benefit in the treatment of what has been described as benzene-related MDS, as this illness appears to be similar to benzene-induced aplastic anemia, which also tends to respond favorably to immunosuppressive therapy [53].

This pattern of immune dysregulation that may be modified by immunosuppressive therapy is not characteristic of more advanced or high-risk cases of MDS. Here, there are increased numbers of regulatory cells, which dampen any type of favorable response to immunosuppressive therapy. This may, in turn, allow for a damaged or dysplastic clone to escape from immune surveillance and progress to a more aggressive expression of the disease [88, 89]. Further, in high-risk examples of MDS, pathological changes include apoptosis resistance, which could allow secondary genetic abnormalities to appear and stimulate an increase in cellular proliferation, thus providing potential growth advances for the aberrant clone and resulting in a much higher propensity for evolution into AML [91].

Immunosuppressive therapy seems to be most effective when applied early in those with low-risk MDS. Many studies have used the combination of anti-thymocyte globulin (ATG) and cyclosporine A (CsA), because of their well-known benefit in forms of aplastic anemia and in the organ transplant field. However, corticosteroids, alemtuzumab, and newer immunosuppressive agents, such as mycofenolate mofetil and TNF-α inhibitors, have also been effective in MDS and may be used on a chronic basis, unlike ATG, which is typically administered as a single infusion because of the potential for severe reactions to additional challenges.

While the fog obscuring the certain diagnosis of MDS is slowly lifting, clinicians must remain alert to the possibility of an alternate disorder in certain cases of AMD. Our therapeutic armamentarium continues to improve along with efforts to define in which examples of MDS and in which clinical settings they are most likely to initiate a favorable response. While it is clear that immunosuppressive therapy may be beneficial in a subset of individuals with MDS, the most effective types of immunosuppressive regimens and the duration of such therapy remain to be determined. Moreover, such favorable response does not necessarily imply a causative autoimmune illness or exclude a neoplasm.

References

[1] A. A. N. Giagounidis, "Myelodysplasia or myelodysplastic syndrome?" *Leukemia Research*, vol. 33, no. 8, p. 1019, 2009.

[2] M. A. Lichtman, "Myelodysplasia or myeloneoplasia: thoughts on the nosology of clonal myeloid diseases," *Blood Cells, Molecules, and Diseases*, vol. 26, no. 6, pp. 572–581, 2000.

[3] U. Germing, N. Gattermann, M. Aivado, B. Hildebrandt, and C. Aul, "Two types of acquired idiopathic sideroblastic anaemia (AISA): a time-tested distinction," *The British Journal of Haematology*, vol. 108, no. 4, pp. 724–728, 2000.

[4] R. Garand, J. Gardais, T. M. Bizet et al., "Heterogeneity of acquired idiopathic sideroblastic anaemia (AISA)," *Leukemia Research*, vol. 16, no. 5, pp. 463–468, 1992.

[5] L. Malcovati, U. Germing, A. Kuendgen et al., "Time-dependent prognostic scoring system for predicting survival and leukemic evolution in myelodysplastic syndromes," *Journal of Clinical Oncology*, vol. 25, no. 23, pp. 3503–3510, 2007.

[6] R. D. Irons, S. A. Gross, A. Le et al., "Integrating WHO 2001–2008 criteria for the diagnosis of Myelodysplastic syndrome (MDS): a case-case analysis of benzene exposure," *Chemico-Biological Interactions*, vol. 184, no. 1-2, pp. 30–38, 2010.

[7] E. A. Natelson, "Benzene exposure and refractory sideroblastic erythropoiesis: is there an association?" *The American Journal of the Medical Sciences*, vol. 334, no. 5, pp. 356–360, 2007.

[8] U. Germing and A. Kundgen, "Prognostic scoring systems in MDS," *Leukemia Research*, vol. 36, no. 12, pp. 1463–1469, 2012.

[9] S. Parmentier, J. Schetelig, K. Lorenz et al., "Assessment of dysplastic hematopoiesis: lessons from healthy bone marrow donors," *Haematologica*, vol. 97, no. 5, pp. 723–730, 2012.

[10] J. W. Vardiman, "Hematopathological concepts and controversies in the diagnosis and classification of myelodysplastic syndromes," *ASH Education Book*, no. 1, pp. 199–204, 2006.

[11] H. L. Fred, *Elephant Medicine and More: Musings of a Medical Educator*, Mercer University Press, Macon, Ga, USA, 1989.

[12] K. L. Chang, M. R. O'Donnell, M. L. Slovak et al., "Primary myelodysplasia occurring in adults under 50 years old: a clinicopathologic study of 52 patients," *Leukemia*, vol. 16, no. 4, pp. 623–631, 2002.

[13] M. Breccia, A. Mengarelli, M. Mancini et al., "Myelodysplastic syndromes in patients under 50 years old: a single institution experience," *Leukemia Research*, vol. 29, no. 7, pp. 749–754, 2005.

[14] A. Kuendgen, C. Strupp, M. Aivado et al., "Myelodysplastic syndromes in patients younger than age 50," *Journal of Clinical Oncology*, vol. 24, no. 34, pp. 5358–5365, 2006.

[15] J. Irwin, A. D'Souza, L. Johnson, and J. Carter, "Myelodysplasia in the Wellington region 2002–2007: disease incidence and treatment patterns," *Internal Medicine Journal*, vol. 41, no. 5, pp. 399–407, 2011.

[16] D. E. Rollison, N. Howlader, M. T. Smith et al., "Epidemiology of myelodysplastic syndromes and chronic myeloproliferative disorders in the United States, 2001–2004, using data from the NAACCR and SEER programs," *Blood*, vol. 112, no. 1, pp. 45–52, 2008.

[17] U. Germing, C. Aul, C. M. Niemeyer, R. Haas, and J. M. Bennett, "Epidemiology, classification and prognosis of adults and children with myelodysplastic syndromes," *Annals of Hematology*, vol. 87, no. 9, pp. 691–699, 2008.

[18] E. A. Natelson and H. L. Fred, "Lead poisoning from cocktail glasses. Observation on 2 patients," *The Journal of the American Medical Association*, vol. 236, no. 22, p. 2527, 1976.

[19] W. N. Rezuke, C. Anderson, W. T. Pastuszak, S. R. Conway, and S. I. Firshein, "Arsenic intoxication presenting as a myelodysplastic syndrome: a case report," *The American Journal of Hematology*, vol. 36, no. 4, pp. 291–293, 1991.

[20] H. Gill, W. W. Choi, and Y. L. Kwong, "Refractory anemia with ringed sideroblasts: more than meets the eye," *Journal of Clinical Oncology*, vol. 28, no. 32, pp. e654–e655, 2010.

[21] E. Koca, Y. Buyukasik, D. Cetiner et al., "Copper deficiency with increased hematogones mimicking refractory anemia with excess blasts," *Leukemia Research*, vol. 32, no. 3, pp. 495–499, 2008.

[22] J. D. Huff, Y. Keung, M. Thakuri et al., "Copper deficiency causes reversible myelodysplasia," *The American Journal of Hematology*, vol. 82, no. 7, pp. 625–630, 2007.

[23] A. L. Summerfield, F. U. Steinberg, and J. G. Gonzalez, "Morphologic findings in bone marrow precursor cells in zinc-induced copper deficiency anemia," *The American Journal of Clinical Pathology*, vol. 97, no. 5, pp. 665–668, 1992.

[24] N. Saini, J. O. Jacobson, S. Jha, V. Saini, and R. Weinger, "The perils of not digging deep enough-uncovering a rare cause of acquired anemia," *The American Journal of Hematology*, vol. 87, no. 4, pp. 413–416, 2012.

[25] R. J. Piso, K. Kriz, and M. Desax, "Severe isoniazid related sideroblastic anemia," *Hematology Reviews*, vol. 3, no. 1, article e2, 2011.

[26] R. Colella and S. C. Hollensead, "Understanding and recognizing the Pelger-Huët anomaly," *The American Journal of Clinical Pathology*, vol. 137, no. 3, pp. 358–366, 2012.

[27] J. M. Cunningham, M. M. Patnaik, D. E. Hammerschmidt, and G. M. Vercellotti, "Historical perspective and clinical implications of the Pelger-Huët cell," *The American Journal of Hematology*, vol. 84, no. 2, pp. 116–119, 2009.

[28] J. E. Etzell and E. Wang, "Acquired Pelger-Huët anomaly in association with concomitant tacrolimus and mycophenolate mofetil in a liver transplant patient: a case report and review of the literature," *Archives of Pathology and Laboratory Medicine*, vol. 130, no. 1, pp. 93–96, 2006.

[29] E. Wang, E. Boswell, I. Siddiqi et al., "Pseudo-Pelger-Huët anomaly induced by medications: a clinicopathologic study in comparison with myelodysplastic syndrome-related pseudo-Pelger-Huët anomaly," *The American Journal of Clinical Pathology*, vol. 135, no. 2, pp. 291–303, 2011.

[30] D. Liu, Z. Chen, Y. Xue et al., "The significance of bone marrow cell morphology and its correlation with cytogenetic features in the diagnosis of MDS-RA patients," *Leukemia Research*, vol. 33, no. 8, pp. 1029–1038, 2009.

[31] L. Lv, G. Lin, X. Gao et al., "Case-control study of risk factors of myelodysplastic syndromes according to World Health Organization classification in a Chinese population," *The American Journal of Hematology*, vol. 86, no. 2, pp. 163–169, 2011.

[32] S. Y. Kristinsson, M. Björkholm, M. Hultcrantz, A. R. Derolf, O. Landgren, and L. R. Goldin, "Chronic immune stimulation might act as a trigger for the development of acute myeloid leukemia or myelodysplastic syndromes," *Journal of Clinical Oncology*, vol. 29, no. 21, pp. 2897–2903, 2011.

[33] J. Zervas, C. G. Geary, and S. Oleesky, "Sideroblastic anemia treated with immunosuppressive therapy," *Blood*, vol. 44, no. 1, pp. 117–123, 1974.

[34] P. Fenaux and L. Ades, "How we treat lower-risk myelodysplastic syndromes," *Blood*, vol. 121, no. 21, pp. 4280–4286, 2013.

[35] J. Vardiman, "The classification of MDS: from FAB to WHO and beyond," *Leukemia Research*, vol. 36, no. 12, pp. 1453–1458, 2012.

[36] M. Cazzola, M. G. Della Porta, E. Travaglino, and L. Malcovati, "Classification and prognostic evaluation of Myelodysplastic syndromes," *Seminars in Oncology*, vol. 38, no. 5, pp. 627–634, 2011.

[37] M. Voulgarelis, S. Giannouli, K. Ritis, and A. G. Tzioufas, "Myelodysplasia-associated autoimmunity: clinical and pathophysiologic concepts," *European Journal of Clinical Investigation*, vol. 34, no. 10, pp. 690–700, 2004.

[38] D. Farmakis, E. Polymeropoulos, A. Polonifi et al., "Myelodysplastic syndrome associated with multiple autoimmune disorders," *Clinical Rheumatology*, vol. 24, no. 4, pp. 428–430, 2005.

[39] S. M. Ramadan, T. M. Fouad, V. Summa, S. Hasan, and F. Lo-Coco, "Acute myeloid leukemia developing in patients with autoimmune diseases," *Haematologica*, vol. 97, no. 6, pp. 805–817, 2012.

[40] M. J. Olnes and E. M. Sloand, "Targeting immune dysregulation in myelodysplastic syndromes," *The Journal of the American Medical Association*, vol. 305, no. 8, pp. 814–819, 2011.

[41] M. Vignon-Pennamen, C. Juillard, M. Rybojad et al., "Chronic recurrent lymphocytic sweet syndrome as a predictive marker of myelodysplasia: a report of 9 cases," *Archives of Dermatology*, vol. 142, no. 9, pp. 1170–1176, 2006.

[42] P. R. Cohen, "Sweet's syndrome—a comprehensive review of an acute febrile neutrophilic dermatosis," *Orphanet Journal of Rare Diseases*, vol. 2, no. 1, article 34, 2007.

[43] H. Enright and W. Miller, "Autoimmune phenomena in patients with myelodysplastic syndromes," *Leukemia and Lymphoma*, vol. 24, no. 5-6, pp. 483–489, 1997.

[44] A. G. Tristano, "Acquired amegakaryocytic thrombocytopenic purpura: review of a not very well-defined disorder," *European Journal of Internal Medicine*, vol. 16, no. 7, pp. 477–481, 2005.

[45] J. Latvala, S. Parkkila, and O. Niemelä, "Excess alcohol consumption is common in patients with cytopenia: studies in blood and bone marrow cells," *Alcoholism: Clinical and Experimental Research*, vol. 28, no. 4, pp. 619–624, 2004.

[46] E. A. Natelson, "Pregnancy-induced pancytopenia with cellular bone marrow: distinctive hematologic features," *The American Journal of the Medical Sciences*, vol. 332, no. 4, pp. 205–207, 2006.

[47] Y. Li, P. Lin, Y. Ge, and G. Garcia-Manero, "Myelodysplastic syndromes should been renamed as myelodysplastic neoplasms," *Leukemia Research*, vol. 37, no. 4, pp. 463–464, 2013.

[48] N. Tanaka, J. S. Kim, J. D. Newell et al., "Rheumatoid arthritis-related lung diseases: CT findings," *Radiology*, vol. 232, no. 1, pp. 81–91, 2004.

[49] R. D. Irons, L. Lv, S. A. Gross et al., "Chronic exposure to benzene results in a unique form of dysplasia," *Leukemia Research*, vol. 29, no. 12, pp. 1371–1380, 2005.

[50] L. Lv, P. Kerzic, G. Lin et al., "The TNF-α 238A polymorphism is associated with susceptibility to persistent bone marrow dysplasia following chronic exposure to benzene," *Leukemia Research*, vol. 31, no. 11, pp. 1479–1485, 2007.

[51] M. A. Ruiz, L. G. S. Augusto, J. Vassallo, A. C. Vigorito, I. Lorand-Metze, and C. A. Souza, "Bone marrow morphology in patients with neutropenia due to chronic exposure to organic solvents (benzene): early lesions," *Pathology Research and Practice*, vol. 190, no. 2, pp. 151–154, 1994.

[52] M. Aksoy, "Different types of malignancies due to occupational exposure to benzene: a review of recent observations in Turkey," *Environmental Research*, vol. 23, no. 1, pp. 181–190, 1980.

[53] Z. N. Singh, D. Huo, J. Anastasi et al., "Therapy-related myelodysplastic syndrome: morphologic subclassification may not be clinically relevant," *The American Journal of Clinical Pathology*, vol. 127, no. 2, pp. 197–205, 2007.

[54] Y. Song, X. Du, F. Hao et al., "Immunosuppressive therapy of cyclosporin A for severe benzene-induced haematopoietic disorders and a 6-month follow-up," *Chemico-Biological Interactions*, vol. 186, no. 1, pp. 96–102, 2010.

[55] L. Li, X. Liu, L. Nie et al., "Unique cytogenetic features of primary myelodysplastic syndromes in Chinese patients," *Leukemia Research*, vol. 33, no. 9, pp. 1194–1198, 2009.

[56] Y. Cheng, Y. Wang, H. Wang et al., "Cytogenetic profile of de novo acute myeloid leukemia: a study based on 1432 patients in a single institution of China," *Leukemia*, vol. 23, no. 10, pp. 1801–1806, 2009.

[57] D. Gómez-Almaguer, M. Solano-Genesta, L. Tarín-Arzaga et al., "Low-dose rituximab and alemtuzumab combination therapy for patients with steroid-refractory autoimmune cytopenias," *Blood*, vol. 116, no. 23, pp. 4783–4785, 2010.

[58] E. A. Natelson, "Myelodysplasia with isolated trisomy 15: a 15-year follow-up without specific therapy," *The American Journal of the Medical Sciences*, vol. 331, no. 3, pp. 157–158, 2006.

[59] E. M. Sloand, "Hypocellular myelodysplasia," *Hematology/Oncology Clinics of North America*, vol. 23, no. 2, pp. 347–360, 2009.

[60] P. K. Epling-Burnette, J. McDaniel, S. Wei, and A. F. List, "Emerging immunosuppressive drugs in myelodysplastic syndromes," *Expert Opinion on Emerging Drugs*, vol. 17, no. 4, pp. 519–541, 2012.

[61] A. A. van de Loosdrecht and T. M. Westers, "Cutting edge: flow cytometry in myelodysplastic syndromes," *Journal of the National Comprehensive Cancer Network*, vol. 11, no. 7, pp. 892–902, 2013.

[62] R. Bejar, R. V. Tiu, M. Sekeres, and R. S. Komrokji, "Myelodysplastic syndromes: recent advancements in risk stratification and unmet therapeutic challenges," *The American Society of Clinical Oncology Educational Book*, no. 1, pp. 256–270, 2013.

[63] A. Maassen, C. Strupp, A. Giagounidis et al., "Validation and proposals for a refinement of the WHO, 2008 classification of myelodysplastic syndromes without excess of blasts," *Leukemia Research*, vol. 37, no. 1, pp. 64–70, 2013.

[64] R. Invernizzi, A. Pecci, L. Bellotti, and E. Ascari, "Expression of p53, Bcl-2 and ras oncoproteins and apoptosis levels in acute leukaemias and myelodysplastic syndromes," *Leukemia and Lymphoma*, vol. 42, no. 3, pp. 481–489, 2001.

[65] M. Kitagawa, S. Yamaguchi, M. Takahashi, T. Tanizawa, K. Hirokawa, and R. Kamiyama, "Localization of Fas and Fas ligand in bone marrow cells demonstrating myelodysplasia," *Leukemia*, vol. 12, no. 4, pp. 486–492, 1998.

[66] A. Orazi, M. Kahsai, K. John, and R. S. Neiman, "p53 Overexpression in myeloid leukemic disorders is associated with increased apoptosis of hematopoietic marrow cells and ineffective hematopoiesis," *Modern Pathology*, vol. 9, no. 1, pp. 48–52, 1996.

[67] A. Parcharidou, A. Raza, T. Economopoulos et al., "Extensive apoptosis of bone marrow cells as evaluated by the in situ end-labelling (ISEL) technique may be the basis for ineffective haematopoiesis in patients with myelodysplastic syndromes," *European Journal of Haematology*, vol. 62, no. 1, pp. 19–26, 1999.

[68] S. D. Mundle, S. Reza, A. Ali et al., "Correlation of tumor necrosis factor α (TNFα) with high caspase 3-like activity in myelodysplastic syndromes," *Cancer Letters*, vol. 140, no. 1-2, pp. 201–207, 1999.

[69] J. E. Parker, G. J. Mufti, F. Rasool, A. Mijovic, S. Devereux, and A. Pagliuca, "The role of apoptosis, proliferation, and the Bcl-2-related proteins in the myelodysplastic syndromes and acute myeloid leukemia secondary to MDS," *Blood*, vol. 96, no. 12, pp. 3932–3938, 2000.

[70] S. D. Mundle, A. Ali, J. D. Cartlidge et al., "Evidence for involvement of tumor necrosis factor-α in apoptotic death of bone marrow cells in myelodysplastic syndromes," *The American Journal of Hematology*, vol. 60, no. 1, pp. 36–47, 1999.

[71] S. D. Mundle, V. T. Shetty, and A. Raza, "Is excessive spontaneous intramedullary apoptosis unique to myelodysplasia?" *Experimental Hematology*, vol. 26, no. 11, pp. 1014–1017, 1998.

[72] A. Raza, S. Gezer, S. Mundle et al., "Apoptosis in bone marrow biopsy samples involving stromal and hematopoietic cells in 50 patients with myelodysplastic syndromes," *Blood*, vol. 86, no. 1, pp. 268–276, 1995.

[73] A. Raza, S. Mundle, A. Iftikhar et al., "Simultaneous assessment of cell kinetics and programmed cell death in bone marrow biopsies of myelodysplastics reveals extensive apoptosis as the probable basis for ineffective hematopoiesis," *The American Journal of Hematology*, vol. 48, no. 3, pp. 143–154, 1995.

[74] V. Shetty, S. Mundle, S. Alvi et al., "Measurement of apoptosis, proliferation and three cytokines in 46 patients with myelodysplastic syndromes," *Leukemia Research*, vol. 20, no. 11-12, pp. 891–900, 1996.

[75] S. Aggarwal, A. A. van de Loosdrecht, C. Alhan, G. J. Ossenkoppele, T. M. Westers, and H. J. Bontkes, "Role of immune responses in the pathogenesis of low-risk MDS and high-risk MDS: implications for immunotherapy," *The British Journal of Haematology*, vol. 153, no. 5, pp. 568–581, 2011.

[76] D. Bouscary, J. de Vos, M. Guesnu et al., "Fas/Apo-1(CD95) expression and apoptosis in patients with myelodysplastic syndromes," *Leukemia*, vol. 11, no. 6, pp. 839–845, 1997.

[77] M. E. D. Chamuleau, T. M. Westers, L. van Dreunen et al., "Immune mediated autologous cytotoxicity against hematopoietic precursor cells in patients with myelodysplastic syndrome," *Haematologica*, vol. 94, no. 4, pp. 496–506, 2009.

[78] P. K. Epling-Burnette, F. Bai, J. S. Painter et al., "Reduced natural killer (NK) function associated with high-risk myelodysplastic syndrome (MDS) and reduced expression of activating NK receptors," *Blood*, vol. 109, no. 11, pp. 4816–4824, 2007.

[79] M. Kitagawa, R. Kamiyama, and T. Kasuga, "Increase in number of bone marrow macrophages in patients with myelodysplastic syndromes," *European Journal of Haematology*, vol. 51, no. 1, pp. 56–58, 1993.

[80] J. Wu and L. L. Lanier, "Natural killer cells and cancer," *Advances in Cancer Research*, vol. 90, pp. 127–156, 2003.

[81] M. Wetzler, R. Kurzrock, Z. Estrov, E. Estey, and M. Talpaz, "Cytokine expression in adherent layers from patients with myelodysplastic syndrome and acute myelogenous leukemia," *Leukemia Research*, vol. 19, no. 1, pp. 23–34, 1995.

[82] P. R. Crocker, S. Freeman, S. Gordon, and S. Kelm, "Sialoadhesin binds preferentially to cells of the granulocytic lineage," *Journal of Clinical Investigation*, vol. 95, no. 2, pp. 635–643, 1995.

[83] E. M. Sloand and K. Rezvani, "The role of the immune system in myelodysplasia: implications for therapy," *Seminars in Hematology*, vol. 45, no. 1, pp. 39–48, 2008.

[84] P. A. Miescher, H. Favre, and P. Beris, "Autoimmune myelodysplasias," *Seminars in Hematology*, vol. 28, no. 4, pp. 322–330, 1991.

[85] M. J. Smyth, G. P. Dunn, and R. D. Schreiber, "Cancer immunosurveillance and immunoediting: the roles of immunity in suppressing tumor development and shaping tumor immunogenicity," *Advances in Immunology*, vol. 90, no. 1, pp. 1–50, 2006.

[86] L. B. Travis, C. Y. Li, Z. N. Zhang et al., "Hematopoietic malignancies and related disorders among benzene-exposed workers in China," *Leukemia and Lymphoma*, vol. 14, no. 1-2, pp. 91–102, 1994.

[87] L. Lv, H. J. Zou, G. W. Lin, and R. R. Irons, "Genetic polymorphism of tumor necrosis factor-alpha in patients with chronic benzene poisoning," *Zhonghua Lao Dong Wei Sheng Zhi Ye Bing Za Zhi*, vol. 23, no. 3, pp. 195–198, 2005.

[88] S. Y. Kordasti, B. Afzali, Z. Lim et al., "IL-17-producing CD4$^+$ T cells, pro-inflammatory cytokines and apoptosis are increased in low risk myelodysplastic syndrome," *The British Journal of Haematology*, vol. 145, no. 1, pp. 64–72, 2009.

[89] S. Y. Kordasti, W. Ingram, J. Hayden et al., "CD4$^+$CD25^{high} Foxp3$^+$ regulatory T cells in myelodysplastic syndrome (MDS)," *Blood*, vol. 110, no. 3, pp. 847–850, 2007.

[90] P. J. Kerzic, D. W. Pyatt, J. H. Zheng, S. A. Gross, A. Le, and R. D. Irons, "Inhibition of NF-κB by hydroquinone sensitizes human bone marrow progenitor cells to TNF-α-induced apoptosis," *Toxicology*, vol. 187, no. 2-3, pp. 127–137, 2003.

[91] C. Acquaviva, V. Gelsi-Boyer, and D. Birnbaum, "Myelodysplastic syndromes: lost between two states," *Leukemia*, vol. 24, no. 1, pp. 1–5, 2010.

9

MicroRNAs as Haematopoiesis Regulators

Ram Babu Undi, Ravinder Kandi, and Ravi Kumar Gutti

Hematologic Oncology, Stem Cells and Blood Disorders Laboratory, Department of Biochemistry, School of Life Sciences, University of Hyderabad, Gachibowli, Hyderabad, Andhra Pradesh 500046, India

Correspondence should be addressed to Ravi Kumar Gutti; guttiravi@gmail.com

Academic Editor: Aldo Roccaro

The production of different types of blood cells including their formation, development, and differentiation is collectively known as haematopoiesis. Blood cells are divided into three lineages erythriod (erythrocytes), lymphoid (B and T cells), and myeloid (granulocytes, megakaryocytes, and macrophages). Haematopoiesis is a complex process regulated by several mechanisms including microRNAs (miRNAs). miRNAs are small RNAs which regulate the expression of a number of genes involved in commitment and differentiation of hematopoietic stem cells. Evidence shows that miRNAs play an important role in haematopoiesis; for example, myeloid and erythroid differentiation is blocked by the overexpression of miR-15a. miR-221, miR-222, and miR-24 inhibit the erythropoiesis, whereas miR-150 plays a role in B and T cell differentiation. miR-146 and miR-10a are downregulated in megakaryopoiesis. Aberrant expression of miRNAs was observed in hematological malignancies including chronic myelogenous leukemia, chronic lymphocytic leukemia, multiple myelomas, and B cell lymphomas. In this review we have focused on discussing the role of miRNA in haematopoiesis.

1. Background

MicroRNAs (miRNAs) are 20–22 nucleotides long small noncoding RNAs that can bind to the $3'$UTR or $5'$UTR or in ORF of target mRNA resulting in translational repression or mRNA degradation based on degree of homology. It is believed that miRNAs regulate gene expression in multicellular organisms, but miRNAs are also identified in unicellular algae *Chlamydomonas reinhardtii* [1]. Interestingly it has been shown that miRNAs can activate the translation. miRNA-122 is specifically expressed in liver where; it plays vital role in fatty acid metabolism and enhances the replication of hepatitis C virus (HCV) RNA by binding to its $5'$UTR [2–4]. Ørom et al. found that miR-10a binds to the messenger RNAs (mRNAs) encoding ribosomal proteins to enhance the translation of proteins and ribosomal biogenesis [5]. Due to increase in cloning and computational approaches, there has been a tremendous increase in the number of newly found miRNAs. A total of 9169 miRNAs have been found in different species among which human genome codes for 1424 miRNAs [5]. It has been found that 60% of the human mRNA contains miRNA binding sites. Each mRNA is targeted by many miRNAs conversely and each miRNA can target many mRNAs. miRNAs exhibit different characteristics in plants and mammals. In plants, miRNAs require perfect match with their target mRNAs, whereas in mammals miRNA complementarily covers 2–7 bases, also known as the seed region [6, 7]. In mammals, miRNA target sites are mostly in the $3'$UTR region and rarely in $5'$UTR and coding regions also, whereas, in case of plants target sites are mostly in the coding region. The mechanism by which a miRNA can diminish protein expression is unclear, but several proposals are there from different experimental evidences. miRNAs can interfere with translation process at the stage of initiation (Figure 2) or elongation (Figure 3), or target mRNA may be affected by isolating it from ribosomal machinery [8–10].

The experimental evidences indicate that miRNA regulates translation inhibition at initiation (Figure 2) or later stages of translation (Figure 3). Binding of eIF4E to the cap region of mRNA is the initiation of the assembly of the initiation complex; it is identified that miRNA interfere with the eIF4E and impairs its function and poly(A) tail function is also inhibited [11]. There are other evidences suggesting that miRNAs repress translation at later stages of

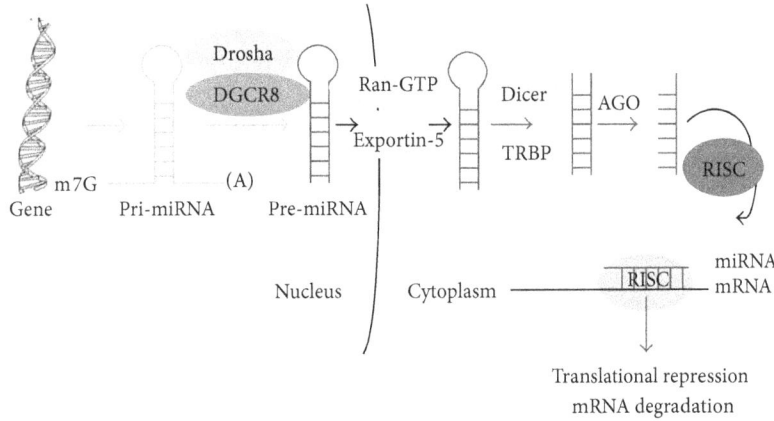

FIGURE 1: Biogenesis of miRNA. miRNAs are transcribed into pri-miRNA and are capped and polyadenylated. This pri-miRNA is processed by Drosha and DGCR8 into pre-miRNA, which by Ran-GTP and Exportin-5 are transported into the cytoplasm and further processed by Dicer. The miRNA dissociates and with help of RISC gets involved in gene silencing by translation repression or degradation of target mRNA.

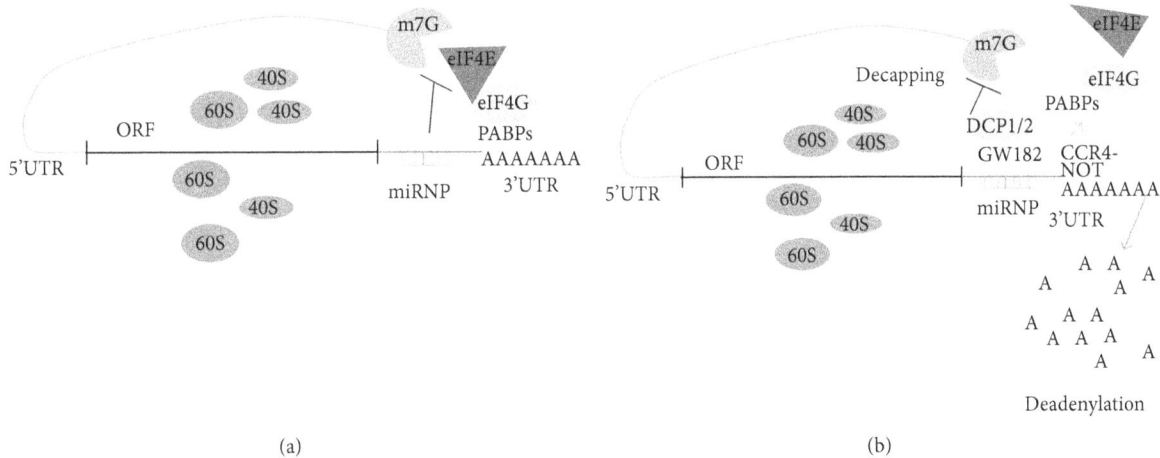

FIGURE 2: miRNA mediated translation repression. (a) At initiation stage the miRNP (miRNA ribonucleoprotein complex) impairs the recognition of cap by eIF4E there by inhibiting the recruitment of ribosomal subunits onto the mRNA. (b) miRNA mediated degradation of mRNA by deadenylation of $3'$–$5'$ exonuclease after recruiting CCR4-NOT to the polyadenylation site where GW182 is required to bind to miRNPs. Replacement of cap by decapping enzymes DCP1/2 hampers the translation initiation.

initiation. miRNA lin-4 target the lin-14 and lin-28 mRNAs, but under inhibitory conditions mRNAs of lin-14, lin-28 are not altered indicating that miRNAs inhibit translation after the initiation stage. Interestingly in both cap dependent and cap independent translation mRNAs are inhibited by synthetic miRNA suggesting postinitiation inhibition. Another mechanism by which miRNA inhibit translation is by ribosome drop off, in which ribosomes which are engaged in translation are directed to terminate translation prematurely (Figure 3(a)). There is other proposed mechanisms that miRNAs are degrading the nascent polypeptides by recruiting the proteolytic enzymes (Figure 3(b)) [12, 13].

2. Biogenesis of miRNA

There are various proteins involved in miRNA biogenesis (Table 2). miRNAs are synthesised from coding or noncoding part of genes (promoter, introns, and exons) by RNA

polymerase II into a precursor called pri-miRNA. The pri-miRNA is processed by the enzyme Drosha and cleaved into 70–120 nucleotides called precursor miRNA (pre-miRNA). The recombinant Drosha is unable to produce pre-miRNA suggesting that other cofactors may be required for its action. DGCR8 an important cofactor is required for the processing of pri-miRNA and is believed to recognize the cleavage site between ssRNA and stem of pri-miRNA. It is approximately 11 base pairs away from the dsRNA-ssRNA junction [79]. Interestingly some miRNAs are processed independent of Drosha to generate pre-miRNA from introns with the association of debranching enzyme and spliceosome [80]. Pre-miRNA is exported from the nucleus to the cytoplasm [81] by Exportin-5 and it is processed to 19–22 nucleotide duplex by Dicer [82]. Like Drosha, Dicer contains associated proteins TRBP, PACT which increases Dicer stability and activity. There are various isoforms of Dicer and the roles of these isoforms are not known [83, 84]. The mature miRNA then associates with a protein complex known as RNA induced

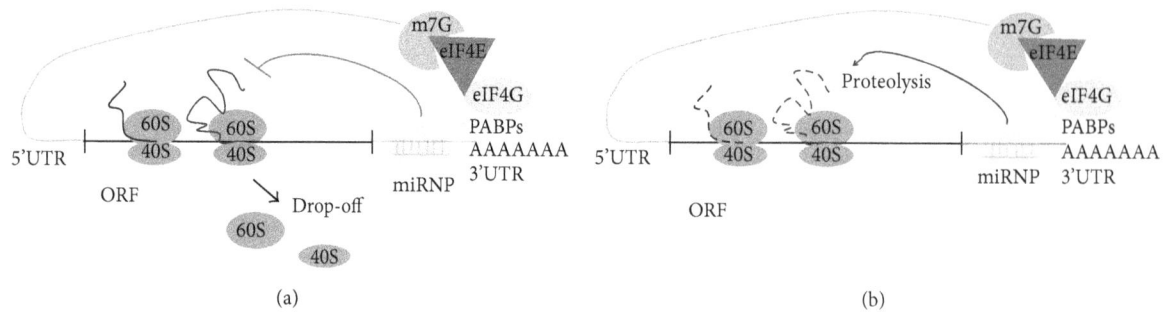

FIGURE 3: miRNA mediated regulation of translation at postinitiation stage. (a) Ribosome drop-off is the proposed mechanism where translation is initiated and miRNA directed ribosomes to inhibit the translation prematurely. (b) Other possible mechanisms of miRNA mediated translation repression are nascent polypeptides which are degraded by proteosomes.

TABLE 1: miRNA nomenclature.

Notation	Description
"hsa" (Eg. hsa-miR-21)	Species name (*Homo sapiens*) Eg. Mmu—mus musculus rno—*Rattus norvegicus* cel—*Caenorhabditis elegans* ath—*Arabidopsis thaliana* dme-*Drosophila melanogaster*
"miR" (Eg. hsa-mir-17)	Denotes immature form of miRNA (pre-miRNA) or primary transcript or genomic locus
"miR" (Eg. has-miR-10)	Refers to the mature form of miRNA
a and b notation (Eg. miR-147a, miR-147b)	When two miRNAs are similar except in 2 or 3 nt, then they are denoted by lowercased letters
Additional numbers in names (Eg. miR-16-1, miR-16-2)	In case of two miRNAs are 100% similar, but they are located on different chromosomes and then they are denoted by extra dash followed by number
"*" notation (Eg. miR-56/ miR-56*)	If the same precursor miRNA produces two miRNAs, then the less predominant one is denoted by*
3p- and 5p- notation (Eg. miR-56-3p, miR-56-5p)	If the data is not sufficient to know which one is predominant, then it is written as 3p- or 5p-. 3p- and 5p- indicate that it is derived from $3'$, $5'$ arms, respectively.

silencing complex (RISC) at $3'$UTR or $5'$UTR or in ORF of target genes [10] (Figure 1). Complementarity between target mRNA and miRNA particularly in seed region is important in determining the miRNA target sites. The mechanism of miRNA mediated gene silencing is not clearly explored till now and it has been known that miRNA suppresses the expression of a gene by inhibiting the translation of its mRNA. Other major functions of the miRNA are removal of mRNA from translation machinery and associating it with processing bodies (P-bodies) where mRNA is degraded [85]. It has been reported that miRNA association with mRNA degrades the mRNA through decapping and deadenylation of mRNA [86]. By repressing the mRNAs, miRNAs are involved in gene expression changes leading to regulation of different biological aspects including proliferation, differentiation, apoptosis, immune response, ageing, and metabolism.

3. Detection of miRNA

miRNA detection enable us to study the regulation of miRNA in various biological processes. There are various methods to detect the mature forms of miRNA which include deep sequencing [87], microarrays [88], northern blot [89], and real-time PCR [90]. In microarray analysis the first step is

isolation of the total RNA which contains miRNA and here enrichment of small RNA enhances the sensitivity of the detection. This RNA is labeled and hybridized to designed probes specific for a miRNA and later studying the signal intensities we can measure the levels of miRNA in a sample. Microarray analysis can give the data of known miRNAs and it cannot be quantified, but it is useful to assess the miRNA in two different samples relatively. To find new miRNAs deep sequencing can be used, but it is not very established technique; it includes sequencing RNA and analyzing the folding properties and validating the data by northern blot or real-time PCR [87].

4. Prediction of miRNA Targets

Many studies indicate that deregulation of miRNAs results in various disorders including cancer, diabetes, metabolic disorders, and cardiovascular disorders, so understanding of miRNA regulation in various pathologies enables us to solve the diagnostic and therapeutic challenges. To understand the association of miRNA and mRNA many computational based databases have been developed which predict possible targets of miRNAs by using different algorithms (Table 3). All these tools recognize miRNA targets based on seed

TABLE 2: Proteins involved in miRNA biogenesis.

Gene	Description	Location	Function	Domains	Reference
Dicer	Dicer 1, ribonuclease type II	14q31	miRNA processing	Type III restriction enzyme, RNase3, DEAH, helicase, dsRBD, PAZ	[14]
AGO3	Argonaute 3	1p34-p34	Short-interfering-RNA-mediated gene silencing	PAZ, PIWI, DUF1785, DUF2344, DUF2678	[15]
Gemin3	DEAD (Asp-Glu-Ala-Asp) box polypeptide 20	1p13.2	RNA helicase	DEAD, Type III restriction enzyme, helicase C	[16]
Drosha	Drosha, ribonuclease type II	5p14-p13	Pri-miRNA processing	RNase3 domain, Double-stranded RNA binding motif	[17]
Exportin-5	Karyopherin family	6p21.1	Transport of small RNAs	Importin-beta N-terminal domain, exportin 1-like protein	[18]
FMRP	Fragile X mental retardation 1	Xq27.3	mRNA trafficking	KH domain	[19]
ADAR	Adenosine deaminase, RNA-specific	1q21.3	RNA and miRNA editing	z-Alpha, Dsrm, Editase	[20]
TRBP	TAR (HIV-1) RNA binding protein	12q12, q-13	Dicer stabilization	DZF, dsRBD	[21]
Importin-8	GTPase Ran mediate nuclear import	12p11.21	Nuclear localization of Argonaute proteins	Cse1	[22]
ELAV1	(Embryonic lethal, abnormal vision, *Drosophila*-like 1)	19p13.2	Repression of target sites	RBD	[23]
Dnd1	Dead end homolog 1	5q31.3	Inhibiting miRNA-mediated repression	PMP-22	[24]

sequence of miRNA and $3'$ UTR of target genes. Hence it becomes necessary to validate these targets by experimental approaches such as luciferase assay, RNA interference, microarray, pulsed (p) SILAC, and Argonaute HITS-CLIP [88–91]. The nomenclature of miRNA is a sequential process given in Table 1.

4.1. Ago HITS-CLIP. Genome-wide functional protein-RNA interaction sites on RNA can be identified by HITS-CLIP, high throughput sequencing of RNAs isolated by cross linking, and immunoprecipitation (Figure 4). In this method RNA and bound protein Argonaute are cross linked by ultraviolet light which gives Arg-miRNA and Arg-RNA binding sites. The remaining RNA is digested and then the RNA and RNA complexes are isolated by immunoprecipitation which are sequenced by next generation sequencers. Comparison of these two datasets helps us to know the miRNA target sites [91].

4.2. Microarray and qRT-PCR. miRNAs target the corresponding mRNA and reduce its stability by degrading it. miRNA target can be detected by overexpressing the miRNA in a cell line that does not express the miRNA. Comparison of control and miRNA overexpression in cell lines using qRT-PCR and microarray will enable the detection of miRNA target or its associated pathway [87].

4.3. SILAC. Baek et al. have shown the use of stable isotope labeling using amino acids in cell culture (SILAC) in the identification of miRNA targets [92]. In this method proteins of the culture medium are labeled with radio-labeled amino acids. For the identification of miRNA targets SILAC method is slightly modified, instead of radio-labeled amino acid, and heavy isotope is added to the growth medium for short time to know the newly synthesized proteins. Heavy and medium heavy isotope signal intensities are measured, if the mRNA is the target of a miRNA, the heavy medium isotope signal intensity is decreased; otherwise there is no change in the intensities (i.e., normal and malignant tissue). Protein analysis by mass spectrometry combined with SILAC has strong correlation with miRNA activity [93] (Figure 5).

5. Biological Roles of miRNA

miRNAs regulate several biological processes such as apoptosis, insulin secretion, lipid metabolism, stem cell

TABLE 3: miRNA target prediction tools.

Database	Description	URL	Reference
miRSystem	Predict the target genes and pathways	http://mirsystem.cgm.ntu.edu.tw/	[25]
miRanda	Predict targets by finding high complementarity regions in 3'UTR	http://www.microrna.org	[26]
TargetScan	Detect target genes by perfect complementarity to the seed region	http://www.targetscan.org	[27]
PicTar	Seed match, binding energy, conservation	http://pictar.mdc-berlin.de/	[28]
DIANA-microT	Based on affinity interaction between miRNA and mRNA	http://diana.cslab.ece.ntua.gr/	[29]
Mire	Based on miRNA; mRNA duplex stability properties	http://didattica-online.polito.it/eda/miREE/	[30]
RNA22	Detect targets by pattern recognition and folding energy	http://cbcsrv.watson.ibm.com/rna22.html	[31]
Tar Base	Curated database for experimentally tested miRNA targets	http://diana.cslab.ece.ntua.gr/tarbase/	[32]
miRNA MAP	Collection of experimentally verified miRNA targets	http://mirnamap.mbc.nctu.edu.tw/	[33]
MiRSel	Extraction of miRNA; gene interactions from the literature	http://services.bio.ifi.lmu.de/mirsel/	[34]
miRecords	Targets identified by 11 target prediction programmes	http://mirecords.biolead.org/	[35]
MiRTarBase	Targets collected manually from the literature	http://mirtarbase.mbc.nctu.edu.tw/	[36]
miRWalk	Target identification by complimentarity (perl language)	http://www.umm.uni-heidelberg.de/apps/zmf/mirwalk/	[37]
Star Base	Use CLIP-Seq and Degradome-Seq data for miRNA target identification	http://starbase.sysu.edu.cn/	[38]
VHoT	It gives information of viral miRNA relation with host	http://acl.snu.ac.kr/vhot/	[39]
OMIT	Based on ontology design, data integration	http://bioportal.bioontology.org/ontologies/OMIT	[40]
MiRPara	It uses support vector machine based software	http://159.226.126.177/mirpara/	[41]

differentiation, heart development, muscle differentiation, cardiomyocyte hypertrophy, antigen presentation, and ageing. In this section biological roles of miRNA are described briefly.

5.1. Apoptosis. Apoptosis is a regulated process of cell death necessary for normal development and homeostasis. Aberrant expression of miRNA leads to failure of apoptosis finally resulting in evolution of cancer. Even though the exact role of miRNA in the apoptosis is not well understood, there are several instances of its role in apoptosis. Cimmino et al. showed that miR-15 and miR-16 induce apoptosis by targeting Bcl2 [94], whereas miR-330 induces apoptosis in PC-3 cells by reducing the E2F1 mediated Akt phosphorylation [95]. Interestingly, miR-21 acts as an antiapoptotic factor and its knockdown activates caspase activity and increased apoptotic cell death in glioblastoma cells [96].

5.2. Insulin Secretion. Diabetes is the most common metabolic disorder in the world. miRNAs have been found to

be involved in the several physiological processes including glucose homeostasis. It was reported that some miRNAs are important for the release of insulin. miR-375 is essential for β-cell survival, proliferation, and division. The expression level of transcription factor Onecut-2 was reduced, whereas the level of granuphilin was increased by miR-9 which is a negative regulator of insulin release [97]. Surprisingly, knockdown of miR-24, miR-26, miR-182, or miR-148 in cultured β-cells also resulted in reduced insulin mRNA level [98].

5.3. Lipid Metabolism. miRNAs have been shown to be important regulators of lipid metabolism also. miR-33 downregulates ABC transporters there by controlling the cholesterol efflux and HDL biogenesis. Decreased serum cholesterol levels were observed due to miR-122 inhibition and it has been shown that it maintains the hepatic cell phenotype [99, 100]. In addition, miR-33a is involved in the cholesterol export and β-oxidation of fatty acids. Its inhibition leads to increased levels of HDL in mice [101, 102].

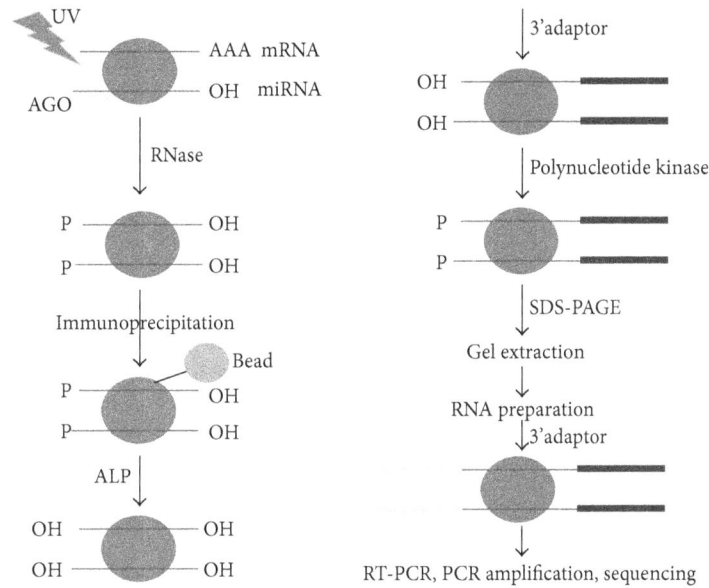

FIGURE 4: Scheme of Argonaute high-throughput sequencing of RNAs by cross linking and immunoprecipitation. RNA and protein are cross linked by UV and then RNA is digested by RNase, a treatment which is finally immunoprecipated. $5'$ ends are dephosphorylated and $3'$ ends are adapter ligated followed by phosphate addition at $5'$ ends. The complexes of RNA and protein are separated by SDS-PAGE and RNA are amplified after $5'$-adaptor ligation. These amplified products will be sequenced by next generation sequencers and finally computational approaches will help identify the miRNA target.

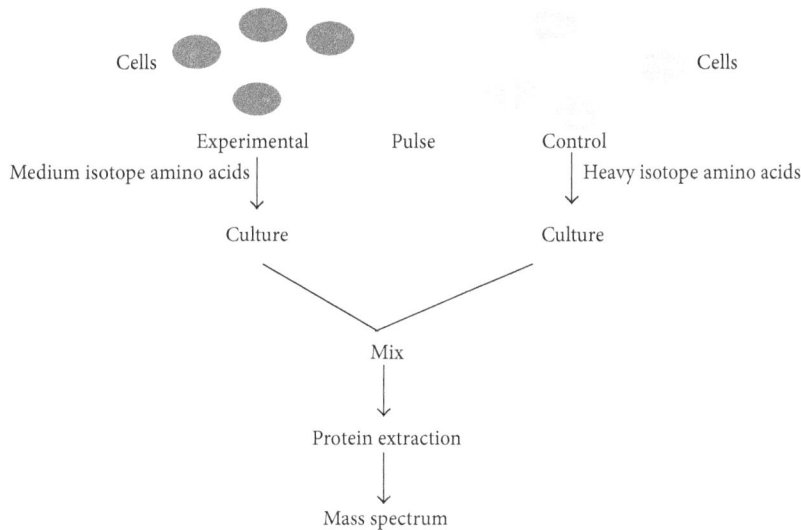

FIGURE 5: Schematic representation of pulsed SILAC. Proteins of the culture medium of control and experimental sample are labelled with heavy and medium isotopes, respectively, by adding them to growth medium. After short time comparison of heavy and medium isotope signal intensities miRNA target mRNA will be detected.

5.4. *Immunity.* It has been reported that CD34$^+$ hematopoietic stem cells express 33 miRNAs, among which miR-155 regulates both myelopoiesis and erythropoiesis [103]. In ES (expand) cells, miRNAs regulate Sox2, Nanog, and Oct-4 pluripotency transcription factors [104]. They play major role in immunity where overexpression of miR-181a results in reduction in CD8$^+$ T cells and removal of Dicer in early B cell development leads to prevention of pre-B cell to pro-B cell transition [105, 106]. Liu et al. showed that miR-148

and miR-152 negatively regulate the antigen presentation of DCs and inhibited the production of cytokines [107]. Antigen specific T-cell mediated immunity is suppressed by miR-155 and inhibition of miR-155 reversed this effect [108].

6. Haematopoiesis

The production of different types of blood cells including their formation, development, and differentiation of blood

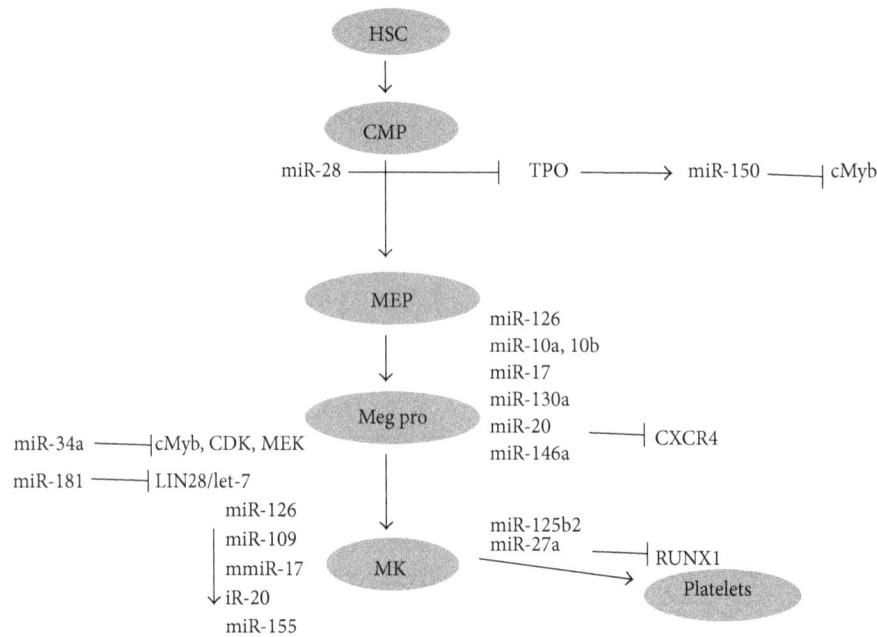

FIGURE 6: miRNA in megakaryopoiesis. miRNAs playing crucial role in the development of megakaryocyte (MegP-megakaryocyte progenitor, CMP-common myeloid progenitor, MEP-megakaryocyte erythroid progenitor).

cells is collectively known as haematopoiesis. Blood cells are divided into three lineages erythroid cells, lymphocytes, and myeloid cells. From many studies on miRNA expression including murine and hematopoietic system, it has been shown that miRNAs are not only involved in the normal haematopoiesis but also play a vital role in every stage of haematopoiesis. Dicer is an enzyme essential for miRNA biogenesis, whose deficiency leads to embryonic death and lack of stem cells in hematopoietic system [109]. Pro-B cell to pre-B cell transition is blocked due to removal of Dicer in B-cell progenitors [106]. T-cell development and differentiation is impaired in conditional deletion of Dicer and reduction in the number of CD8[+], CD 4[+]T cells in thymus [110].

6.1. Megakaryopoiesis. From the hematopoietic stem cells through series of commitment steps megakaryocytes (MKs) are generated. MKs undergo a unique maturation process including megakaryoblast formation and polyploidization to produce proplatelets (Figure 6). Platelets are shed from these proplatelets into bone marrow sinusoids. Earlier studies have shown that miRNAs control the MK development and release of platelets (Table 4). Opalinska et al. studied miRNA expression in murine system where they examined 435 miRNAs among them 13 were upregulated and 81 were downregulated [46]. Overexpressing the miR-155 in K562 cells decreased the differentiation of megakaryocyte and erythroid cells by regulating the targets Meis-1 and Ets-1 [44]. The miR-34a contributes to MK differentiation by targeting cMyb, CDKs and it targets MEK1, thereby repressing proliferation [42, 43]. Interestingly, miR-146a, miR-145 are involved in megakaryopoiesis by activating innate immunity targets TIRAP and TRAF6 [111] which mediates the 5q syndrome phenotype

[45]. During megakaryocyte development increase in miR-146a levels is repressed by PLZF transcription factor and its target CXCR4 [112]. miR-150 favors the differentiation of megakaryocyte-erythroid progenitors into megakaryocyte lineage rather than erythroid lineage. TPO induces miR-150 expression which in turn targets cMyb in TPO cells [47, 48]. It was detected in myeloproliferative neoplasm patient platelets that miRNA-28 is overexpressed which prevents megakaryocyte differentiation from CD34[+]cells by targeting TPO receptor [49]. RUNX1 upregulates miR-27a by binding to it and miR-27a targets RUNX1 and decreases its levels and miR181a inhibit Ca2[+] induced differentiation and accelerates apoptosis [50, 51]. LIN28 is repressed by miR-181, thereby interrupting the LIN28/let-7 and axis then let-7 is upregulated; finally it promotes megakaryocyte differentiation identifying that miR-130 targets MAFB and miR-10a expression inversely correlate with HOX A1 in differentiated megakaryocytes [53, 113].

6.2. Erythropoiesis. The term erythropoiesis refers to the process of production of red blood cells. In humans erythropoiesis occurs in red bone marrow. Kidneys respond to low levels of oxygen by releasing a hormone erythropoietin, which triggers erythropoiesis. It has been identified that certain miRNAs play crucial role in erythroid homeostasis (Figure 7). miR-144 and miR-451 are required for erythroid homeostasis (Table 5). Mice deficient of miR-144 and miR-451 have shown to undergo impairment in late erythrocyte maturation which further leads to splenomegaly, mild anaemia, and erythroid hyperplasia. GATA1 controls the erythropoiesis through regulating the two conserved miRNAs, miR-451 and miR-144, which in turn regulate GATA1 expression [54]. Defect in erythroid differentiation and reduction

TABLE 4: miRNA involved in megakaryopoiesis.

miRNA	Function	Putative targets	Reference
miR-34a	MK differentiation of K562 cells, targets cMyb, CDKs, and MEK1	HMGN4, CCDC52, KLRK1, RGS17, NFATCG	[42, 43]
miR-155	Downregulated in megakaryopoiesis, targets Meis-1 and Ets-1	MMP16, SLC11A2, C2orf18	[44]
miR-146a, miR-145	Involved in megakaryopoiesis by activating innate immunity and mediates 5q syndrome phenotype	SOX11, SP1	[45]
miR-146a	Increased in MK development and targets CXCR4	CREBL2, NOTCH2, TRAK2, TBX18, RIN2, RAD23B, SLC1A2	[46, 47]
miR-150	Favours megakaryocyte lineage differentiation; it targets cMyb, induced by TPO	SLC24A4	[47, 48]
miR-28	It targets TPO receptor and prevents MK differentiation from CD34$^+$ cells		[49]
miR-27a	miR-27a targets and decrease RUNX1 levels	TRIM9, CYB5B, EGR2, BASP1	[50]
miR-181a	miR-181a inhibit Ca2$^+$ induced differentiation of MKs		[51]
miR-125b-2	Induces proliferation and differentiation of MKs	RAD98, ZNF100, PDS5B, SHE, CDR2	[52]
miR-181	Mediates MK differentiation by disrupting LIN28/let-7 axis	FOXP1, CCN8, HOXA1	[53]

TABLE 5: miRNAs involved in erythropoiesis.

MiRNA	Function	Putative targets	Reference
miR-144, miR-451	Erythroid homeostasis, deficiency leads to splenomegaly, mild anaemia, and erythroid hyperplasia, controlled by GATA1	TSPAN12, HMGCR, FBN2, MAP3K8, CXCL16, EREG, ATF2, CDKN2B	[54, 55]
miR-451	Erythroid differentiation defect and reduction in haematocrit in miRNA-451$^{-/-}$ mice	CDKN2B, CXCL16, EREG, ATF2	[56]
miR-223	Reduces the commitment of erythroid progenitors	LIN54, FOXO1, USP42, ALCAM, BCLAF1, SLC11A2	[57, 58]
miR-15b, mi16, miR-22	Positive correlation with erythroid markers CD36, CD235a, and CD71	PRDM4, KIF1B, LAMP3, SWAP70, LIN7C, AKT3, LAMC1	[59, 60]
miR-28	Negatively correlate with CD71		[59, 60]
miR-320	Favours CD71 transcriptional activities		[60]
miR-221, miR-222	Inhibit normal erythropoiesis	TAF9B, MYLIP, RAB18, CYP7A1, KIF16B, MAT2A, NXN	[61]
miR-24	Targets ALK4	TRIB3, CBX5, KCNJ2, DGA52	[62]
miR-15a	Transition from BFU-E to CFU-E stage	GFAP, SLC9A8, ZNRF2, FAM81A	[63]

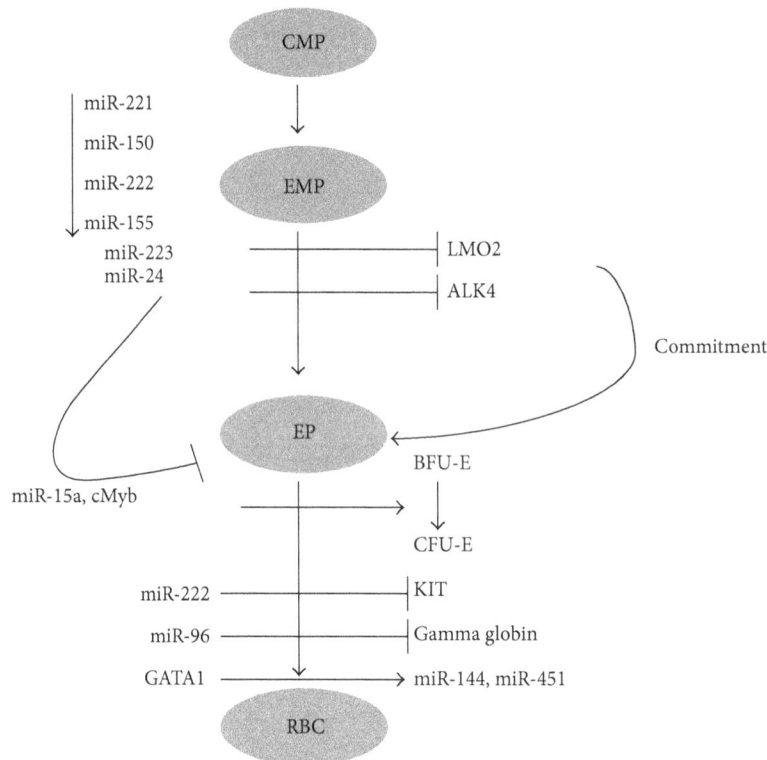

FIGURE 7: miRNA in erythropoiesis. miRNA in the erythrocyte development. (EP-erythroid progenitor, BFU-E-burst forming unit erythroid, CFU-E-colony forming unit erythroid).

in hematocrit are observed in miR-451$^{-/-}$ mice. miR-451 upregulation rescued the defect in erythroid differentiation by targeting 14-3-3ζ [56]. LMO2 is a transcriptional regulator which is important for HSC development and erythropoiesis. Blood formation is affected in mice lacking this gene and miR-223. LMO2 levels inversely correlated to this miRNA and transduction of miR-223 reduces the commitment of erythroid progenitors [57, 58]. miR-15b, miR-16, and miR-22 have shown strong correlation with the erythroid surface markers CD36, CD235a, and CD71, whereas miR-28 was negatively correlated and CD71 transcriptional activities favour miR-320 in reticulocytes [59, 60]. miR-221, miR-222, and miR-24 inhibit normal erythropoiesis and miR-24 targets ALK4. cMyb and miR-15a are involved in the transition from BFU-E to CFU-E stage [61–63]. Fetal haemoglobin ($\alpha 2 \gamma 2$) is the crucial oxygen carrying protein from 2nd to 3rd trimester development stage which has been observed to be completely replaced by ($\alpha 2 \beta 2$) in adults. It was identified that miR-96 inhibits the γ-globin gene expression, thereby repressing the erythropoiesis [114].

6.3. Mast Cells. Mast cells are resident cells of tissues throughout body and contain granules rich in histamine and heparin. Mast cells are bone marrow derived and their survival depends on stem cell factor. Biological roles of mast cells include wound healing, innate immunity defense against pathogens, and angiogenesis. miRNAs play important role in mast cells; for example, miR-221 is involved in the adhesion of mast cells, degranulation, and migration towards

SCF (expand) and cytokine production [115]. miR-126 favors mast cell proliferation and cytokine production by targeting Spred1. miR-221 and 222 are upregulated after mast cell activation; overexpression of these miRNAs causes defect in cell morphology and cell cycle regulation without affecting viability [116, 117].

6.4. Myelopoiesis. Myelopoiesis is the formation of myeloid cells including granulocytes, monocytes, eosinophils, basophiles, and neutrophils. Many studies reported the role of miRNA in myelopoiesis and in myeloid malignancies. Eva et al. showed that miR-125b affects myelopoiesis in several ways and finally cause of blocking the G-CSF induced differentiation of granulocytes. They found that the Stat3 and Bak1 are the direct targets of miR-125b [118]. AML1 regulates myelopoiesis by recruiting chromatin remodeling enzymes on pre-miR-223 gene and silencing cell differentiation [119]. NF1-A negatively regulates granulocyte and monocyte differentiation. miR-223 and miR-424 repress NF1- A and these miRNA are activated by C/EBPα and PU.1, respectively. AML1 is known to be targeted by miR-17-5p-92 cluster, where this cluster is downregulated in monocytopoiesis and thereby AML1 is upregulated causing induction of M-CSF [120]. Zinc finger protein growth factor independent-1 (Gfi-1) is essential for normal granulocyte differentiation. A mutation in GFI1 causes severe congenital neutropenia (SCN). miR-196B and miR-21 are downregulated in SCN and up- or down- regulation of these miRNAs severely affects myelopoiesis [121]. miR-299-5p is involved in the CD34^{+} progenitor cell regulation and also in the modulation of monocyte differentiation [122].

Granulocytes. Granulocytes are classified as basophils, eosinophils, and neutrophils based on their morphology and staining properties of their cytoplasm. Basophils are comprised of <1% of white blood cells and eosinophils 1–3% and neutrophils constitute 50–70% of white blood cells. Basophils are nonphagocytic and release certain pharmacologically active substances from their cytoplasmic granules which are involved in certain allergic reactions. These granulocytes have lobed nucleus, granular cytoplasm, and stains with methylene blue which is a basic dye. There are no reports on miRNA regulation of basophils but identified that miR-31, miR-107, and miR-222 are highly expressed in basophils [123].

Eosinophils. Eosinophils are motile phagocytic cells that can migrate from blood to tissue spaces. They have bilobed nucleus, granular cytoplasm and can be stained with compounds like eosin red, an acidic dye. Very few studies have been reported on the miRNA regulation of eosinophils. miR-126 inhibition has been found to cause blockade of the recruitment of eosinophils at the airway walls in allergic asthma, which results in suppressing the development of airway disease [124]. miR-935 is found to be upregulated in eosinophils (5.6 fold) compared to DCs. Inhibition of miR-145 suppresses the eosinophil inflammation and mucous secretion. On treating mice with anti-miR-145 and dexamethasone, a similar effect was shown by both reducing eosinophils infiltration and suppression of mucous secretion in air ways [125, 126]. Wong et al. reported that miR-21* regulate the eosinophil apoptosis by enhancing GM-CSF (expand) which activates and sustains the survival of eosinophils through ERK pathway. Inhibition of miR-21* diminishes its survival activity and activates apoptosis in eosinophils [127].

Neutrophils. Neutrophils are called as polymorph nuclear leucocyte and they have multilobed nucleus. The granulated cytoplasm can stain with both acidic and basic stains. After being produced in bone marrow these are released into the peripheral blood and circulate 7–10 hours after which these migrate into the tissues. miR-29B regulates the neutrophil differentiation and PU1, Myc are the transcriptional regulators of miR-29B [128]. miR-223 is highly expressed in neutrophils and it plays a crucial role in granulocyte progenitor proliferation and function [129]. miRNA clusters regulate apoptosis and survival of several cancers recently. Ward et al. showed that miRNA clusters are expressed in human neutrophils. miR-17-92 cluster (miR-17, miR-19a, miR-19b, miR-20a, miR-92a, miR-18a, and miR-17*) contains seven mature miRNAs five of them (miR-17, miR-19a, miR-19b, miR-20a, miR-92a) are expressed in human neutrophils, whereas miR-18a, miR-17* were not detected in human neutrophils. This suggests that these clusters may play a crucial role in regulating neutrophil functions [130]. Proinflammatory signals upregulate miR-9 in neutrophils through NF-κb [131]. Neutrophil elastase (NE), a serine protease, stimulates

the secretion of mucus in pulmonary tracts by inducing MUC5AC. miR-146a negatively regulates the hypersecretion of the mucus by MUC5AC [132]. After spinal cord injury miR-223 was upregulated and highly expressed after 12 hours. Immunohistochemistry revealed that this miR-223 observed in Gr-1 positive neutrophil which indicates that miR-223 regulates neutrophil after spinal cord injury [133]. miR-133a and miR-1 are downregulated in myeloproliferative disorder neutrophils; these have also been reported previously in certain cancers [134]. Radom-Aizik et al. showed the neutrophil miRNA expression pattern after exercise, interestingly 20 of 38 miRNAs downregulated immediately after exercise; remaining 18 miRNAs were upregulated. These miRNAs which were affected are regulating the genes that are involved in the apoptosis and immune processes [135].

Mononuclear Phagocytes. Mononuclear phagocytes are comprised of monocytes and macrophages and monocytes are present in blood and macrophages reside in tissues. In bone marrow granulocyte-monocyte progenitors differentiate into promonocytes and on entering the blood stream these mature into monocytes. After being circulated in blood for 8 hours these enlarge and enter into tissues and differentiate into tissue specific macrophages. MiRNAs have been found to play a crucial role in regulation of monocyte/macrophages. miR-146a increases in monocytes/macrophages upon induction of LPS and it negatively regulates innate immune response as it targets TRAF6 which is involved in TLR signalling, this regulation is dependent on Relb [136, 137]. Pauley et al. showed that in Sjogren's syndrome miR-146a increases the phagocytic activity of monocytes and it suppresses the inflammatory cytokine production [138]. On treating monocytes and U937 cell lines with LPS it was found that there is an upregulation of miR-525-5p and its putative target VPAC1 was shown to be down-regulated suggesting that miR-525-5p regulates the control of immune homeostasis [139]. miR-124 has been found to have role in macrophage activation and its overexpression in bone marrow macrophages leads to inhibition of TNFα [140]. In human monocytes, resveratrol increases miR-663 which target genes such as JunD and JunB decreasing the AP1 activity induced by LPS, hence altering the immune response [141]. Sharbati et al. showed that miR-21, miR-222, miR-23b, miR-24, and miR-27a are upregulated in monocyte differentiation and miR-29 in monocyte infection which suggests that these miRNAs may regulate monocyte defence mechanisms through TGF-β signalling [142].

T-Lymphocytes. T-lymphocytes belonging to white blood cells are produced in bone marrow and mature in thymus and express T cell receptors. T cell receptors recognize an antigen which is bound to major histocompatibility protein, a membrane protein by the process known as antigen presentation. When a T-cell recognizes an antigen which is bound to MHC on a cell it proliferates and differentiates into memory cell and effector cells (Figure 8). There are three subpopulations of T cells they are T helper cell (Th), T-cytotoxic cell (Tc), and T suppressor cell (Ts). T helper cells can be distinguished from T-cytotoxic cells based on the membrane protein CD4 and CD8, respectively. Like other biological processes regulated

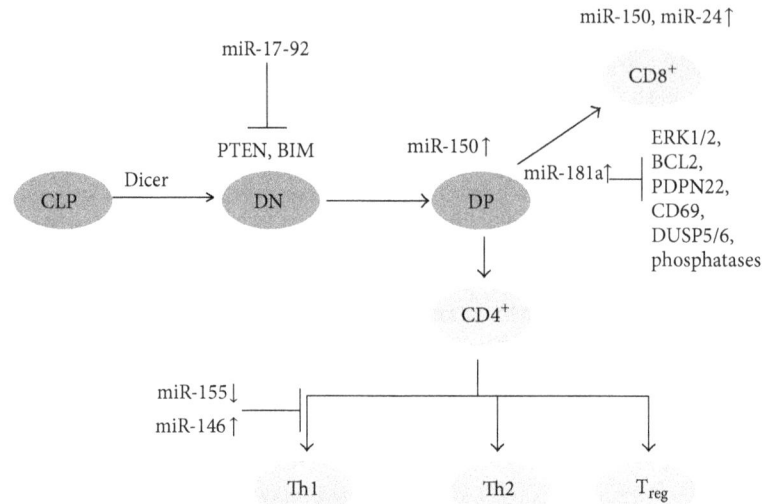

FIGURE 8: miRNA in T cell development. miRNA regulation at different developmental stages of T-cell development (CLP-common lymphoid progenitor, DN-double negative, DP-bouble positive).

by miRNA T-cell development in thymus and their activation is controlled by miRNAs. Wu et al. studied the miRNA profiling of naive, effector, and CD8 memory T-cells and they found that miR-16, miR-21, miR-142-3p, miR-142-5p, miR-150, miR-15b, and let-7f are upregulated sevenfold than other miRNAs. They also observed that miRNA expression in effector T-cells was down-regulated compared to naive T cells but their levels are restored back in memory T-cells, suggesting that miRNA may have important in regulation of T-cell development and differentiation [143]. Proliferating T cells contain shorter $3'$UTR compared to the normal cells due to which they have less miRNA targeting sites; hence proliferating cells are resistant to regulation by miRNA [144]. Deletion of Dicer in T-cell lineage results in reduction in the number of Treg cells and its suppressor activity. Since Dicer is required for miRNA biogenesis and absence of Dicer is found to hinder in Treg cell development in thymus, it indicates that miRNAs are required for the T-cell development [145, 146]. miRNA-181a is involved in the T and B cell differentiation; the miRNA expression is found to be low in matured and peripheral T-cells, whereas it is highly expressed in the double positive T lymphocytes which are sensitive to low affinity peptide antigens, indicating that miRNA regulates the sensitivity of T-cell receptor [147]. Virts and Thoman showed the age related expression of miRNA in thymopoiesis and they observed that 53% of miRNAs are upregulated in the aged TN1 cells [148]. Ohyashiki et al. showed that miR-92a reduced in CD8$^+$ T-cells progressively with age [149]. miRNA-146a is upregulated, whereas miR-363, miR-498 are downregulated in rheumatoid arthritis CD4$^+$ T-cells and miR-146a is involved in the suppression of apoptosis and play a role in rheumatoid arthritis pathogenesis [150]. Almanza et al. showed that cell fate determination takes place based on the balancing effects of different miRNAs such as miR-150,

the let-7, and miR-155 and they found that miR-150 targets KChIP which is upregulated in CD8 T-cell [151].

B Lymphocytes. B lymphocytes produced in the bone marrow as immature cells and migrate to the secondary lymphoid organs where they transformed into mature B cell. They express a membrane bound antibody, molecule called B-cell receptor. When a naive B-cell finds an antigen which matches its membrane bound antibody then it starts proliferating and they differentiate into memory B-cell and effector B-cell which produce antibody molecules. Antibodies are glycoproteins and they consist of two light chain polypeptides and two heavy chain polypeptides. Several observations suggest that the role of miRNA in B-cell development and function (Figure 9). Tan et al. studied the miRNA profiling of germinal center, memory, and naive B cells. They observed that several miRNAs are elevated in germinal center of B-cell, which include miR-106a, miR-181b, and miR-17-5p. miR-150 is upregulated in all the three subsets and found that it is the target of survivin, cMyb which is critical for B Cell development and its premature expression inhibits the B- cell early development [152]. These results suggest that miRNAs regulate B-cell maturation and development and very little is known about their regulation in B-cell. MiR-150 reduces the mature B cell levels in circulation but has little effect on myeloid lineage cells. It blocks the transition from pro-B cell to pre-B cell by targeting cMyb, which is crucial for the lymphocyte maturation [153]. miR-155 is required for the B-Cell responses to both thymic dependent and independent antigens and the B-Cell which lacks miR-155 decreases in its response to antigen and production of high affinity IgG1 antibody; interestingly it has been found that miR-155 targets the PU1 transcription factor [154]. miR-15 and miR-16 are deleted (13q14) or downregulated in most of the B-CLLs indicating their involvement in the pathogenesis of B-cell chronic lymphocytic leukemias [155]. Chen et al. identified

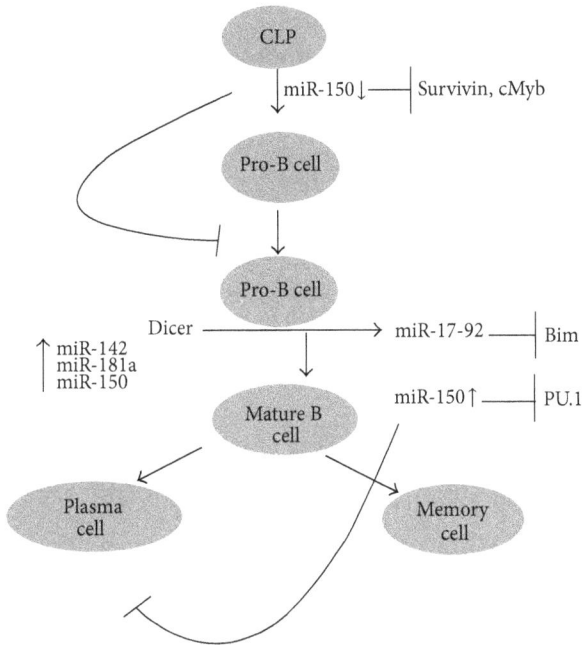

FIGURE 9: miRNA in B cell development and miRNA regulation of B-cell development from common lymphoid progenitor cell to produce memory and plasma cell.

that miR-181 increase the B lineage cells suggesting that it may play a crucial role in B-cell differentiation [105].

7. miRNA in Haematological Malignancies

Haematological malignancies are malignant neoplasms that affect blood, lymph node, bone marrow, and other parts of the lymphatic system. These malignancies may arise from myeloid and lymphoid cell lineages lymphoma. Lymphocytic leukaemia and myeloma arise from lymphoid lineage cells, whereas AML, CML, and myelodisplastic syndromes arise from myeloid lineage cells. Haematological malignancies account for 9.5% and lymphomas are more common than any other malignancies in the USA. Leukemias are classified into acute myelogenous leukemia (AML), chronic myelogenous leukemia (CML), acute lymphocytic leukemia (ALL), chronic lymphocytic leukemia (CLL), acute monocytic leukemia (AMOL), and so forth. Lymphomas are classified into Hodgkin's lymphomas and non-Hodgkin's lymphomas [156]. Expression profiles of miRNAs have shown that they are involved in the haematological malignancies.

7.1. Acute Myeloid Leukemia. Acute myelogenous leukemia is the most common type of leukemia in adults also known as acute myeloblastic leukemia, acute nonlymphocytic leukemia, and acute granulocytic leukemia and is a rapidly growing malignant neoplasm in which many WBCs are found in blood and bone marrow. In acute myeloid leukemia more immature cells are produced abruptly and progression is very fast. Many studies have shown deregulation of miRNAs in AMLs (Table 6). Li et al. showed that

miR-126/126* upregulation is associated with chromosomal translocations and inhibited apoptosis and enhances cell viability and proliferation. They also observed that miR-126 targets the tumour suppressor protein PLK2 (polo-like kinase2) which is involved in the cell cycle checkpoint [64]. Transcription factor C/EBPα regulates miR-223 expression. miR-223 inhibits the cell cycle regulator protein E2F1 which leads to suppression of granulopoiesis. They also found that E2F1 binds to the miR-223 promoter in AML cells and blocks its expression indicating that E2F1 is a transcriptional inhibitor of miR-223 in AML. miRNA-221 has been shown to be overexpressed in several solid tumours and it is highly expressed in AML showing its significant role in oncogenesis. miRNAs are epigenetically deregulated in AML. miR-223 is silenced by the hypermethylation of its upstream elements [65]. Cammarata et al. described the oncogenic role of miRNA-221 in AML and it has been found that it inhibits the CDK inhibitor p27. They also observed that the tumour suppressor miRNA let-7b is down-regulated in AML [66]. C/EBPα is epigenetically silenced in AML, thereby blocking the myeloid differentiation and leads to leukemia. It was identified by computational approach that miR-124a target the C/EBPα [67]. Hypoxia-inducible factor 1 (HIF-1) is also playing a crucial role in the miRNA signaling network by modulating the miR-20a and miR-17 which can inhibit the p21 [68]. Garzon et al. suggested miR-29b as a tumour suppressor miRNA in AML. Its expression is low in AML restoration which leads to reduction in the tumorigenicity and have shown the relation between miRNA and DNA hypermethylation [69]. miR-29b overexpression resulted in the reduced expression of DNA methyl transferases DNMT1, DNMT3B, and DNMT3A. ERG is an oncogene which is deregulated in AML and T-ALL. It has been shown that miR-196a and miR-196b regulate the ERG mRNA; its aberrant expression indicates its role in AML [70]. Protooncogene c-Kit overexpress in AML and it has been shown that miR-193b is downregulated in AML and its overexpression resulted in downregulation of c-Kit. It clearly indicated that c-Kit is direct target of miR-193b and it may be therapeutic target in c-Kit positive AML cases [71].

7.2. Chronic Myelogenous Leukemia. Chronic myelogenous leukemia or chronic granulocytic leukemia is a neoplasm of blood cells especially myeloid cells in which uncontrolled growth of granulocytes (eosinophils, basophils, and neutrophils) is observed. This leukemia is characterized by Philadelphia chromosome translocation and it is a translocation between two chromosomes chromosome 9 and 22, it is denoted as t(9; 22)(q34; q11) [157]. Due to this translocation BCR gene on chromosome 22 and ABL gene on chromosome 9 is fused and this fusion product of BCR-ABL protein is a tyrosine kinase. It causes genomic instability by inhibiting DNA repair and finally leads to accumulation of genetic abnormalities [157]. Recently it has been shown that miR-203 inhibits the expression of BCR-ABL and thereby inhibited cell growth and colony formation. In another study it is shown that overexpression of miR-29b inhibited cell growth and colony formation by inhibiting ABL1 and

TABLE 6: miRNAs involved in AML.

miRNA	Function	Putative targets	Reference
miR-126*	Upregulation leads to chromosomal translocations and inhibits apoptosis	ADAT2,FOF1, LMO7,	[64]
miR-126	Targets tumour suppressor PLK2	TOM1, CKMT2, ZNF131, RGS3,	[64]
miR-223	C/EBPα regulates its expression in turn it inhibits E2F1 in AML cells	ANKH, SCN1A, SCN3A, CBFB, CDH11, NEBL, RILPL1, CENPN	[65]
miR-221	Oncogenic miRNA, it inhibits the CDK inhibitor p27	HIPK1, RAB18, DNM3, ZNF547,	[66]
miR-124a	Target the C/EBPα, silenced and block differentiation gives leukemia phenotype		[67]
miR-20a and miR-17	Inhibits the p21	POLQ, KLF12, STK38, CENTD1, NUP35, GNB5, CTSK	[68]
miR-29b	Tumour suppressor in AML and reduce tumorigenicity	SCML2, C1orf96, COL3A1, COL7A1, COL11A1	[69]
miR-29b	Reduced expression of DNA methyltransferases	CD93, HBP1, SNX21, GNS, HMGCR, HNF4G, DNMT3B	[69]
miR-196a and miR-196b	They target ERG expression	FOS, GATA6, HOXB6, HOXC8, ZNF24, CCDC47	[70]
miR-193b	Downregulated in AML and it targets c-Kit	MMP19, ARMC1, ARPC5	[71]

BCR/ABL1 [76]. Xu et al. showed the feedback regulation between BCR, BCR/ABL1, GATA1 and miR-138. In this study they demonstrated that overexpression of miR-138 represses BCR/ABL1 and CCND3 by binding to the coding and 3′UTR regions, respectively [77]. Interestingly, miR-138 expression is increased by GATA1, and repressed by BCR/ABL in addition to imatinib resistance in CML.Turrini et al. suggested that miRNA may play a role in imatinib distribution in CML therapy and they found that miR-212 increases the ABCG2 expression upon treatment with imatinib in CML [78]. To study the pathology of CML it is essential to study the signaling pathways. Specific miRNAs miR-155, miR-564, and miR-31 are downregulated in CML and extrapolation of these results suggested that VEGF, mTOR, ErbB, and MAPK are the main signaling pathways related to the miRNAs [158]. In a different study it was shown that miR-181a, miR-221, miR-20a, miR-17, miR-19a, miR-103, miR-144, miR-155, miR-150, and miR-222 are downregulated in CML and the targets of these miRNAs are associated with EGFR, ERBB, TGFB1, MAPK, and p53 pathways [159]. RalA is a downstream molecule of Bcr-Abl in Ras signalling pathway and is targeted by miR-181a which plays an important role in CML [160]. Bcr-Abl decreases the tumor suppressor miRNAs and increases the oncogenic miRNAs that leads to leukemic transformation. It was confirmed that knockdown of BCR-ABL results in reduction of miR-212, miR-425-5p, miR-130a, miR-130b and

miR-148a. Interestingly, overexpression of these miRNAs is correlated with reduction in CCND3 suggesting that BCR-ABL induced oncogenic miRNAs are involved in the downregulation of CCND3 in CML [161]. miRNAs which are involved in CML pathogenesis are described in Table 7.

7.3. Multiple Myeloma. Myeloma is a clonal B-cell malignancy characterized by the aberrant accumulation of plasma cells (PCs) within bone marrow (BM) and extramedullary sites [162, 163]. Myeloma arises from the multifocal proliferation of long-lived PCs and, despite all available therapies, remains invariably fatal [164]. Several studies have identified miRNAs that are deregulated during myelomagenesis, and subsequent studies have explored the role of miRNAs as diagnostics to detect disease or to monitor myeloma progression [165, 166]. These studies have found that the vast majority of miRNAs that are aberrantly expressed in MM cells are upregulated compared with their expression in normal PCs [165]. Zhou et al. compared miRNA expression profiles (miREP) of 52 newly diagnosed MM patients with that obtained from PCs of two healthy donors. Among 464 miRNAs analyzed, 95 had a higher mean expression in PC samples of MM patients compared with those of healthy donors [167]. In related studies, miRNA-15a was downregulated in relapsed and/or refractory MM and found to regulate tumor progression in MM cell lines (MMCLs)

TABLE 7: miRNAs involved in CML.

miRNA	Function	Putative targets	Reference
miR-17-92	Down-regulated in imatinib treated CML cells	IRF9, RAB10, TXNIP, TET2	[72]
miR-21	Antisense inhibition leads to inhibition of migration and cell growth and induces apoptosis	TXPAN2, LUM, SUZ12, MSH2, PDZD2	[73]
miR-203	Methylated in AML, CML, ALL, CLL. Inhibit the expression of BCR-ABL	RTKN2, AAK1, MYST4 CD109, IL21, PLD2	[74]
miR-451	Associated with Bcr-Abl	TSC1, ACADSB, GRSF1, MAML1, GDI1, NAMPT	[75]
miR-29b	Inhibits ABL1 and BCR/ABL1 there by inhibiting cell growth and colony formation	HAS3, SNX24, CD93, SCML2, COL7A1, ZNF396, HMGCR, ICOS	[76]
miR-138	Represses BCR/ABL1 and CCND3, increases by GATA1	KLF12, H3F3B, MYO5C, NXN, NEBL, PDPN, STK38	[77]
miR-212	Increases the ABCG2 expression	APAF1, EP300, EDNRA, CFL2, NOS1, SOX4, SOX11	[78]

[168]. Separately, it was found that miRNAs-15a and miRNAs-16 expression levels were often elevated in the PCs from newly diagnosed MM patients in comparison with healthy PCs [169]. The miRNA-17-92 cluster, which targets the apoptosis facilitator Bcl-2, was also reported to confer tumourigenicity in MM [170]. miRNA-29b has been reported to downregulate Mcl-1 and to induce apoptosis of myeloma cells [171]. The miRNA-193b-365 cluster is overexpressed in MM and three miRNAs-720, 1308, and 1246 were significantly higher in PCs of myeloma patients than healthy controls [166, 172]. HOX9, c-Myc, Bcl-2, and SHP1/SHP2 represent targets of miRNA-146b, 140, 145, 125a, 151, 223, 155, and Let-7f, and changes in expression of these miRNAs may be involved in myelomagenesis and associated with overall prognosis [173]. miRNA-17-92 clusters are other pivotal miRNAs activated by Myc and are highly linked to the progression of MM. Gao et al. reported that in addition to miRNA-17-92 cluster expression; miRNA-15a and 16-1 are also linked to poor prognosis in MM patients [174]. Those with elevated miRNA-17, 20, and 92 levels had shorter progression-free survival than those with reduced miRNA levels. Higher miRNA-20a and 148a levels in myeloma patients are associated with a shorter relapse-free survival, to suggest a possible association between miRNA-20a and poor prognosis [175]. Expression of miRNAs-153, 490, 455, 642, 500, and 296 is associated with a better event-free survival, whereas miRNAs-548d, 373, 554, and 888 expression correlates with a poorer outcome [175]. The precise role of miRNAs in myeloma needs to be further elucidated, although they are predicted to be involved in PC growth, survival, growth factor response, homing, drug resistance, and BM interaction.

8. Conclusions

miRNAs are important regulators of haematopoiesis and control the gene expression of several transcription factors essential for the commitment, proliferation, differentiation,

and apoptosis of hematopoietic stem cells. Hematological malignancies arise not only due to the aberrant expression of proteins but also by the regulators of the genes such as miRNAs. Deregulation of miRNA expression results in haematological malignancies. A single miRNA targets many genes and it is not clear whether targeting a single gene or multiple genes leads to hematological malignancies. miRNAs can function through several pathways which are involved in disease manifestations. Gain of function and loss of function experiments will give a better idea about the clinical use of miRNAs. In future more studies need to be focussed on the animal models for the consistent and reliable results which will enable us to understand the pathophysiology of haematological malignancies.

Conflict of Interests

The authors declare that there is no conflict of interests regarding the publication of this paper.

Acknowledgments

This work was supported by DBT-IYBA, DBT-RGYI, DBT-NIAB, DST, ICMR, UPE-UoH, and UGC grants of Government of India. The authors appreciate the funding in form of CSIR and UGC fellowships from Government of India.

References

[1] A. Molnár, F. Schwach, D. J. Studholme, E. C. Thuenemann, and D. C. Baulcombe, "miRNAs control gene expression in the single-cell alga Chlamydomonas reinhardtii," *Nature*, vol. 447, no. 7148, pp. 1126–1129, 2007.

[2] R. C. Lee, R. L. Feinbaum, and V. Ambros, "The C. elegans heterochronic gene lin-4 encodes small RNAs with antisense complementarity to lin-14," *Cell*, vol. 75, no. 5, pp. 843–854, 1993.

[3] A. Molnár, F. Schwach, D. J. Studholme, E. C. Thuenemann, and D. C. Baulcombe, "miRNAs control gene expression in the single-cell alga Chlamydomonas reinhardtii," *Nature*, vol. 447, no. 7148, pp. 1126–1129, 2007.

[4] C. L. Jopling, M. Yi, A. M. Lancaster, S. M. Lemon, and P. Sarnow, "Modulation of hepatitis C virus RNA abundance by a liver-specific MicroRNA," *Science*, vol. 309, no. 5740, pp. 1577–1581, 2005.

[5] U. A. Ørom, F. C. Nielsen, and A. H. Lund, "MicroRNA-10a Binds the $5'$UTR of ribosomal protein mRNAs and enhances their translation," *Molecular Cell*, vol. 30, no. 4, pp. 460–471, 2008.

[6] R. C. Friedman, K. K.-H. Farh, C. B. Burge, and D. P. Bartel, "Most mammalian mRNAs are conserved targets of MicroRNAs," *Genome Research*, vol. 19, no. 1, pp. 92–105, 2009.

[7] H. Siomi and M. C. Siomi, "Posttranscriptional regulation of MicroRNA biogenesis in animals," *Molecular Cell*, vol. 38, no. 3, pp. 323–332, 2010.

[8] S. Nottrott, M. J. Simard, and J. D. Richter, "Human let-7a miRNA blocks protein production on actively translating polyribosomes," *Nature Structural and Molecular Biology*, vol. 13, no. 12, pp. 1108–1114, 2006.

[9] R. S. Pillai, S. N. Bhattacharyya, and W. Filipowicz, "Repression of protein synthesis by miRNAs: how many mechanisms?" *Trends in Cell Biology*, vol. 17, no. 3, pp. 118–126, 2007.

[10] F. Moretti, R. Thermann, and M. W. Hentze, "Mechanism of translational regulation by miR-2 from sites in the $5'$ untranslated region or the open reading frame," *RNA*, vol. 16, no. 12, pp. 2493–2502, 2010.

[11] D. T. Humphreys, B. J. Westman, D. I. K. Martin, and T. Preiss, "MicroRNAs control translation initiation by inhibiting eukaryotic initiation factor 4E/cap and poly(A) tail function," *Proceedings of the National Academy of Sciences of the United States of America*, vol. 102, no. 47, pp. 16961–16966, 2005.

[12] P. H. Olsen and V. Ambros, "The lin-4 regulatory RNA controls developmental timing in Caenorhabditis elegans by blocking LIN-14 protein synthesis after the initiation of translation," *Developmental Biology*, vol. 216, no. 2, pp. 671–680, 1999.

[13] C. P. Petersen, M.-E. Bordeleau, J. Pelletier, and P. A. Sharp, "Short RNAs repress translation after initiation in mammalian cells," *Molecular Cell*, vol. 21, no. 4, pp. 533–542, 2006.

[14] E. Bernstein, A. A. Caudy, S. M. Hammond, and G. J. Hannon, "Role for a bidentate ribonuclease in the initiation step of RNA interference," *Nature*, vol. 409, no. 6818, pp. 363–366, 2001.

[15] J. Liu, M. A. Carmell, F. V. Rivas et al., "Argonaute2 is the catalytic engine of mammalian RNAi," *Science*, vol. 305, no. 5689, pp. 1437–1441, 2004.

[16] Z. Mourelatos, J. Dostie, S. Paushkin et al., "miRNPs: a novel class of ribonucleoproteins containing numerous MicroRNAs," *Genes and Development*, vol. 16, no. 6, pp. 720–728, 2002.

[17] Y. Lee, C. Ahn, J. Han et al., "The nuclear RNase III Drosha initiates MicroRNA processing," *Nature*, vol. 425, no. 6956, pp. 415–419, 2003.

[18] M. T. Bohnsack, K. Czaplinski, and D. Görlich, "Exportin 5 is a RanGTP-dependent dsRNA-binding protein that mediates nuclear export of pre-miRNAs," *RNA*, vol. 10, no. 2, pp. 185–191, 2004.

[19] A. A. Caudy, M. Myers, G. J. Hannon, and S. M. Hammond, "Fragile X-related protein and VIG associate with the RNA interference machinery," *Genes and Development*, vol. 16, no. 19, pp. 2491–2496, 2002.

[20] S. W. Knight and B. L. Bass, "The role of RNA editing by ADARs in RNAi," *Molecular Cell*, vol. 10, no. 4, pp. 809–817, 2002.

[21] Y. Lee, I. Hur, S.-Y. Park, Y.-K. Kim, R. S. Mi, and V. N. Kim, "The role of PACT in the RNA silencing pathway," *The EMBO Journal*, vol. 25, no. 3, pp. 522–532, 2006.

[22] L. Weinmann, J. Höck, T. Ivacevic et al., "Importin 8 is a gene silencing factor that targets argonaute proteins to distinct mRNAs," *Cell*, vol. 136, no. 3, pp. 496–507, 2009.

[23] S. N. Bhattacharyya, R. Habermacher, U. Martine, E. I. Closs, and W. Filipowicz, "Relief of MicroRNA-mediated translational repression in human cells subjected to stress," *Cell*, vol. 125, no. 6, pp. 1111–1124, 2006.

[24] M. Kedde, M. J. Strasser, B. Boldajipour et al., "RNA-binding protein Dnd1 inhibits MicroRNA access to target mRNA," *Cell*, vol. 131, no. 7, pp. 1273–1286, 2007.

[25] T. P. Lu, C. Y. Lee, M. H. Tsai et al., "miRSystem: an integrated system for characterizing enriched functions and pathways of MicroRNA targets," *PLoS ONE*, vol. 7, no. 8, Article ID e42390, 2012.

[26] B. John, A. J. Enright, A. Aravin, T. Tuschl, C. Sander, and D. S. Marks, "Human MicroRNA targets," *PLoS Biology*, vol. 2, no. 11, article e363, 2004.

[27] B. P. Lewis, C. B. Burge, and D. P. Bartel, "Conserved seed pairing, often flanked by adenosines, indicates that thousands of human genes are MicroRNA targets," *Cell*, vol. 120, no. 1, pp. 15–20, 2005.

[28] A. Krek, D. Grün, M. N. Poy et al., "Combinatorial MicroRNA target predictions," *Nature Genetics*, vol. 37, no. 5, pp. 495–500, 2005.

[29] M. Maragkakis, M. Reczko, V. A. Simossis et al., "DIANA-MicroT web server: elucidating MicroRNA functions through target prediction," *Nucleic Acids Research*, vol. 37, supplement 2, pp. W273–W276, 2009.

[30] P. H. Reyes-Herrera, E. Ficarra, A. Acquaviva, and E. Macii, "miREE: miRNA recognition elements ensemble," *BMC Bioinformatics*, vol. 12, article 454, 2011.

[31] K. C. Miranda, T. Huynh, Y. Tay et al., "A pattern-based method for the identification of MicroRNA binding sites and their corresponding heteroduplexes," *Cell*, vol. 126, no. 6, pp. 1203–1217, 2006.

[32] T. Vergoulis, I. S. Vlachos, P. Alexiou et al., "TarBase 6.0: capturing the exponential growth of miRNA targets with experimental support," *Nucleic Acids Research*, vol. 40, no. D1, pp. D222–D229, 2012.

[33] S.-D. Hsu, C.-H. Chu, A.-P. Tsou et al., "miRNAMap 2.0: genomic maps of MicroRNAs in metazoan genomes," *Nucleic Acids Research*, vol. 36, supplement 1, pp. D165–D169, 2008.

[34] H. Naeem, R. Küffner, G. Csaba, and R. Zimmer, "miRSel: automated extraction of associations between MicroRNAs and genes from the biomedical literature," *BMC Bioinformatics*, vol. 11, article 135, 2010.

[35] F. Xiao, Z. Zuo, G. Cai, S. Kang, X. Gao, and T. Li, "miRecords: an integrated resource for MicroRNA-target interactions," *Nucleic Acids Research*, vol. 37, supplement 1, pp. D105–D110, 2009.

[36] S.-D. Hsu, F.-M. Lin, W.-Y. Wu et al., "miRTarBase: a database curates experimentally validated MicroRNA-target interactions," *Nucleic Acids Research*, vol. 39, supplement 1, pp. D163–D169, 2011.

[37] H. Dweep, C. Sticht, P. Pandey, and N. Gretz, "miRWalk—database: prediction of possible miRNA binding sites by

" walking" the genes of three genomes," *Journal of Biomedical Informatics*, vol. 44, no. 5, pp. 839–847, 2011.

[38] J.-H. Yang, J.-H. Li, P. Shao, H. Zhou, Y.-Q. Chen, and L.-H. Qu, "StarBase: a database for exploring MicroRNA-mRNA interaction maps from Argonaute CLIP-Seq and Degradome-Seq data," *Nucleic Acids Research*, vol. 39, supplement 1, pp. D202–D209, 2011.

[39] H. Kim, S. Park, H. Min, and S. Yoon, "vHoT: a database for predicting interspecies interactions between viral MicroRNA and host genomes," *Archives of Virology*, vol. 157, no. 3, pp. 497–501, 2012.

[40] J. Huang, C. Townsend, D. Dou, H. Liu, and M. Tan, "OMIT: a domain-specific knowledge base for MicroRNA target prediction," *Pharmaceutical Research*, vol. 28, no. 12, pp. 3101–3104, 2011.

[41] Y. Wu, B. Wei, H. Liu, T. Li, and S. Rayner, "miRPara: a SVM-based software tool for prediction of most probable MicroRNA coding regions in genome scale sequences," *BMC Bioinformatics*, vol. 12, article 107, 2011.

[42] F. Navarro, D. Gutman, E. Meire et al., "miR-34a contributes to megakaryocytic differentiation of K562 cells independently of p53," *Blood*, vol. 114, no. 10, pp. 2181–2192, 2009.

[43] A. Ichimura, Y. Ruike, K. Terasawa, K. Shimizu, and G. Tsujimoto, "MicroRNA-34a inhibits cell proliferation by repressing mitogen-activated protein kinase kinase 1 during megakaryocytic differentiation of K562 cells," *Molecular Pharmacology*, vol. 77, no. 6, pp. 1016–1024, 2010.

[44] P. Romania, V. Lulli, E. Pelosi, M. Biffoni, C. Peschle, and G. Marziali, "MicroRNA 155 modulates megakaryopoiesis at progenitor and precursor level by targeting Ets-1 and Meis1 transcription factors," *British Journal of Haematology*, vol. 143, no. 4, pp. 570–580, 2008.

[45] D. T. Starczynowski, F. Kuchenbauer, B. Argiropoulos et al., "Identification of miR-145 and miR-146a as mediators of the 5q-syndrome phenotype," *Nature Medicine*, vol. 16, no. 1, pp. 49–58, 2010.

[46] J. B. Opalinska, A. Bersenev, Z. Zhang et al., "MicroRNA expression in maturing murine megakaryocytes," *Blood*, vol. 116, no. 23, pp. e128–e138, 2010.

[47] J. Lu, S. Guo, B. L. Ebert et al., "MicroRNA-mediated control of cell fate in megakaryocyte-erythrocyte progenitors," *Developmental Cell*, vol. 14, no. 6, pp. 843–853, 2008.

[48] C. F. Barroga, H. Pham, and K. Kaushansky, "Thrombopoietin regulates c-Myb expression by modulating micro RNA 150 expression," *Experimental Hematology*, vol. 36, no. 12, pp. 1585–1592, 2008.

[49] M. Girardot, C. Pecquet, S. Boukour et al., "miR-28 is a thrombopoietin receptor targeting MicroRNA detected in a fraction of myeloproliferative neoplasm patient platelets," *Blood*, vol. 116, no. 3, pp. 437–445, 2010.

[50] O. Ben-Ami, N. Pencovich, J. Lotem, D. Levanon, and Y. Groner, "A regulatory interplay between miR-27a and Runx1 during megakaryopoiesis," *Proceedings of the National Academy of Sciences of the United States of America*, vol. 106, no. 1, pp. 238–243, 2009.

[51] C. Guimaraes-Sternberg, A. Meerson, I. Shaked, and H. Soreq, "MicroRNA modulation of megakaryoblast fate involves cholinergic signaling," *Leukemia Research*, vol. 30, no. 5, pp. 583–595, 2006.

[52] J.-H. Klusmann, Z. Li, K. Böhmer et al., "miR-125b-2 is a potential oncomiR on human chromosome 21 in megakaryoblastic leukemia," *Genes and Development*, vol. 24, no. 5, pp. 478–490, 2010.

[53] X. Li, J. Zhang, L. Gao et al., "miR-181 mediates cell differentiation by interrupting the Lin28 and let-7 feedback circuit," *Cell Death and Differentiation*, vol. 19, no. 3, pp. 378–386, 2012.

[54] L. C. Dore, J. D. Amigo, C. O. Dos Santos et al., "A GATA-1-regulated MicroRNA locus essential for erythropoiesis," *Proceedings of the National Academy of Sciences of the United States of America*, vol. 105, no. 9, pp. 3333–3338, 2008.

[55] K. D. Rasmussen, S. Simmini, C. Abreu-Goodger et al., "The miR-144/451 locus is required for erythroid homeostasis," *Journal of Experimental Medicine*, vol. 207, no. 7, pp. 1351–1358, 2010.

[56] D. M. Patrick, C. C. Zhang, Y. Tao et al., "Defective erythroid differentiation in miR-451 mutant mice mediated by 14-3-3ζ," *Genes and Development*, vol. 24, no. 15, pp. 1614–1619, 2010.

[57] A. J. Warren, W. H. Colledge, M. B. L. Carlton, M. J. Evans, A. J. H. Smith, and T. H. Rabbitts, "The oncogenic cysteine-rich LIM domain protein rbtn2 is essential for erythroid development," *Cell*, vol. 78, no. 1, pp. 45–57, 1994.

[58] N. Felli, F. Pedini, P. Romania et al., "MicroRNA 223-dependent expression of LMO2 regulates normal erythropoiesis," *Haematologica*, vol. 94, no. 4, pp. 479–486, 2009.

[59] M. L. Choong, H. H. Yang, and I. McNiece, "MicroRNA expression profiling during human cord blood-derived CD34 cell erythropoiesis," *Experimental Hematology*, vol. 35, no. 4, pp. 551–564, 2007.

[60] S.-Y. Chen, Y. Wang, M. J. Telen, and J.-T. Chi, "The genomic analysis of erythrocyte MicroRNA expression in sickle cell diseases," *PLoS ONE*, vol. 3, no. 6, Article ID e2360, 2008.

[61] N. Felli, L. Fontana, E. Pelosi et al., "MicroRNAs 221 and 222 inhibit normal erythropoiesis and erythroleukemic cell growth via kit receptor down-modulation," *Proceedings of the National Academy of Sciences of the United States of America*, vol. 102, no. 50, pp. 18081–18086, 2005.

[62] Q. Wang, Z. Huang, H. Xue et al., "MicroRNA miR-24 inhibits erythropoiesis by targeting activin type I receptor ALK4," *Blood*, vol. 111, no. 2, pp. 588–595, 2008.

[63] H. Zhao, A. Kalota, S. Jin, and A. M. Gewirtz, "Autoregulatory feedback loop in human hematopoietic cells the c-myb proto-oncogene and MicroRNA-15a comprise an active," *Blood*, vol. 113, no. 3, pp. 505–516, 2009.

[64] Z. Li, J. Lu, M. Sun et al., "Distinct MicroRNA expression profiles in acute myeloid leukemia with common translocations," *Proceedings of the National Academy of Sciences of the United States of America*, vol. 105, no. 40, pp. 15535–15540, 2008.

[65] M. Eyholzer, S. Schmid, J. A. Schardt, S. Haefliger, B. U. Mueller, and T. Pabst, "Complexity of miR-223 regulation by CEBPA in human AML," *Leukemia Research*, vol. 34, no. 5, pp. 672–676, 2010.

[66] G. Cammarata, L. Augugliaro, D. Salemi et al., "Differential expression of specific MicroRNA and their targets in acute myeloid leukemia," *The American Journal of Hematology*, vol. 85, no. 5, pp. 331–339, 2010.

[67] B. Hackanson, K. L. Bennett, R. M. Brena et al., "Epigenetic modification of CCAAT/enhancer binding protein α expression in acute myeloid leukemia," *Cancer Research*, vol. 68, no. 9, pp. 3142–3151, 2008.

[68] M. He, Q. Y. Wang, Q. Q. Yin et al., "HIF-1alpha downregulates miR-17/20a directly targeting p21 and STAT3: a role in myeloid leukemic cell differentiation," *Cell Death Differentiation*, vol. 20, no. 3, pp. 408–418, 2013.

[69] R. Garzon, S. Liu, M. Fabbri et al., "MicroRNA-29b induces global DNA hypomethylation and tumor suppressor gene reexpression in acute myeloid leukemia by targeting directly DNMT3A and 3B and indirectly DNMT1," *Blood*, vol. 113, no. 25, pp. 6411–6418, 2009.

[70] E. Coskun, E. K. von der Heide, C. Schlee et al., "The role of MicroRNA-196a and MicroRNA-196b as ERG regulators in acute myeloid leukemia and acute T-lymphoblastic leukemia," *Leukemia Research*, vol. 35, no. 2, pp. 208–213, 2011.

[71] X.-N. Gao, J. Lin, L. Gao, Y.-H. Li, L.-L. Wang, and L. Yu, "MicroRNA-193b regulates c-Kit proto-oncogene and represses cell proliferation in acute myeloid leukemia," *Leukemia Research*, vol. 35, no. 9, pp. 1226–1232, 2011.

[72] L. Venturini, K. Battmer, M. Castoldi et al., "Expression of the miR-17-92 polycistron in chronic myeloid leukemia (CML) CD34+ cells," *Blood*, vol. 109, no. 10, pp. 4399–4405, 2007.

[73] H. Hu, Y. Li, J. Gu et al., "Antisense oligonucleotide against miR-21 inhibits migration and induces apoptosis in leukemic K562 cells," *Leukemia and Lymphoma*, vol. 51, no. 4, pp. 694–701, 2010.

[74] C. S. Chim, K. Y. Wong, C. Y. Leung et al., "Epigenetic inactivation of the hsa-miR-203 in haematological malignancies," *Journal of Cellular and Molecular Medicine*, vol. 15, no. 12, pp. 2760–2767, 2011.

[75] T. Lopotová, M. Žáčková, H. Klamová, and J. Moravcová, "MicroRNA-451 in chronic myeloid leukemia: miR-451-BCR-ABL regulatory loop?" *Leukemia Research*, vol. 35, no. 7, pp. 974–977, 2011.

[76] Y. Li, H. Wang, K. Tao et al., "miR-29b suppresses CML cell proliferation and induces apoptosis via regulation of BCR/ABL1 protein," *Experimental Cell Research*, vol. 319, no. 8, pp. 1094–1101, 2013.

[77] C. Xu, H. Fu, L. Gao et al., "BCR-ABL/GATA1/miR-138 mini circuitry contributes to the leukemogenesis of chronic myeloid leukemia," *Oncogene*, 2012.

[78] E. Turrini, S. Haenisch, S. Laechelt, T. Diewock, O. Bruhn, and I. Cascorbi, "MicroRNA profiling in K-562 cells under imatinib treatment: influence of miR-212 and miR-328 on ABCG2 expression," *Pharmacogenetics and Genomics*, vol. 22, no. 3, pp. 198–205, 2012.

[79] J. Han, Y. Lee, K.-H. Yeom, Y.-K. Kim, H. Jin, and V. N. Kim, "The Drosha-DGCR8 complex in primary MicroRNA processing," *Genes and Development*, vol. 18, no. 24, pp. 3016–3027, 2004.

[80] J. G. Ruby, C. H. Jan, and D. P. Bartel, "Intronic MicroRNA precursors that bypass Drosha processing," *Nature*, vol. 448, no. 7149, pp. 83–86, 2007.

[81] E. Lund, S. Güttinger, A. Calado, J. E. Dahlberg, and U. Kutay, "Nuclear export of MicroRNA precursors," *Science*, vol. 303, no. 5654, pp. 95–98, 2004.

[82] T. P. Chendrimada, R. I. Gregory, E. Kumaraswamy et al., "TRBP recruits the Dicer complex to Ago2 for MicroRNA processing and gene silencing," *Nature*, vol. 436, no. 7051, pp. 740–744, 2005.

[83] A. D. Haase, L. Jaskiewicz, H. Zhang et al., "TRBP, a regulator of cellular PKR and HIV-1 virus expression, interacts with Dicer and functions in RNA silencing," *EMBO Reports*, vol. 6, no. 10, pp. 961–967, 2005.

[84] S. Singh, S. C. Bevan, K. Patil, D. C. Newton, and P. A. Marsden, "Extensive variation in the 5′-UTR of Dicer mRNAs influences translational efficiency," *Biochemical and Biophysical Research Communications*, vol. 335, no. 3, pp. 643–650, 2005.

[85] D. P. Bartel, "MicroRNAs: target recognition and regulatory functions," *Cell*, vol. 136, no. 2, pp. 215–233, 2009.

[86] I. Behm-Ansmant, J. Rehwinkel, T. Doerks, A. Stark, P. Bork, and E. Izaurralde, "mRNA degradation by miRNAs and GW182 requires both CCR4:NOT deadenylase and DCP1:DCP2 decapping complexes," *Genes and Development*, vol. 20, no. 14, pp. 1885–1898, 2006.

[87] E. van Rooij, "The art of MicroRNA research," *Circulation Research*, vol. 108, no. 2, pp. 219–234, 2011.

[88] L. F. Sempere, S. Freemantle, I. Pitha-Rowe, E. Moss, E. Dmitrovsky, and V. Ambros, "Expression profiling of mammalian MicroRNAs uncovers a subset of brain-expressed MicroRNAs with possible roles in murine and human neuronal differentiation," *Genome Biology*, vol. 5, no. 3, article R13, 2004.

[89] O. Barad, E. Meiri, A. Avniel et al., "MicroRNA expression detected by oligonucleotide Microarrays: system establishment and expression profiling in human tissues," *Genome Research*, vol. 14, no. 12, pp. 2486–2494, 2004.

[90] C. Chen, D. A. Ridzon, A. J. Broomer et al., "Real-time quantification of MicroRNAs by stem-loop RT-PCR," *Nucleic Acids Research*, vol. 33, no. 20, article e179, 2005.

[91] S. W. Chi, J. B. Zang, A. Mele, and R. B. Darnell, "Argonaute HITS-CLIP decodes MicroRNA-mRNA interaction maps," *Nature*, vol. 460, no. 7254, pp. 479–486, 2009.

[92] D. Baek, J. Villén, C. Shin, F. D. Camargo, S. P. Gygi, and D. P. Bartel, "The impact of MicroRNAs on protein output," *Nature*, vol. 455, no. 7209, pp. 64–71, 2008.

[93] J. Vinther, M. M. Hedegaard, P. P. Gardner, J. S. Andersen, and P. Arctander, "Identification of miRNA targets with stable isotope labeling by amino acids in cell culture," *Nucleic Acids Research*, vol. 34, no. 16, article e107, 2006.

[94] A. Cimmino, G. A. Calin, M. Fabbri et al., "miR-15 and miR-16 induce apoptosis by targeting BCL2," *Proceedings of the National Academy of Sciences of the United States of America*, vol. 102, no. 39, pp. 13944–13949, 2005.

[95] K.-H. Lee, Y.-L. Chen, S.-D. Yeh et al., "MicroRNA-330 acts as tumor suppressor and induces apoptosis of prostate cancer cells through E2F1-mediated suppression of Akt phosphorylation," *Oncogene*, vol. 28, no. 38, pp. 3360–3370, 2009.

[96] J. A. Chan, A. M. Krichevsky, and K. S. Kosik, "MicroRNA-21 is an antiapoptotic factor in human glioblastoma cells," *Cancer Research*, vol. 65, no. 14, pp. 6029–6033, 2005.

[97] V. Plaisance, A. Abderrahmani, V. Perret-Menoud, P. Jacquemin, F. Lemaigre, and R. Regazzi, "MicroRNA-9 controls the expression of Granuphilin/Slp4 and the secretory response of insulin-producing cells," *Journal of Biological Chemistry*, vol. 281, no. 37, pp. 26932–26942, 2006.

[98] T. Melkman-Zehavi, R. Oren, S. Kredo-Russo et al., "miRNAs control insulin content in pancreatic β-cells via downregulation of transcriptional repressors," *The EMBO Journal*, vol. 30, no. 5, pp. 835–845, 2011.

[99] C. Esau, S. Davis, S. F. Murray et al., "miR-122 regulation of lipid metabolism revealed by in vivo antisense targeting," *Cell Metabolism*, vol. 3, no. 2, pp. 87–98, 2006.

[100] J. Elmén, M. Lindow, A. Silahtaroglu et al., "Antagonism of MicroRNA-122 in mice by systemically administered LNA-antimiR leads to up-regulation of a large set of predicted target mRNAs in the liver," *Nucleic Acids Research*, vol. 36, no. 4, pp. 1153–1162, 2008.

[101] K. J. Rayner, F. J. Sheedy, C. C. Esau et al., "Antagonism of miR-33 in mice promotes reverse cholesterol transport and regression

of atherosclerosis," *Journal of Clinical Investigation*, vol. 121, no. 7, pp. 2921–2931, 2011.

[102] K. J. Rayner, Y. Suárez, A. Dávalos et al., "miR-33 contributes to the regulation of cholesterol homeostasis," *Science*, vol. 328, no. 5985, pp. 1570–1573, 2010.

[103] R. W. Georgantas III, R. Hildreth, S. Morisot et al., "CD34+ hematopoietic stem-progenitor cell MicroRNA expression and function: a circuit diagram of differentiation control," *Proceedings of the National Academy of Sciences of the United States of America*, vol. 104, no. 8, pp. 2750–2755, 2007.

[104] A. Marson, S. S. Levine, M. F. Cole et al., "Connecting MicroRNA genes to the core transcriptional regulatory circuitry of embryonic stem cells," *Cell*, vol. 134, no. 3, pp. 521–533, 2008.

[105] C.-Z. Chen, L. Li, H. F. Lodish, and D. P. Bartel, "MicroRNAs modulate hematopoietic lineage differentiation," *Science*, vol. 303, no. 5654, pp. 83–86, 2004.

[106] S. B. Koralov, S. A. Muljo, G. R. Galler et al., "Dicer ablation affects antibody diversity and cell survival in the B lymphocyte lineage," *Cell*, vol. 132, no. 5, pp. 860–874, 2008.

[107] X. Liu, Z. Zhan, L. Xu et al., "MicroRNA-148/152 impair innate response and antigen presentation of TLR-triggered dendritic cells by targeting CaMKIIα," *The Journal of Immunology*, vol. 185, no. 12, pp. 7244–7251, 2010.

[108] C.-P. Mao, L. He, Y.-C. Tsai et al., "In vivo MicroRNA-155 expression influences antigen-specific T cell-mediated immune responses generated by DNA vaccination," *Cell and Bioscience*, vol. 1, no. 1, article 3, 2011.

[109] E. Bernstein, S. Y. Kim, M. A. Carmell et al., "Dicer is essential for mouse development," *Nature Genetics*, vol. 35, no. 3, pp. 215–217, 2003.

[110] B. S. Cobb, T. B. Nesterova, E. Thompson et al., "T cell lineage choice and differentiation in the absence of the RNase III enzyme Dicer," *Journal of Experimental Medicine*, vol. 201, no. 9, pp. 1367–1373, 2005.

[111] K. D. Taganov, M. P. Boldin, K.-J. Chang, and D. Baltimore, "NF-κB-dependent induction of MicroRNA miR-146, an inhibitor targeted to signaling proteins of innate immune responses," *Proceedings of the National Academy of Sciences of the United States of America*, vol. 103, no. 33, pp. 12481–12486, 2006.

[112] C. Labbaye, I. Spinello, M. T. Quaranta et al., "A three-step pathway comprising PLZF/miR-146a/CXCR4 controls megakaryopoiesis," *Nature Cell Biology*, vol. 10, no. 7, pp. 788–801, 2008.

[113] R. Garzon, F. Pichiorri, T. Palumbo et al., "MicroRNA fingerprints during human megakaryocytopoiesis," *Proceedings of the National Academy of Sciences of the United States of America*, vol. 103, no. 13, pp. 5078–5083, 2006.

[114] I. Azzouzi, H. Moest, J. Winkler et al., "Microrna-96 directly inhibits γ-globin expression in human erythropoiesis," *PLoS ONE*, vol. 6, no. 7, Article ID e22838, 2011.

[115] R. J. Mayoral, L. Deho, N. Rusca et al., "miR-221 influences effector functions and actin cytoskeleton in mast cells," *PLoS ONE*, vol. 6, no. 10, Article ID e26133, 2011.

[116] T. Ishizaki, T. Tamiya, K. Taniguchi et al., "miR126 positively regulates mast cell proliferation and cytokine production through suppressing Spred1," *Genes to Cells*, vol. 16, no. 7, pp. 803–814, 2011.

[117] R. J. Mayoral, M. E. Pipkin, M. Pachkov, E. van Nimwegen, A. Rao, and S. Monticelli, "MicroRNA-221-222 regulate the cell cycle in mast cells," *The Journal of Immunology*, vol. 182, no. 1, pp. 433–445, 2009.

[118] E. Surdziel, M. Cabanski, I. Dallmann et al., "Enforced expression of miR-125b affects myelopoiesis by targeting multiple signaling pathways," *Blood*, vol. 117, no. 16, pp. 4338–4348, 2011.

[119] F. Fazi, S. Racanicchi, G. Zardo et al., "Epigenetic silencing of the myelopoiesis regulator MicroRNA-223 by the AML1/ETO oncoprotein," *Cancer Cell*, vol. 12, no. 5, pp. 457–466, 2007.

[120] A. Ventura, A. G. Young, M. M. Winslow et al., "Targeted deletion reveals essential and overlapping functions of the miR-17~92 family of miRNA clusters," *Cell*, vol. 132, no. 5, pp. 875–886, 2008.

[121] C. S. Velu, A. M. Baktula, and H. L. Grimes, "Gfi1 regulates miR-21 and miR-196b to control myelopoiesis," *Blood*, vol. 113, no. 19, pp. 4720–4728, 2009.

[122] E. Tenedini, E. Roncaglia, F. Ferrari et al., "Integrated analysis of MicroRNA and mRNA expression profiles in physiological myelopoiesis: role of hsa-miR-299-5p in CD34+ progenitor cells commitment," *Cell Death and Disease*, vol. 1, no. 2, article e28, 2010.

[123] S. Kuchen, W. Resch, A. Yamane et al., "Regulation of MicroRNA expression and abundance during lymphopoiesis," *Immunity*, vol. 32, no. 6, pp. 828–839, 2010.

[124] J. Mattes, A. Collison, M. Plank, S. Phipps, and P. S. Foster, "Antagonism of MicroRNA-126 suppresses the effector function of T H2 cells and the development of allergic airways disease," *Proceedings of the National Academy of Sciences of the United States of America*, vol. 106, no. 44, pp. 18704–18709, 2009.

[125] A. Collison, J. Mattes, M. Plank, and P. S. Foster, "Inhibition of house dust mite-induced allergic airways disease by antagonism of MicroRNA-145 is comparable to glucocorticoid treatment," *Journal of Allergy and Clinical Immunology*, vol. 128, no. 1, pp. 160–167, 2011.

[126] F. Allantaz, D. T. Cheng, T. Bergauer et al., "Expression profiling of human immune cell subsets identifies miRNA-mRNA regulatory relationships correlated with cell type specific expression," *PLoS ONE*, vol. 7, no. 1, Article ID e29979, 2012.

[127] C. K. Wong, K. M. Lau, I. H. S. Chan et al., "MicroRNA-21* regulates the prosurvival effect of GM-CSF on human eosinophils," *Immunobiology*, vol. 218, no. 2, pp. 255–262, 2013.

[128] J. Batliner, E. Buehrer, E. A. Federzoni et al., "Transcriptional regulation of miR29B by PU.1 (SPI1) and MYC during neutrophil differentiation of acute promyelocytic leukaemia cells," *British Journal of Haematology*, vol. 157, no. 2, pp. 270–274, 2012.

[129] J. B. Johnnidis, M. H. Harris, R. T. Wheeler et al., "Regulation of progenitor cell proliferation and granulocyte function by MicroRNA-223," *Nature*, vol. 451, no. 7182, pp. 1125–1129, 2008.

[130] J. R. Ward, P. R. Heath, J. W. Catto, M. K. B. Whyte, M. Milo, and S. A. Renshaw, "Regulation of neutrophil senescence by MicroRNAs," *PLoS ONE*, vol. 6, no. 1, Article ID e15810, 2011.

[131] F. Bazzoni, M. Rossato, M. Fabbri et al., "Induction and regulatory function of miR-9 in human monocytes and neutrophils exposed to proinflammatory signals," *Proceedings of the National Academy of Sciences of the United States of America*, vol. 106, no. 13, pp. 5282–5287, 2009.

[132] T. Zhong, J. M. Perelman, V. P. Kolosov, and X.-D. Zhou, "miR-146a negatively regulates neutrophil elastase-induced MUC5AC secretion from 16HBE human bronchial epithelial cells," *Molecular and Cellular Biochemistry*, vol. 358, no. 1-2, pp. 249–255, 2011.

[133] B. Izumi, T. Nakasa, N. Tanaka et al., "MicroRNA-223 expression in neutrophils in the early phase of secondary damage after spinal cord injury," *Neuroscience Letters*, vol. 492, no. 2, pp. 114–118, 2011.

[134] S. Slezak, P. Jin, L. Caruccio et al., "Gene and MicroRNA analysis of neutrophils from patients with polycythemia vera and essential thrombocytosis: down-regulation of MicroRNA-1 and -133a," *Journal of Translational Medicine*, vol. 7, article 39, 2009.

[135] S. Radom-Aizik, F. Zaldivar Jr., S. Oliver, P. Galassetti, and D. M. Cooper, "Evidence for MicroRNA involvement in exercise-associated neutrophil gene expression changes," *Journal of Applied Physiology*, vol. 109, no. 1, pp. 252–261, 2010.

[136] C. Schmelzer, M. Kitano, G. Rimbach et al., "Effects of ubiquinol-10 on MicroRNA-146a expression in vitro and in vivo," *Mediators of Inflammation*, vol. 2009, Article ID 415437, 7 pages, 2009.

[137] M. Etzrodt, V. Cortez-Retamozo, A. Newton et al., "Regulation of monocyte functional heterogeneity by miR-146aand Relb," *Cell Reports*, vol. 1, no. 4, pp. 317–324, 2012.

[138] K. M. Pauley, C. M. Stewart, A. E. Gauna et al., "Altered miR-146a expression in Sjögren's syndrome and its functional role in innate immunity," *European Journal of Immunology*, vol. 41, no. 7, pp. 2029–2039, 2011.

[139] E. Cocco, F. Paladini, G. Macino, V. Fulci, M. T. Fiorillo, and R. Sorrentino, "The expression of vasoactive intestinal peptide receptor 1 is negatively modulated by MicroRNA 525-5p," *PLoS ONE*, vol. 5, no. 8, Article ID e12067, 2010.

[140] A. T. Conrad and B. N. Dittel, "Taming of macrophage and Microglial cell activation by MicroRNA-124," *Cell Research*, vol. 21, no. 2, pp. 213–216, 2011.

[141] E. Tili, J.-J. Michaille, B. Adair et al., "Resveratrol decreases the levels of miR-155 by upregulating miR-663, a MicroRNA targeting JunB and JunD," *Carcinogenesis*, vol. 31, no. 9, pp. 1561–1566, 2010.

[142] S. Sharbati, J. Sharbati, L. Hoeke, M. Bohmer, and R. Einspanier, "Quantification and accurate normalisation of small RNAs through new custom RT-qPCR arrays demonstrates Salmonella-induced MicroRNAs in human monocytes," *BMC Genomics*, vol. 13, no. 1, article 23, 2012.

[143] H. Wu, J. R. Neilson, P. Kumar et al., "miRNA profiling of naïve, effector and memory CD8 T cells," *PLoS ONE*, vol. 2, no. 10, Article ID e1020, 2007.

[144] R. Sandberg, J. R. Neilson, A. Sarma, P. A. Sharp, and C. B. Burge, "Proliferating cells express mRNAs with shortened 3′ untranslated regions and fewer MicroRNA target sites," *Science*, vol. 320, no. 5883, pp. 1643–1647, 2008.

[145] B. S. Cobb, A. Hertweck, J. Smith et al., "A role for Dicer in immune regulation," *Journal of Experimental Medicine*, vol. 203, no. 11, pp. 2519–2527, 2006.

[146] A. Liston, L.-F. Lu, D. O'Carroll, A. Tarakhovsky, and A. Y. Rudensky, "Dicer-dependent MicroRNA pathway safeguards regulatory T cell function," *Journal of Experimental Medicine*, vol. 205, no. 9, pp. 1993–2004, 2008.

[147] T. M. Laufer, "T-cell sensitivity: a MicroRNA regulates the sensitivity of the T-cell receptor," *Immunology and Cell Biology*, vol. 85, no. 5, pp. 346–347, 2007.

[148] E. L. Virts and M. L. Thoman, "Age-associated changes in miRNA expression profiles in thymopoiesis," *Mechanisms of Ageing and Development*, vol. 131, no. 11-12, pp. 743–748, 2010.

[149] M. Ohyashiki, J. H. Ohyashiki, A. Hirota, C. Kobayashi, and K. Ohyashiki, "Age-related decrease of miRNA-92a levels in human CD8+ T-cells correlates with a reduction of naïve T lymphocytes," *Immunity & Ageing*, vol. 8, article 11, 2011.

[150] J. Li, Y. Wan, Q. Guo et al., "Altered MicroRNA expression profile with miR-146a upregulation in CD4+ T cells from patients with rheumatoid arthritis," *Arthritis Research & Therapy*, vol. 12, no. 3, article R81, 2010.

[151] G. Almanza, A. Fernandez, S. Volinia, X. Cortez-Gonzalez, C. M. Croce, and M. Zanetti, "Selected MicroRNAs define cell fate determination of murine central memory CD8 T cells," *PLoS ONE*, vol. 5, no. 6, Article ID e11243, 2010.

[152] L. P. Tan, M. Wang, J.-L. Robertus et al., "miRNA profiling of B-cell subsets: specific miRNA profile for germinal center B cells with variation between centroblasts and centrocytes," *Laboratory Investigation*, vol. 89, no. 6, pp. 708–716, 2009.

[153] C. Xiao, D. P. Calado, G. Galler et al., "miR-150 controls B cell differentiation by targeting the transcription factor c-Myb," *Cell*, vol. 131, no. 1, pp. 146–159, 2007.

[154] E. Vigorito, K. L. Perks, C. Abreu-Goodger et al., "MicroRNA-155 regulates the generation of immunoglobulin class-switched plasma cells," *Immunity*, vol. 27, no. 6, pp. 847–859, 2007.

[155] G. A. Calin, C. D. Dumitru, M. Shimizu et al., "Frequent deletions and down-regulation of Micro-RNA genes miR15 and miR16 at 13q14 in chronic lymphocytic leukemia," *Proceedings of the National Academy of Sciences of the United States of America*, vol. 99, no. 24, pp. 15524–15529, 2002.

[156] "Cancer Facts & Figures 2012," 2012, http://www.cancer.org/research/cancerfactsfigures/cancerfactsfigures/cancer-facts.

[157] S. Faderl, M. Talpaz, Z. Estrov, and H. M. Kantarjian, "Chronic myelogenous leukemia: biology and therapy," *Annals of Internal Medicine*, vol. 131, no. 3, pp. 207–219, 1999.

[158] O. H. Rokah, G. Granot, A. Ovcharenko et al., "Downregulation of miR-31, miR-155, and miR-564 in chronic myeloid leukemia cells," *PLoS ONE*, vol. 7, no. 4, Article ID e35501, 2012.

[159] K. Machova Polakova, T. Lopotova, H. Klamova et al., "Expression patterns of MicroRNAs associated with CML phases and their disease related targets," *Molecular Cancer*, vol. 10, article 41, 2011.

[160] J. Fei, Y. Li, X. Zhu, and X. Luo, "miR-181a post-transcriptionally downregulates oncogenic rala and contributes to growth inhibition and apoptosis in chronic myelogenous leukemia (CML)," *PLoS ONE*, vol. 7, no. 3, Article ID e32834, 2012.

[161] S. Suresh, L. McCallum, W. Lu, N. Lazar, B. Perbal, and A. E. Irvine, "MicroRNAs 130a/b are regulated by BCR-ABL and downregulate expression of CCN3 in CML," *Journal of Cell Communication and Signaling*, vol. 5, no. 3, pp. 183–191, 2011.

[162] K. Bommert, R. C. Bargou, and T. Stühmer, "Signalling and survival pathways in multiple myeloma," *European Journal of Cancer*, vol. 42, no. 11, pp. 1574–1580, 2006.

[163] A. Mahindra, T. Hideshima, and K. C. Anderson, "Multiple myeloma: biology of the disease," *Blood Reviews*, vol. 24, supplement 1, pp. S5–S11, 2010.

[164] R. A. Kyle and S. V. Rajkumar, "Multiple myeloma," *Blood*, vol. 111, no. 6, pp. 2962–2972, 2008.

[165] S. L. Corthals, S. M. Sun, R. Kuiper et al., "MicroRNA signatures characterize multiple myeloma patients," *Leukemia*, vol. 25, no. 11, pp. 1784–1789, 2011.

[166] C. I. Jones, M. V. Zabolotskaya, A. J. King et al., "Identification of circulating MicroRNAs as diagnostic biomarkers for use in multiple myeloma," *British Journal of Cancer*, vol. 107, no. 12, pp. 1987–1996, 2012.

[167] Y. Zhou, L. Chen, B. Barlogie et al., "High-risk myeloma is associated with global elevation of miRNAs and overexpression of EIF2C2/AGO2," *Proceedings of the National Academy of*

Sciences of the United States of America, vol. 107, no. 17, pp. 7904–7909, 2010.

[168] A. M. Roccaro, A. Sacco, B. Thompson et al., "MicroRNAs 15a and 16 regulate tumor proliferation in multiple myeloma," *Blood*, vol. 113, no. 26, pp. 6669–6680, 2009.

[169] S. L. Corthals, M. Jongen-Lavrencic, Y. de Knegt et al., "Micro-RNA-15a and Micro-RNA-16 expression and chromosome 13 deletions in multiple myeloma," *Leukemia Research*, vol. 34, no. 5, pp. 677–681, 2010.

[170] L. Chen, C. Li, R. Zhang et al., "miR-17-92 cluster MicroRNAs confers tumorigenicity in multiple myeloma," *Cancer Letters*, vol. 309, no. 1, pp. 62–70, 2011.

[171] Y.-K. Zhang, H. Wang, Y. Leng et al., "Overexpression of MicroRNA-29b induces apoptosis of multiple myeloma cells through down regulating Mcl-1," *Biochemical and Biophysical Research Communications*, vol. 414, no. 1, pp. 233–239, 2011.

[172] K. Unno, Y. Zhou, T. Zimmerman, L. C. Platanias, and A. Wickrema, "Identification of a novel MicroRNA cluster miR-193b-365 in multiple myeloma," *Leukemia and Lymphoma*, vol. 50, no. 11, pp. 1865–1871, 2009.

[173] S. Adamia, H. Avet-Loiseau, S. B. Amin et al., "Clinical and biological significance of MicroRNA profiling in patients with myeloma," *Journal of Clinical Oncology*, vol. 27, supplement 15, p. 8539, 2009.

[174] X. Gao, R. Zhang, X. Qu et al., "miR-15a, miR-16-1 and miR-17-92 cluster expression are linked to poor prognosis in multiple myeloma," *Leukemia Research*, vol. 36, no. 12, pp. 1505–1509, 2012.

[175] J. Chi, E. Ballabio, X.-H. Chen et al., "MicroRNA expression in multiple myeloma is associated with genetic subtype, isotype and survival," *Biology Direct*, vol. 6, article 23, 2011.

10

Development and Characterization of Anti-Nitr9 Antibodies

Radhika N. Shah,[1,2] Ivan Rodriguez-Nunez,[1] Donna D. Eason,[3,4]
Robert N. Haire,[3] Julien Y. Bertrand,[5] Valērie Wittamer,[6] David Traver,[6]
Shila K. Nordone,[1,2] Gary W. Litman,[3,4,7] and Jeffrey A. Yoder[1,2]

[1] Department of Molecular Biomedical Sciences and Center for Comparative Medicine and Translational Research,
   College of Veterinary Medicine, North Carolina State University, 1060 William Moore Drive, Raleigh, NC 27607, USA
[2] Immunology Program, College of Veterinary Medicine, North Carolina State University, 1060 William Moore Drive,
   Raleigh, NC 27607, USA
[3] Children's Research Institute, Department of Pediatrics, University of South Florida College of Medicine, 140 Seventh Avenue South,
   St. Petersburg, FL 33701, USA
[4] Immunology Program, H. Lee Moffitt Cancer Center and Research Institute, 12902 Magnolia Avenue, Tampa, FL 33612, USA
[5] Department of Pathology and Immunology, University of Geneva School of Medicine, Rue Michel-Servet 1, 1211 Geneva 4, Switzerland
[6] Department of Cellular and Molecular Medicine and Section of Cell and Developmental Biology, University of California at San Diego,
   9500 Gilman Drive, La Jolla, CA 92093-0380, USA
[7] Department of Molecular Genetics, All Children's Hospital, 501 Sixth Avenue South, St. Petersburg, FL 33701, USA

Correspondence should be addressed to Jeffrey A. Yoder, jeff_yoder@ncsu.edu

Academic Editor: Christopher Hall

The novel immune-type receptors (NITRs), which have been described in numerous bony fish species, are encoded by multigene families of inhibitory and activating receptors and are predicted to be functional orthologs to the mammalian natural killer cell receptors (NKRs). Within the zebrafish NITR family, *nitr9* is the only gene predicted to encode an activating receptor. However, alternative RNA splicing generates three distinct *nitr9* transcripts, each of which encodes a different isoform. Although *nitr9* transcripts have been detected in zebrafish lymphocytes, the specific hematopoietic lineage(s) that expresses Nitr9 remains to be determined. In an effort to better understand the role of NITRs in zebrafish immunity, anti-Nitr9 monoclonal antibodies were generated and evaluated for the ability to recognize the three Nitr9 isoforms. The application of these antibodies to flow cytometry should prove to be useful for identifying the specific lymphocyte lineages that express Nitr9 and may permit the isolation of Nitr9-expressing cells that can be directly assessed for cytotoxic (e.g., NK) function.

1. Introduction

Mammalian natural killer (NK) cells are large, granular lymphocytes of the innate immune system that express several cell surface receptors to regulate cytotoxic function through a complex network of signaling pathways. NK cell receptors include both activating and inhibitory forms that are proficient in distinguishing neoplastic or virally infected cells from normal host cells [1, 2]. The regulation of NK cell cytotoxicity is dependent on the integration of signals from activating and inhibitory receptors [3]. Although it is postulated that NK cell receptors arose early in vertebrate phylogeny, functional data are based primarily on studies of mammalian NK cell receptors [4].

In order to appreciate the origins and evolution of NK cell receptors and their function, it is critical to define equivalent receptor forms in nonmammalian species. The bony fish represent one of the earliest vertebrate lineages with a functional innate and adaptive immune response that closely parallels that of humans and other mammals [5]. A large multigene family of recently and rapidly evolving inhibitory and activating novel immune-type receptors (NITRs) that share structural and functional characteristics with mammalian NK cell receptors has been identified in multiple fish species [6, 7]. Complete analyses of the NITR gene clusters at the sequence level only have been performed with the zebrafish and medaka genomes [8–11]. Although transcripts of various catfish NITRs have been detected in NK-like, T, B, and macrophage cell lines [12], transcripts of all zebrafish NITRs are detectable in the lymphoid, but not the myeloid, lineage [13]. Of the 39 NITR genes that have been identified within the zebrafish genome, *nitr9* is the only NITR gene that is predicted to encode an activating receptor [10, 11, 14]. Three alternatively spliced transcripts of *nitr9* have been characterized: Nitr9-long (Nitr9L), Nitr9-short (Nitr9S), and Nitr9-supershort (Nitr9SS), which differ in their extracellular domains [13, 14]. Nitr9L is the most similar to other NITRs in that it possesses two extracellular Ig domains: one of the variable (V) type and one of the intermediate (I) type [6]. Nitr9S arises through cryptic splice donor and acceptor sites within the exon encoding the V domain. Nitr9SS lacks the entire V domain exon. The transmembrane domain of all Nitr9 isoforms possesses a positively charged residue: this feature permits Nitr9L to associate with and signal through the adaptor protein Dap12 [14]. Based on protein structures, Nitr9S and Nitr9SS also are expected to signal via Dap12; however, this has not been verified experimentally.

Although *nitr9* transcripts have been detected in zebrafish lymphocytes, the identification and recovery of Nitr9-expressing cells has not been possible. Herein we describe the derivation of two anti-Nitr9 monoclonal antibodies, demonstrate their utility to recognize recombinant Nitr9 by indirect immunofluorescence, flow cytometry, and Western blot analyses, and subsequently identify all three Nitr9 isoforms in zebrafish tissues by Western blot analyses. These antibodies should prove useful for: (1) evaluating Nitr9 protein levels within tissues by Western blot, (2) evaluating the distribution of Nitr9 expressing cells within tissues by indirect immunofluorescence, (3) defining the specific hematopoietic lineage(s) that express Nitr9 by flow cytometry, and (4) purifying Nitr9 expressing cells by fluorescence-activated cell sorting (FACS) for functional characterization.

2. Materials and Methods

2.1. Zebrafish. All experiments involving live zebrafish (*Danio rerio*) were performed in accordance with relevant institutional and national guidelines and regulations and were approved by the North Carolina State University Institutional Animal Care and Use Committee. Adult zebrafish (EkkWill Waterlife Resources, Ruskin, FL) were maintained and sacrificed as described [15].

2.2. Reverse Transcriptase-PCR. Total RNA from dissected zebrafish tissues (2 μg) was reverse transcribed (SuperScript III Reverse Transcriptase, Life Technologies, Carlsbad, CA), and cDNAs were subjected to thermal cycling with gene-specific primers (Table 1) and Titanium *Taq* DNA polymerase (Clontech, Mountain View, CA). The number of PCR cycles used for detecting nitr9 and β-actin (both annealing at 65∘C) was 40 and 25, respectively.

Lymphoid and myeloid cell populations were purified from the kidney of multiple zebrafish and pooled as described [16]. Total RNA from isolated cells (1 μg) was reverse transcribed (SuperScript III Reverse Transcriptase). cDNAs from tissues and isolated cells were subjected to quantitative PCR (Q-PCR) with TaqMan primers and probes (Life Technologies, Carlsbad, CA) (Table 1). Q-PCR was performed on a single-color MyiQ real-time PCR detection system (Bio-Rad, Hercules, CA) using the protocol: 50∘C for 2 min, 95∘C for 10 min, followed by 55 cycles at 95∘C for 15 s and at 60∘C for 1 min. The threshold cycle (C_T) value was calculated by the iQ5 Optical System Software (Bio-Rad). Relative transcript levels of nitr9 were normalized to β-actin and calculated using the $2^{-\Delta\Delta C_T}$ method [17]. All reactions were carried out as technical triplicates.

2.3. Antibody Development and Purification. The coding sequence of the Nitr9 I domain (nucleotides 298–623 of GenBank NM_001005576.1) was amplified by PCR (Table 1) and cloned into pETBlue-1 (EMD Millipore, Billerica, MA), and *E. coli* Tuner cells (EMD Millipore) were transformed employing a standard procedure. Cells were induced, and the Nitr9 I domain was recovered from inclusion bodies.

Swiss Webster mice were immunized with the Nitr9 I domain expressed in *E. coli* and splenocytes were fused with P3X63Ag8.653 cells (CRL-1580, ATCC, Manassas, VA). Approximately 3,000 individual hybridoma supernatants were screened by an enzyme-linked immunosorbent assay (ELISA) against the denatured recombinant Nitr9 I domain (Immunology Core Facility, University of North Carolina, Chapel Hill). The most strongly reactive ~100 supernatants in turn were screened by parallel Western blot analyses and indirect immunofluorescence. Two single clones, 19.1.1 (herein referred to as anti-Nitr9[19]) and 90.10.5 (herein referred to as anti-Nitr9[90]), were selected for additional characterization based on their ability to recognize recombinant Nitr9. Antibody isotypes were determined (IsoStrips: Roche; Indianapolis, IN) to be IgG2b, κ light chain (90.10.5), and IgG2a, κ light chain (19.1.1). Antibodies were purified via protein A agarose columns (Upstate Cell Signaling Solutions; Lake Placid, NY).

2.4. Plasmids and Cell Culture. Nitr9 expression cassettes (without epitope tags) were constructed with *pcDNA3* (Life Technologies). Epitope (FLAG)-tagged Nitr9 (FLAG-Nitr9) expression cassettes were constructed with the *pLF* plasmid which incorporates an amino-terminal leader sequence and FLAG epitope [14]. The coding sequences of zebrafish *nitr9L*, *nitr9S*, and *nitr9SS* were amplified by PCR and cloned into *pcDNA3* or *pLF*. Nitr9 and FLAG-Nitr9 cassettes were then shuttled into *pIRES2-EGFP* (Clontech) generating: *pNitr9L/EGFP*, *pNitr9S/EGFP*, *pNitr9SS/EGFP*, *pFLAG-Nitr9L/EGFP*, *pFLAG-Nitr9S/EGFP*, and *pFLAG-Nitr9SS/EGFP* plasmids (Figure 1). Primer sequences that were used in cloning steps are included in Table 1. Plasmids were transfected into human HEK293T cells using Fugene 6 (Roche) according to the manufacturer's instructions and were harvested 48 hr after transfection.

TABLE 1: Oligonucleotide primer sequences.

Purpose	Primer sequence
Reverse transcriptase—PCR: *nitr9*	GGATTTTTGGACTTTTCTGTC TCCACATGCGGTAACTGTAC
Reverse transcriptase—PCR: *β-actin*	GGTATGGAATCTTGCGGTATCCAC ATGGGCCAGACTCATCGTACTCCT
TaqMan Q-PCR: *nitr9* (probe = CAAGGTTTGGAAAAGCAC)	GTCAAAGGGACAAGGCTGATAGTT GTTCAAAACAGTGCATGTAAGACTCA
TaqMan Q-PCR: *β-actin* (probe = CCCATGCCATCCTGC)	CCATCTATGAGGGTTACGCTCTTC AGGATCTTCATCAGGTAGTCTGTCA
Amplify *nitr9* I domain for bacterial expression construct	<u>ATG</u>GAAAAGCACACTGTAGTA[a] **TTA**TTTAGAGCCATTCCTGTCC[b]
Amplify *nitr9L* for FLAG-tagged expression cassette	CACCCAAATGCACCACCTGTGTTTGTTAAAC[c] gactgcggccgcTTACTGCTGGTTAGAAAC[d]
Amplify *nitr9S* for FLAG-tagged expression cassette	CACCCAAATGCACCACCTGTG[c] gactgcggccgcTTACTGCTGGTTAGAAAC[d]
Amplify *nitr9SS* for FLAG-tagged expression cassette	CATGATTTAATTCCATCCCA[c] gactgcggccgcTTACTGCTGGTTAGAAAC[d]
Amplify wild type *nitr9L*, *nitr9S* and *nitr9SS* for expression cassettes	gatcggatccgacATGATCAACTTTTGGATTT[e] gatcgaattcTTACTGCTGGTTAGAAACCGAG[f]

[a]An artificial start codon is underlined.
[b]An artificial stop codon is bold.
[c]These primers are designed for blunt PCR cloning into the *Eco*RV site of pLF.
[d]Overhang (5′) sequences are in lower case text and include a *Not* I site for cloning into pLF.
[e]Overhang (5′) sequences are in lower case text and include a *Bam*HI site for cloning into pcDNA3.
[f]Overhang (3′) sequences are in lower case text and include an *Eco*RI site for cloning into pcDNA3.

2.5. Indirect Immunofluorescence. HEK293T cells were transfected in four well chamber slides (Thermo Fisher Scientific, Rochester, NY). Transfected cells were washed in phosphate buffered saline (PBS), fixed with 3% paraformaldehyde for 20 min and treated with 50 mM NH$_4$Cl, PBS for 5 minutes. Cells were then permeabilized with 1.0% Triton-X-100 in PBS for 5 min, rinsed and blocked with 1% BSA in PBS for 5 min. Permeabilized cells were incubated with the anti-Nitr9[19], anti-Nitr9[90], or anti-FLAG antibody for 1 hr, rinsed with PBS, incubated with a phycoerythrin (PE) anti-mouse IgG antibody and DAPI (1:1000) for 1 hr, and washed with PBS. Chambers were removed from the slides, and coverslips were mounted using immunomount (Thermo Shandon, Pittsburgh, PA). Cells were photographed at 40x magnification using a Leica DM5000 microscope.

2.6. Flow Cytometry. Transfected HEK293T cells were incubated with the anti-Nitr9[19], anti-Nitr9[90], or anti-FLAG monoclonal antibody for 1 hr, washed in PBS, and incubated for 30 min with an allophycocyanin- (APC-) conjugated anti-mouse IgG secondary antibody. Labeled cells were washed and then fixed with 3% paraformaldehyde and subjected to flow cytometric analysis (BD FACSCalibur, BD Biosciences, San Jose, CA).

2.7. Western Analyses. Transfected HEK293T cells were washed with PBS and lysed with mammalian protein extraction reagent (M-PER, Pierce, Rockford, IL). Kidney, spleen, intestine, and gills were removed from sacrificed adult zebrafish and collected directly into tissue protein extraction reagent (T-PER, Pierce) supplemented with protease inhibitors (Pierce) and homogenized. Lysates were centrifuged to remove nuclei, and cell debris and protein concentrations were determined (BCA Protein Assay, Pierce). Proteins were resolved on 12% SDS-polyacrylamide gels and transferred to polyvinylidene difluoride (PVDF) membranes for Western analyses. Membranes were washed in Tris-buffered saline with 0.1% Tween 20 (TBST) and incubated in blocking buffer (100 mM boric acid, 25 mM Na-Borate, 75 mM NaCl, 5% goat serum, and 5% dry milk powder) for 1 hr. Membranes were incubated overnight with primary antibodies in blocking buffer at 4°C. Primary antibodies include anti-Nitr9[90], anti-FLAG (M2) mouse monoclonal antibody (Sigma-Aldrich, St. Louis, MO), anti-GFP mouse monoclonal antibody (Roche), and anti-GAPDH rabbit polyclonal antibody (AnaSpec, Fremont, CA). Membranes were washed in TBST, followed by incubation with blocking buffer and either horseradish peroxidase-conjugated anti-mouse IgG secondary antibody (Roche) or horseradish

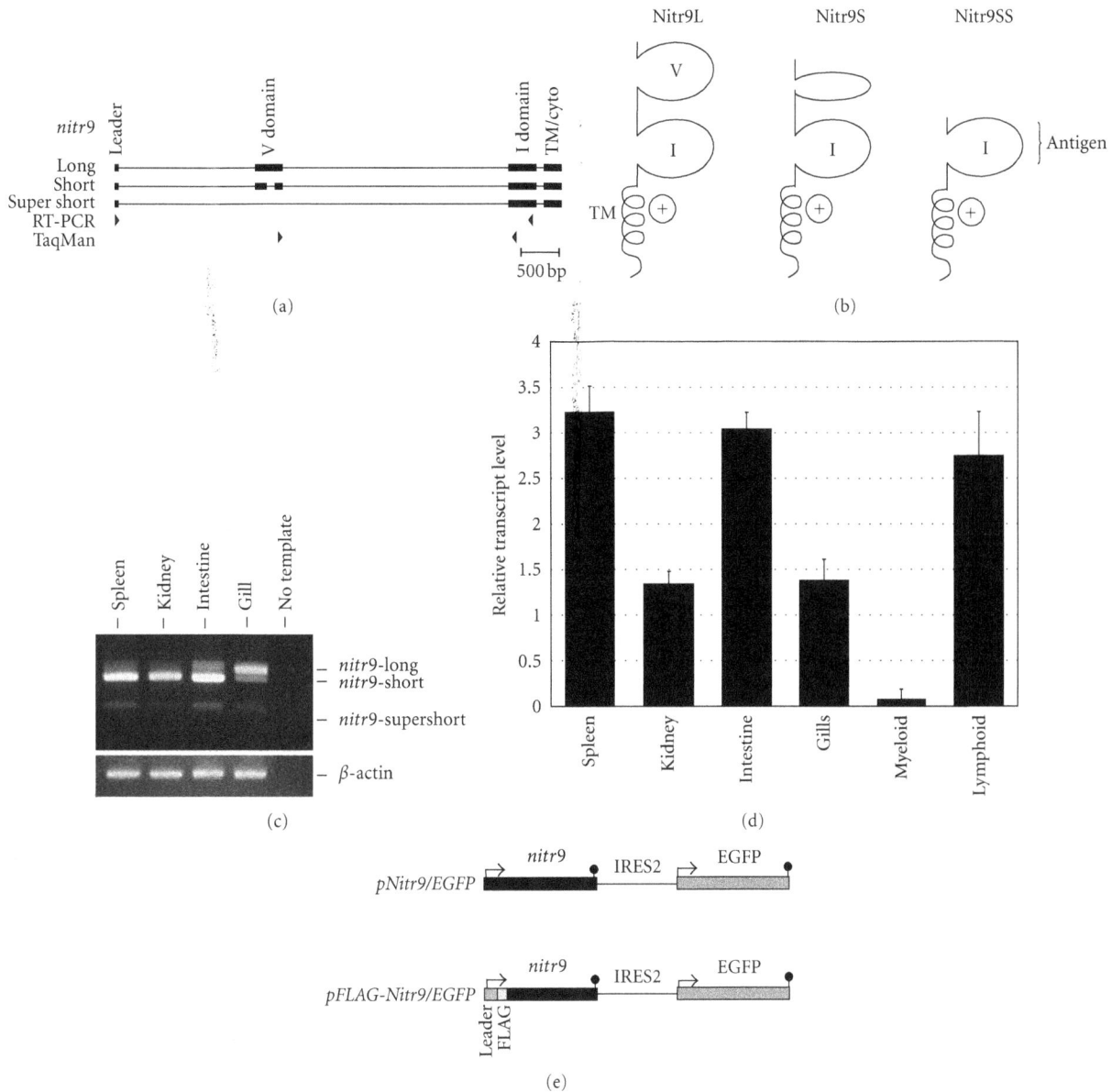

FIGURE 1: Transcriptional variation and expression of Nitr9. (a) Exon organization of the *nitr9* gene depicting the three transcript variants. Primer positions for PCR are indicated below. (b) The predicted Nitr9 protein isoforms encoded by the three *nitr9* transcripts. Transmembrane (TM) and immunoglobulin domains (of the variable (V) and intermediate (I) types) of Nitr9 are indicated. The I domain of Nitr9 was used as the antigen for antibody production. The positive charge within the TM domain of Nitr9 is represented by a plus sign. (c) RT-PCR with primers whose positions are depicted in (a) detects transcripts of all three *nitr9* isoforms. (d) Quantitative RT-PCR with *nitr9* primers (Table 1), whose positions are depicted in (a), and a TaqMan probe that spans an exon-exon boundary reveal relative levels of *nitr9L/S* transcripts in different tissues. (e) Schematic representation of the recombinant Nitr9 expression constructs used in this paper. Constructs include an internal ribosomal entry sequence (IRES2) permitting the expression of two proteins from a single transcript.

peroxidase-conjugated anti-rabbit IgG secondary antibody (Santa Cruz Biotechnology, Santa Cruz, CA). After washing with TBST, the Lumi-Light^PLUS western blotting substrate and detection system (Roche) was used to visualize reactivity.

2.8. Endoglycosidase Treatment. Cleared lysates (20 μg) from transfected cells were incubated with N-Glycosidase F (PNGase F, New England Biolabs, Ipswich, MA) for 1 hr at 37°C. Cleared lysates (25 μg) from zebrafish tissues were

precipitated with OrgoSOL buffer (G-Biosciences, St. Louis, MO) and resuspended in PNGase buffer for treatment with PNGase F.

3. Results and Discussion

3.1. Nitr9 Isoforms. The genomic organization and predicted protein structures of Nitr9L, Nitr9S, and Nitr9SS are shown in Figures 1(a) and 1(b). All three isoforms are predicted to

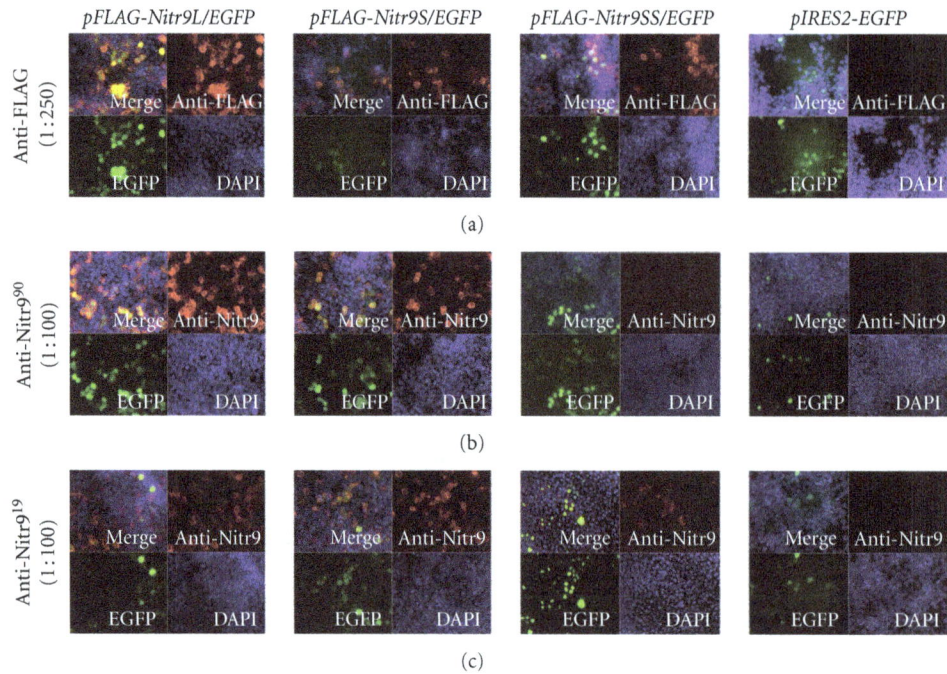

FIGURE 2: Detection of FLAG-tagged isoforms of Nitr9 from transfected cells by indirect immunofluorescence. HEK293T cells were transfected with plasmids encoding FLAG-tagged Nitr9 isoforms and EGFP as indicated on top of the panels. FLAG-tagged Nitr9 proteins were detected with (a) an anti-FLAG antibody, (b) anti-Nitr9[90] or (c) anti-Nitr9[19], and a PE conjugated secondary antibody (red). Transfected cells can be identified by EGFP expression (green). DAPI labels the nuclei of all cells (blue). The pIRES2-EGFP parental plasmid was included as a negative control.

encode type I transmembrane cell surface receptors that possess a positively charged residue within the transmembrane domain. The *nitr9S* isoform is expressed at higher levels in the zebrafish spleen, kidney, and intestine than the *nitr9L* and *nitr9SS* isoforms, whereas, *nitr9L* transcripts are the most abundant isoform expressed in gills. Transcripts of *nitr9SS* are detected in all four tissues at reduced levels relative to the other isoforms (Figure 1(c)). Q-PCR (Table 1) was employed to determine the combined relative levels of *nitr9L* and *nitr9S* transcripts in these same tissues as well as in purified lymphoid and myeloid cells (the TaqMan primer/probe set employed in this paper does not detect *nitr9SS* transcripts). The combined relative expression level of *nitr9L* and *nitr9S* transcripts is consistently higher in intestine than in kidney and gill (Figure 1(d)). However, the relative expression level of *nitr9L* and *nitr9S* in spleen varied between biological replicates, ranging from levels matching those in intestine to lower levels as observed in kidney and gill. As reported previously, *nitr9* transcripts are present at much higher levels in zebrafish lymphocytes as compared to myeloid cells [13]. In order to generate monoclonal antibodies that could detect all three Nitr9 isoforms, mice were immunized with a bacterially expressed Nitr9 I domain (see Figure 1(b)), and hybridomas were screened for the production of antibodies that recognize recombinant Nitr9 by ELISA, Western blot and indirect immunofluorescence. Two clones, 19.1.1 (herein referred to as anti-Nitr9[19]) and 90.10.5 (herein referred to as anti-Nitr9[90]), were selected for further evaluation.

3.2. Detection of Nitr9 Isoforms in Transfected Cells by Indirect Immunofluorescence. In order to determine if anti-Nitr9[19] and anti-Nitr9[90] could detect all three isoforms of Nitr9 by indirect immunofluorescence, HEK293T cells were transfected with plasmids that coexpress EGFP and either a FLAG-tagged or endogenous isoform of Nitr9; in this way, any cell expressing Nitr9 also expresses EGFP (Figure 1(e)). To ensure that the recombinant Nitr9 proteins could be detected by immunofluorescence, an anti-FLAG antibody was used to detect all three FLAG-tagged isoforms of Nitr9 in transfected cells (Figure 2(a)). It was then shown that both anti-Nitr9[19] and anti-Nitr9[90] recognize FLAG-Nitr9L and FLAG-Nitr9S by immunofluorescence, but either fail to bind (anti-Nitr9[90]) or bind less effectively (anti-Nitr9[19]) to FLAG-Nitr9SS (Figures 2(b) and 2(c)). In contrast, both anti-Nitr9[19] and anti-Nitr9[90] effectively recognize all three isoforms of endogenous Nitr9 when expressed in transfected cells albeit with an apparent higher background labeling of cells with anti-Nitr9[19] (Figure 3). It is possible that the FLAG-tag disrupts folding of Nitr9SS or sterically interferes with antibody recognition of the I domain of FLAG-Nitr9SS; this also was observed with Western analyses (discussed below).

3.3. Detection of Nitr9 Isoforms in Transfected Cells by Flow Cytometry. In order to determine if anti-Nitr9[19] and anti-Nitr9[90] could detect all three isoforms of Nitr9 by flow cytometry, HEK293T cells were transfected with plasmids encoding an endogenous or FLAG-tagged isoform of Nitr9

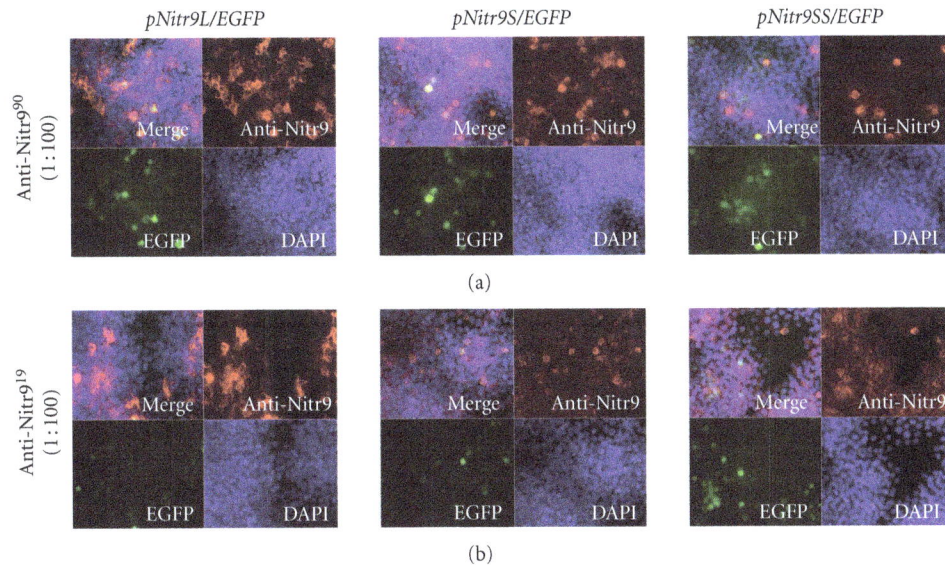

FIGURE 3: Detection of endogenous isoforms of Nitr9 from transfected cells by indirect immunofluorescence. HEK293T cells were transfected with plasmids encoding endogenous isoforms of Nitr9 and EGFP as indicated on top of the panels. Nitr9 proteins were detected with (a) anti-Nitr9^{90} or (b) anti-Nitr9^{19} and a PE conjugated secondary antibody (red). Transfected cells can be identified by EGFP expression (green). DAPI labels the nuclei of all cells (blue).

and EGFP (Figure 1(e)). Flow cytometry was performed using the anti-FLAG, anti-Nitr9^{19}, and anti-Nitr9^{90} antibodies to detect Nitr9 expressing cells. The percentage of double positive FLAG-Nitr9L expressing cells (i.e., EGFP^{+} and Nitr9^{+}) was similar (55–63% of EGFP^{+} cells) when the anti-FLAG or the anti-Nitr9 antibodies were employed (Figure 4(a)). Both anti-Nitr9 antibodies recognize transfected cells expressing the endogenous isoform of Nitr9L with a similar efficiency (61–73% of EGFP^{+} cells) (Figure 4(b)).

The anti-FLAG monoclonal antibody failed to bind FLAG-Nitr9S and the anti-Nitr9^{19} antibody failed to detect the Nitr9S- or FLAG-Nitr9S-expressing cells (2–9% of EGFP^{+} cells) (Figures 4(c) and 4(d)). Although the anti-Nitr9^{90} antibody detects FLAG-Nitr9S (31% of EGFP^{+} cells), it does not recognize endogenous Nitr9S (~5% of EGFP^{+} cells). Although the Nitr9S and FLAG-Nitr9S proteins are produced by transfected cells (see Figures 2 and 3 and Western blot results below) they may not be expressed effectively on the cell surface. To determine if cell surface expression of Nitr9S requires coexpression of the signaling adaptor protein Dap12, cells were cotransfected with plasmids encoding Nitr9S and zebrafish Dap12. No increase was observed in cell surface labeling by the anti-Nitr9 antibodies (data not shown).

The anti-FLAG and anti-Nitr9^{19} antibodies effectively bound FLAG-Nitr9SS (57% and 31% of EGFP^{+} cells, resp.). The anti-Nitr9^{90} antibody failed to bind FLAG-Nitr9SS, possibly due to steric hindrance by the FLAG tag (Figure 4(e)) since both anti-Nitr9 antibodies were effective at recognizing Nitr9SS (65–75% of EGFP^{+} cells; Figure 4(f)).

3.4. Anti-Nitr9^{90} Binds All Three Isoforms of Nitr9 in Western Analyses. In order to evaluate the ability of the anti-Nitr9^{90} antibody to detect the three isoforms of Nitr9 in Western

analyses, HEK293T cells were transfected with plasmids encoding endogenous and FLAG-tagged isoforms of Nitr9 (Figure 1(e)). Cell lysates were subjected to Western blot analyses using the anti-Nitr9^{90} antibody. All three isoforms of the endogenous Nitr9 as well as the FLAG-tagged Nitr9L and Nitr9S proteins were detected. A binding pattern equivalent to that seen with the anti-FLAG monoclonal antibody positive control is apparent (Figure 5(a)). However, anti-Nitr9^{90} failed to bind the FLAG-tagged Nitr9SS. As mentioned above, this may be a result of the FLAG-tag blocking access to the specific epitope recognized by this antibody.

Two proteins bands were detected by anti-Nitr9^{90} in both endogenous and FLAG-tagged Nitr9L and Nitr9S transfections that were also bound by the anti-FLAG antibody. Both observed Nitr9L proteins migrated at a higher molecular weight than the predicted size of Nitr9L (34 kD), and one of the observed Nitr9S proteins was larger than the predicted size of Nitr9S (30 kD). The differences are consistent with differential glycosylation (see below). Based on the chemiluminescence exposure times required for detecting the different isoforms of Nitr9, anti-Nitr9^{90} appears to exhibit a higher affinity for Nitr9L as compared to Nitr9S and Nitr9SS. In parallel experiments, the anti-Nitr9^{19} antibody did not bind endogenous Nitr9S and Nitr9SS proteins (data not shown) and was not characterized further in the Western blot analyses.

3.5. Nitr9 Glycosylation in Transfected Cells. Nitr9L, Nitr9S and Nitr9SS possess three (NMSC, NDSR, and NGSK), two (NMSC and NGSK), and one (NGSK) candidate N-linked glycosylation sites, respectively. Treatment of lysates from Nitr9 transfected cells with endoglycosidase (PNGase F) results in the detection of only a single protein of

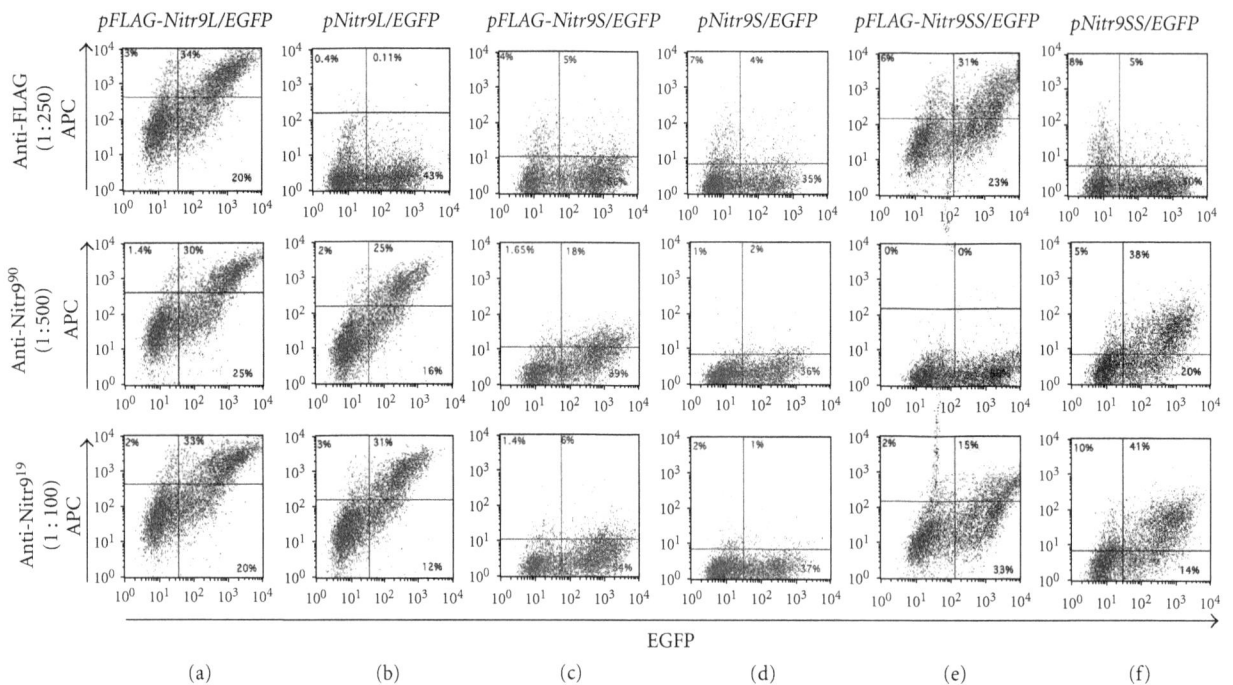

FIGURE 4: Detection of Nitr9 isoforms by flow cytometry. HEK293T cells were transfected with plasmids encoding FLAG-tagged (a, c, and e) or endogenous (b, d, and f) isoforms of Nitr9 and EGFP as indicated above the panels. Cells were labeled with an anti-FLAG antibody (top row), anti-Nitr9[90] (middle row) or anti-Nitr9[19] (bottom row), and an APC conjugated secondary antibody. Flow cytometric analyses were employed to detect EGFP positive (X axis) and APC positive (Y axis) cells. Isotype-matched antibodies were evaluated as controls for both anti-Nitr9 antibodies and displayed no labeling of transfected cells (data not shown).

the expected size for both Nitr9L and Nitr9S (Figure 5(b)). Both sets of results are consistent with *in vivo* glycosylation. The observed size of Nitr9SS in transfected cells does not appear to be altered by endoglycosidase treatment, with the limitations of detection, suggesting that it may not be glycosylated.

3.6. Nitr9 Proteins Are Differentially Expressed in Different Tissues of Zebrafish. In order to determine if the anti-Nitr9[90] antibody can recognize endogenous Nitr9, lysates from adult zebrafish tissues were treated with endoglycosidase and subjected to Western blot analyses (Figure 5(c)). Nitr9L and Nitr9S were detected at varying levels in the spleen, kidney, gills, and intestine. Nitr9SS was detected only in the spleen, although faint bands also have been observed in intestine (data not shown). A nonspecific band of approximately 28 kD is detected in zebrafish tissues as well as in HEK293T cells when the anti-Nitr9[90] antibody is used with large total protein loads (e.g., 25 μg lysate; Figure 5(c)).

4. Conclusions

Three different transcript variants from *nitr9*, the single putative activating NITR gene in zebrafish, and their corresponding protein isoforms have been identified and characterized. The utility of the anti-Nitr9[19] and anti-Nitr9[90] monoclonal antibodies for detecting recombinant Nitr9 was demonstrated by indirect immunofluorescence, flow

cytometry, and Western blot analyses. The antibodies exhibit profound differences in recognizing the three different Nitr9 isoforms. When employed for indirect immunofluorescence, both anti-Nitr9 antibodies bound efficiently and specifically to cells-expressing all three Nitr9 isoforms. Both anti-Nitr9 antibodies are effective for detecting cell surface expression of Nitr9L and Nitr9SS by flow cytometry. The anti-Nitr9[90] antibody recognized all three Nitr9 isoforms by Western blot analyses, although a higher affinity for Nitr9L is noted. When using anti-Nitr9[90] in Western blot analyses with high levels of protein, a nonspecific band was identified. Although the identity of this protein remains unknown, it may represent a well-conserved member of the Ig superfamily.

Marked differences in the relative levels of Nitr9 transcripts and protein isoforms are apparent. Although the PCR analyses (Figure 1(c)) suggest that *nitr9S* may be the predominant mRNA isoform in spleen, kidney, and intestine, Western analyses demonstrate that Nitr9L is the predominant protein isoform expressed in kidney. This discrepancy may reflect differing transcript and protein stability in different tissues or the preferred reactivity of the antibody with Nitr9L (Figure 5(a)).

The monoclonal antibodies described here should be useful for further evaluation of Nitr9 protein levels in zebrafish tissues by Western blot analyses and identifying Nitr9 expressing cells in tissue sections by indirect immunofluorescence. Efforts are underway to purify Nitr9-expressing zebrafish cells employing FACS in order to characterize their morphology and cytotoxic properties.

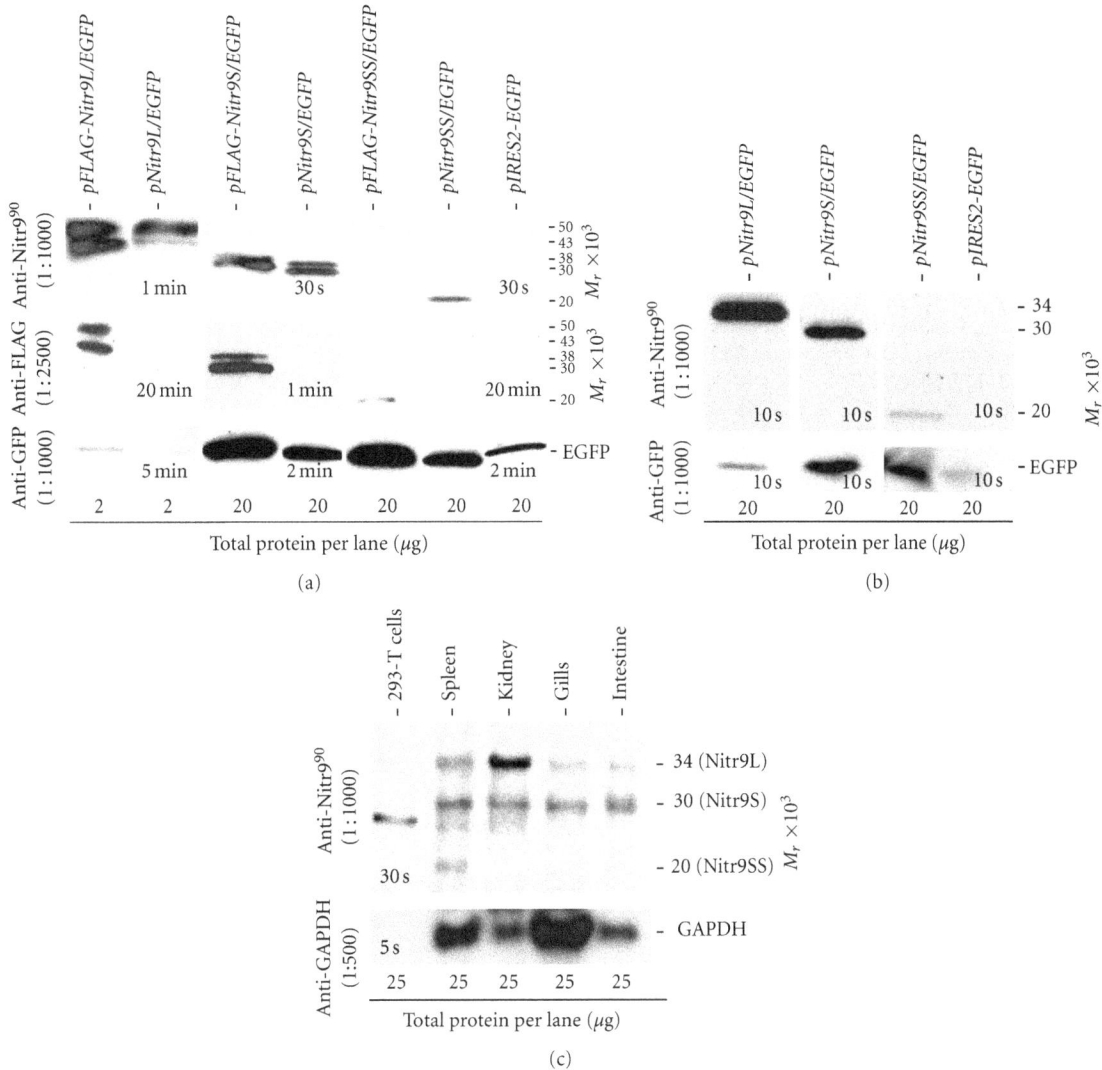

FIGURE 5: Detection of Nitr9 protein by Western analyses. (a) Western blot analyses of total protein lysates from HEK293T cells transiently transfected with plasmids expressing a Nitr9 isoform and EGFP. Plasmids encode either an endogenous isoform of Nitr9 or a FLAG-tagged Nitr9 as indicated above each lane. The primary antibodies utilized are shown on the left, and the molecular weights of identified bands are shown on the right. The anti-FLAG antibody serves as a positive control for Nitr9 detection, and the anti-GFP antibody indicates transfection efficiency of each plasmid. Note the total protein loaded (bottom) for the Nitr9L isoform is ten times less than that for Nitr9S and Nitr9SS plasmids. Exposure times for chemiluminescence detection are indicated in each panel. (b) Nitr9L and Nitr9S are glycosylated. Western blot analyses of endoglycosidase-treated total protein lysates from HEK293T cells that were transfected with plasmids encoding endogenous Nitr9 isoforms. The anti-Nitr9⁹⁰ antibody recognizes all three Nitr9 isoforms at the predicted size (right). (c) Detection of Nitr9 protein from zebrafish tissues. Western blot analyses of 25 μg of endoglycosidase-treated total protein from zebrafish tissues and HEK293T cells. Note that a nonspecific band (~28 kD) is detected in HEK293T cells as well as in zebrafish kidney and spleen, with high protein loads. Bottom panel indicates loading control using an anti-GAPDH polyclonal antibody.

These antibodies may also prove to be useful for activating (crosslinking) or blocking Nitr9 function in both cell culture and *ex-vivo* functional assays as well as in dissecting isoform-specific functions of NITRs.

Acknowledgments

The authors are grateful to Bradley Bone and Karen Marcus for assistance with generating hybridomas and performing ELISAs, Janet Dow for assistance with flow cytometry, and Barb Pryor for editorial assistance. This paper was supported by grants awarded by the National Science Foundation (MCB-0505585 to J. A. Yoder) and the National Institutes of Health (R01 AI057559 to G. W. Litman and J. A. Yoder).

References

[1] R. Biassoni, "Human natural killer receptors, co-receptors, and their ligands," *Current Protocols in Immunology*, chapter 14, unit 14.10, 2009.

[2] L. L. Lanier, "Up on the tightrope: natural killer cell activation and inhibition," *Nature Immunology*, vol. 9, no. 5, pp. 495–502, 2008.

[3] L. L. Lanier, "NK cell recognition," *Annual Review of Immunology*, vol. 23, pp. 225–274, 2005.

[4] J. A. Yoder and G. W. Litman, "The phylogenetic origins of natural killer receptors and recognition: relationships, possibilities, and realities," *Immunogenetics*, vol. 63, no. 3, pp. 123–141, 2011.

[5] G. W. Litman, J. P. Cannon, and L. J. Dishaw, "Reconstructing immune phylogeny: new perspectives," *Nature Reviews Immunology*, vol. 5, no. 11, pp. 866–879, 2005.

[6] J. A. Yoder, "Form, function and phylogenetics of NITRs in bony fish," *Developmental and Comparative Immunology*, vol. 33, no. 2, pp. 135–144, 2009.

[7] S. Ferraresso, H. Kuhl, M. Milan et al., "Identification and characterisation of a novel immune-type receptor (NITR) gene cluster in the European sea bass, Dicentrarchus labrax, reveals recurrent gene expansion and diversification by positive selection," *Immunogenetics*, vol. 61, no. 11-12, pp. 773–788, 2009.

[8] S. Desai, A. K. Heffelfinger, T. M. Orcutt, G. W. Litman, and J. A. Yoder, "The medaka novel immune-type receptor (NITR) gene clusters reveal an extraordinary degree of divergence in variable domains," *BMC Evolutionary Biology*, vol. 8, no. 1, article 177, 2008.

[9] J. A. Yoder, M. G. Mueller, S. Wei et al., "Immune-type receptor genes in zebrafish share genetic and functional properties with genes encoded by the mammalian leukocyte receptor cluster," *Proceedings of the National Academy of Sciences of the United States of America*, vol. 98, no. 12, pp. 6771–6776, 2001.

[10] J. A. Yoder, R. T. Litman, M. G. Mueller et al., "Resolution of the novel immune-type receptor gene cluster in zebrafish," *Proceedings of the National Academy of Sciences of the United States of America*, vol. 101, no. 44, pp. 15706–15711, 2004.

[11] J. A. Yoder, J. P. Cannon, R. T. Litman, C. Murphy, J. L. Freeman, and G. W. Litman, "Evidence for a transposition event in a second NITR gene cluster in zebrafish," *Immunogenetics*, vol. 60, no. 5, pp. 257–265, 2008.

[12] J. Evenhuis, E. Bengtén, C. Snell, S. M. Quiniou, N. W. Miller, and M. Wilson, "Characterization of additional novel immune type receptors in channel catfish, Ictalurus punctatus," *Immunogenetics*, vol. 59, no. 8, pp. 661–671, 2007.

[13] J. A. Yoder, P. M. Turner, P. D. Wright et al., "Developmental and tissue-specific expression of NITRs," *Immunogenetics*, vol. 62, no. 2, pp. 117–122, 2010.

[14] S. Wei, J.-M. Zhou, X. Chen et al., "The zebrafish activating immune receptor Nitr9 signals via Dap12," *Immunogenetics*, vol. 59, no. 10, pp. 813–821, 2007.

[15] D. D. Jima, R. N. Shah, T. M. Orcutt et al., "Enhanced transcription of complement and coagulation genes in the absence of adaptive immunity," *Molecular Immunology*, vol. 46, no. 7, pp. 1505–1516, 2009.

[16] J. A. Yoder, T. M. Orcutt, D. Traver, and G. W. Litman, "Structural characteristics of zebrafish orthologs of adaptor molecules that associate with transmembrane immune receptors," *Gene*, vol. 401, no. 1-2, pp. 154–164, 2007.

[17] K. J. Livak and T. D. Schmittgen, "Analysis of relative gene expression data using real-time quantitative PCR and the $2^{-\Delta\Delta C_T}$ method," *Methods*, vol. 25, no. 4, pp. 402–408, 2001.

11

Clinically Significant Minor Blood Group Antigens amongst North Indian Donor Population

Divjot Singh Lamba, Ravneet Kaur, and Sabita Basu

Department of Transfusion Medicine, Block D, Level II, Government Medical College & Hospital, Chandigarh 160030, India

Correspondence should be addressed to Ravneet Kaur; rkbedi15@yahoo.com

Academic Editor: Mark R. Litzow

Background. Racial differences in blood group antigen distribution are common and may result in striking and interesting findings. These differences in blood group antigen distribution are important due to their influence on the clinical practice of transfusion medicine. *Study Design and Methods*. This is a prospective study, involving 1000 healthy regular repeat voluntary blood donors associated with the department. The clinically significant minor blood group antigens of these donors were studied. *Results*. Out of 1000 healthy regular repeat voluntary blood donors, 93% were D positive and 2.8% were K positive. Amongst the Rh antigens, e was the most common (99%), followed by D (93%), C (85.1%), c (62.3%), and E (21.5%). Within the MNS blood group system, antigen frequency was M (88%), N (57.5%), S (57.8%), and s (87.5%). Within the Duffy blood group system, antigen frequency was Fy^a (87.3%) and Fy^b (58.3%). *Conclusions*. This data base will help us to prevent alloimmunisation in young females, pregnant women, and patients who are expected to require repeated transfusions in life by providing them with antigen matched blood. Antigen negative blood can also be made available without delay to already alloimmunized multitransfused patients.

1. Introduction

A total of 30 blood group systems are recognized by the International Society of Blood Transfusion (ISBT). Nine blood group systems (ABO, Rhesus, Kell, Kidd, Duffy, MNS, P, Lewis, and Lutheran) are considered to be clinically significant as these are known to cause hemolytic transfusion reactions (HTR) and hemolytic disease of fetus and newborn (HDFN) [1–4].

In developing countries like India only ABO and D status of blood donor and recipients are taken into account for compatibility testing. However, the phenotype of clinically significant blood group antigens on the donor red blood cells (RBCs) is required to be known at times when alloimmunization is particularly undesirable, such as in young females, pregnant women, and patients who are expected to require repeated transfusions in life, such as thalassemia or sickle cell disease patients. When selecting blood for transfusion to such patients, it would be useful if we have access to already phenotyped RBCs of donor population so that particular antigen typed blood can be given to such patients to prevent alloimmunization [5]. Furthermore, these are beneficial for already immunized patients if the transfusion is urgent and/or if clinically significant alloantibodies to particular antigen/antigens are present in the patient's serum. In such situations, corresponding antigen negative blood can be given to such recipients without much delay [5].

Racial differences in blood group antigen distributions are common and may result in striking and interesting findings. Very little information is available regarding distribution of various clinically significant minor blood group antigens in northern region of our country. The previous studies are done with limited number donors [6–8]. The present study was done to get an insight of frequency of clinically significant minor blood group antigens amongst regular voluntary blood donors and also to lay foundation of starting a donor database on RBC antigens.

2. Material and Methods

This prospective study was conducted in the department of transfusion medicine of a tertiary care hospital after approval

TABLE 1: Comparison of antigen frequency of Rh subgroup antigens.

Antigens	Antigen frequency in total 1000 donors (%)	Antigen frequency in Indians by Thakral et al. [7]	Antigen frequency in Indians by Chaudhary et al. [6]	Antigen frequency in whites [9–11]	Antigen frequency in blacks [9–11]
D	930 (93.0%)	93.4%	ND	85%	92%
C	851 (85.1%)	84.8%	95.2%	68%	27%
c	623 (62.3%)	52.8%	69.2%	80%	96%
E	215 (21.5%)	17.9%	15.4%	29%	22%
e	990 (99.0%)	98.3%	98.1%	98%	98%

TABLE 2: Comparison of antigen frequency of Rh subgroup antigens in D positive and D negative donors.

Antigens	Antigen frequency in D positive donors	Antigen frequency in D negative donors	Antigen frequency in total 1000 donors (%)
C	90.8%	10%	851 (85.1%)
c	59.6%	98.6%	623 (62.3%)
E	22.8%	4.3%	215 (21.5%)
e	98.9%	100%	990 (99.0%)

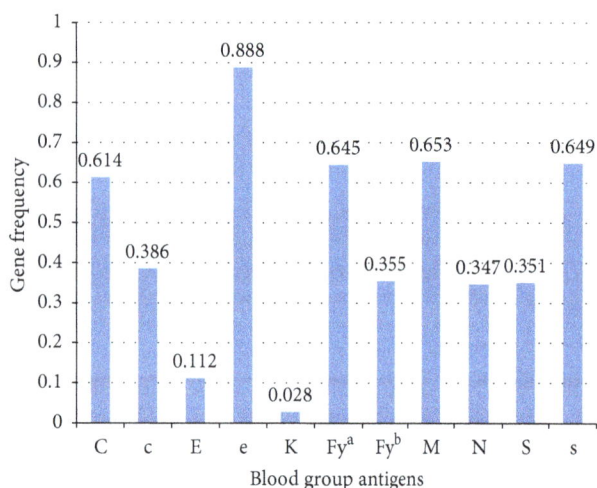

FIGURE 1: Gene frequency of minor blood group antigens.

by the Institutional Ethics Committee and a written informed consent given by the donors.

Blood samples were collected from 1,000 healthy regular repeat voluntary blood donors (who have donated two or more than two times before) between September 2010 and July 2011. Donors to be studied were arranged group-wise, that is, O positive: 34%, A positive: 22%, B positive: 32%, AB positive: 5%, and negatives: 7% as per the frequency of these blood groups in North Indian population [12, 13]. The clinically significant minor blood antigens of the Rh blood group system—C, c, E, and e; Kell blood group system—K; Duffy blood system—Fy^a and Fy^b; MNS blood group system—M, N, S, and s were studied using DIAMED (Bio-Rad Laboratories, DiaMed Switzerland) gel cards.

3. Statistical Analysis

The statistical analysis was carried out using Statistical Package for Social Sciences (SPSS Inc., Chicago, IL, version

15.0 for Windows). Qualitative or categorical variables were described as frequencies and proportions. Proportions for gender were compared using chi-square test. Gene frequencies were calculated using the Hardy Weinberg principle where $p + q = 1$ and $p = \{2 \times obs(AA) + obs(Aa)\}/2 \times \{obs(AA) + obs(Aa) + obs(aa)\}$; thus $q = 1 - p$.

4. Results

The study included 1,000 healthy regular repeat voluntary blood donors of which 947 were males and 53 were females. The males were significantly more than females with $P < 0.001$. The mean age for donors was 35.30 ± 9.86. Of the 1,000 blood donors 930 were D positive and 70 were D negative. The gene frequency for various blood group systems is depicted in Figure 1.

4.1. Antigen Frequencies

4.1.1. Rh Antigens. Amongst Rh antigens, e was the most common (99%) followed by D (93%), C (85.1%), c (62.3%), and E (21.5%) (Table 1).

4.1.2. Rh Subgroup Antigens in D Positive and D Negative Donors. 98.6% D negative donors had c antigen and 100% D negative donors had e antigen on their red cells. Thus, there is strong association of c antigen and e antigen with D negative donors. C antigen was found to be more associated with presence of D antigen as compared to its absence (90.8% and 10%, resp.) (Table 2).

4.1.3. Minor Blood Group Antigen Frequencies. Amongst minor blood group antigens Kell antigen frequency was 2.8%, Duffy (Fy^a) 7.3%, Duffy (Fy^b) 58.3%, M 88%, N 57.5%, S 57.8%, and s 87.5% (Table 3).

4.2. Phenotype Frequencies

4.2.1. Duffy Blood Group System. Most common phenotypes in Duffy system were $Fy^a+Fy^b+ = 45.6\%$ and $Fy^a+Fy^b- = 41.7\%$ (Table 4).

TABLE 3: Antigen frequency of clinically significant minor blood group antigens.

Blood group antigen	In 1000 cases (%)	Indian study by Thakral et al. [7]	Indian study by Chaudhary et al. [6]	In whites [6]	In blacks [6]
Kell (K)	28 (2.8%)	5.56%	1.92%	0.2%	<0.1%
Fy^a	873 (87.3%)	86.8%	73.1%	17%	9%
Fy^b	583 (58.3%)	56.2%	53.8%	34%	22%
M	880 (88%)	75.4%	77.9%	28%	24%
N	575 (57.5%)	61.5%	73.1%	22%	30%
S	578 (57.8%)	56.5%	63.5%	11%	3%
s	875 (87.5%)	87.4%	45.2%	45%	69%

TABLE 4: Phenotype frequencies of Duffy blood group system.

Phenotype	In 1000 cases (%)	Indian study by Thakral et al. [7]	Indian study by Chaudhary et al. [6]	Indian study by Nanu and Thapliyal [8]	In whites [9–11]	In blacks [9–11]
Fy^a+Fy^b−	**417 (41.7%)**	**43.9%**	**43%**	**40.8%**	**17%**	**9%**
Fy^a−Fy^b+	127 (12.7%)	13.3%	24%	16.2%	34%	22%
Fy^a+Fy^b+	**456 (45.6%)**	**42.9%**	**30%**	**42.6%**	**49%**	**1%**
Fy^a−Fy^b−	0 (0%)	0%	3%	0.44%	<0.1%	68%

TABLE 5: Phenotype frequencies of MN and Ss in MNS blood group system.

Phenotype	In 1000 cases (%)	Indian study by Thakral et al. [7]	Indian study by Nanu and Thapliyal [8]	In Europeans [14, 15]	In African Americans [14, 15]
M+N−	**425 (42.5%)**	**38.5%**	**42.3%**	**28%**	**26%**
M−N+	120 (12.0%)	24.6%	14.6%	22%	30%
M+N+	**455 (45.5%)**	**36.9%**	**43.1%**	**50%**	**44%**
S+s−	124 (12.4%)	12.6%	10%	11%	03%
S−s+	**421 (42.1%)**	**43.5%**	**62.1%**	**45%**	**69%**
S+s+	**454 (45.4%)**	**43.9%**	**26.8%**	**44%**	**28%**
S−s−	1 (0.1%)	0%	1.2%	0%	01%

4.2.2. MNS Blood Group System. Most common phenotypes were M+N− (42.5%), M+N+ (45.5%), S−s+ (42.1%), and S+s+ (45.4%). (Table 5) The frequency of M+N−S+s+, M+N+S+s+, and M+N+S−s+ phenotypes was comparable in our study (Table 6).

5. Discussion

Besides ABO and Rh antibodies, antibodies to other clinically significant antigens are also known to cause HTR, HDFN, or shortened survival of transfused red cells [3]. The knowledge of these clinically significant antigens can help in prevention and appropriate management of pregnancies at risk of HDFN and multitransfused patients with alloimmunization. The frequency of such antigens is available for Caucasians and Black races [9–11, 14, 15]. Very limited information is available on antigen and phenotype frequencies in North India. Other studies are either of small sample size or done in particular blood group donors [6–8]. This is the first study where frequency of clinically significant antigens is studied in 1,000 voluntary blood donors. All the antigen and phenotype frequencies reported in our study were compared with that of

White and Black population [9–11] and with the other studies from North India [6–8].

In the present study the frequency of D and other Rh antigens was comparable with that of other studies from the region but was markedly different when compared to Whites and Blacks (Table 1).

The antigen frequencies of Duffy and MNS antigens were comparable to antigen frequencies of other studies in this region but were different from that of white and black population (Table 3). The Kell antigen frequency in our study was less (2.8% versus 5.56%) compared to those of another study from this region and is higher than that reported in blacks and in whites (Table 3). The difference in Kell antigen frequency in our study compared to the another study from this region may be due to the fact that donor population in our study includes donors of all blood groups as compared to "O blood group" donors in their study. Thus there is a need to perform more studies with a much larger sample size to know more accurately the antigen frequency of Kell antigen in the population of this region.

The phenotype frequencies of Duffy and MNS blood group systems were compared with those of other studies

TABLE 6: Combined phenotype frequencies of MNSs in MNS blood group system.

Phenotype	In 1000 cases (%)	Indian study by Thakral et al. [7]	Indian study by Nanu and Thapliyal [8]	In Europeans [14, 15]	In African Americans [14, 15]
M+N−S+s−	65 (6.5%)	7.9%	5.5%	5.7%	2.1%
M+N−S+s+	**208 (20.8%)**	**14.8%**	**13.3%**	**14%**	**7%**
M+N−S−s+	151 (15.1%)	15.8%	22.6%	10.1%	15.5%
M+N+S+s−	50 (5%)	3.5%	4.6%	3.9%	2.2%
M+N+S+s+	**201 (20.1%)**	**19.6%**	**10.7%**	**22.4%**	**13%**
M+N+S−s+	**204 (20.4%)**	**13.9%**	**27.8%**	**22.6%**	**33.4%**
M−N+S+s−	9 (0.9%)	1.3%	1.2%	0.3%	1.6%
M−N+S+s+	45 (4.5%)	9.5%	3.5%	5.4%	4.5%
M−N+S−s+	66 (6.6%)	13.9%	9.3%	15.6%	19.2%
M−N+S−s−	0 (0%)	0%	0.3%	0%	0.7%

from the region and with that of white and black population (Tables 4, 5, and 6). These results support the fact that there is variation in the distribution of antigens in the Duffy and MNS blood group system even in North Indian population [7]. Thus there is a need to perform more studies with a much larger sample size to know more accurately the phenotype frequency of Duffy and MNS antigens in the population of this region.

The beta thalassemia carrier rate in India is around 3–7% with higher frequency in northwest India. Approximately 10,000 thalassemia major cases are added each year [16]. The prevalence of alloimmunization in multitransfused patients in India is approximately 3–10% [17, 18]. This study has provided us with donor database of regular repeat voluntary blood donors with known antigenic profile which is referred to, to provide antigen matched blood to young females, pregnant women, and patients who are expected to require repeated transfusions in life. Antigen negative blood is also being provided to already alloimmunized multitransfused patients. This has helped us to prevent alloimmunisation in these groups of patients and prevent already alloimmunised patients from further alloimmunisation.

6. Limitations

Kidd antigen evaluation in donors was not done due to cost constraints.

Conflict of Interests

No author has a direct financial relation with the commercial identities mentioned in the paper that might lead to conflict of interests for any of the authors.

References

[1] G. Daniels, L. Castilho, W. A. Flegel et al., "International society of blood transfusion committee on terminology for red blood cell surface antigens: macao report," *Vox Sanguinis*, vol. 96, no. 2, pp. 153–156, 2009.

[2] E. Smart and B. Armstrong, "Blood group systems," *International Society of Blood Transfusion Science Series*, vol. 3, pp. 68–92, 2008.

[3] J. Poole and G. Daniels, "Blood group antibodies and their significance in transfusion medicine," *Transfusion Medicine Reviews*, vol. 21, no. 1, pp. 58–71, 2007.

[4] J. M. Bowman, "Intrauterine transfusion," in *Anderson and Ness Scientific Basis of Transfusion Medicine: Implications for Clinical Practice*, K. C. Anderson and P. M. Ness, Eds., pp. 403–420, WB Saunders, Philadelphia, PA, USA, 2nd edition, 1994.

[5] B. Diedrich, J. Andersson, S. Sallander, and A. Shanwell, "K, Fya and Jka phenotyping of donor RBCs on microplates," *Transfusion*, vol. 41, no. 10, pp. 1263–1267, 2001.

[6] R. K. Chaudhary, J. S. Shukla, and V. Ray, "Minor Red cell antigens in north Indian blood donor population," *Indian Journal of Hematology and Blood Transfusion*, vol. 21, pp. 34–35, 2003.

[7] B. Thakral, K. Saluja, R. R. Sharma, and N. Marwaha, "Phenotype frequencies of blood group systems (Rh, Kell, Kidd, Duffy, MNS, P, Lewis, and Lutheran) in North Indian blood donors," *Transfusion and Apheresis Science*, vol. 43, no. 1, pp. 17–22, 2010.

[8] A. Nanu and R. M. Thapliyal, "Blood group gene frequency in a selected north Indian population," *Indian Journal of Medical Research*, vol. 106, pp. 242–246, 1997.

[9] M. E. Brecher, *Technical Manual*, American Association of Blood Banks, Bethesda, Md, USA, 15th edition, 2005.

[10] G. Daniels, *Human Blood Groups*, Blackwell Science, Oxford, UK, 2nd edition, 2002.

[11] D. M. Harmening, *Modern Blood Banking and Transfusion Practices*, FA Davis Company, Philadelphia, PA, USA, 5th edition, 2005.

[12] N. A. Bhat, M. A. Kammili, S. A. Kadla, and A. Nafae, "Frequency of blood groups in donors and recipients," *The Indian Practitioner*, vol. 52, pp. 160–164, 1999.

[13] J. A. Latoo, N. A. Masoodi, N. A. Bhat, G. Q. Khan, and S. A. Kadla, "The ABO and Rh blood groups in Kashmiri population," *Indian Journal for the Practising Doctor*, vol. 3, no. 2, 2 pages, 2006, http://www.indmedica.com/journals.php.

[14] T. E. Cleghorn, "MNSs gene frequencies in English blood donors," *Nature*, vol. 187, no. 4738, p. 701, 1960.

[15] R. R. Race and R. Sanger, *Blood Groups in Man*, Blackwell Scientific Publications, Oxford, UK, 4th edition, 1975.

[16] I. Panigrahi and R. K. Marwaha, "Common queries in thalassemia care," *Indian Pediatrics*, vol. 43, no. 6, pp. 513–518, 2006.

[17] B. Thakral, K. Saluja, N. Marwaha, and R. R. Sharma, "Red cell alloimmunization in a transfused patient population: a study from a tertiary care hospital in north India," *Hematology*, vol. 13, no. 5, pp. 313–318, 2008.

[18] R. Gupta, D. K. Singh, B. Singh, and U. Rusia, "Alloimmunization to red cells in thalassemics: emerging problem and future strategies," *Transfusion and Apheresis Science*, vol. 45, no. 2, pp. 167–170, 2011.

12

Ethical and Clinical Aspects of Intensive Care Unit Admission in Patients with Hematological Malignancies: Guidelines of the Ethics Commission of the French Society of Hematology

Sandra Malak,[1,2] **Jean-Jacques Sotto,**[2,3] **Joël Ceccaldi,**[2,4] **Philippe Colombat,**[2,5] **Philippe Casassus,**[2,6] **Dominique Jaulmes,**[2,7] **Henri Rochant,**[2,8] **Morgane Cheminant,**[2,9] **Yvan Beaussant,**[2,10] **Robert Zittoun**[2,11] **and Dominique Bordessoule**[2,12]

[1] *Hematology Department of the René Huguenin Hospital, Institut Curie, 35 rue Dailly, 92210 Saint-Cloud, France*
[2] *Ethics Commission of the French Society of Hematology, France*
[3] *Hematology Department of the University of Grenoble, 38043 Grenoble, France*
[4] *Hematology Department of the Robert Boulin Hospital, 33505 Libourne, France*
[5] *Hematology Department of the University of Tours, 37044 Tours, France*
[6] *Hematology Department of the University of Bobigny, 93000 Bobigny, France*
[7] *Hematology Department of the University of Saint-Antoine, 75012 Paris, France*
[8] *Hematology Department of the University of Créteil, 94010 Créteil, France*
[9] *Hematology Department of the University of Necker, 75015 Paris, France*
[10] *Hematology Department of the University of Besançon, 25030 Besançon, France*
[11] *Hematology Department of the Hôtel-Dieu Hospital, 75001 Paris, France*
[12] *Hematology Department of the University of Limoges, 87042 Limoges, France*

Correspondence should be addressed to Sandra Malak; sandra.malak@curie.fr

Academic Editor: Emili Montserrat

Admission of patients with hematological malignancies to intensive care unit (ICU) raises recurrent ethical issues for both hematological and intensivist teams. The decision of transfer to ICU has major consequences for end of life care for patients and their relatives. It also impacts organizational human and economic aspects for the ICU and global health policy. In light of the recent advances in hematology and critical care medicine, a wide multidisciplinary debate has been conducted resulting in guidelines approved by consensus by both disciplines. The main aspects developed were (i) clarification of the clinical situations that could lead to a transfer to ICU taking into account the severity criteria of both hematological malignancy and clinical distress, (ii) understanding the process of decision-making in a context of regular interdisciplinary concertation involving the patient and his relatives, (iii) organization of a collegial concertation at the time of the initial decision of transfer to ICU and throughout and beyond the stay in ICU. The aim of this work is to propose suggestions to strengthen the collaboration between the different teams involved, to facilitate the daily decision-making process, and to allow improvement of clinical practice.

1. Current Situation

Therapeutic advances regarding hematological malignancies allow the care of an increased number and older patients and improve the chances of cure or prolonged remissions [1–7]. At the same time, aggressiveness of therapeutics is often associated with a high risk of clinical distress [8–10].

It has been reported that 7% of all new cases of hematological malignancies and up to 15% of acute myeloid leukemia may justify a transfer to ICU [11, 12]. The main reasons for ICU admission include acute respiratory failure, septic shock, acute kidney injury, and coma [13].

Advances in life-sustaining therapies improve the management of these patients, with increased knowledge of the chances of reversibility and of the risk factors of unfavorable outcomes [14–20], but mortality in this group of patients still ranges from 33 to 58% [14, 21–25]. Intensive care treatments may even allow, if necessary, continuing hematological treatments in the most appropriate environment [26–28].

The human and economic costs of critical care should prompt the reflection on the justification of each admission to ICU [29–32]. The information due to patients and relatives implies that they are informed and that their views are taken into account [33, 34]. The collaboration of the teams of hematology and intensive care should improve the necessary collegial decision-making process whose traceability is mandatory.

2. The Views of Hematologists

The clinical distress, particularly when it is not related to the expected evolution of the disease, is a situation where decision-making is of high importance for the hematologic team and where interpersonal difficulties can appear [35, 36].

The hematologists may have difficulties to estimate the severity of the sudden acute clinical condition and its chances of reversibility. Whereas some early warning scoring systems have been established to detect patients at risk of rapid deterioration and critical illness among general medical patients, they have been found inconsistently reliable in the hematological setting [37–39]. The risk could be to maintain the patient in hematology department instead of organizing an early transfer to ICU. On the other hand, increased requests for transfer to ICU for patients who will not benefit from this highly technological environment are not desirable [32, 40, 41].

To avoid these extreme situations, we propose to distinguish medical situations when hematologists should consider a transfer to intensive care units according to the expected evolution of the underlying condition, while knowing that there can be no rigid criteria to send patients to ICU and that this decision has to be individualized [13, 20].

It is usually admitted that characteristics of the underlying disease fail to predict short term survival [20, 42–49] but do influence longer term survival [50–52]. But recently, a large study demonstrated that remission status was correlated with in-hospital mortality [13].

The prognosis and the chances of reversibility depending on the nature and the extent of the organ failure are less predictable.

From the hematologists' point of view, we identified four admission situations (Figure 1).

(1) (a) The hematologic underlying condition is at a palliative stage or (b) the patient suffers from an end-stage progressive condition unresponsive to any undertaken therapeutic measure, even if in remission of the hematologic disease (e.g., severe GVHD or progressive pulmonary failure). The acute illness is, then, the ultimate manifestation of an ineluctable deterioration. Usually, the transfer to ICU should not be proposed. It would be considered as an unreasonable and futile option. The decision of nontransfer

should be anticipated, discussed with the members of staff, communicated clearly to the teams and the families, and recorded in the medical file.

(2) The patient is (a) in first-line treatment and the therapeutic response cannot be assessed yet, (b) in complete remission or (c) showing a very good response to treatment; in those cases, the objectives of care are curative. The admission to ICU is necessary and the arguments must be presented to the intensivists so that they admit those patients regardless of the severity of the acute condition.

(3) The patient is showing (a) a partial response, (b) a chemosensitive relapse, or (c) refractory to first-line treatments but with reasonable chances of efficacy with innovative further-line treatments. This represents the most difficult case in the decision-making process and justifies a thorough collegial concertation. The arguments to take into account include the patient himself (age, performance status, and comorbidities), the severity of the clinical distress, and the prognosis of the underlying malignancy.

(4) The patient is involved in therapeutics with high-risk mortality and iatrogenic morbidities such as complications of allogeneic bone marrow transplant or experimental treatments. The decision-making process is usually complex and it should include the most recent prognosis assessment. The decision is not only technical and medical but also deals with the ethical and personal context that engages the responsibility of the hematologists prescribing procedures with potentially severe adverse consequences and for whom it may be difficult to assume disengagement.

3. The Views of Intensivist Physicians

In the past, the Society of Critical Care Medicine (SCCM) and the American Medical Association (AMA) [53, 54] clearly discouraged the admission of patients with oncological or hematological diseases to intensive care. This was especially true for patients requiring mechanical ventilation, with studies reporting more than 90% mortality in this population [55–58]. This led intensivists to have a negative image of patients with oncohematological conditions. These recommendations have been widely applied to adult patients for nearly ten years [59, 60].

Meanwhile considerable progress has improved the survival of these patients in ICU with an average mortality reduced to 40% including those requiring mechanical ventilation, dialysis, or shock therapy [15, 16, 22, 23, 43, 61]. As a result, the number of patients candidate for transfer to ICU increased considerably over the past years with the constant worry of doing the appropriate selection [62].

In the past, it has been reported that hematologic patients presented to the French intensivists for transfer to ICU had only 50% chances of being admitted [8]. More recently, 75% of patients considered for ICU admissions were finally admitted, but with 10% requiring more than one request before admission [13]. Interestingly, repeated requests were

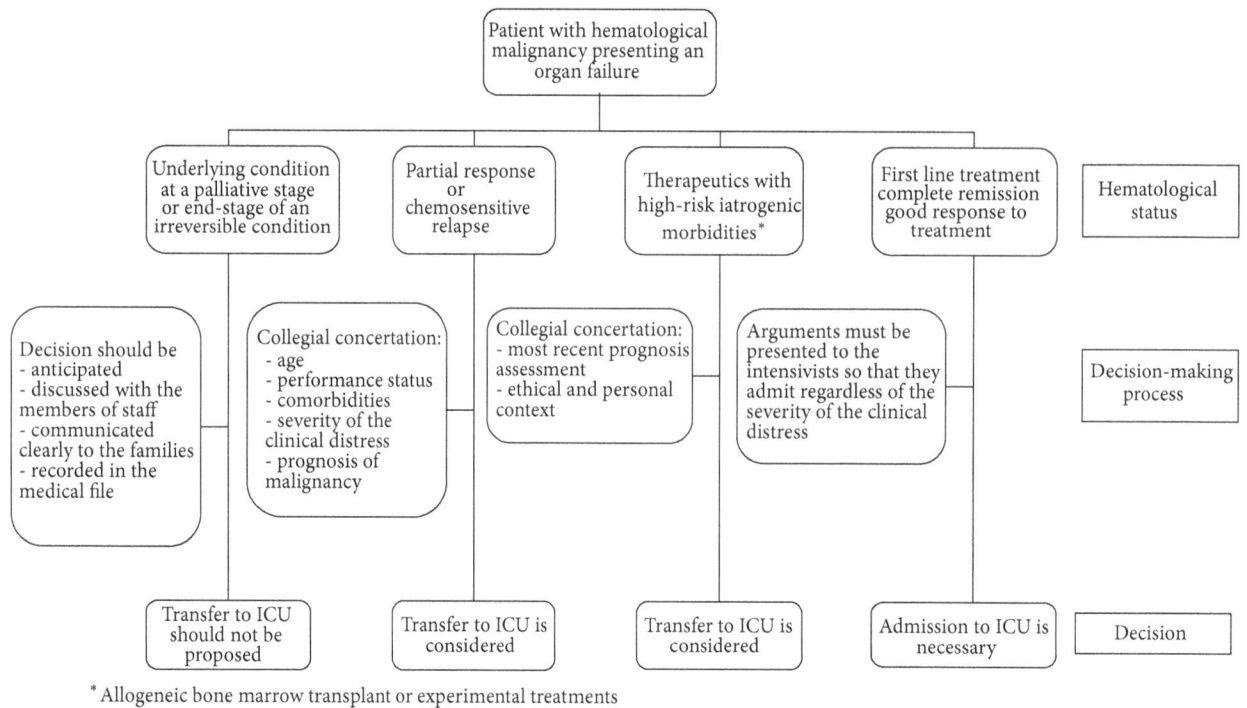

FIGURE 1: Decision model of ICU transfer of patients with hematological malignancies.

more frequent in patients admitted later, which may suggest a persistent reluctance to admit certain hematological patients. Besides a possible persistent negative image of the prognosis of hematological patients, this might be related to selection criteria that motivate refusal of admission to ICU.

These selection criteria differ between hematologists and intensivists. Hematologists consider in priority the underlying hematologic condition, the age of the patient, the performance status, and the availability of potentially life-prolonging treatments. Moreover, the concern about the infectious risk of neutropenic patients can lead to delaying the transfer, to maintain the patient in a protected environment. On the other hand, intensivists take into account the nature and the extent of multiple organ failures and favor early transfer to ICU so that patients can benefit from noninvasive diagnostic and therapeutic strategies before a potential deterioration of their clinical status [26, 63–65].

The difficulties arise from the fact that the information available at the admission to ICU is insufficient to discriminate the patients that will survive from those that will die [52, 66].

In order to maximize the chances of survival of the patients who may benefit from intensive care, different admission policies have been proposed. They are not necessarily exclusive of each other.

(i) Agreement on the level of care: also a single life-supporting intervention is associated with good survival; organ dysfunction appearing during the stay in ICU is associated with increased mortality [13, 25]. Consequently, in some cases, in particular when multiple variables predict a poor outcome, the intensivists

and the hematologists may agree on the limitations of the level of care to deliver during the first days in ICU (e.g., noninvasive ventilation rather than endotracheal or nonactive treatment of a new organ failure such as dialysis in renal failure of a patient ventilated after a bone marrow transplant).

(ii) ICU trial: a new strategy for admission of onco-hematologic patients to intensive care entitled ICU trial as a politics of "do everything that can be done" [62], but for a limited period, has been elaborated instead of the well-known old strategy "just say no" [67, 68]. The ICU trial is an alternative to ICU refusal for hematologic patients that consists of unlimited ICU support during a limited period of time, where everything is done for at least 3 to 5 days [24, 63]. Considering the seriousness of such decisions and their potential impact on the patients' outcome, the ICU trial could be a solution that takes into account the ethical tension between utility and futility.

(iii) Early transfer: this strategy favors early transfer to ICU so that patients can benefit from noninvasive diagnostic and therapeutic strategies before a potential deterioration of their clinical status. This approach is proactive rather than reactive and has been associated with improved outcomes [13, 61, 69].

4. Decision-Making Process

A structured process of decision making is critical to ensure consistency and the moral defensibility of these difficult decisions. The decision of transfer should arise from regular

TABLE 1: Multistep decision-making approach.

Before initiating any high-risk treatment	Possibility of a transfer to ICU should be discussed
As soon as a clinical distress appears	Intensivists must be consulted; they should participate in the early detection of critical states.
Transfer to ICU	Decision must arise from an interdisciplinary concertation between intensivists and hematologists. The need to document patient preferences is crucial.
Decision of nontransfer to ICU	Falls within the general context of limitations of treatments in hematology. Palliative care is required to guarantee end-of-life quality. The views of intensivists can be sought to help in symptom control.
3 to 5 days after admission to ICU	Concerted reevaluation must be programmed, especially in case of an ICU trial. Need to decide whether to maintain the same intensity of life-sustaining therapies or to consider withdrawal.
During stay in ICU	Hematologists have to visit regularly their patients in ICU and should take part actively in the decision to maintain the patient in ICU.
Regular scheduled multidisciplinary meetings	The objective is to discuss clinical situations involving intensivists and hematologists. It should be open to palliative care specialists and psychologists. The aim is to identify areas of improvement.
In case of limitation or withdrawal of active treatments	Collegial concertation has to be maintained to initiate palliative care and patient accompaniment and to provide the appropriate support to the relatives. At this stage, a transfer back to hematology can be discussed.

concertations between hematologists, intensivists, and their medical teams. The staff should be trained to be at a proactive interface with the patients and their relatives and to collect their consent for care and advance care planning [33, 34, 70].

The broad admission policies described earlier should lead to ICU admission for most patients within the scope of medical conditions 2, 3, and 4 described above that require life sustaining therapies because of at least one organ failure (other than hematologic failure) to define conditions of nontransfer (patients in palliative care, situation 1, or do-not-resuscitate order).

This project implies a multistep approach (Table 1).

(i) Early, when discussing the intensive hematological therapy, patients and their relatives must be informed of the risk of life-threatening evolutions, the consent for care must be obtained, and the patient's views about advance care planning should be reviewed.

(ii) Intensivists must be consulted as soon as a clinical situation may require a transfer and they have to participate in the early detection of critical states to avoid taking decisions in emergency.

(iii) The decision of transfer to ICU must arise from an interdisciplinary and collegial concertation between intensivists and hematologists, preferably in the day-time to avoid decisions taken in emergency or by a single physician as it could happen during the nighttime. The need to document patient preferences for resuscitation and end-of-life procedures is crucial before and at the admission to ICU.

(iv) The decision of nontransfer falls within the general context of limitations of treatments in hematology. This involves mainly patients with poor life expectancy regardless of treatments and palliative care is then required to guarantee end-of-life quality [71–74]. The views of intensivists can be sought in critical situations even if hematologists do not consider formally the transfer to ICU.

(v) When a patient has been admitted in ICU, a concerted reevaluation must be programmed regularly. This assessment specifies the number of organ failures and redefines the objectives of care. Hematologists have to visit regularly their patients in ICU and should take part actively in the decision to maintain the patient in ICU.

Apart from patients who improved rapidly and are transferred back to hematology ward and those who died, the active collaboration between intensivists and hematologists mainly concerns the issue of extension of stay in intensive care that arises for other patients.

Different evolutions are possible [24, 44].

(i) The clinical state of the patient improves partially. Life support is pursued without limit, subject to regular concerted assessment.

(ii) The clinical status deteriorates. The decision to withhold life-sustaining therapy should be considered. This is where the threshold between reasonable and nonreasonable stubbornness becomes an issue.

(iii) Some of these patients will neither improve nor deteriorate with active life-sustaining therapies, with the same persistent organ failure as at admission. Those patients ultimately raise major issues for intensivists and hematologic teams but also for their family [75]. The medical decision has to be individual. Most often, life support is pursued with continuation of active hematological treatment if required, while indicating the relatives in an adequate way that any deterioration will not necessarily lead to therapeutic escalation. In all cases, it is essential to ensure that all means are sought to guarantee patient comfort and support for their families.

In case of limitation or withdrawal of active treatments, collegial concertation has to be maintained to initiate palliative care and patient accompaniment and to provide the appropriate support to the relatives [34, 76, 77]. At this stage, a transfer back to hematology ward could be organized for non-ventilated patients. It is not there to abandon the patient but rather to facilitate the end-of-life in a quiet and comfortable environment, surrounded by the multidisciplinary team and the known caregivers, to allow his relatives to be free from the constraints of the ICU, and to facilitate psychological support. According to each situation, a transfer can be organized from hematology ward either towards a palliative care unit or back to the patient's home in collaboration with the family doctor.

5. Organization of the Concertation and Beyond

It is recommended to organize the concertation by integrating when possible the following procedures.

(i) On request of the hematologists, an intensivist can attend meetings in the department of hematology where high-risk procedures will be decided for the patients.

(ii) It may be useful to appoint a referent intensivist that will be at a privileged interface with the department of hematology.

(iii) Regular scheduled multidisciplinary meetings should be organized to evaluate the decisions and the collaboration, even retrospectively. The objective is to analyze clinical situations involving intensivists and hematologists, and their attitudes before the transfer to ICU, during the stay in critical care, after the release, and remotely beyond. These meetings would be opened to physicians and caregivers of both teams as well as to the palliative care specialists and psychologists. The aim is to identify areas of improvement.

(iv) Multidisciplinary meetings of morbimortality conferences should be organized periodically.

All centers of hematology should establish a framework agreement according to their specificities with their referent ICU to define the rules of functioning, including staff training, as recommended by the Joint Accreditation Committee of the International Society for Cellular Therapy (ISCT) and the European Group for Blood and Marrow Transplantation (EBMT) [78]. Facilitating this collaborative work and the involvement of highly qualified personnel should be one of the priorities of the institutional management.

The organization of multidisciplinary concertation ahead of the admission decision as well as the development of

information and communication should help in most cases to limit potential conflicts by anticipating them. Conflicts between physicians and patients or relatives may occur when there are decisions concerning the immediate future of the patient. Decisions to transfer or not to ICU may be perceived either as an aggressive treatment "*too much is done*" or on the contrary as abandonment and loss of chance "*not enough is done*" [75, 79, 80].

Immediate management of conflict and candid explanation to the patient or his relatives with a reasoned justification of the decision should help resolve the issues. If tension persists, it would be desirable to design a mediator to resolve the conflict. This mediator could be a member of the palliative care team, an ethicist, or a psychologist.

Investigations are still needed in the hematology units to monitor and evaluate the behavior and the factors influencing the primary decision of the hematologists to propose or not an admission to ICU, where selection criteria may vary according to the decision-making habits and the environment of each department. As a result, the only available research comes from ICU and includes only patients proposed to them. The objective would be to associate intensivists in the preliminary analyses of patients hospitalized in hematology, to organize a multidisciplinary dialogue, to anticipate the decisions, and thus to improve the identification of the patients that justify a transfer to ICU.

6. Conclusion

This work is the result of a collective reflection at the interface of two disciplines: hematology and intensive care and involves a common medical situation with decisions eminently difficult to manage in everyday life. Clarifying the medical conditions that may lead to a transfer to ICU, the relevant and consensual criteria of the decision-making process, and the concept of "ICU trial" represents an original aspect of this work.

The transfer of a patient has to respond to well-defined process on the basis of regular interdisciplinary collaboration before, during, and after the stay in intensive care. Decisions in this context have to comply with the principles of collegiality, with the involvement of the patient and his family and priority is given to anticipation approach. Traceability of decisions should also enable the individual and collective evaluation of these evolving professional practices. The evaluations of activities and regular meetings will allow maintaining communication between the professionals working in these departments and should lead to future collaborative research studies.

Conflict of Interests

The authors declare that there is no conflict of interests regarding the publication of this paper.

Acknowledgments

The authors would like to thank the members of the institutions involved in this work: (1) the members of the

Ethics Commission of the French Society of Hematology: Bastard Christian (Rouen), Beaussant Yvan (Besançon), Bauchetet Chantal (Paris, Necker), Cahn Jean-Yves (Grenoble), Cassassus Philippe (Paris, Avicennes), Ceccaldi Joël (Libourne), Cheminant Morgane (Paris), Colombat Philippe (Tours), Damotte Diane (Paris, Hôtel-Dieu), Gervaise Sylvie (Paris, Trousseau), Fiat Eric (Paris), Jaulmes Dominique (Paris, Saint-Antoine), Jouet Jean-Pierre (Lille), Margueritte Geneviève (Montpellier), Morin Sarah (Paris), Polomeni Alice (Paris, Saint-Antoine), Rochant Henri (Paris, Henri Mondor), Sotto Jean-Jacques (Grenoble), Zandecki Marc (Angers), and Zittoun Robert (Paris, Hôtel-Dieu), (2) the members of the Société de Réanimation en Langue Française: Azoulay Elie (Paris, Saint-Louis), Guidet Bertrand (Paris, Saint-Antoine), Rabbat Antoine (Paris, Hôtel-Dieu), and Timsit Jean-François (Grenoble), (3) the Members of the Groupe Francophone de Réanimation et Urgences Pédiatrique: Emeriaud Guillaume (Grenoble), Hubert Philippe (Paris, Necker), Valla Frédéric (Lyon), and (4) the members invited: Legrand Ollivier (Hématologie, Paris Hôtel-Dieu), and Leverger Guy (Pédiatrie, Paris Trousseau). The authors thank them for their participation, reflections, and contributions.

References

[1] D. Pulte, A. Gondos, and H. Brenner, "Improvements in survival of adults diagnosed with acute myeloblastic leukemia in the early 21st century," *Haematologica*, vol. 93, no. 4, pp. 594–600, 2008.

[2] D. Pulte, A. Gondos, and H. Brenner, "Ongoing improvement in outcomes for patients diagnosed as having non-Hodgkin lymphoma from the 1990s to the early 21st century," *Archives of Internal Medicine*, vol. 168, no. 5, pp. 469–476, 2008.

[3] S. Y. Kristinsson, P. W. Dickman, W. H. Wilson, N. Caporaso, M. Björkholm, and O. Landgren, "Improved survival in chronic lymphocytic leukemia in the past decade: a population-based study including 11,179 patients diagnosed between 1973–2003 in Sweden," *Haematologica*, vol. 94, no. 9, pp. 1259–1265, 2009.

[4] N. Pemmaraju, H. Kantarjian, J. Shan et al., "Analysis of outcomes in adolescents and young adults with chronic myelogenous leukemia treated with upfront tyrosine kinase inhibitor therapy," *Haematologica*, vol. 97, no. 7, pp. 1029–1035, 2012.

[5] R. Gurion, L. Vidal, A. Gafter-Gvili, Y. B. Yeshurun, P. Raanani, and O. Shpilberg, "5-Azacitidine prolongs overall survival in patients with myelodysplastic syndrome—a systematic review and meta-analysis," *Haematologica*, vol. 95, no. 2, pp. 303–310, 2010.

[6] E. Estey, "Acute myeloid leukemia and myelodysplastic syndromes in older patients," *Journal of Clinical Oncology*, vol. 25, no. 14, pp. 1908–1915, 2007.

[7] B. J. Roth, L. Krilov, S. Adams et al., "Clinical cancer advances 2012: annual report on progress against cancer from the American Society of Clinical Oncology," *Journal of Clinical Oncology*, vol. 31, no. 1, pp. 131–161, 2013.

[8] G. Thiéry, É. Azoulay, M. Darmon et al., "Outcome of cancer patients considered for intensive care unit admission: a hospital-wide prospective study," *Journal of Clinical Oncology*, vol. 23, no. 19, pp. 4406–4413, 2005.

[9] C. Morgan, T. Tillett, J. Braybrooke, and T. Ajithkumar, "Management of uncommon chemotherapy-induced emergencies," *The Lancet Oncology*, vol. 12, no. 8, pp. 806–814, 2011.

[10] S. Vento, F. Cainelli, and Z. Temesgen, "Lung infections after cancer chemotherapy," *The Lancet Oncology*, vol. 9, no. 10, pp. 982–992, 2008.

[11] A. C. Gordon, H. E. Oakervee, B. Kaya et al., "Incidence and outcome of critical illness amongst hospitalised patients with haematological malignancy: a prospective observational study of ward and intensive care unit based care," *Anaesthesia*, vol. 60, no. 4, pp. 340–347, 2005.

[12] P. Schellongowski, T. Staudinger, M. Kundi et al., "Prognostic factors for intensive care unit admission, intensive care outcome, and post-intensive care survival in patients with de novo acute myeloid leukemia: a single center experience," *Haematologica*, vol. 96, no. 2, pp. 231–237, 2011.

[13] E. Azoulay, D. Mokart, F. Pène et al., "Outcomes of critically ill patients with hematologic malignancies: prospective multicenter data from France and Belgium—a groupe de recherche respiratoire en réanimation onco-hématologique study," *Journal of Clinical Oncology*, vol. 31, no. 22, pp. 2810–2818, 2013.

[14] S. A. Namendys-Silva, M. O. Gonzalez-Herrera, F. J. Garcia-Guillen, J. Texcocano-Becerra, and A. Herrera-Gomez, "Outcome of critically ill patients with hematological malignancies," *Annals of Hematology*, vol. 92, no. 5, pp. 699–705, 2013.

[15] J. Larché, É. Azoulay, F. Fieux et al., "Improved survival of critically ill cancer patients with septic shock," *Intensive Care Medicine*, vol. 29, no. 10, pp. 1688–1695, 2003.

[16] É. Azoulay, G. Thiéry, S. Chevret et al., "The prognosis of acute respiratory failure in critically ill cancer patients," *Medicine*, vol. 83, no. 6, pp. 360–370, 2004.

[17] P. A. Hampshire, C. A. Welch, L. A. McCrossan, K. Francis, and D. A. Harrison, "Admission factors associated with hospital mortality in patients with haematological malignancy admitted to UK adult, general critical care units: a secondary analysis of the ICNARC Case Mix Programme Database," *Critical Care*, vol. 13, no. 4, article R137, 2009.

[18] W. M. Townsend, A. Holroyd, R. Pearce et al., "Improved intensive care unit survival for critically ill allogeneic haematopoietic stem cell transplant recipients following reduced intensity conditioning," *British Journal of Haematology*, vol. 161, no. 4, pp. 578–586, 2013.

[19] C. D. Yeo, J. W. Kim, S. C. Kim et al., "Prognostic factors in critically ill patients with hematologic malignancies admitted to the intensive care unit," *Journal of Critical Care*, vol. 27, no. 6, pp. 739.e1–739.e6, 2012.

[20] Q. A. Hill, "Intensify, resuscitate or palliate: decision making in the critically ill patient with haematological malignancy," *Blood Reviews*, vol. 24, no. 1, pp. 17–25, 2010.

[21] B. Y. Khassawneh, P. White Jr., E. J. Anaissie, B. Barlogie, and F. Charles Hiller, "Outcome from mechanical ventilation after autologous peripheral blood stem cell transplantation," *Chest*, vol. 121, no. 1, pp. 185–188, 2002.

[22] V. Peigne, K. Rusinová, L. Karlin et al., "Continued survival gains in recent years among critically ill myeloma patients," *Intensive Care Medicine*, vol. 35, no. 3, pp. 512–518, 2009.

[23] F. Pene, S. Percheron, V. Lemiale et al., "Temporal changes in management and outcome of septic shock in patients with malignancies in the intensive care unit," *Critical Care Medicine*, vol. 36, no. 3, pp. 690–696, 2008.

[24] G. T. Bird, P. Farquhar-Smith, T. Wigmore, M. Potter, and P. C. Gruber, "Outcomes and prognostic factors in patients

with haematological malignancy admitted to a specialist cancer intensive care unit: a 5 yr study," *British Journal of Anaesthesia*, vol. 108, no. 3, pp. 452–459, 2012.

[25] D. A. Geerse, L. F. R. Span, S.-J. Pinto-Sietsma, and W. N. K. A. van Mook, "Prognosis of patients with haematological malignancies admitted to the intensive care unit: sequential Organ Failure Assessment (SOFA) trend is a powerful predictor of mortality," *European Journal of Internal Medicine*, vol. 22, no. 1, pp. 57–61, 2011.

[26] M. Darmon, G. Thiery, M. Ciroldi et al., "Intensive care in patients with newly diagnosed malignancies and a need for cancer chemotherapy," *Critical Care Medicine*, vol. 33, no. 11, pp. 2488–2493, 2005.

[27] D. M. Vandijck, D. D. Benoit, P. O. Depuydt et al., "Impact of recent intravenous chemotherapy on outcome in severe sepsis and septic shock patients with hematological malignancies," *Intensive Care Medicine*, vol. 34, no. 5, pp. 847–855, 2008.

[28] J.-U. Song, G. Y. Suh, M. P. Chung et al., "Risk factors to predict outcome in critically ill cancer patients receiving chemotherapy in the intensive care unit," *Supportive Care in Cancer*, vol. 19, no. 4, pp. 491–495, 2011.

[29] S. G. Oeyen, D. D. Benoit, L. Annemans et al., "Long-term outcomes and quality of life in critically ill patients with hematological or solid malignancies: a single center study," *Intensive Care Medicine*, vol. 39, no. 5, pp. 889–898, 2013.

[30] T. M. Merz, P. Schär, M. Bühlmann, J. Takala, and H. U. Rothen, "Resource use and outcome in critically ill patients with hematological malignancy: a retrospective cohort study," *Critical Care*, vol. 12, no. 3, article R75, 2008.

[31] C. C. Earle, M. B. Landrum, J. M. Souza, B. A. Neville, J. C. Weeks, and J. Z. Ayanian, "Aggressiveness of cancer care near the end of life: is it a quality-of-care issue?" *Journal of Clinical Oncology*, vol. 26, no. 23, pp. 3860–3866, 2008.

[32] A. Giannini and D. Consonni, "Physicians' perceptions and attitudes regarding inappropriate admissions and resource allocation in the intensive care setting," *British Journal of Anaesthesia*, vol. 96, no. 1, pp. 57–62, 2006.

[33] A. A. Wright, B. Zhang, A. Ray et al., "Associations between end-of-life discussions, patient mental health, medical care near death, and caregiver bereavement adjustment," *Journal of the American Medical Association*, vol. 300, no. 14, pp. 1665–1673, 2008.

[34] M. J. Loscalzo, "Palliative care and psychosocial contributions in the ICU," *Hematology*, vol. 2008, no. 1, pp. 481–490, 2008.

[35] T. Shanafelt and L. Dyrbye, "Oncologist burnout: causes, consequences, and responses," *Journal of Clinical Oncology*, vol. 30, no. 11, pp. 1235–1241, 2012.

[36] D. A. Whippen and G. P. Canellos, "Burnout syndrome in the practice of oncology: results of a random survey of 1,000 oncologists," *Journal of Clinical Oncology*, vol. 9, no. 10, pp. 1916–1920, 1991.

[37] S. W. I. Bokhari, T. Munir, S. Memon, J. L. Byrne, N. H. Russell, and M. Beed, "Impact of critical care reconfiguration and track-and-trigger outreach team intervention on outcomes of haematology patients requiring intensive care admission," *Annals of Hematology*, vol. 89, no. 5, pp. 505–512, 2010.

[38] T. Cooksley, E. Kitlowski, and P. Haji-Michael, "Effectiveness of Modified Early Warning Score in predicting outcomes in oncology patients," *QJM: An International Journal of Medicine*, vol. 105, no. 11, Article ID hcs138, pp. 1083–1088, 2012.

[39] M. von Lilienfeld-Toal, K. Midgley, S. Lieberbach et al., "Observation-based early warning scores to detect impending

critical illness predict in-hospital and overall survival in patients undergoing allogeneic stem cell transplantation," *Biology of Blood and Marrow Transplantation*, vol. 13, no. 5, pp. 568–576, 2007.

[40] D. C. Angus, A. E. Barnato, W. T. Linde-Zwirble et al., "Use of intensive care at the end of life in the United States: an epidemiologic study," *Critical Care Medicine*, vol. 32, no. 3, pp. 638–643, 2004.

[41] R. D. Truog, M. L. Campbell, J. R. Curtis et al., "Recommendations for end-of-life care in the intensive care unit: a consensus statement by the American College of Critical Care Medicine," *Critical Care Medicine*, vol. 36, no. 3, pp. 953–963, 2008.

[42] F. Blot, M. Guiguet, G. Nitenberg, B. Leclercq, B. Gachot, and B. Escudier, "Prognostic factors for neutropenic patients in an intensive care unit: respective roles of underlying malignancies and acute organ failures," *European Journal of Cancer*, vol. 33, no. 7, pp. 1031–1037, 1997.

[43] E. Azoulay, C. Alberti, C. Bornstain et al., "Improved survival in cancer patients requiring mechanical ventilatory support: impact of noninvasive mechanical ventilatory support," *Critical Care Medicine*, vol. 29, no. 3, pp. 519–525, 2001.

[44] L. Lecuyer, S. Chevret, G. Thiery, M. Darmon, B. Schlemmer, and É. Azoulay, "The ICU trial: a new admission policy for cancer patients requiring mechanical ventilation," *Critical Care Medicine*, vol. 35, no. 3, pp. 808–814, 2007.

[45] A. O. Soubani, E. Kseibi, J. J. Bander et al., "Outcome and prognostic factors of hematopoietic stem cell transplantation recipients admitted to a medical ICU," *Chest*, vol. 126, no. 5, pp. 1604–1611, 2004.

[46] C. Ferrà, P. Marcos, M. Misis et al., "Outcome and prognostic factors in patients with hematologic malignancies admitted to the intensive care unit: a single-center experience," *International Journal of Hematology*, vol. 85, no. 3, pp. 195–202, 2007.

[47] S. R. Jackson, M. G. Tweeddale, M. J. Barnett et al., "Admission of bone marrow transplant recipients to the intensive care unit: outcome, survival and prognostic factors," *Bone Marrow Transplantation*, vol. 21, no. 7, pp. 697–704, 1998.

[48] H. Y. Park, G. Y. Suh, K. Jeon et al., "Outcome and prognostic factors of patients with acute leukemia admitted to the intensive care unit for septic shock," *Leukemia & Lymphoma*, vol. 49, no. 10, pp. 1929–1934, 2008.

[49] F. Kroschinsky, M. Weise, T. Illmer et al., "Outcome and prognostic features of intensive care unit treatment in patients with hematological malignancies," *Intensive Care Medicine*, vol. 28, no. 9, pp. 1294–1300, 2002.

[50] A. Rabbat, D. Chaoui, D. Montani et al., "Prognosis of patients with acute myeloid leukaemia admitted to intensive care," *British Journal of Haematology*, vol. 129, no. 3, pp. 350–357, 2005.

[51] J.-P. Sculier, M. Paesmans, E. Markiewicz, and T. Berghmans, "Scoring systems in cancer patients admitted for an acute complication in a medical intensive care unit," *Critical Care Medicine*, vol. 28, no. 8, pp. 2786–2792, 2000.

[52] P. B. Massion, A. M. Dive, C. Doyen et al., "Prognosis of hematologic malignancies does not predict intensive care unit mortality," *Critical Care Medicine*, vol. 30, no. 10, pp. 2260–2270, 2002.

[53] "American College of Chest Physicians/Society of Critical Care Medicine Consensus Conference: definitions for sepsis and organ failure and guidelines for the use of innovative therapies in sepsis," *Critical Care Medicine*, vol. 20, no. 6, pp. 864–874, 1992.

[54] "Guidelines for intensive care unit admission, discharge, and triage. Task Force of the American College of Critical Care Medicine, Society of Critical Care Medicine," *Critical Care Medicine*, vol. 27, no. 3, pp. 633–638, 1999.

[55] L. N. Tremblay, R. H. Hyland, B. D. Schouten, and P. J. Hanly, "Survival of acute myelogenous leukemia patients requiring intubation/ventilatory support," *Clinical and Investigative Medicine*, vol. 18, no. 1, pp. 19–24, 1995.

[56] F. Brunet, J. J. Lanore, J. F. Dhainaut et al., "Is intensive care justified for patients with haematological malignancies?" *Intensive Care Medicine*, vol. 16, no. 5, pp. 291–297, 1990.

[57] A. R. Lloyd-Thomas, I. Wright, T. A. Lister, and C. J. Hinds, "Prognosis of patients receiving intensive care for lifethreatening medical complications of haematological malignancy," *British Medical Journal*, vol. 296, no. 6628, pp. 1025–1029, 1988.

[58] G. D. Rubenfeld and S. W. Crawford, "Withdrawing life support from mechanically ventilated recipients of bone marrow transplants: a case for evidence-based guidelines," *Annals of Internal Medicine*, vol. 125, no. 8, pp. 625–633, 1996.

[59] M. Garrouste-Orgeas, L. Montuclard, J.-F. Timsit et al., "Predictors of intensive care unit refusal in French intensive care units: a multiple-center study," *Critical Care Medicine*, vol. 33, no. 4, pp. 750–755, 2005.

[60] C. L. Sprung, D. Geber, L. A. Eidelman et al., "Evaluation of triage decisions for intensive care admission," *Critical Care Medicine*, vol. 27, no. 6, pp. 1073–1079, 1999.

[61] M. Legrand, A. Max, V. Peigne et al., "Survival in neutropenic patients with severe sepsis or septic shock," *Critical Care Medicine*, vol. 40, no. 1, pp. 43–49, 2012.

[62] É. Azoulay and B. Afessa, "The intensive care support of patients with malignancy: do everything that can be done," *Intensive Care Medicine*, vol. 32, no. 1, pp. 3–5, 2006.

[63] E. Azoulay, M. Soares, M. Darmon, D. Benoit, S. Pastores, and B. Afessa, "Intensive care of the cancer patient: Recent achievements and remaining challenges," *Annals of Intensive Care*, vol. 1, no. 1, pp. 1–13, 2011.

[64] M. Soares, J. I. F. Salluh, N. Spector, and J. R. Rocco, "Characteristics and outcomes of cancer patients requiring mechanical ventilatory support for > 24 hrs," *Critical Care Medicine*, vol. 33, no. 3, pp. 520–526, 2005.

[65] F. Neumann, O. Lobitz, R. Fenk et al., "The sepsis-related Organ Failure Assessment (SOFA) score is predictive for survival of patients admitted to the intensive care unit following allogeneic blood stem cell transplantation," *Annals of Hematology*, vol. 87, no. 4, pp. 299–304, 2008.

[66] J. Timsit, J. Fosse, G. Troché et al., "Accuracy of a composite score using daily SAPS II and LOD scores for predicting hospital mortality in ICU patients hospitalized for more than 72 h," *Intensive Care Medicine*, vol. 27, no. 6, pp. 1012–1021, 2001.

[67] G. C. Carlon, "Just say no," *Critical Care Medicine*, vol. 17, no. 1, pp. 106–107, 1989.

[68] J. S. Groeger and P. B. Bach, "Consider saying yes," *Critical Care Medicine*, vol. 31, no. 1, pp. 320–321, 2003.

[69] E. Lengliné, E. Raffoux, V. Lemiale et al., "Intensive care unit management of patients with newly diagnosed acute myeloid leukemia with no organ failure," *Leukemia and Lymphoma*, vol. 53, no. 7, pp. 1352–1359, 2012.

[70] J. W. Mack, A. Cronin, N. L. Keating et al., "Associations between end-of-life discussion characteristics and care received near death: a prospective cohort study," *Journal of Clinical Oncology*, vol. 30, no. 35, pp. 4387–4395, 2012.

[71] C. Bastard, D. Bordessoule, P. Casassus et al., "Les limitations thérapeutiques en hématologie: réflexions et propositions éthiques de la Société Française d'Hématologie," *Hématologie*, vol. 11, no. 1, pp. 71–79, 2005.

[72] A. A. Wright, N. L. Keating, T. A. Balboni, U. A. Matulonis, S. D. Block, and H. G. Prigerson, "Place of death: correlations with quality of life of patients with cancer and predictors of bereaved caregivers' mental health," *Journal of Clinical Oncology*, vol. 28, no. 29, pp. 4457–4464, 2010.

[73] Y. H. Yun, Y. C. Kwon, M. K. Lee et al., "Experiences and attitudes of patients with terminal cancer and their family caregivers toward the disclosure of terminal illness," *Journal of Clinical Oncology*, vol. 28, no. 11, pp. 1950–1957, 2010.

[74] D. W. Frost, D. J. Cook, D. K. Heyland, and R. A. Fowler, "Patient and healthcare professional factors influencing end-of-life decision-making during critical illness: a systematic review," *Critical Care Medicine*, vol. 39, no. 5, pp. 1174–1189, 2011.

[75] M. A. Cesta, M. Cardenas-Turanzas, C. Wakefield, K. J. Price, and J. L. Nates, "Life-supportive therapy withdrawal and length of stay in a large oncologic intensive care unit at the end of life," *Journal of Palliative Medicine*, vol. 12, no. 8, pp. 713–718, 2009.

[76] J. J. Strand and J. A. Billings, "Integrating palliative care in the intensive care unit," *The Journal of Supportive Oncology*, vol. 10, no. 5, pp. 180–187, 2012.

[77] D. Cook and G. Rocker, "Dying with dignity in the intensive care unit," *The New England Journal of Medicine*, vol. 370, no. 26, pp. 2506–2514, 2014.

[78] C. Chabannon, D. Pamphilon, C. Vermylen et al., "Ten years after the first inspection of a candidate European centre, an EBMT registry analysis suggests that clinical outcome is improved when hematopoietic SCT is performed in a JACIE accredited program," *Bone Marrow Transplantation*, vol. 47, no. 1, pp. 15–17, 2012.

[79] K. H. Abbott, J. G. Sago, C. M. Breen, A. P. Abernethy, and J. A. Tulsky, "Families looking back: one year after discussion of withdrawal or withholding of life-sustaining support," *Critical Care Medicine*, vol. 29, no. 1, pp. 197–201, 2001.

[80] T. T. Levin, B. Moreno, W. Silvester, and D. W. Kissane, "End-of-life communication in the intensive care unit," *General Hospital Psychiatry-Journal*, vol. 32, no. 4, pp. 433–442, 2010.

13

Therapy with Interleukin-22 Alleviates Hepatic Injury and Hemostasis Dysregulation in Rat Model of Acute Liver Failure

Tariq Helal Ashour

Department of Laboratory Medicine, Faculty of Applied Medical Sciences, Umm Al-Qura University, P.O. Box 7607, Makkah 7152, Saudi Arabia

Correspondence should be addressed to Tariq Helal Ashour; thaashour@hotmail.com

Academic Editor: Myriam Labopin

The therapeutic efficacy of interleukin-22 (IL-22) on liver injury and hematological disturbances was studied in rat model of acute liver failure (ALF) induced by D-galactosamine/lipopolysaccharide (D-GalN/LPS). The following parameters were investigated: (1) survival rate, (2) serum levels of liver function enzymes (aspartate aminotransferase (AST), alanine aminotransferase (ALT), and alkaline phosphatase (ALP)), total bilirubin (TBILI), and total albumen (ALB), (3) blood clotting tests (prothrombin time (PT), activated partial thromboplastin time (aPTT), and fibrinogen level (FIB)) and white blood cells (WBCs), red blood cells (RBCs), and platelet counts, (4) hepatic levels of tumor necrosis factor-α (TNF-α) and cyclooxygenase-2 (COX-2), and (5) liver histopathology. After 48 hours of D-GalN/LPS, the rats exhibited 20% mortality, significant increases in AST, ALT, ALP, TBILI, PT, and aPTT, TNF-α, and COX-2 and significant decreases in FIB, WBCs, and RBCs. By contrast, therapy with IL-22 prevented the lethal effect of D-GalN/LPS by 100% and efficiently alleviated all the biochemical and hematological abnormalities that were observed in ALF untreated group. Furthermore, IL-22 treatment decreased the hepatic contents of TNF-α and COX-2. The histopathological findings also supported the hepatoprotective effect of IL-22. Taken together, therapy with IL-22 can represent a promising therapeutic tool against liver injury and its associated hemostasis disturbances.

1. Introduction

Acute liver failure (ALF) and fulminant hepatitis (FH) are devastating liver diseases with multiple etiologies, coagulability dysfunctions, poor prognosis, and 90% overall mortality rate [1]. Up till now there are no effective treatment therapies for this disease and its highly fatal complications [2]. Coherently, development of more effective and highly selective therapeutic strategy is a paramount medical need.

IL-22 is a newly emerged cytokine with unique biological activities. Various cell types of hematopoietic origin produce IL-22, such as innate lymphoid cells, NK, NKT, and $\gamma\delta$ T cells [3]. IL-22 exerts its biological functions via activation of membrane-bound heterodimeric receptor complex consisting of IL-22R1 and IL-10R2, which is predominantly expressed by epithelial cells including gut and liver cells [4, 5]. In addition to its defense role against infectious pathogens, numerous studies demonstrated the favorable tissue protective properties of either exogenously administered or endogenously overexpressed IL-22. In this concept, hepatocytes abundantly express IL-22R and its stimulation via IL-22 promotes hepatocyte growth and survival [5].

The hepatoprotective effects of IL-22 have recently been suggested in a variety of hepatocellular damages [6–9]. For example, IL-22 promotes liver regeneration after hepatectomy [7], protects against acute alcohol-induced hepatotoxicity [8], and ameliorates liver fibrogenesis via induction of the senescence of hepatic stellate cell [9], suggesting a therapeutic implication of this cytokine in liver transplantation or patients undergoing hepatic surgery. IL-22 has been shown to promote proliferation of liver stem/progenitor cells in mice and patients with chronic HBV infection [10]. Furthermore, an inverse correlation between the degree of liver fibrosis and IL-22 concentration was recently detected in the liver tissues of patients with chronic HBV infection [11].

Based on these observations, an application of exogenous IL-22 or induction of its endogenous production may represent an innovative therapeutic option in human patients with acute or chronic liver disease [5, 11, 12]. Therefore, the present study was designed to investigate the therapy efficacy or IL-22 therapy against ALF and its associated hemostasis and hematological alterations that are induced rats by D-GalN/LPS.

2. Materials and Methods

2.1. Chemicals and Reagents. Recombinant rat interleukin-22 (rIL-22) was purchased from R&D Systems (Minneapolis, MN, USA). Commercial enzyme-linked immunosorbent assay (ELISA) kits of rat COX-2 rat TNF-α were purchased from R&D Systems and IBL International (GmbH, Hamburg, Germany), respectively. D-Galactosamine (D-GalN) and phenol extracted lipopolysaccharide from *Escherichia coli* (LPS) were obtained from Sigma-Aldrich (St. Louis, MO, USA). Other used chemicals and reagents are stated under the sections of their applications.

2.2. Animals and Experimental Approach. All experimental protocols were approved by the Committee for the Care and Use of Laboratory Animals at Umm Al-Qura University and were in accordance with the Guide for the Care and Use of Laboratory Animals published by the U.S. National Institutes of Health [13].

In this study, thirty adult male Wistar rats weighing 230 ± 15 g were randomly and equally assigned into 3 groups: group I; control rats did not receive any treatment; group II; D-GalN/LPS group in which rats were intraperitoneally (i.p.) injected with a nonhighly lethal dose of D-GalN (400 mg/kg BW) and LPS (40 μg/kg BW) dissolved in 1 mL of sterile saline as described previously [14]; and group III: D-GalN/LPS + rIL-22 group in which the rats were treated with two doses of rIL-22 (1 μg/g BW/dose, dissolved in 0.5 mL saline; i.p.) at time 0 and 6 hrs after D-GalN/LPS injection, respectively.

All animals were observed for 48 hrs for survivability, and two rats from group II only were dead. At the end of the experiments, all animal groups were sacrificed under ether anesthesia and their blood specimens were collected and their livers were harvested for the target examinations.

2.3. Blood Sampling and Analysis. During scarification process, three blood samples were immediately withdrawn from the vena cava of each rat and used for blood coagulation, hematology, and biochemical analyses. The first sample was collected in a tube that contained 0.11 M sodium citrate anticoagulant (1 : 9, v : v) and used for plasma preparation for screening of the following blood coagulation tests: prothrombin time (PT), activated partial thromboplastin time (aPTT), and fibrinogen concentrations (FIB), by using Dade Behring reagents and following manufacturer's instructions as previously described [15]. The second sample was collected in a tube that contained disodium salt of ethylene diamine tetra acetic acid (EDTA) anticoagulant and used for determination of the following hematology parameters: erythrocyte

count (RBC), leukocyte count (WBC), and platelet count (PLT). The last portion of the collected blood was placed in a plain centrifuge tube without any anticoagulant and used for assessment of the serum concentrations of liver function enzymes (aspartate aminotransferase (AST), alanine aminotransferase (ALT), and alkaline phosphatase (ALP)), albumin (ALB), and total bilirubin (TBILI) using commercially available diagnostic kits (Biomerieux SA, France), and according to manufacturer's instructions.

2.4. ELISA Assays of TNF-α and COX-2 Concentrations in Liver. After blood withdrawal, the livers were harvested quickly, and a portion of each isolated liver was homogenized in RIPA lysis buffer (1 : 6, w : v) and then centrifuged at 10,000 rpm for 10 min at 4°C. The obtained supernatant was used for measurement the intrahepatic concentrations of TNF-α and COX-2 proteins by using ELISA kits and an automated ELISA analyzer (HUMAN, Biochemica und Diagnostica, MBH, Germany). All samples were processed in duplicate and according the manufacturer's instructions.

2.5. Histological Analysis. For histopathological investigations, blocks of all isolated livers were fixed in 10% buffered formalin, embedded in paraffin, sectioned into 5 μm-thickness slices, stained with hematoxylin and eosin (H&E), and examined with a light microscopy in a blinded fashion for the presence of the hallmarks of hepatic injury.

2.6. Statistical Analysis. The results were expressed as the mean ± standard deviation and statistical analysis was carried out using SPSS software, version 16.0 (SPSS Inc., Chicago, IL, USA). One-way analysis of variance (ANOVA) followed by Student's *t*-test was used to analyze the statistical differences. Moreover, the statistical significance of survival rate among the groups was determined by using *Chi-square* test. $P < 0.05$ was considered to represent a statistically significant difference.

3. Results

3.1. Hepatoprotective Effect of IL-22 Therapy. All animal groups were monitored over 48 h after D-GalN/LPS injection to determine their survival rate. As shown in Table 1, the injected D-GalN (400 mg/kg) plus LPS (40 μg/kg) resulted in 20% mortality rate associated with severe hepatic injury reflected by significant increases in serum levels of liver function enzymes (AST, ALT, and ALP) and TBILI and significant decreases in serum ALB. On the other hand, administration of IL-22 after D-GalN/LPS kept the rats survivability by 100% and markedly protected their livers, as evidenced by returning the serum levels of AST, ALT, ALP, TBILI, and ALB almost near their baseline control values (Table 1). The histopathological findings also supported the biochemical observations. As illustrated in Figure 1, livers of D-GalN/LPS group showed a high degree of hepatocellular necrosis, apoptosis, and inflammatory cell infiltration; however, rats that were injected with D-GalN/LPS and treated

(a)

(b)

(c)

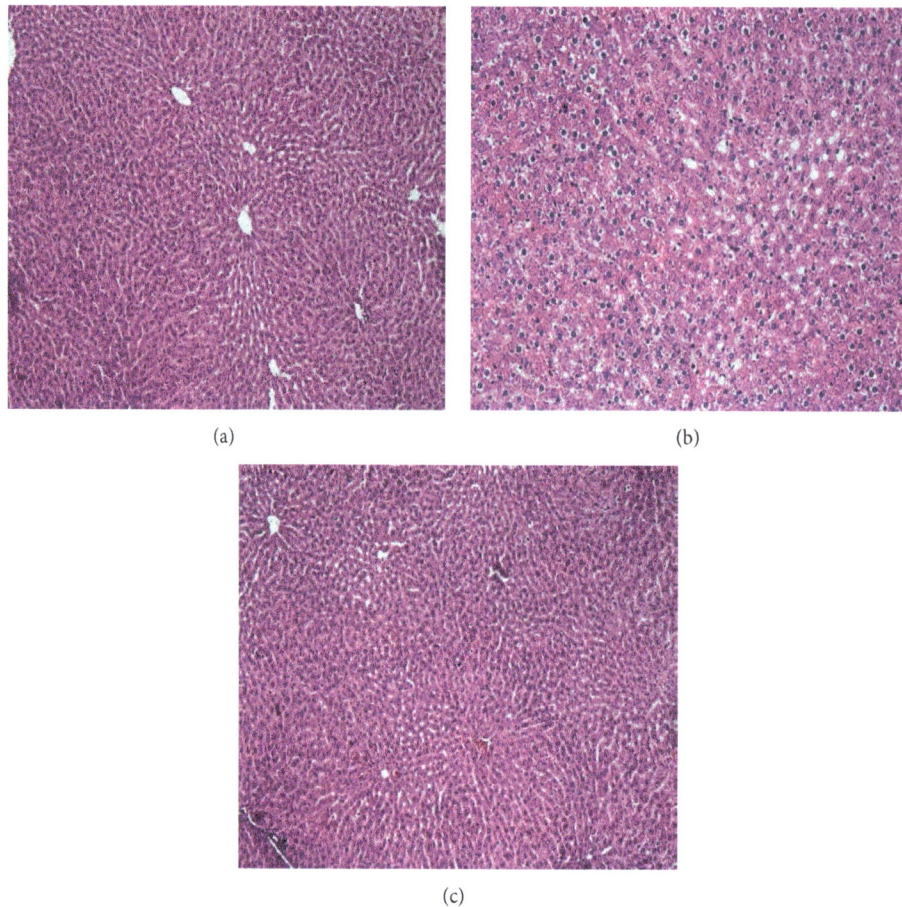

FIGURE 1: Hepatoprotective effect of IL-22 therapy against D-GalN/LPS-induced acute liver injury in rats. In comparison with livers of normal control rats (a), after 48 h from injection of D-GalN/LPS, there was severe hepatic injury that reflected a high degree of hepatocellular necrosis, apoptosis, and inflammatory cell infiltration (b); however, livers of rats injected with D-GalN/LPS and then treated with IL-22 (c) showed scant pathological foci and undetectable inflammatory cell infiltration.

TABLE 1: Effects of IL-22 therapy on the survival rate and liver function serobiomarkers of rats 48 h after D-GalN/LPS injection.

Groups	AST (IU/L)	ALT (IU/L)	ALP (IU/L)	TBILI (mg/dL)	ALB (g/dL)	Mortality (%)
Control	105 ± 15.1	53.7 ± 8.9	211 ± 39.3	0.08 ± 0.01	4.4 ± 0.9	0
D-GalN/LPS	$410 \pm 45.8^*$	$172 \pm 31^*$	$853 \pm 214^*$	$1.1 \pm 0.02^*$	$1.7 \pm 0.3^*$	20^*
D-GalN/LPS + IL-22	$143 \pm 23.3^\#$	$62.6 \pm 11.9^\#$	$259 \pm 41^\#$	$0.1 \pm 0.02^\#$	$4.1 \pm 0.7^\#$	$0^\#$

Values are represented as mean ± SD. $^*P < 0.05$ versus control group; $^\#P < 0.05$ versus D-GalN/LPS group.

with IL-22 showed scant pathological foci and undetectable inflammatory cell infiltration in their lives.

3.2. Blood Coagulation Tests and Hematological Findings. Coagulation and hematological abnormalities are common in human patients with acute liver injury. In consistency, rats with acute liver injury caused by D-GalN/LPS showed significant alterations of blood clotting tests: PT, aPTT, and FIB, indicating the influence on the intrinsic, extrinsic, and common pathway of coagulation. As shown in Figure 2, PT and aPTT values were prolonged more than 2 times, and FIB values were reduced to ≥2-folds after 48 h of injection of D-GalN/LPS relative to their control values. Also, as compared with control values, D-GalN/LPS significantly decreased the

blood counts of WBCs, RBCs, and PLT (Figure 2). By contrast, treatment of D-GalN/LPS-injected rats with IL-22 had significantly succeeded in reversion of all these abnormalities in blood coagulation tests and counts of WBCs, RBCs, and PLT (Figure 2).

3.3. Hepatic Levels of TNF-α and COX-2. There is strong evidence that D-GalN/LPS-induced acute liver injury and fulminant hepatitis are associated with liver infiltration with inflammatory immune cells with subsequent abundant increase in the production of proinflammatory mediators including TNF-α and COX-2. To confirm this fact, the concentrations of these two molecules were measured in the livers of all animal groups after 48 h form D-GalN/LPS. As

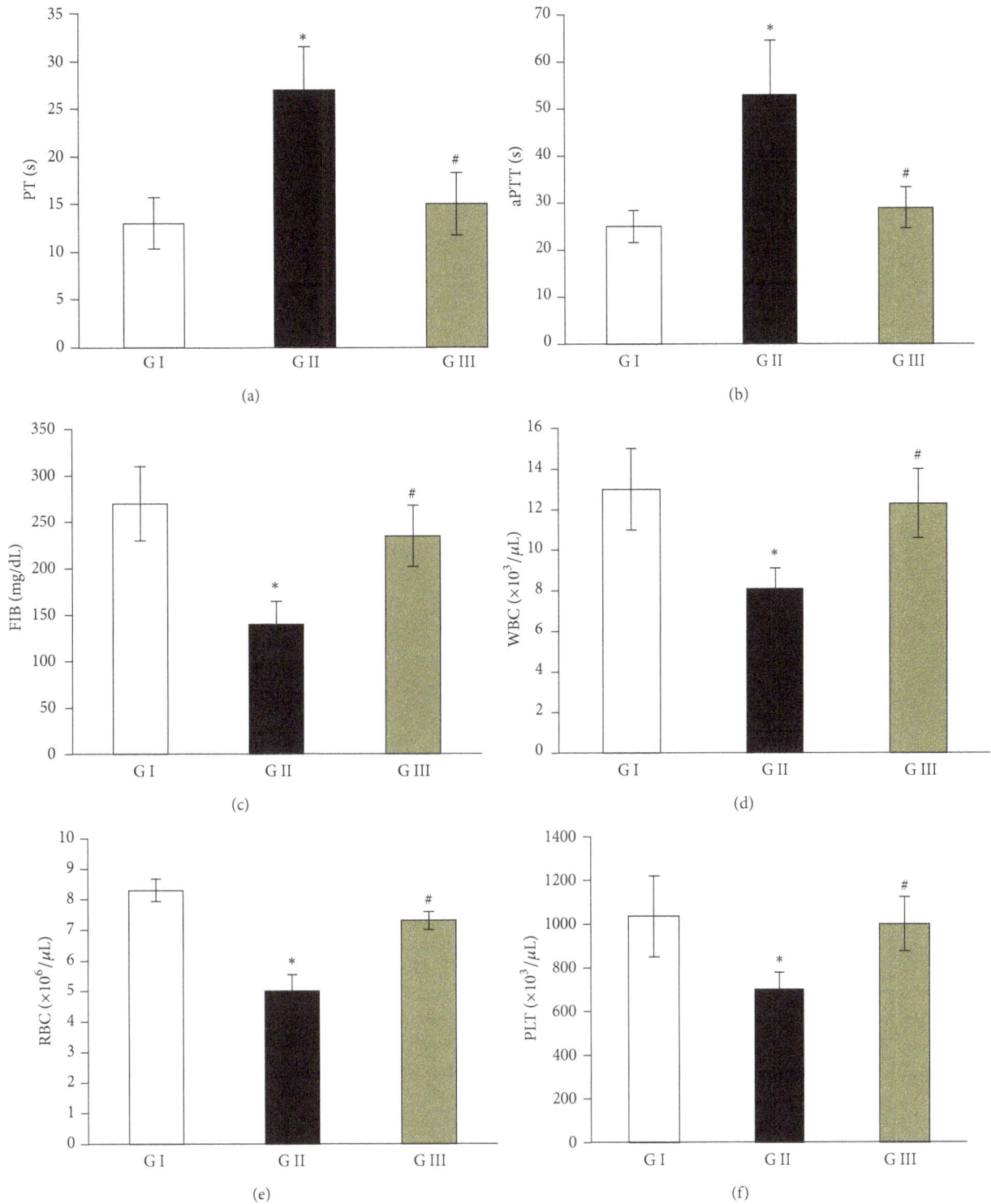

FIGURE 2: Alleviatived effects of IL-22 therapy on the alterations of blood coagulation tests and blood cell counts in D-GalN/LPS injected rats. GI: control group, GII: D-GalN/LPS group, and GIII: D-GalN/LPS + IL-22 group. Values are represented as mean ± SD. $^{*}P < 0.05$ versus control group; $^{#}P < 0.05$ versus D-GalN/LPS untreated group.

demonstrated in Figure 3, livers of normal control group contain extremely very low or even undetectable levels of TNF-α and COX-2; however, after 48 h of D-GalN/LPS injection there was a significant increase in the intrahepatic levels of these two proinflammatory molecules. In contrast, therapy with IL-22 was efficiently succeeded in inhibiting the stimulating effects of D-GalN/LPS on TNF-α and COX-2 production in liver tissues (Figure 3).

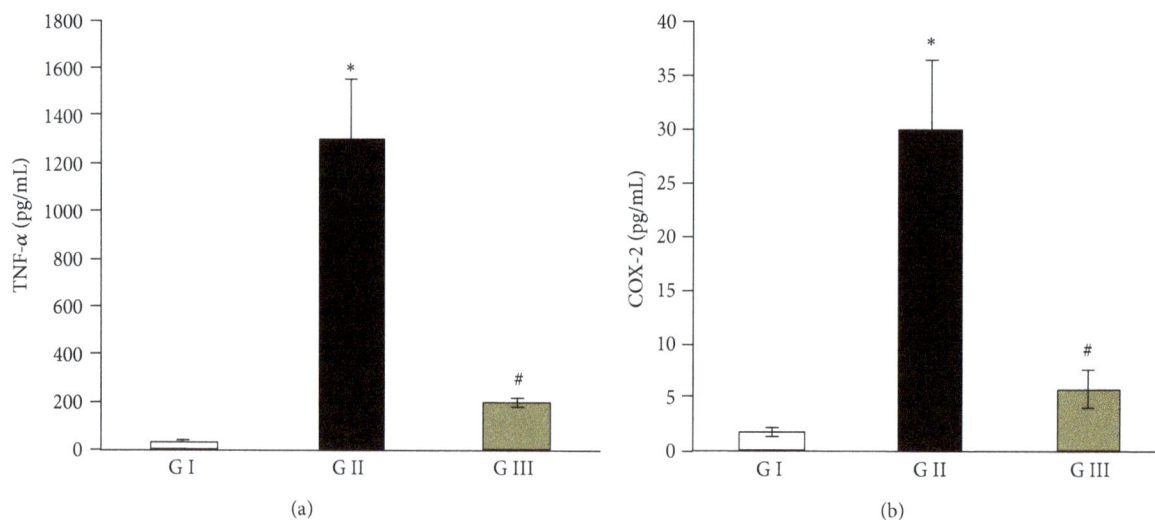

FIGURE 3: Levels of proinflammatory mediators; tumor necrosis factor-α (TNF-α), and cyclooxygenase-2 (COX-2), in the liver tissues. GI: control group, GII: D-GalN/LPS group, and GIII: D-GalN/LPS + IL-22 group. Values are represented as mean ± SD. $^*P$ < 0.05 versus control group; $^\#P$ < 0.05 versus D-GalN/LPS untreated group.

4. Discussion

Despite the substantial advances in controlling of human diseases, the impact of liver diseases is still worldwide a major health problem. Bacterial endotoxin (LPS) derived from intestinal bacteria is implicated in the pathogenesis of several acute and chronic inflammatory liver diseases [1, 16]. At the experimental level, LPS/D-GalN-induced liver injury is a well-established animal model of acute liver failure (ALF) and fulminant hepatitis. In this model D-GalN blocks gene transcription in the liver and LPS in turn induces an acute cytokine-dependent liver inflammation accompanied by massive liver necrosis, hemostasis disturbances, and death of the animals [17–19]. The current study showed that therapy with IL-22 completely prevented the mortality and significantly alleviated the hepatic damage and the deteriorated blood cell counts and coagulation tests in a rat model of ALF induced by D-GalN/LPS. Moreover, it also significantly suppressed the production of TNF-α and COX-2 in the liver tissues of rats injected with D-GalN/LPS. Coherently, IL-22 may be a promising therapeutic agent that can reverse the hepatic injury and subsequent coagulation dysfunction in patients with acute hepatitis.

IL-22 is a recently discovered cytokine with pivotal biological activities that its hepatoprotective effects have recently been suggested in a variety of hepatocellular damages [6]. In this concept, it has been postulated that IL-22 is a survival factor for hepatocytes and induces antiapoptotic and mitogenic gene expression in the liver cells [20, 21]. IL-22 was found to enhance liver regeneration [7] and protect the liver against fatty liver disease [22], as well as against ethanol-, concanavalin A-, carbon tetrachloride-, and Fas ligand-induced liver injury [8, 20, 21]. Additionally, an inverse correlation between the degree of liver fibrosis and IL-22 concentration was recently observed in the liver tissues of patients with chronic HBV infection, hypothesizing that

IL-22 may also play an antifibrotic role in human liver diseases [9–12]. In agreement with these previous findings, the remarkable hepatoprotective effects of IL-22 against D-GalN/LPS-induced acute liver injury in rats were significantly detected at the biochemical and histopathological levels (Table 1 and Figure 1).

The liver is the major organ for synthesis of blood clotting factors and blood proteins. Consequently, coagulation and hematological abnormalities are common in human patients with acute liver injury [19]. Consistent with this fact, rats injected with D-GalN/LPS had developed severe hepatic injury, as evidenced by elevations in the serum levels of liver function enzymes (AST, ALT, and ALP) and total bilirubin and a significant decrease in total albumen, which were associated with coagulation dysfunction reflected by prolonged PT and aPTT, and decreased fibrinogen levels. Moreover, there was a significant reduction in the blood WBCs, RBCs, and platelet counts in rats received D-GalN/LPS. Similar findings of hemostasis disturbances in D-GalN/LPS-induced ALF have also been previously reported by Korish [19]. Interestingly, therapy with IL-22 after D-GalN/LPS injection had not only reversed the abnormal liver functions and blood coagulation tests but also numbers of WBCs, RBSc, and platelets almost near to their normal control values (Figure 2). In support, Liang et al. [23] revealed that injection of IL-22 into mice modulates the factors involved in coagulation, including fibrinogen levels and platelet numbers, and cellular constituents of blood, such as neutrophil and RBC counts. In their study, mice treated with IL-22 showed significant increases in platelets and neutrophils counts in their blood, and an enhanced fibrinogen transcript in their liver [23]. Collectively, these findings indicate that IL-22 can alleviate the hepatic damage and disturbances in blood hemostasis and cellularity that were observed in acute liver injury as in D-GalN/LPS model.

There is ample evidence of the central pathogenic role of TNF-α in development of a variety of liver disease modalities, particularly in mortality, acute liver injury, and fulminant hepatitis induced by D-GalN/LPS [17, 18, 24]. TNF-α causing fatal hepatic failure and septic shock in humans has also been reported [25]. Blocking of TNF-α synthesis or activity can attenuate LPS-induced liver injury, and this confirms the pivotal role of TNF-α in sepsis-related liver toxicity [26, 27]. Interestingly, the results of the current study are in harmony with these facts, whereas rats injected with D-GalN/LPS and left without treatment exhibited abundant release of TNF-α in their liver tissues, and this phenomenon was markedly inhibited via IL-222 therapy (Figure 3).

In the present study, D-GalN/LPS significantly induced the hepatic COX-2 production, and treatment of these animals with IL-22 was efficiently succeeded to counteract this effect (Figure 3). In support, Chang and his colleagues demonstrated that therapy with IL-22 directly suppressed the production of COX-2 in injured myocardial cells [28]. COX-2 has a crucial role in the pathogenesis of inflammation by synthesis of potent inflammatory mediators (prostanoids) in inflamed tissues. LPS has been shown to stimulate the expression of COX-2 in various human cells including hepatocytes [29], and intrahepatic expression of COX-2 is induced in liver injury by LPS [30]. More interestingly, to evaluate the effect of hepatocyte COX-2 in D-GalN/LPS-induced liver injury, Han et al. [31] had generated transgenic mice with targeted expression of COX-2 in the liver, and then the animals were injected with D-GalN/LPS. In comparison with wild type mice, the COX-2 transgenic mice exhibited earlier mortality, higher serum ALT and AST levels, and more prominent liver tissue damage. Moreover, pretreatment of these COX-2 transgenic mice with a selective COX-2 inhibitor markedly attenuated D-GalN/LPS-induced liver damage, suggesting that hepatocyte COX-2 and its downstream signaling pathway accelerate LPS-induced liver injury [31].

5. Conclusions

The present data indicate that therapy with IL-22 has a potent protective effect against D-GalN/LPS-induced liver injury, coagulation, and hematological disturbances in rats. The beneficial effects of IL-22 could, at least in part, be due to the direct and/or indirect inhibition of proinflammatory factors, such as TNF-α and COX-2. These findings can also suggest the potential therapeutic application of IL-22 for the treatment of acute liver damage and its associated coagulation dysfunction.

Conflict of Interests

The author declares that there is no conflict of interests regarding the publication of this paper.

Acknowledgment

The author gratefully acknowledges the help of Dr. Adel Galal El-Shemi (Departments of Lab Medicine, UQU, Saudi Arabia, and Pharmacology, Assiut University-Egypt) through the different phases of this study.

References

[1] W. M. Lee, "Acute liver failure," *Seminars in Respiratory and Critical Care Medicine*, vol. 33, pp. 36–45, 2012.

[2] F. Wu, M. Wang, and D. Tian, "Serum from patients with hepatitis E virus-related acute liver failure induces human liver cell apoptosis," *Experimental and Therapeutic Medicine*, vol. 7, no. 1, pp. 300–304, 2014.

[3] P. L. Simonian, F. Wehrmann, C. L. Roark, W. K. Born, R. L. O'Brien, and A. P. Fontenot, "$\gamma\delta$ T cells protect against lung fibrosis via IL-22," *Journal of Experimental Medicine*, vol. 207, no. 10, pp. 2239–2253, 2010.

[4] P. W. Wu, J. Li, S. R. Kodangattil et al., "IL-22R, IL-10R2, and IL-22BP binding sites are topologically juxtaposed on adjacent and overlapping surfaces of IL-22," *Journal of Molecular Biology*, vol. 382, no. 5, pp. 1168–1183, 2008.

[5] P. Kumar, K. Rajasekaran, J. M. Palmer, M. S. Thakar, and S. Malarkannan, "IL-22: an evolutionary missing-link authenticating the role of the immune system in tissue regeneration," *Journal of Cancer*, vol. 4, no. 1, pp. 57–65, 2013.

[6] L. A. Zenewicz and R. A. Flavell, "Recent advances in IL-22 biology," *International Immunology*, vol. 23, no. 3, pp. 159–163, 2011.

[7] X. Ren, B. Hu, and L. M. Colletti, "IL-22 is involved in liver regeneration after hepatectomy," *The American Journal of Physiology: Gastrointestinal and Liver Physiology*, vol. 298, no. 1, pp. G74–G80, 2010.

[8] W.-W. Xing, M.-J. Zou, S. Liu, T. Xu, J.-X. Wang, and D.-G. Xu, "Interleukin-22 protects against acute alcohol-induced hepatotoxicity in mice," *Bioscience, Biotechnology and Biochemistry*, vol. 75, no. 7, pp. 1290–1294, 2011.

[9] X. Kong, D. Feng, H. Wang et al., "Interleukin-22 induces hepatic stellate cell senescence and restricts liver fibrosis," *Hepatology*, vol. 56, no. 3, pp. 1150–1159, 2012.

[10] D. Feng, X. Kong, H. Weng et al., "Interleukin-22 promotes proliferation of liver stem/progenitor cells in mice and patients with chronic HBV infection," *Gastroenterology*, vol. 143, no. 1, pp. 188.e7–198.e7, 2012.

[11] X. Xiang, H. Gui, N. J. King et al., "IL-22 and non-ELR-CXC chemokine expression in chronic hepatitis B virus-infected liver," *Immunology and Cell Biology*, vol. 90, pp. 611–619, 2012.

[12] X. Kong, D. Feng, S. Mathews, and B. Gao, "Hepatoprotective and anti-fibrotic functions of interleukin-22: therapeutic potential for the treatment of alcoholic liver disease," *Journal of Gastroenterology and Hepatology*, vol. 28, no. 1, pp. 56–60, 2013.

[13] Institute of Laboratory Animal Resources, *Guide for the Care and Use of Laboratory Animals*, Institute of Laboratory Animal Resources, Commission on Life Sciences, National Research Council, Washington, DC, USA, 7th edition, 1996.

[14] L.-M. Liu, J.-X. Zhang, J. Luo et al., "A role of cell apoptosis in lipopolysaccharide (LPS)-induced nonlethal liver injury in D-galactosamine (D-GalN)-sensitized rats," *Digestive Diseases and Sciences*, vol. 53, no. 5, pp. 1316–1324, 2008.

[15] C. Lemini, R. Jaimez, and Y. Franco, "Gender and inter-species influence on coagulation tests of rats and mice," *Thrombosis Research*, vol. 120, no. 3, pp. 415–419, 2007.

[16] D.-W. Han, "Intestinal endotoxemia as a pathogenetic mechanism in liver failure," *World Journal of Gastroenterology*, vol. 8, no. 6, pp. 961–965, 2002.

[17] L. Dong, L. Zuo, S. Xia et al., "Reduction of liver tumor necrosis factor-α expression by targeting delivery of antisense oligonucleotides into Kupffer cells protects rats from fulminant hepatitis," *Journal of Gene Medicine*, vol. 11, no. 3, pp. 229–239, 2009.

[18] G. Sass, S. Heinlein, A. Agli, R. Bang, J. Schümann, and G. Tiegs, "Cytokine expression in three mouse models of experimental hepatitis," *Cytokine*, vol. 19, no. 3, pp. 115–120, 2002.

[19] A. A. Korish, "Effect of caffeic acid phenethyl ester on the hemostatic alterations associated with toxic-induced acute liver failure," *Blood Coagulation and Fibrinolysis*, vol. 21, no. 2, pp. 158–163, 2010.

[20] H. Pan, F. Hong, S. Radaeva, and B. Gao, "Hydrodynamic gene delivery of interleukin-22 protects the mouse liver from concanavalin A-, carbon tetrachloride-, and Fas ligand-induced injury via activation of STAT3," *Cellular & Molecular Immunology*, vol. 1, no. 1, pp. 43–49, 2004.

[21] S. Radaeva, R. Sun, H.-N. Pan, F. Hong, and B. Gao, "Interleukin 22 (IL-22) plays a protective role in T cell-mediated murine hepatitis: IL-22 is a survival factor for hepatocytes via STAT3 activation," *Hepatology*, vol. 39, no. 5, pp. 1332–1342, 2004.

[22] L. Yang, Y. Zhang, L. Wang et al., "Amelioration of high fat diet induced liver lipogenesis and hepatic steatosis by interleukin-22," *Journal of Hepatology*, vol. 53, no. 2, pp. 339–347, 2010.

[23] S. C. Liang, C. Nickerson-Nutter, D. D. Pittman et al., "IL-22 induces an acute-phase response," *Journal of Immunology*, vol. 185, no. 9, pp. 5531–5538, 2010.

[24] Z. Wu, X. Kong, T. Zhang, J. Ye, Z. Fang, and X. Yang, "Pseudoephedrine/ephedrine shows potent anti-inflammatory activity against TNF-alpha-mediated acute liver failure induced by lipopolysaccharide/d-galactosamine," *European Journal of Pharmacology*, vol. 724, pp. 112–121, 2014.

[25] A. Waage, "Presence and involvement of TNF-alpha in septic shock," in *Tumor Necrosis Factors: The Molecules and Their Emerging Role in Medicine*, B. Beutler, Ed., pp. 275–283, Raven Press, New York, NY, USA, 1993.

[26] H. Jaeschke, G. J. Gores, A. I. Cederbaum, J. A. Hinson, D. Pessayre, and J. J. Lemasters, "Mechanisms of hepatotoxicity," *Toxicological Sciences*, vol. 65, no. 2, pp. 166–176, 2002.

[27] L. Dejager and C. Libert, "Tumor necrosis factor alpha mediates the lethal hepatotoxic effects of poly(I:C) in d-galactosamine-sensitized mice," *Cytokine*, vol. 42, no. 1, pp. 55–61, 2008.

[28] H. Chang, H. Hanawa, H. Liu et al., "Hydrodynamic-based delivery of an interleukin-22-Ig fusion gene ameliorates experimental autoimmune myocarditis in rats," *Journal of Immunology*, vol. 177, no. 6, pp. 3635–3643, 2006.

[29] Y.-J. Kang, B. A. Wingerd, T. Arakawa, and W. L. Smith, "Cyclooxygenase-2 gene transcription in a macrophage model of inflammation," *Journal of Immunology*, vol. 177, no. 11, pp. 8111–8122, 2006.

[30] P. E. Ganey, Y.-W. Barton, S. Kinser, R. A. Sneed, C. C. Barton, and R. A. Roth, "Involvement of cyclooxygenase-2 in the potentiation of allyl alcohol-induced liver injury by bacterial lipopolysaccharide," *Toxicology and Applied Pharmacology*, vol. 174, no. 2, pp. 113–121, 2001.

[31] C. Han, G. Li, K. Lim, M. C. DeFrances, C. R. Gandhi, and T. Wu, "Transgenic expression of cyclooxygenase-2 in hepatocytes accelerates endotoxin-induced acute liver failure," *Journal of Immunology*, vol. 181, no. 11, pp. 8027–8035, 2008.

14

Outcome of Adolescents with Acute Lymphoblastic Leukemia Treated by Pediatrics versus Adults Protocols

Abeer Ibrahim,[1] Amany Ali,[2] and Mahmoud M. Mohammed[2]

[1] *Department of Medical Oncology and Hematological Malignancy, South Egypt Cancer Institute, Assiut University,*
 El Methaq Street, Assiut, Egypt
[2] *Department of Pediatrics Oncology and Hematological Malignancy, South Egypt Cancer Institute, Assiut University, Egypt*

Correspondence should be addressed to Abeer Ibrahim; abelsayed40@gmail.com

Academic Editor: Myriam Labopin

Objective. Several studies showed better outcome in adolescents and young adults with acute lymphoblastic leukemia (ALL) treated with pediatrics protocols than similarly aged patients treated with adults protocols, while other studies showed similar outcome of both protocols. We conducted this study to compare the outcome of our pediatrics and adults therapeutic protocols in treatment of adolescents ALL. *Patients and Methods.* We retrospectively reviewed files of 86 consecutive adolescent ALL patients aged 15–18 years who attended to outpatients clinic from January 2003 to January 2010. 32 out of 86 were treated with pediatrics adopted BFM 90 high risk protocol while 54 were treated with adults adopted BFM protocol. We analyzed the effect of different treatment protocols on achieving complete remission (CR), disease-free survival (DFS), and overall survival (OS). *Results.* The 2 patients groups have almost similar characteristics. The CR was significantly higher in pediatrics protocol 96% versus 89% ($P = 0.001$). Despite the fact that the toxicity profiles were higher in pediatrics protocol, they were tolerable. Moreover, the pediatrics protocol resulted in superior outcome in EFS 67% versus 39% ($P = 0.001$), DFS 65% versus 41% ($P = 0.000$), and OS 67% versus 45% ($P = 0.000$). *Conclusion.* Our study's findings recommend using intensified pediatrics inspired protocol to treat adolescents with acute lymphoblastic leukemia.

1. Introduction

Acute lymphoblastic leukemia (ALL) remains one of the most challenging adults' hematological malignancies [1]. With respect to therapy, the use of multiagent chemotherapy regimens for the treatment of acute lymphoblastic leukemia (ALL) is considered as a cancer success story in the pediatric setting [2], which have offered patients who once had a dismal prognosis a cure rate that approaches or exceeds 90% [3, 4]. For adults, the same magnitude of success has not been realized using similar strategies, and the cure rate of adults ALL is estimated to be between 20 and 40% [5, 6]. Adults' patients tend to present with higher risk features at diagnosis, predisposing to chemotherapy resistance and disease relapses after initial achievement of complete remission (CR) [7]. On the other hand, within childhood ALL, older children have shown inferior outcomes, and within adults ALL, younger adults have shown superior outcomes. Retrospective studies focusing on patient's age 15 to 21 years showed that "Adolescents and Young Adults" (AYA) treated with adults ALL protocols have poorer outcomes than similarly aged patients treated with pediatric protocols [8–16]. Five-year event-free survival (EFS) for AYA treated with pediatric regimens ranges from 64% to 69% while in adult regimen it ranges from 34% to 49% [17–20].

In our country, adolescents aged between 15 and 18 years of age are referred either to pediatrics or to adults departments according to physician who firstly made the diagnoses either pediatrician or internist. This study was conducted to assess the outcome of different protocols applied by 2 different teams, namely, pediatrics and adults oncologists in the same age group (adolescent).

2. Patients and Methods

2.1. Study Eligibility. We retrospectively reviewed files of 86 consecutive adolescent ALL patients aged 15–18 years old

TABLE 1: Adults adopted BFM regimen.

Prephase if (TLC > 2.500 cells/mm^3 and/or oraganomegaly)			
Vincristine	2 mg	IV	D1
Dexamethasone	10 mg/m^2	IV	(D1–7)
Phase I induction			
Vincristine	2 mg	IV	(D1, 8, 15, 22)
Doxorubicin	45 mg/m^2	IV	(D1, 8, 15, 22)
L-asparaginase	5000 u/m^2	IM	(D15–28)
Dexamethasone	10 mg/m^2	IV	11 days (if patients received prophase 7 days so to complete 4 more days only)
Methotrexate	15 mg	IT	D1
Phase II induction			
Cyclophosphamide	650 mg/m^2	IV	(D1, 14, 28)
Cytarabine	75 mg/m^2	IV	(D3, 4, 5, 6 and 9, 10, 11, 12 and 16, 17, 18, 19 and 23, 24, 25, 26)
Methotrexate	15 mg	IT	Given as 4 weekly (D1, 8, 15, 22)
Cranial prophylaxis			Irradiation (24 Gy)
Phase I consolidation			
Vincristine	2 mg	IV	(D1, 8, 15, 22)
Doxorubicin	45 mg/m^2	IV	(D1, 8, 15, 22)
Dexamethasone	10 mg/m^2	IV	For 11 days
Phase II consolidation			
Cyclophosphamide	650 mg/m^2	IV	(D1, 14, 28)
Cytarabine	75 mg/m^2	IV	(D3, 4, 5, 6 and 9, 10, 11, 12 and 16, 17, 18, 19 and 23, 24, 25, 26)
Methotrexate	15 mg	IT	4 weekly (D1, 8, 15, 22)
Maintenance will be given for two years			
6-Mercaptopurine	75 mg/m^2	PO	Daily PO
Methotrexate	20 mg/m^2	IV	Once weekly
Triple IT cytarabine 40 mg, MTX 15 mg, Dexamethasone 4 mg			Every 2 months till the end of maintenance

D: Day, Gy: Gray, IT: intrathecal, MTX: Methotrexate, PO: per oral, TLC: total leucocytes count.

attended to outpatients clinic of pediatrics and adults medical oncology and hematological malignancy departments, South Egypt Cancer institute and pediatric oncology department in Sohag Cancer center, Egypt, from January 2003 to January 2010. We divided them into 2 groups according to their different treatment protocols. Group 1 (pediatrics protocol group) included patients treated with the adopted regimen from pediatric BFM90 high risk protocol (BFM90 HR). Since all the patients were above the age of 10, they were all considered as high risk patients (Table 1).

Group 2 (adults protocol group) included patients treated with the adopted regimen from adults BFM protocol (BFM) (Table 2). The 2 protocols were adopted from original protocols by replacing the Daunorubicin (which is not available in our country) with another form of anthracycline. Epirubicin was used in pediatrics protocol whereas Doxorubicin was used in adults' protocol. Also in pediatrics protocol they changed the high dose Methotrexate from 5 mg/m^2 to 3 g/m^2 because they found our pediatrics patients cannot tolerate the original dose. All patients enrolled in the study had complete morphological and immunophenotypical data. Patients who previously received antileukemic treatment or had uncontrolled or severe cardiovascular, hepatic, or renal disease not resulting from ALL and/or severe psychiatric condition were

excluded. Also we excluded patients with ALL-L3 (Burkitt's-type ALL), t(9 : 22), and T-cell lymphoblastic lymphoma.

The study was approved by the institutional review board, in accordance with the ethical standards of the responsible committee on human experimentation and with the Helsinki Declaration of 1975.

2.2. Diagnostic Procedure. Morphologic analysis for bone marrow (BM) and peripheral-blood specimens were stained by May-Grünwald-Giemsa. Immunophenotyping was performed by flow cytometry with monoclonal antibodies reactive with B-(CD10, CD19, CD22, sIg, cIg), T-(CD1, CD2, CD3, CD4, CD5, CD7, CD8), and precursor-cell (TdT, HLA-DR, and CD34)-associated antigens. Chromosomal analyses using FISH on BM samples were performed at diagnosis for t(9 : 22) only.

2.3. Treatment and Criteria for Response. The treatment regimens are shown in Tables 1 and 2. Patients who achieved CR received consolidation followed by maintenance for 2 years. Hospitalization, management of infections, and transfusion policies were carried out according to the institutional discretion.

TABLE 2: Pediatric adopted BFM90 high risk.

Prephase			
Prednisolone	60 mg/m^2	PO	(D1–7)
Induction			
Prednisolone	60 mg/m^2	PO	(D1–28)
Vincristine	1.5 mg/m^2	IV	(D8, 15, 22, 29)
Epirubicin	30 mg/m^2	IV	(D8, 15, 22, 29)
L-asparaginase	10.000 u/m^2	IM	(D19, 22, 25, 28, 31, 34, 37, 40)
Triple age adjusted IT		IT	(D8, 15, 22, 29)
High risk I (HRI)			
Dexamethasone	20 mg/m^2	PO	(D1–5)
Vincristine	1.5 mg/m^2	IV	(D1–5)
6-Mercaptopurine	25 mg/m^2	PO	(D1–5)
MTX (6 HR infusion)	3 g/m^2	IV	(D1)
L-asparaginase	25.000 u/m^2	IM	(D6)
Triple age adjusted IT		IT	(D1)
High risk II (HRII)			
Dexamethasone	20 mg/m^2	PO	(D1–5)
Vincristine	1.5 mg/m^2	IV	(D1)
Ifosfamide	400 mg/m^2	IV	(D1–5)
MTX (6 HR infusion)	3 g/m^2	IV	(D1)
Epirubicin	50 mg/m^2	IV	(D5)
L-asparaginase	25.000 u/m^2	IM	(D6)
Triple age adjusted IT		IT	(D1)
High risk III (HRIII)			
Dexamethasone	20 mg/m^2	PO	(D1–5)
Vincristine	5 mg/m^2	IV	(D1)
Cytarabine	1 g/m^2/12 h	IV	(D2–5)
Etoposide	150 mg/m^2	IV	(D2–5)
L-asparaginase	25.000 u/m^2	IM	(D6)
Triple age adjusted IT		IT	(D1)
Total number of HR are 9 cycles; then if the patient is in CR after the 9th, cranial prophylaxis (18 g) will be given			
Maintenance maximum two years with pulses of			
Vincristine	1.5 mg/m^2	IV	(D1)
Prednisolone	40 mg/m^2	PO	For 7 days every two months
6-Mercaptopurine	25 mg/m^2	PO	Daily
MTX	20 mg/m^2	IM	Weekly
Triple intrathecal (Methotrexate, Ara-C, hydrocortisone)		IT	Every 2 months till the end of maintenance

D: Day, HR: high risk, Gy: gray, MTX: Methotrexate, PO: per oral.

CR was defined as the absence of clinical manifestations of ALL accompanied with neutrophil count higher than 1.5×10^9/L, platelet count higher than 150×10^9/L, and hemoglobin levels higher than 100 g/L and morphological examination of bone marrow shows less than 5% of blast cells.

Patients with blast cells in BM greater than 5% at the end of the induction phase were considered induction failures.

Overall survival was defined as the time from diagnosis until date of death or censoring patients alive at last follow-up date. Disease-free survival (DFS) was defined as survival without relapse or death from the date of first CR or censoring patients alive in continuous complete remission at last follow-up date. Event-free survival (EFS) was defined as time from diagnosis to the date failure of induction course, the date of relapse,

TABLE 3: Patients' characteristics.

Characteristics	Adopted BFM 90 high risk		Adopted BFM for adults		
	Number	%	Number	%	
Sex					
Male	21	66	36	67	NS
Female	11	34	18	33	
Performance status (ECOG)					
0-1	15	47	27	50	0.049
>1	17	53	26		
Median age	16		17		0.931
Phenotype					
B lineage	26	81	44	82	0.999
Early pre-B	4	15	3	7	0.001
Common	4	15	12	27	0.032
Pre-B	18	70	29	66	0.047
T lineage	6	19	10	18	0.919
Total leucocyte count					
Median					
T lineage > 100	2	33	4	40	0.045
B lineage > 50	18	56	26	59	0.049
Serum LDH level					
Normal	7	22	4	6	0.920
Elevated	25	78	50	92	0.051
Induction death	1		3		0.009
CR	27	96	48	89	0.001

CR: complete remission.

or death or censoring patients alive in continuous complete remission at last follow-up date [9].

3. Statistical Analysis

Bivariate tests, Mann-Whitney test, and variance analysis were used to compare quantitative variables when appropriate and the X^2 test was used to assess differences in proportions. All comparisons were two-tailed.

Actuarial curves for DFS and OS were plotted according to the Kaplan-Meier method [21] and were compared by the log-rank test. The statistically significant variables identified in univariate analysis were included in multivariable analyses.

4. Results

4.1. Patient Characteristics. We reviewed retrospectively data of 86 patients who received treatment from January 2003 to January 2010; the characteristics of the patients were summarized in Table 3.

The B lineage was accounted for 81% in pediatrics protocol group and 82% in adults protocol group whereas the T lineage was accounted for 19% in the pediatrics protocols group and 18% in the adults one ($P = 0.091$).

The total leucocytes count (TLC) in B lineage ALL was $> 50 \times 10^9$ cells/L in 56% in pediatrics protocol group, and 59% in adults protocol group ($P = 0.049$). On the other hand, T lineage ALL showed total TLC count of $>100 \times 10^9$ cells/L

in 30% in pediatrics protocol group, and 33% in adults one ($P = 0.045$). No significant difference was remarked between the 2 groups regarding other variables like median age and distribution of sex.

4.2. CR Rates. Our results showed higher percentage of patients who achieved CR in the pediatrics protocol group than the adults' protocol group after first induction (96% versus 89%) (Table 3); only one death was reported during induction in pediatrics protocol group whereas 3 patients died during induction in adults protocol group ($P = 0.009$). No other treatment related deaths were reported in the other phases in both regimens.

Sepsis was the main cause of death in the patient treated with pediatrics protocol and in the 2 patients treated with adults one; however, the third patient in adults protocol group died from CNS hemorrhage.

4.3. Relapse Rate. In pediatrics protocol group, 10 patients (31%) had relapsed after median followup of 39 months with cumulative incidence of relapse "CIR" (0.401) and standard error "SE" (0.1), 6 patients (60%) had isolated BM relapse, 2 patients (20%) had CNS relapse, and 2 patients (22%) had testicular relapse. Timing of relapse was as follows: 1 patient relapsed during consolidation phases, 1 patient relapsed during the first of year of maintenance, 2 patients relapsed in the second years of maintenance, 3 patients relapsed after one

TABLE 4: Toxicity profile difference between 2 regimens during induction.

Toxicity	aBFM 90-HR (%)	aBFM standard (%)	P value
Neutropenia			
GI-II	60	70	0.049
GIII-IV	40	30	0.049
Thrombocytopenia GIV	40	25	0.003
Mucositis GIII-GIV	30	20	0.005
Thrombotic events	7	6	0.010
Liver impairment			
Elevated bilirubin	37	20	0.001
Elevated enzyme	28	11	0.003

TABLE 5: Survival evaluation according to different protocols.

	aBFM 90-HR (%)	aBFM standard (%)	P value
EFS	67	39	0.001
DFS	65	41	0.000
OS	67	45	0.000

CR: complete remission, EFS: event-free survival, DFS: disease-free survival, OS: overall survival.

year of finishing maintenance, and 3 patients relapsed after 2 years of maintenance.

During the same period of followup for the adults protocol group, 30 patients had relapsed (55%) with CIR 0.631 and SE 0.06. 24 patients (80%) had isolated BM relapse, 3 patients (10%) had CNS relapse, 3 patients (10%) had CNS and BM relapse, and none of the patients had testicular relapse. Timing of relapse was as follows: 4 patients relapsed during the consolidation phases, 5 patients during maintenance, 4 patients relapsed shortly after maintenance, and 7 patients relapsed after one year of maintenance, 5 patients after 2 years of finishing maintenance, and 4 patients after 3 years of finishing maintenance.

4.4. Dose Intensity. In pediatrics protocol group, the L-asparaginase dose was 8 times higher than the one used in adults protocol. The cytarabine dose was 4 times higher than the adults' doses; the Dexamethasone was double the dose used in adults protocol and the vincristine dose is almost the same in the 2 protocols; however the vincristine was included in maintenance phase in the pediatrics protocol but not in the adults one. The Etoposide, Ifosfamide, and high dose of Methotrexate are included in the pediatrics protocol but not in the adults one. The duration of treatment was longer in the pediatrics protocol than it was in the adults one due to the fact that induction and consolidation take about 8 months in pediatrics protocol, while they take 3.5 months in the adults. Also, the duration of admission to hospital was also longer in pediatric protocol and also supportive treatment was more in pediatric regimen.

4.5. Toxicity. The study showed higher incidence grade III and IV neutropenia (Table 4) in pediatrics protocol group which resulted in higher episodes of grade III and IV mucositis; also the frequency of grade III and IV thrombocytopenia

was more in pediatrics protocol group. Liver impairment due to L-asparaginase, either in the form of elevated bilirubin levels or in elevated liver enzymes, was significantly higher in pediatrics protocol group. The elevated bilirubin levels occurred in 12 patients (37.5%) in pediatrics protocol group, and in 11 (20.3%) patients in adults protocol group ($P = 0.001$). The elevated liver enzymes occurred in 9 patients (28%) in pediatrics protocol group and in 6 patients (11%) in adults protocol group ($P = 0.003$). However, the liver function tests retained normal levels after median 14 days in pediatric protocol group and 9 days in adults protocol group.

Additionally, there was no significant difference in the number of thromboses related to L-asparaginase that occurred in one patient in pediatric protocol 3% and 2 patients in adults protocol 3.7% in adults group ($P = 0.091$).

4.6. Survival Outcome. After median 39 months of followup, EFS was significantly higher in patients treated in pediatric protocol group 67% (95% CI, 50%–73%) versus 39% (95% CI, 30%–55%) in the adults protocol group $P = 0.001$; the estimated 5-year DFS was 65% (95% CI, 59%–70%) in pediatrics protocol group versus 41% (95% CI, 35%–48%) in adults protocol group $P = 0.000$ (Figure 1). Consequently, OS was higher in pediatric protocol group 67% (95% CI, 60%–72%) than adults protocol group 45% (95% CI, 40%–51%) $P = 0.000$ (Figure 2) (Table 5).

We carried out subanalysis regarding the T lineage groups; the DFS and OS in T-ALL were found to be more than double in pediatrics protocol group compared to that in the adults protocol group 61% versus 25% ($P = 0.001$) and 65% versus 26% ($P = 0.001$), respectively.

5. Discussion

Adolescent and young adults AYAs constitute a particular group of patients who find themselves sandwiched between children and adults and who may be referred to either pediatrics or adults oncologists. Several studies comparing the outcome of AYAs on pediatric and adult protocols demonstrated improved survival for AYAs, who were treated by pediatrics protocols; these findings triggered intense interest in the differences with respect to ALL biology and protocol designs in that age group [22–24]. However, because the results are controversial [25], we conducted this study to compare the efficacy and outcome of our institute adopted

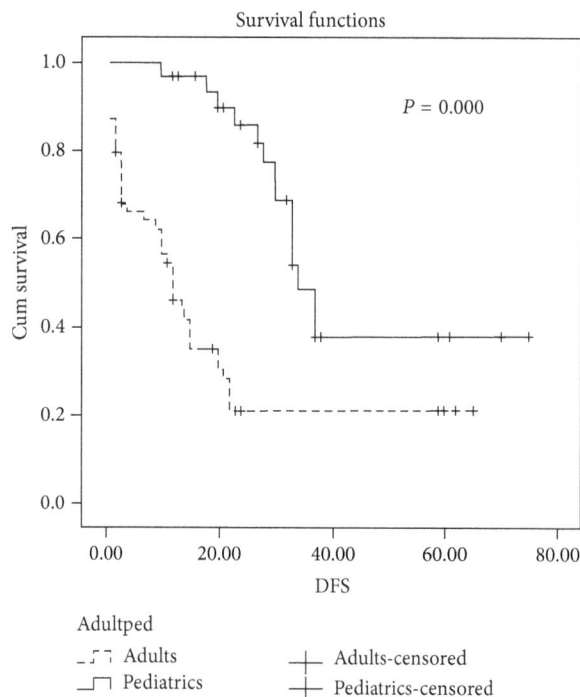

FIGURE 1: Disease-free survival difference between using pediatrics and adults protocols.

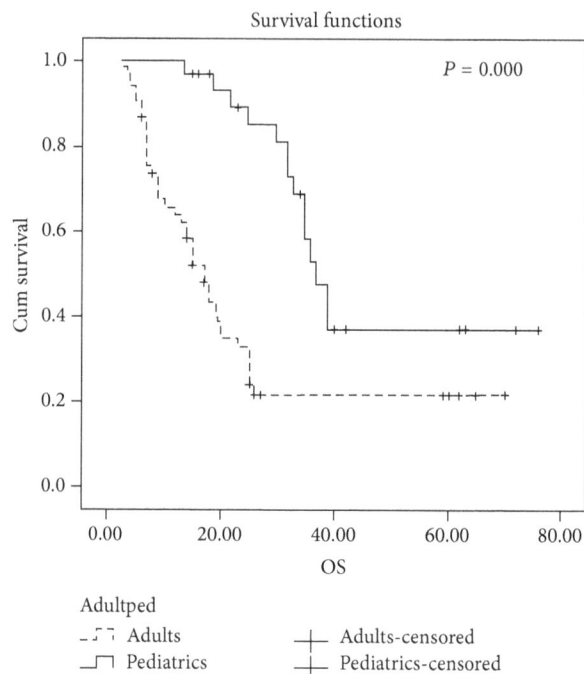

FIGURE 2: Overall survival difference between using pediatrics and adults' protocols.

pediatrics and adults protocols (adult BFM and pediatric BFM90-HR).

The clinical characteristics between 2 groups were quite similar regarding B and T phenotype distribution and the number of patients who had elevated TLC.

Our results showed significant high remission rate 96% and significant difference in EFS ($P = 0.001$) and DFS ($P = 0.000$) in pediatric protocol group. This difference was attributed mainly to high CR rate and lower relapse rate in the pediatrics group. This could be explained based on the differences in induction and consolidation courses, between the 2 protocols since pediatrics protocol has double doses of L-asparaginase and it was repeated in higher doses in all 9 phases of consolidation in pediatrics protocol. Our results are in line with Dana-Farber Consortium study, which showed that children aged 9 to 18 years may have benefited from higher doses of L-asparaginase especially those with T-ALL despite the increased related toxicity [26]. Moreover, the pediatrics protocol is more intensified regimen as it contains higher doses of cytarabine than the adults' protocol in addition to the high doses of Methotrexate which were not included in adults' protocol. The benefit of this strategy was initially proposed by the Berlin-Frankfurt-Munster study group and then it was established by several other studies [27–29]. We noted that the incidence of chemotherapy-related toxicity showed higher significant difference in pediatrics protocol due to the use of more intensified regimen especially in the number of episodes of neutropenia, mucositis, and liver impairment. However, these episodes were reversible and they did not increase the number of deaths. The significant difference which we found in the toxicity profile might contradict the results of similar study conducted by Huguet

et al. [20] because they used more intensified regimen in adults than the regimen we used, which resulted in similar toxicity profile when compared to their center pediatrics protocol. Moreover, our results disagree with the results from Finland, which showed no significant difference regarding DFS and OS between their pediatrics and adults protocols; we also found that they used more intensified regimen in adults which was very similar to their pediatrics protocol [25].

6. Conclusion

We recommend using intensified pediatrics inspired protocol to treat adolescents with acute lymphoblastic leukemia.

Conflict of Interests

The authors declare that there is no conflict of interests regarding the publication of this paper.

References

[1] C.-H. Pui, L. L. Robison, and A. T. Look, "Acute lymphoblastic leukaemia," The Lancet, vol. 371, no. 9617, pp. 1030–1043, 2008.

[2] C.-H. Pui, C. G. Mullighan, W. E. Evans, and M. V. Relling, "Pediatric acute lymphoblastic leukemia: where are we going and how do we get there?" Blood, vol. 120, no. 6, pp. 1165–1174, 2012.

[3] E. J. Freireich, "The history of leukemia therapy—a personal journey," Clinical Lymphoma Myeloma and Leukemia, vol. 12, no. 6, pp. 386–392, 2012.

[4] C.-H. Pui, D. Campana, D. Pei et al., "Treating childhood acute lymphoblastic leukemia without cranial irradiation," The New

England Journal of Medicine, vol. 360, no. 26, pp. 2730–2741, 2009.

[5] J. I. Sive, G. Buck, A. Fielding et al., "Outcomes in older adults with acute lymphoblastic leukaemia (ALL): results from the international MRC UKALL XII/ECOG2993 trial," British Journal of Haematology, vol. 157, no. 4, pp. 463–471, 2012.

[6] D. A. Thomas, S. O'Brien, S. Faderl et al., "Chemoimmunotherapy with a modified hyper-CVAD and rituximab regimen improves outcome in de novo Philadelphia chromosome—negative precursor B-lineage acute lymphoblastic leukemia," Journal of Clinical Oncology, vol. 28, no. 24, pp. 3880–3889, 2010.

[7] C.-H. Pui and W. E. Evans, "Treatment of acute lymphoblastic leukemia," The New England Journal of Medicine, vol. 354, no. 2, pp. 166–178, 2006.

[8] W. Stock, H. Satjer, R. K. Dodge, C. D. Bloomfield, R. A. Larson, and J. Nachman, "Outcome of adolescents and young adults with ALL: a comparison of Children's Cancer Group (CCG) and Cancer and Leukemia Group B (CALGB) regimens," Blood, vol. 96, abstract 476, 2000.

[9] N. Boissel, M.-F. Auclerc, V. Lhéritier et al., "Should adolescents with acute lymphoblastic leukemia be treated as old children or young adults? Comparison of the French FRALLE-93 and LALA-94 trials," Journal of Clinical Oncology, vol. 21, no. 5, pp. 774–780, 2003.

[10] J. M. de Bont, B. van der Holt, A. W. Dekker, A. van der Does-van den Berg, R. Sonneveld, and R. Pieters, "Significant difference in outcome for adolescents with acute lymphoblastic leukemia treated on pediatric vs adult protocols in the Netherlands," Leukemia, vol. 18, no. 12, pp. 2032–2035, 2004.

[11] R. Ramanujachar, S. Richards, I. Hann, and D. Webb, "Adolescents with acute lymphoblastic leukaemia: emerging from the shadow of paediatric and adult treatment protocols," Pediatric Blood and Cancer, vol. 47, no. 6, pp. 748–756, 2006.

[12] R. Ramanujachar, S. Richards, I. Hann et al., "Adolescents with acute lymphoblastic leukaemia: outcome on UK National Paediatric (ALL97) and adult (UKALLXII/E2993) trials," Pediatric Blood & Cancer, vol. 48, no. 3, pp. 254–261, 2007.

[13] H. Schrøder, M. Kjeldahl, A. M. Boesen et al., "Acute lymphoblastic leukemia in adolescents between10 and 19 years of age in Denmark," Danish Medical Bulletin, vol. 53, no. 1, pp. 76–79, 2006.

[14] A. M. Testi, M. G. Valsecchi, V. Conter et al., "Difference in outcome of adolescents with acute lymphoblastic leukemia (ALL) enrolled in pediatric (AIEOP) and adult (GIMEMA) protocols," Blood, vol. 104, p. 1954, 2004.

[15] H. Hallböök, G. Gustafsson, B. Smedmyr, S. Söderhäll, and M. Heyman, "Treatment outcome in young adults and children > 10 year of age with acute lymphoblastic leukemia in Sweden: a comparison between a pediatric protocol and an adult protocol," Cancer, vol. 107, no. 7, pp. 1551–1561, 2006.

[16] C. A. Schiffer, "Differences in outcome in adolescents with acute lymphoblastic leukemia: a consequence of better regimens? Better doctors? Both?" Journal of Clinical Oncology, vol. 21, no. 5, pp. 760–761, 2003.

[17] D. J. De Angelo, "The treatment of adolescents and young adults with acute lymphoblastic leukemia," Hematology/the Education Program of the American Society of Hematology, pp. 123–130, 2005.

[18] S. E. Sallan, "Myths and lessons from the adult/pediatric interface in acute lymphoblastic leukemia," Hematology/the Education Program of the American Society of Hematology:

American Society of Hematology, vol. 2006, no. 1, pp. 128–132, 2006.

[19] D. J. DeAngelo, L. B. Silverman, S. Couban et al., "A multicenter phase II study using a dose intensified pediatric regimen in adults with untreated acute lymphoblastic leukaemia," Blood, vol. 108, p. 526a, 2006.

[20] F. Huguet, T. Leguay, E. Raffoux et al., "Pediatric-inspired therapy in adults with philadelphia chromosome-negative acute lymphoblastic leukemia: the GRAALL-2003 study," Journal of Clinical Oncology, vol. 27, no. 6, pp. 911–918, 2009.

[21] E. L. Kaplan and P. Meier, "Nonparametric estimation from incomplete observations," Journal of the American Statistical Association, vol. 53, pp. 457–481, 1958.

[22] W. Stock, M. La, B. Sanford et al., "What determines the outcomes for adolescents and young adults with acute lymphoblastic leukemia treated on cooperative group protocols? A comparison of Children's Cancer Group and Cancer and Leukemia Group B studies," Blood, vol. 112, no. 5, pp. 1646–1654, 2008.

[23] N. Boissel, M.-F. Auclerc, V. Lhéritier et al., "Should adolescents with acute lymphoblastic leukemia be treated as old children or young adults? Comparison of the French FRALLE-93 and LALA-94 trials," Journal of Clinical Oncology, vol. 21, no. 5, pp. 774–780, 2003.

[24] R. Ramanujachar, S. Richards, I. Hann et al., "Adolescents with acute lymphoblastic leukaemia: outcome on UK National Paediatric (ALL97) and adult (UKALLXII/E2993) trials," Pediatric Blood and Cancer, vol. 48, no. 3, pp. 254–261, 2007.

[25] A. Usvasalo, R. Räty, S. Knuutila et al., "Acute lymphoblastic leukemia in adolescents and young adults in Finland," Haematologica, vol. 93, no. 8, pp. 1161–1168, 2008.

[26] L. B. Silverman, R. D. Gelber, V. K. Dalton et al., "Improved outcome for children with acute lymphoblastic leukemia: results of Dana-Farber Consortium Protocol 91-01," Blood, vol. 97, no. 5, pp. 1211–1218, 2001.

[27] H. Riehm, H. Gadner, G. Henze et al., "Results and significance of six randomized trials in four consecutive ALL-BFM studies," Haematology and Blood Transfusion, vol. 33, pp. 439–450, 1990.

[28] J. B. Nachman, H. N. Sather, M. G. Sensel et al., "Augmented post-induction therapy for children with high-risk acute lymphoblastic leukemia and a slow response to initial therapy," The New England Journal of Medicine, vol. 338, no. 23, pp. 1663–1671, 1998.

[29] J.-M. Ribera, A. Oriol, M.-A. Sanz et al., "Comparison of the results of the treatment of adolescents and young adults with standard-risk acute lymphoblastic leukemia with the programa Español de tratamiento en hematología pediatric-based protocol ALL-96," Journal of Clinical Oncology, vol. 26, no. 11, pp. 1843–1849, 2008.

15

DNMT3A Mutations in Patients with Acute Myeloid Leukemia in South Brazil

Annelise Pezzi,[1,2] **Lauro Moraes,**[1] **Vanessa Valim,**[1,2] **Bruna Amorin,**[1,2] **Gabriela Melchiades,**[1]
Fernanda Oliveira,[1] **Maria Aparecida da Silva,**[1,2] **Ursula Matte,**[3]
Maria S. Pombo-de-Oliveira,[4] **Rosane Bittencourt,**[5] **Liane Daudt,**[5] **and Lúcia Silla**[1,2,5,6]

[1] *Cellular Therapy Center, Center for Experimental Research, Hospital de Clinicas de Porto Alegre,*
 90035-903 Porto Alegre, RS, Brazil
[2] *Postgraduate Course of Medical Sciences, Federal University of Rio Grande do Sul, 90035-903 Porto Alegre, RS, Brazil*
[3] *Gene Therapy Center, Center for Experimental Research, Hospital de Clinicas de Porto Alegre, 90035-903 Porto Alegre, RS, Brazil*
[4] *Pediatric Hematology and Oncology Program, Research Center, Instituto Nacional de Câncer, 20230-130 Rio de Janeiro, RJ, Brazil*
[5] *Hematology and Bone Marrow Transplantation, Hospital de Clinicas de Porto Alegre, 90035-903 Porto Alegre, RS, Brazil*
[6] *Laboratory of Cell Culture and Molecular Analysis of Hematopoietic Cells, Center for Experimental Research,*
 Hospital de Clínicas de Porto Alegre, 2350 Ramiro Barcelos, 90035-903 Porto Alegre, RS, Brazil

Correspondence should be addressed to Lúcia Silla, lsilla@hcpa.ufrgs.br

Academic Editor: Helen A. Papadaki

Acute myeloid leukemia (AML) is a complex and heterogeneous hematopoietic tissue neoplasm. Several molecular markers have been described that help to classify AML patients into risk groups. DNA methyltransferase 3A (*DNMT3A*) gene mutations have been recently identified in about 22% of AML patients and associated with poor prognosis as an independent risk factor. Our aims were to determine the frequency of somatic mutations in the gene *DNMT3A* and major chromosomal translocations in a sample of patients with AML. We investigated in 82 samples of bone marrow from patients with AML for somatic mutations in *DNMT3A* gene by sequencing and sought major fusion transcripts by RT-PCR. We found mutations in the *DNMT3A* gene in 6 patients (8%); 3 were type R882H. We found fusion transcripts in 19 patients, namely, AML1/ETO ($n = 5$; 6.1%), PML/RARα ($n = 12$; 14.6%), MLL/AF9 (0; 0%), and CBFβ/MYH11 ($n = 2$; 2.4%). The identification of recurrent mutations in the *DNMT3A* gene and their possible prognostic implications can be a valuable tool for making treatment decisions. This is the first study on the presence of somatic mutations of the *DNMT3A* gene in patients with AML in Brazil. The frequency of these mutations suggests a possible ethnogeographic variation.

1. Introduction

Acute myeloid leukemia (AML) is a complex and heterogeneous hematopoietic tissue neoplasm caused by gene mutations, chromosomal rearrangements, deregulation of gene expression, and epigenetic modifications. These changes lead to unregulated proliferation and loss of differentiation capacity of myeloid hematopoietic cells. In recent years, several important prognostic molecular markers have been described for AML which not only improved disease characterization, but also allowed stratification of patients into risk groups and can guide therapeutic decision-making [1]. However, these molecular markers are often unable to provide accurate prognostic and therapeutic information, since the course of the disease varies significantly between patients belonging to the same risk category [2–4].

The traditional view of cancer as a disease caused by some genetic mutation has been replaced by the concept of a complex network of gene deregulation and epigenetic changes. Additionally, although extremely important, those mutations that have been reported are found in only a minority of patients with AML [5–7]. The distinct components of epigenetic machinery such as DNA methylation, covalent modifications of histones, and noncoding RNAs have been described as cocontrollers of gene expression and within a context of cancer may contribute to leukemogenesis [8]. Methyltransferases such as *DNMT1*, *DNMT3A*, and *DNMT3B* are key components of the epigenetic regulation of genes as they catalyze the addition of methyl groups to the cytosine residue of CpG dinucleotides.

Recently, in a study using whole genome sequencing, recurrent somatic mutations have been described in the DNA methyltransferase 3A gene (*DNMT3A*) in 22% of patients with AML [9]. In this study, *DNMT3A* mutations were independently associated with a poor prognosis and more frequent in patients with normal cytogenetics and as such, of utmost clinical relevance. Eighteen different mutations were found, most of them missense mutations. Preliminary data show that the incidence of these mutations in AML ranges from 4.1% in a Japanese study [10], 9% in a study with Chinese patients [11], and about 15–25% in two Western studies [9, 12–14]. Given the association with CN-AML observed in all studies, it is not astonishing that the highest prevalence was reported in the 2 series focusing on CN-AML (29–36%) [15, 16]. These possible ethnogeographic differences in the incidence of *DNMT3A* mutations as well as their prognostic role need, however, to be better characterized. The exact mechanisms by which of *DNMT3A* mutations act in AML are still unclear, since the global pattern of methylation in the genome of such patients with AML does not appear to be significantly changed [9].

The aim of this study was to characterize the frequency and clinical impact of mutations in the *DNMT3A* gene, correlating it with clinical data and with already well defined translocations in AML in a group of patients treated at the Hospital das Clinicas, in Porto Alegre, Rio Grande do Sul, Brazil.

2. Materials and Methods

2.1. Patients. We have studied 87 samples of bone marrow from patients with AML, at diagnosis and prior to any chemotherapy, which had been cryopreserved at the Laboratory of Cell Culture and Molecular Analysis of Hematopoietic Cells belonging to the Center for Experimental Research at the Hospital de Clinicas of Porto Alegre (CPE-HCPA) since 2001 to the present date. The patients' clinical information was obtained from the AML database of the Service of Hematology and Bone Marrow Transplantation of HCPA. Patients were stratified into risk groups—favorable, intermediate, and high—according to the WHO criteria [17]. The favorable subgroup is represented by recurrent reciprocal translocations t(15;17), t(8;21), and inv(16); the intermediate includes patients with a normal karyotype, +8 and t(9;11); and the unfavorable subgroup includes complex karyotypes (≥3 abnormality) −5 and −7 abnormalities, anomalies of chromosome 3, and balanced structural rearrangements as: t(6;9), t(6;11), and t(11;19). Karyotypic characterization of our sample is shown in Table 1.

The procedures were approved by the Ethical Committee of Human Experimentation in Brazil, and are in accordance with the Helsinki Declaration of 1975.

TABLE 1: Karyotypic characterization of our sample.

Result of karyotype result analysis	Number of pts (%)
Normal	38 (61.3%)
t(15;17)	5 (8.0%)
t(8;21)	4 (6.4%)
Complex karyotype	3 (4.8%)
del(11)	1 (1.6%)
del(X)	1 (1.6)%
add(7)	1 (1.6%)
t(6;9)	1 (1.6%)
t(1;2)	1 (1.6%)
t(18;9)	1 (1.6%)
t(3;21)	1 (1.6%)
t(10;11) and del(7)	1 (1.6%)
add(18)(21)(7)	1 (1.6%)
Trisomy 4 and 8	1 (1.6%)
Tetraploid	1 (1.6%)
Polyploidy	1 (1.6%)

2.2. Extraction of DNA and RNA. Samples of cryopreserved bone marrow were thawed, washed with PBS1x with 5% albumin, and then had their DNA and RNA extracted with Trizol Reagent (Invitrogen), according to the manufacturer's recommendations.

2.3. Identification of Fusion Transcripts. After RNA extraction we proceeded to reverse transcription using the *SuperScript III* kit (Invitrogen). The effectiveness of RNA extraction and of cDNA synthesis was monitored by the amplification of the constitutive gene glyceraldehyde-3-phosphate dehydrogenase (*GAPDH*) and negative samples were discarded.

The sequences of interest were amplified by the polymerase chain reaction (PCR) according to BIOMED-1 [18] (Table 2). PCR products were visualized by electrophoresis on 1.5% agarose gel and bands were considered positive in the following sizes: *AML-A/ETO-B*: 395 bp, *PML-A1/RARα-B*: 381 bp, *PML-A2/RARα-B*: 376 bp, *CBFβ-A/MYH11-B2*: 418, and *MLL6S/AF9AS3*: 651 bp [18, 19].

2.4. Identification of Mutations in DNMT3A Gene. The extracted DNA was amplified by PCR at the *DNMT3A* exons 19, 20, 21, 22, and 23, with primers described by Thol et al. [14] (Table 2). After electrophoresis on 1.5 agarose gel, PCR products were subjected to purification using Exonuclease I and Shrimp Alkaline Phosphatase (EXO-SAP, GE Healthcare) and then sequenced.

2.5. Sequencing. Samples were sequenced at the Unidade de Análises Moleculares e de Proteínas (Centro de Pesquisa Experimental, HCPA) using ABI 3500 Genetic Analyzer with 50 cm capillaries and POP7 polymer (Applied Biosystems). PCR products were labeled with 3.2 pmol of the forward primer and 1 μL of BigDye Terminator v3.1 Cycle Sequencing Kit (Applied Biosystems) in a final volume of 10 μL. Labeled samples were purified using BigDye XTerminator

TABLE 2: Primer sequences for genes of interest.

Chromosomal translocation	Fusion transcript	Sequence (5'–3')
t(8;21)	AML1-A	CTACCGCAGCCATGAAGAACC
	ETO-B	AGAGGAAGGCCCATTGCTGAA
t(15;17)	PML-A1	CAGTGTACGCCTTCTCCATCA
	PML-A2	CTGCTGGAGGCTGTGGAC
	RARα-B	GCTTGTAGATGCGGGGTAGA
inv16	CBFβ-A	GCAGGCAAGGTATATTTGAAGG
	MYH11-B2	TCCTCTTCTCCTCATTCTGCTC
t(9;11)	MLL6S	GCAAACAGAAAAAAGTGGCTCCCCG
	AF9AS3	TCACGATCTGCTGCAGAATGTGTCT
Gene	Exon	Sequence (5'–3')
DNMT3A	Exon 19	CACCACTGTCCTATGCAGACA
		ATTAGTGAGCTGGCCAAACC
DNMT3A	Exon 20	CCTTGGCTCATCTTCAAACC
		CACTATGGGTCATCCCACCT
DNMT3A	Exon 21	CCGCTGTTATCCAGGTTTCT
		CCCAGCAGAGGTTCTAGACG
DNMT3A	Exon 22	TTTGGTAGACGCATGACCAG
		AGCACAGCAATCAGAACAGC
DNMT3A	Exon 23	TCCTGCTGTGTGGTTAGACG
		ATGATGTCCAACCCTTTTCG

Purification Kit (Applied Biosystems) and electroinjected in the automatic sequencer. Electropherograms were compared to the reference sequence (NM_022552). Altered sequencing results were confirmed by reverse strand sequencing.

2.6. Statistical Analysis. Statistical analysis was performed using SPSS V18. Overall Survival and Disease-Free Survival curves were calculated using the *Kaplan-Meier* survival function and comparison by the *Long Rank* test. For categorical data *Fisher*'s exact test was used. P value of less than 0.05 was considered statistically significant.

3. Results

3.1. Characterization of the Sample. Of the 87 AML samples taken from the cell bank of the Laboratory of Cell Culture and Molecular Analysis of Hematopoietic Cell, 82 could be analyzed. Of the studied patient population, 58.5% (48) were male with a median age of 42 years. According to the FAB classification, 6.8% (5) were AML M0, 21.9% (16) AML M1, 30.1% (22) AML M2, 19.2% (14) AML M3, 17.8% (13) AML M4, 1.4% (1) AML M5, and 2.7% (2) were classified as AML and not M3. The median white blood cell (WBC) count at diagnosis was 6.6×10^9/L ranging from 0.16 to 374.5×10^9/L. There were 23 (41.8%) cases with karyotype alterations. As for risk stratification, 18 (29%) patients were allocated to the favorable group, 38 (61.3%) to the intermediate group, 6 (9.7%) belonged to the unfavorable risk group, and in 20 (16.4%) karyotypic analysis was not performed and therefore could not be classified (Table 3).

As shown in Table 3, we were able to stratify into risk categories only 62 patients since for 20 of them we did not have enough information. Eighteen (29.0%) were in the favorable, 38 (61.3%) in the intermediate, and 6 (9.7%) in the unfavorable risk group. Except for the group of patients with AML M3 who were treated according to the APL protocol [20], all other patients received remission induction and consolidation using the protocol 7 + 3, and intensification with high doses of AraC. Of these, 8 were subsequently submitted to autologous and 22 to allogeneic bone marrow transplantation (BMT). Of the entire group, 14 (19.2%) were refractory to treatment. Of these, 1 (7.1%) belonged to the favorable, 8 (57.1%) to the intermediate, 2 (14.2%) to the unfavorable, and 3 (21.4%) belonged to the unclassified group. The overall survival (OS) of the 62 categorized patients, with a followup of 120 months, was 54.9%, 39.0%, and 16.7% for favorable, intermediate, and unfavorable risk category, respectively ($P = 0.15$) (Figure 1). The OS and disease-free survival (DFS) of the entire group of patients, with a followup of 120 months, was 41.7% and 23.4%, respectively (Figure 2).

3.2. Fusion Transcripts. Nineteen patients (23.1%) had fusion transcripts identified by RT-PCR. Five (6.1%) presented the *AML1/ETO*, 12 (14.6%) *PML/RARα*, and 2 (2.4%) the *CBFβ/MYH11* fusion genes. The presence of *MLL/AF9* t(9;11) was not found in our series of AML patients. The transcript *PML/RARα* was identified in 78.5% (11) of the cases classified as APL. Of the 12 *PML/RARα* positive patients, only 4 had a compatible karyotype, positive for

TABLE 3: Characteristics of the entire patient population.

Variable	Number of patients (%)
Age—$n = 82$	
Median (SD)	42 (18.5)
Mean (SD)	40.6 (18.5)
Range	3–75
Sex—$n = 82$	
Male	58.5% (48)
Female	41.5% (34)
FAB classification—$n = 73$	
M0	6.8% (5)
M1	21.9% (16)
M2	30.1% (22)
M3	19.2% (14)
M4	17.8% (13)
M5	1.4% (1)
M6	0% (0)
M7	0% (0)
AML not M3	2.4% (2)
Karyotype—$n = 55$	
Normal	58.2% (32)
With alteration	41.8% (23)
Risk classification—$n = 62$	
Favorable	29% (18)
Intermediate	61.3% (38)
Unfavorable	9.7% (6)
Leukocytes ($\times 10^9$/L)—$n = 82$	
Median (SD)	6.6 (51.9)

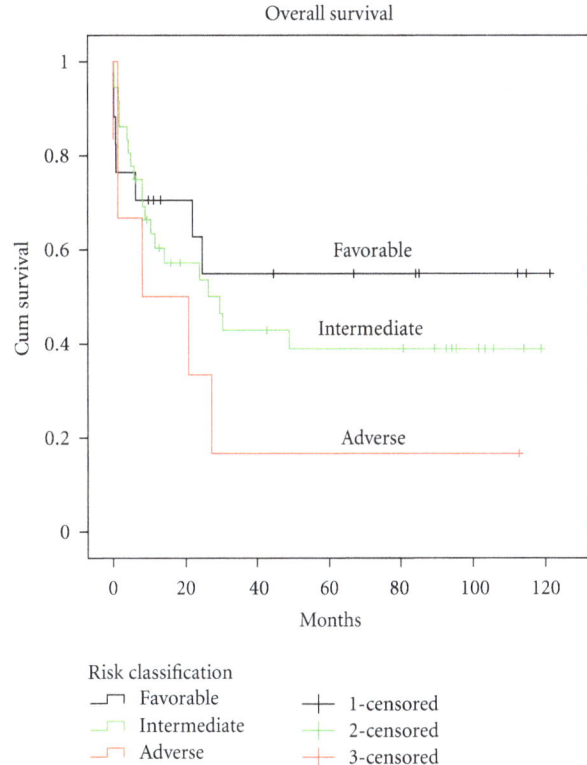

FIGURE 1: Comparison of the estimated overall survival according to the risk category with a followup of 120 months: favorable (54.9%), intermediate (39%), and unfavorable (16.7%) ($P = 0.15$).

t(15;17), and the remaining had either normal (3) or no karyotype (5).

When comparing the overall survival for positive and negative $PML/RAR\alpha$ patients, with a followup of 120 months, we observed that the OS was 72.7% for positive and 37.6% for the negative ($P = 0.19$) (Figure 1). A tendency for prognostic value was also shown for the presence of AML1/ETO with an OS of 22.7% and 60.2% for positive and negative, respectively ($P = 0.19$). Finally, one of the inv16 patients died during remission induction and the other is still alive in continuous complete remission.

3.3. DNMT3A. Somatic mutations were found in 8% (6) of the samples, being 5 missensemutations and one silent mutation, including the p.R882H mutation described by Ley et al. [9] that was identified in 3 patients. All variant sequences were heterozygous and no patient had more than one mutation. The new mutations found were: p.R973Q, p.D748N, and p.H896. The mutations location domains are shown in Figure 3. Of the 6 cases with *DNMT3A* mutations, the majority (5, or 83.3%) were located in exon 23. Four (80.0%) patients with mutations belonged to the intermediate risk group with normal karyotype, 1 to the favorable group, and 1 unclassified. Of the patients with *DNMT3A* mutation, only 1 was positive for the fusion transcript

$PML/RAR\alpha$ and died of coagulopathy during induction; the patient with trisomy 4 and 8 is alive in continuous remission (Table 4).

The characteristics of patients with or without *DNMT3A* gene mutation did not differ significantly, and they are represented in Table 5. Although the sample size does not allow a comparative analysis of survival, with a followup of 120 months, OS for patients with wild *DNMT3A* gene was 41.4% and for patients with mutated *DNMT3A* was 44.4% ($P = 0.59$); the SLD was 22.7% and 0%, respectively ($P = 0.32$).

4. Discussion

Of the 82 patients studied, we were able to classify 73 according to the FAB classification. The frequency of FAB subtypes M0, M1, and M2 was similar to that reported in the literature except for subtypes M4, M5, M6, and M7 whose frequency was lower (Table 3). The M3 subtype was more frequent (19.2%) in our group when compared with international studies; this confirms the results reported by Capra et al. [21] in a study in Rio Grande do Sul, Brazil and is similar to that reported by others for the Latin American population [22, 23]. The frequency distribution of FAB classification subtypes we found in our sample was the same described in 532 AML cases we reported [21] in the same region with patients with the same ethnic background. Based on this finding we can say that although now reporting a smaller sample of patients from a single institution, it

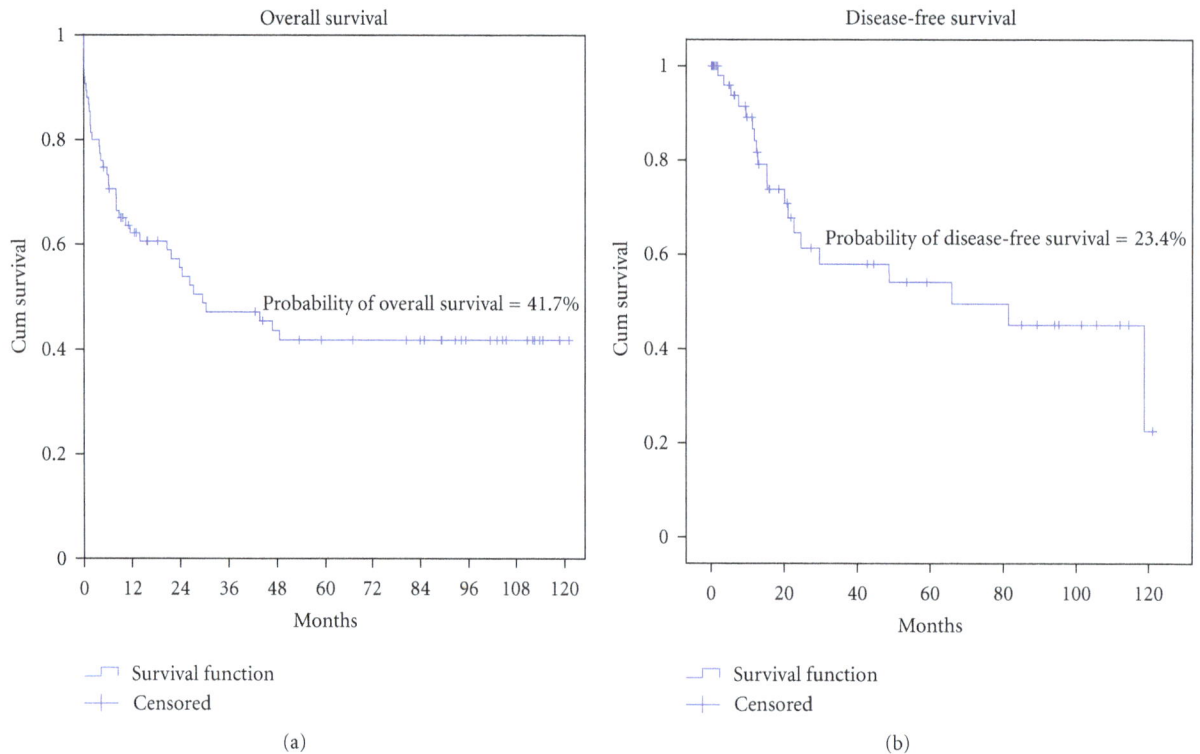

FIGURE 2: (a) Overall survival in a followup of 120 months with an estimated probability of overall survival of 41.7%; (b) disease-free survival in a followup of 120 months with an estimated probability of disease-free survival of 23.4%.

TABLE 4: Description of somatic mutations found in gene *DNMT3A*.

Patient identification	Mutation	Allelic change	Exon	Type of mutation	FAB subtype	PCR	Risk group	Karyotype
39	D748N	G>A	19	*Missense*	M1	Negative	Intermediate	Normal
79	R882H	G>A	23	*Missense*	M1	Negative	Intermediate	Trisomy (8)(9)
4	R882H	G>A	23	*Missense*	M3	Negative	Intermediate	Normal
70	R882H	G>A	23	*Missense*	M2	Negative	Intermediate	Normal
41	H896*	A>G	23	*Silent*	M3	PML/RARα	Favorable	t(15;17)
78	R973Q	G>A	23	*Missense*	—	Negative	—	—

is a representative of our population. Our institution is a university public hospital with one of the most active bone marrow transplantation centers in the country to where AML patients from all over the state are referred for treatment. Regarding the classification of risk found in our sample of 29.0%, 61.3%, and 9.7% for the favorable, intermediate, and unfavorable risk categories, respectively, in spite of having a significant number of cases not classified, in general it agrees with the distribution described in the literature and is virtually identical to that reported in patients in the same region of the country [21].

The frequency of fusion transcripts, particularly the *AML1/ETO* found in 6.1% of our sample, was similar to that described in the literature (6 a 12%) [24, 25], while the relative frequency of *PML/RARα* (14.6%) was higher (5–8%) [26], probably reflecting the higher incidence of AML M3 in our population. For the transcript *CBFβ/MYH11*

we had a relative frequency of 2.4%, slightly lower than the (5–8%) reported by others [27], and none positive for the transcript *MLL/AF9*, which correlates with the literature, which indicates a frequency of approximately 1% [19]. However, in general, the finding of rearrangements in 22% of our patients is consistent with the frequency of 20% found in 1065 patients in the UK [28]. Finally, the analysis of chromosomal translocations by RT-PCR proved to be advantageous in our center since only 7 of the 19 patients with fusion transcripts were detected by karyotype analysis, explaining the frequency of only 41.8% of karyotype abnormalities found in our group of patients, less than the 65% reported by Look [29].

The search for recurrent somatic mutations in the gene DNA methyltransferase 3A (*DNMT3A*) was performed in all our 82 patients. We chose to sequence the last five exons of the gene *DNMT3A* since, as demonstrated by Ley et al. [9],

TABLE 5: Clinical characteristics of patients with acute myeloid leukemia with or without *DNMT3A* mutations.

Characteristics	Number of pts (%) DNMT3A mutated	Number of pts (%) DNMT3A not mutated	P
Age (median)	40.2	44.8	0.56
Sex			
Male	50% (3)	59.3% (45)	0.68
Female	50% (3)	40.7% (31)	
Subtype FAB			
M0	0%	7.2% (5)	
M1	60% (3)	18.8% (13)	
M2	20% (1)	30.4% (21)	0.56
M3	20% (1)	20.3% (14)	
M4	0%	18.8% (13)	
M5	0%	1.4% (1)	
Not M3	0%	2.9% (2)	
Risk groups			
Favorable	20% (1)	29.8% (17)	
Intermediate	80% (4)	59.6% (34)	1.000
Unfavorable	0%	10.5% (6)	
Leukocytes ($\times 10^3$) (median)	20.67	6.41	0.28
Death	50% (3)	51.4% (37)	1.000
Relapses	50% (2)	30.9% (17)	0.58
Refractory	20% (1)	19.1% (13)	0.96

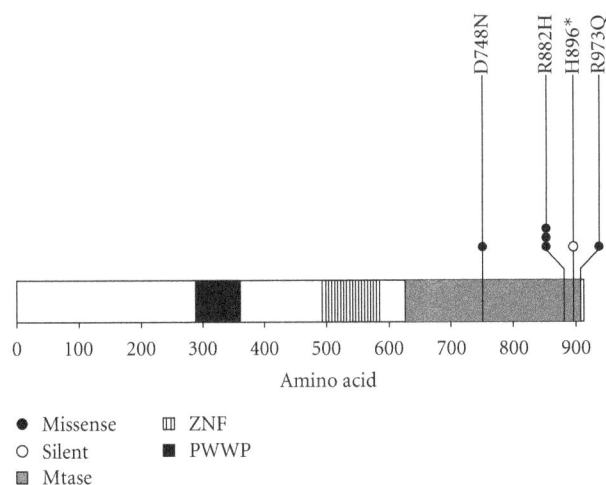

FIGURE 3: Location and classification of gene mutations found in gene *DNMT3A*. Representation of the *DNMT3A* gene and its domains: *methyltransferase* (MTase), *zinc-finger* (ZNF), and *conserved proline-tryptophan-tryptophan-proline* (PWWP).

approximately 80% of the mutations were located in these exons, with 58% of them in the last one (exon 23), where, in fact, most mutations in our study were found (Figure 3). The frequency of somatic *DNMT3A* mutations found in 8% of our 82 cases is lower than the 22% reported in 281 patients by Ley et al. [9], and lower than the 17.8% found by Thol et al. [14], also in Western patients, including about 500 patients. Interestingly, although the first study has sequenced the

entire gene, in the latter only the last nine exons were studied. The lowest frequency of mutations in our sample appears similar to that reported for patients of other ethnic groups. In a Japanese study [10], including 74 patients and sequencing the entire gene, the frequency of mutations was found to be only 4.1%, all located in exon 23, while in a Chinese study [11] including 355 patients and also sequencing the entire gene, the frequency of mutations, predominately affecting exon 23, was approximately 9%.

As for the sequences of *DNMT3A* gene variants, in accordance with a study of Stegelmann et al. [30], all our cases were heterozygous and no patient had more than one mutation; in addition, 3 of 6 mutations were p.R882H, already described by Ley et al. [9] who found a frequency of 59% of such mutation.

Five, or 80%, of our patients harboring a *DNMT3A* mutation belonged to the intermediate risk category, as was reported by others [9]. We also found a tendency ($P = 0.28$) to an increased leukocyte number at diagnosis for patients with mutation (20.7×10^9/L) comparing to the ones without mutation (6.4×10^9/L) which is in agreement with those reported in numerous studies [9–11, 31–33]. Interestingly, and worth mentioning, in our group of patients there was one case of *DNMT3A* mutation that also harbored *PML/RARα*.

Finally, the OS according to risk category in our group of 62 patients showed a prognostic trend similar to that reported in the literature (Figure 1). A prognostic evaluation for *DNMT3A* somatic mutations or its concurrency with fusion transcripts could not be determined in our study due to our sample size.

5. Conclusions

In conclusion, to our knowledge, this is the first study on the presence of somatic mutations of the gene *DNMT3A* in patients with AML in Brazil. Although in a small number of patients, we found the frequency of these mutations to be lower than that reported for Western patients. This could indicate an ethnogeographical variation already suggested in the literature for Eastern and Caucasian patients [34]. The discovery of recurrent mutations in the gene *DNMT3A* and its possible prognostic implications can provide valuable information for risk stratification for patients with AML and represents a valuable tool for making therapeutic decisions. However, the use of mutations in the *DNMT3A* gene as a tool for risk stratification needs to be discussed considering their application in different ethnicgeographic groups.

Acknowledgments

The study received financial support from the Research and Event Incentive Fund of Hospital de Clínicas de Porto Alegre (FIPE-HCPA) and The National Council for Scientific and Technological Development (CNPq) and has been supported by CNPq research scholarship no. 309091/2007-10. This paper has no conflict of interests.

References

[1] S. Fröhling, C. Scholl, D. G. Gilliland, and R. L. Levine, "Genetics of myeloid malignancies: pathogenetic and clinical implications," *Journal of Clinical Oncology*, vol. 23, no. 26, pp. 6285–6295, 2005.

[2] R. D. Brunning and, "Classification of acute leukemias," *Seminars in Diagnostic Pathology*, vol. 20, pp. 142–153, 2003.

[3] T. Szczepanski, V. H. J. van Velden, and J. J. M. van Dongen, "Classification systems for acute and chronic leukemias," *Best Practice & Research Clinical Haematology*, vol. 16, pp. 561–582, 2003.

[4] T. Peter and H. Andrew, "The epigenomics revolution in myelodysplasia: a clinic-pathological perspective," *Hematopathology*, vol. 43, pp. 536–546, 2011.

[5] C. Plass, C. Oakes, W. Blum, and G. Marcucci, "Epigenetics in acute myeloid leukemia," *Seminars in Oncology*, vol. 35, no. 4, pp. 378–387, 2008.

[6] O. Galm, S. Wilop, C. Lüders et al., "Clinical implications of aberrant DNA methylation patterns in acute myelogenous leukemia," *Annals of Hematology, Supplement*, vol. 84, no. 13, pp. 39–46, 2005.

[7] J. Boultwood and J. S. Wainscoat, "Gene silencing by DNA methylation in haematological malignancies," *British Journal of Haematology*, vol. 138, no. 1, pp. 3–11, 2007.

[8] P. A. Jones and S. B. Baylin, "The epigenomics of cancer," *Cell*, vol. 128, no. 4, pp. 683–692, 2007.

[9] T. J. Ley, L. Ding, M. J. Walter et al., "*DNMT3A* mutations in acute myeloid leukemia," *The New England Journal of Medicine*, vol. 363, no. 25, pp. 2424–2433, 2010.

[10] Y. Yamashita, J. Yuan, I. Suetake et al., "Array-based genomic resequencing of human leukemia," *Oncogene*, vol. 29, no. 25, pp. 3723–3731, 2010.

[11] X. J. Yan, J. Xu, Z. H. Gu et al., "Exome sequencing identifies somatic mutations of DNA methyltransferase gene *DNMT3A* in acute monocytic leukemia," *Nature Genetics*, vol. 43, no. 4, pp. 309–315, 2011.

[12] A. F. Ribeiro, M. Pratcorona, and C. Erpelinck-Verschueren, "Mutant *DNMT3A*: a marker of poor prognosis in acute myeloid leukemia," *Blood*, vol. 119, pp. 5824–5831, 2012.

[13] J. P. Patel, M. Gönen, and M. E. Figueroa, "Prognostic relevance of integrated genetic profiling in acute myeloid leukemia," *The New England Journal of Medicine*, vol. 366, no. 12, pp. 1079–1089, 2012.

[14] F. Thol, F. Damm, A. Lüdeking et al., "Incidence and prognostic influence of *DNMT3A* mutations in acute myeloid leukemia," *Journal of Clinical Oncology*, vol. 29, no. 21, pp. 2889–2896, 2011.

[15] G. Marcucci, K. H. Metzeler, S. Schwind et al., "Age related prognostic impact of different types of *DNMT3A* mutations in adults with primary cytogenetically normal acute myeloid leukemia," *Journal of Clinical Oncology*, vol. 30, no. 7, pp. 742–750, 2012.

[16] A. Renneville, N. Boissel, O. Nibourel et al., "Prognostic significance of DNA methyltransferase 3A mutations in cytogenetically normal acute myeloid leukemia: a study by the Acute Leukemia French Association," *Leukemia*, vol. 26, no. 6, pp. 1247–1254, 2011.

[17] S. H. Swerdlow, E. Campo, N. L. Harris et al., *WHO Classification of Tumours of Hematopoietic and Lymphoid Tissues*, International Agency for Research on Cancer (IARC), Lyon, France, 2008.

[18] J. J. M. Van Dongen, E. A. Macintyre, J. A. Gabert et al., "Standardized RT-PCR analysis of fusion gene transcripts from chromosome aberrations in acute leukemia for detection of minimal residual disease. Report of the BIOMED-1 Concerted Action: investigation of minimal residual disease in acute leukemia," *Leukemia*, vol. 13, no. 12, pp. 1901–1928, 1999.

[19] G. Mitterbauer, C. Zimmer, C. Fonatsch et al., "Monitoring of minimal residual leukemia in patients with MLL-AF9 positive acute myeloid leukemia by RT-PCR," *Leukemia*, vol. 13, no. 10, pp. 1519–1524, 1999.

[20] R. H. Jácomo, R. A. M. Melo, F. R. Souto et al., "Clinical features and outcomes of 134 Brazilians with acute promyelocytic leukemia who received ATRA and anthracyclines," *Haematologica*, vol. 92, no. 10, pp. 1431–1432, 2007.

[21] M. Capra, L. Vilella, W. V. Pereira et al., "Estimated number of cases, regional distribution and survival of patients diagnosed with acute myeloid leukemia between 1996 and 2000 in Rio Grande do Sul, Brazil," *Leukemia and Lymphoma*, vol. 48, no. 12, pp. 2381–2386, 2007.

[22] K. J. Phekoo, M. A. Richards, H. Møller, and S. A. Schey, "The incidence and outcome of myeloid malignancies in 2,112 adult patients in south East-England," *Haematologica*, vol. 91, no. 10, pp. 1400–1404, 2006.

[23] D. Douer, S. Preston-Martin, E. Chang, P. W. Nichols, K. J. Watkins, and A. M. Levine, "High frequency of acute promyelocytic leukemia among Latinos with acute myeloid leukemia," *Blood*, vol. 87, no. 1, pp. 308–313, 1996.

[24] C. Schoch, D. Haase, T. Haferlach et al., "Fifty-one patients with acute myeloid leukemia and translocation t(8;21)(q22 q22): an additional deletion in 9q is an adverse prognostic factor," *Leukemia*, vol. 10, no. 8, pp. 1288–1295, 1996.

[25] M. F. Chauffaille, D. Borri, and S. R. Martins, "Leucemia mielóide aguda t(8;21): freqüência em pacientes brasileiros," *Revista Brasileira de Hematologia e Hemoterapia*, vol. 26, no. 2, pp. 99–103, 2004.

[26] D. A. Arber, R. D. Brunning, M. M. Le Beau, S. H. Swerdlow, E. Campo, and N. L. Harris, "Acute myeloid leukaemia with

recurrent genetic abnormalities," in *WHO classification of tumours of haematopoietic and lymphoid tissues*, pp. 110–23, IARC Press, Lyon, 4th edition, 2008.

[27] C. Schoch and T. Haferlach, "Cytogenetics in acute myeloid leukemia," *Current Oncology Reports*, vol. 4, no. 5, pp. 390–397, 2002.

[28] D. Grimwade, H. Walker, G. Harrison et al., "The predictive value of hierarchical cytogenetic classification in older adults with acute myeloid leukemia (AML): analysis of 1065 patients entered into the United Kingdom Medical Research Council AML11 trial," *Blood*, vol. 98, no. 5, pp. 1312–1320, 2001.

[29] A. T. Look, "Oncogenic transcription factors in the human acute leukemias," *Science*, vol. 278, no. 5340, pp. 1059–1064, 1997.

[30] F. Stegelmann, L. Bullinger, R. F. Schlenk et al., "*DNMT3A* mutations in myeloproliferative neoplasms," *Leukemia*, vol. 25, no. 7, pp. 1217–1219, 2011.

[31] J. Marková, P. Michková, and K. Burèková, "Prognostic impact of *DNMT3A* mutations in patients with intermediate cytogenetic risk profile acute myeloid leukemia," *European Journal of Haematology*, vol. 88, no. 2, pp. 10–128, 2012.

[32] F. Thol, C. Winschel, A. Lüdeking et al., "Rare occurrence of *DNMT3A* mutations in myelodysplastic syndromes," *Haematologica*, vol. 96, no. 12, pp. 1870–1873, 2011.

[33] J. Lin, Y. Dm, J. Qian et al., "Recurrent *DNMT3A* R882 mutations in Chinese patients with acute myeloid leukemia and myelodysplastic syndrome," *PLoS ONE*, vol. 6, Article ID e26906, p. 10, 2011.

[34] C. Thiede, "Mutant *DNMT3A*: teaming up to transform," *Blood*, vol. 119, no. 24, Article ID 56157, 2012.

16

Management of Adenovirus in Children after Allogeneic Hematopoietic Stem Cell Transplantation

Winnie WY Ip[1] and Waseem Qasim[1,2]

[1] Molecular Immunology Unit, UCL Institute of Child Health, 30 Guildford Street, London WC1N 1EH, UK
[2] Department of Clinical Immunology, Great Ormond Street Hospital, London WC1N 3JH, UK

Correspondence should be addressed to Winnie WY Ip; w.ip@ucl.ac.uk

Academic Editor: Mark R. Litzow

Adenovirus (ADV) can cause significant morbidity and mortality in children following haematopoietic stem cell transplantation (HSCT), with an incidence of up to 27% and notable associated morbidity and mortality. T-cell depleted grafts and severe lymphopenia are major risk factors for the development of adenovirus disease after HSCT. Current antiviral treatments are at best virostatic and may have significant side effects. Adoptive transfer of donor-derived virus-specific T cells has been shown to be an effective strategy for the prevention and treatment of ADV infection after HSCT. Here we review progress in the field and present a pathway for the management of adenovirus in the posttransplant setting.

1. Introduction

Adenovirus (ADV) causes mild illnesses in immunocompetent hosts but can cause significant morbidity and mortality in the immunocompromised, for example, children in the posthaematopoietic stem cell transplant setting. Haematopoietic stem cell transplantation (HSCT) can offer a cure for many haematological diseases, primary immunodeficiencies, and inborn errors of metabolism. However, not all transplant recipients have fully matched sibling donors and alternative donor sources have to be sought. In HLA-matched or mismatched unrelated donor setting, conditioning regimens will often include serotherapy such as Alemtuzumab (monoclonal anti-CD52 antibody) or thymoglobulin (polyclonal horse or rabbit thymocyte globulin [ATG]) to remove alloreactive T cells in the recipient that can cause acute Graft versus Host Disease (GVHD). During the posttransplant period of reduced T-cell immunity when reconstitution of donor-derived immune system is slow and the use of immunosuppressive agents is necessary, transplant recipients are especially vulnerable to viral reactivations and/or infections.

Whilst antivirals such as ribavirin and cidofovir are available for the treatment of ADV, they are associated with toxicity and have variable efficacy. Over the past decade or so,

adoptive transfer of donor-derived virus-specific T cells has been explored extensively as an alternative method to prevent and treat ADV and other viral infections after HSCT. This review examines recent preclinical and clinical studies on T-cell immunotherapy for ADV and provides a strategy for monitoring and management of ADV in children after allo-HSCT.

2. Adenovirus

Adenoviruses (ADV) were first isolated in 1953 from human adenoid tissues obtained during adenoidectomy [1]. They are nonenveloped, double stranded DNA viruses that range in size from 65 to 80 nm in diameter [2]. To date, over 60 ADV types have been identified, which can be classified into seven subgroups, A–G, on the basis of their haemagglutination properties, their oncogenic potential in rodents and DNA homology, or GC content of their DNA (Table 1) [3–6]. The virion is composed of 252 capsomers: 240 hexons and 12 pentons arranged in an icosahedral shape and a nucleoprotein core that contains the DNA viral genome and internal proteins. The linear, double stranded DNA genome is 34–36 kb in size and encodes for more than 30 structural and nonstructural proteins [5, 6]. Each penton in the capsid

TABLE 1: Classification of human adenoviruses and their sites of infection.

Subgroup	Serotype	Sites of infection
A	12, 18, 31	Gastrointestinal
B1	3, 7, 16, 21, 50	Respiratory
B2	11, 14, 34, 35	Urinary tract/renal
C	1, 2, 5, 6	Respiratory
D	8, 9, 10, 13, 15, 17, 19, 20, 22–30, 32, 33, 36, 37, 38, 39, 42–48, 49, 51	Eye
E	4	Respiratory
F	40, 41	Gastrointestinal

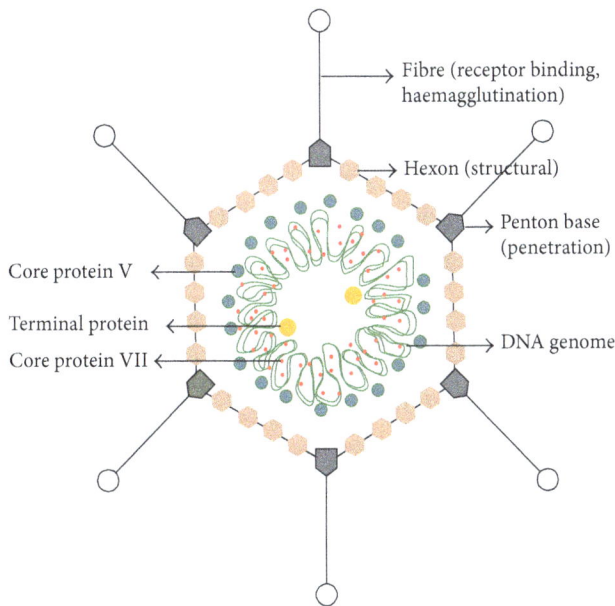

FIGURE 1: Structure of adenovirus.

comprises a base and a rod-like outward fibre projection of variable length depending on serotypes [2, 7]. The hexon contains group-specific antigenic determinants in addition to subgroup-specific determinants and type-specific neutralising epitopes (Figure 1) [7]. Tissue tropism of ADV differs among the different serotypes but generally corresponds to the subgroups. Subgroups C and E and some B viruses typically infect the respiratory tract; other B serotypes infect the urinary tract (B11, B34, and B35); serotypes from subgroups A and F target the gastrointestinal tract and serotypes from species D the eyes [5, 8].

3. Humoral Immunity Against ADV

Hexon, fibre, and to a lesser extent penton have been shown to be the major targets for ADV neutralising antibodies (Nab) [9–12]. After HSCT, subjects who developed ADV viraemia but subsequently cleared the infection have detectable humoral immune responses after a period of several weeks to months after viral clearance, with titres of serotype-specific Nabs increasing by 8–16-fold. Interestingly in some cases, preexisting, high titres of ADV-specific Nabs in serum did

not prevent progression to viraemia [13]. Whilst humoral immunity clearly plays a critical role in anti-ADV immunity, administration of immunoglobulin therapy has not been shown to be effective in preventing ADV reactivation or of proven benefit for the management of established viraemia or organ specific infection [14, 15].

4. Cell-Mediated Immunity Against ADV

Cellular immunity towards adenoviruses has been extensively studied over the past two decades and has been found to be cross-reactive across serotypes, confirming the presence of conserved antigens [16–21]. In a group of 8 healthy subjects with no serologic evidence of prior exposure to the uncommon group B Ad35, specific CD4+ proliferation has been shown to both Ad2- and Ad35-infected cell lysates [16]. In humans the response is predominantly in CD4+ T cells specific for capsid derived antigens [16, 19, 20], but cytotoxic responses are also found in CD8+ T cells against both viral structural and recognition proteins. The immunodominant CD4+ and CD8+ T-cell epitopes are found located in the major capsid protein hexon and have been found to induce T cells that are either broadly cross-reactive or reactive within particular subgroups [20–24]. Healthy adults have low frequencies of ADV hexon-specific CD8+ (38%) and CD4+ (81%) T cells detected in peripheral blood [25]. In a group of 8 healthy subjects with no serologic evidence of prior exposure to the uncommon group B Ad35, specific CD4+ proliferation has been shown to both Ad2- and Ad35-infected cell lysates [16].

5. Adenoviral Infection in the Immunodeficient Host

Adenovirus is endemic in paediatric populations with 80% of children between 1 and 5 years of age having antibody to one or more serotypes. Infections in immunocompetent hosts are usually benign and short-lived and most commonly manifest as upper respiratory tract infections [26]. ADV causes 2–7% of respiratory tract infections in children in the first 5 years of life and is responsible for 5–11% of cases of viral pneumonia and bronchiolitis in infants and children. Illness typically lasts less than 2 weeks, but once infected the virus remains latent in lymphoreticular tissue including tonsils, adenoids, and intestines. In healthy children viral shedding can persist for months or years. In the immunocompromised patients ADV can cause severe and protracted systemic illnesses such as hepatitis, pneumonitis, colitis, haemorrhagic cystitis, and encephalitis [26, 27]. The immunosuppressed paediatric host is particularly susceptible, most notably in the allogeneic transplant setting where cellular immunity is compromised. The incidence of ADV infection reported in bone marrow transplant recipients ranges from 5% to 29% in earlier studies where ADV was detected via routine weekly surveillance cultures up to first 100 days after transplant [7, 26, 28–32]. The advent of robust PCR based detection meant that serial ADV PCR has become the mainstay of routine surveillance, with incidence of viral isolation reported as between 17 and 27% in paediatric transplant recipients [4, 33].

These retrospective and prospective studies have facilitated the identification of several risk factors that are predictive for the development of ADV infection and/or disease in transplant recipients. One risk factor identified is T-cell depletion either *ex vivo* by CD34+ positive selection or *in vivo* with Alemtuzumab or antithymocyte globulin (ATG). In a group of 153 children receiving HSCT, adenoviraemia occurred in 26 children (17%), all of whom had received T-cell depleted grafts. Similarly Lion et al. found a significant increase in incidence of ADV infection in group of paediatric patients transplanted with T-cell depleted grafts [4]. And in a cohort of 76 adult allograft recipients ADV was isolated exclusively in recipients of Alemtuzumab mediated T-cell depleted grafts (15 of 76, 20%) [34].

Detection of ADV infection at multiple sites has also been correlated with increased risk for invasive disease in children [4, 30, 31]. However, the most significant predictor of adenovirus infection identified in the majority of studies was lymphopenia, with all patients who developed adenovirus disease or with persistent adenoviraemia having an absolute lymphocyte count (ALC) of less than $300/\mu L$ [33, 34]. In patients with established adenoviraemia, an increase in lymphocyte counts correlated with clearance of infection and survival of the host whereas those who died of adenoviraemia had continuously increasing ADV DNA loads in plasma with no lymphocyte recovery [13]. To further illustrate the importance of immune reconstitution in clearance of adenoviraemia, 46 children after HSCT were prospectively studied. Children who died (7/21) of ADV infection had no adenovirus-specific T cells and had significantly reduced T-cell reconstitution, although absolute lymphocyte count was above $0.3 \times 10^9/L$ at 30 days after transplant. Ninety-three percent of patients who successfully cleared ADV infection had presence of virus-specific T cells, compared to 54% of children without any ADV infection. They also had good T-cell reconstitution, especially CD8+ T cells ($>0.4 \times 10^9/L$) at 60 days after transplant [35]. In the current era of prospective monitoring, Hiwarkar et al. considered the impact of ADV reactivation in 291 paediatric HSCT procedures and again found reduced CD4 counts of less than $0.15 \times 10^9/L$ in the first 3 months after transplantation as a significant risk factor for developing adenoviraemia [36]. The overall mortality from ADV infection after HSCT ranges from 6% and 60% in studies of mixed populations with adults and children [7, 29, 30, 32] and between 19% to 83% amongst paediatric patients [26, 33, 37].

6. Diagnosis and Monitoring

The development of real-time quantitative PCR assays has allowed for accurate detection of ADV in a variety of tissues, including blood, stool, and urine [2] and allows for prospective monitoring of adenoviraemia in the posttransplantation setting. Kampmann et al. report a median of 21 days after transplant before adenoviraemia was evident [33]. In a prospective study that identified 21 paediatric HSCT patients with ADV infection, 90% of infections occurred during the first 3 months after transplant, with more than 50% of patients having ADV infection within 30 days after HSCT

[35]. The most prevalent group of adenovirus identified had been subgroup C [4, 33, 34], and subtypes 2, 5, 1, 6, 31, and 4 (in decreasing frequency) are the most prevalent [38].

There is a correlation between high plasma viral load and fatal outcome or invasive disease, with those who died of disseminated ADV disease having a much higher ADV DNA load than patients who survived [39, 40]. There is also association between onset of ADV-related disease and mortality. In a study of 132 consecutive paediatric patients undergoing SCT, 91% of those who were ADV positive in peripheral blood died, with adenoviral DNA detected in blood at a median of 29 days before death. And in those who developed disseminated disease, virus was detected in blood by a median of more than 3 weeks before onset of clinical symptoms [4]. These earlier studies all suggest that high viral load precedes symptoms of disseminated disease; therefore prospective monitoring of ADV load is now implemented in many of the paediatric transplant centres.

7. Management of Adenoviral Infection in Immunocompromised Children

7.1. Antiviral Drugs. Cidofovir is an acyclic nucleoside phosphonate derivative of cytosine which is converted to an active intracellular metabolite, cidofovir diphosphate, by cellular kinases [14, 41]. The active intracellular diphosphate form of the drug exerts its mechanism of action as both a competitive inhibitor and an alternative substrate for $2'$-deoxycytidine $5'$-triphosphate in the viral DNA polymerase reaction [42], thus inhibiting viral replication. Antiviral selectivity results from the higher affinity for the viral DNA polymerase compared to cellular DNA polymerases [8].

Several studies have reported on the success of CDV in the treatment of ADV infection in immunocompromised hosts after HSCT [14, 42], especially when given early [43–46] and combined with withdrawal of immunosuppression [33]. At our centre, if blood ADV reaches >1000 copies per mL on two consecutive occasions CDV is started at 5 mg/kg once every week for 2 weeks, followed by maintenance dose of 5 mg/kg once every fortnight. Notable side effects include nephrotoxicity, especially when used in combination with other nephrotoxic drugs such as cyclosporine or tacrolimus [15]. CDV is a dianion that is taken up into the proximal renal tubular cells by an organic anion transporter at the antiluminal membrane. Once taken up into the cells, a slow diffusion rate into the tubule lumen, as well as CDV's long intracellular half-life, can lead to toxic intracellular accumulation and subsequent tubular necrosis. Toxicity can be reduced by concomitant use of oral probenecid and intravenous hyperhydration [41]. Probenecid competes for the kidney anion transporter and along with hyperhydration can help protect tubular cells by decreasing plasma clearance rate of CDV [47, 48]. Ljungman et al. published two studies each on the use of CDV as therapy for ADV and cytomegalovirus infection in 126 stem cell transplant patients combined [44]. The risk of renal toxicity in both studies was 26% and most of the renal toxicity was mild (low-degree proteinuria or mild elevation of serum creatinine), but approximately half had remaining signs of renal impairment after discontinuation of CDV [44].

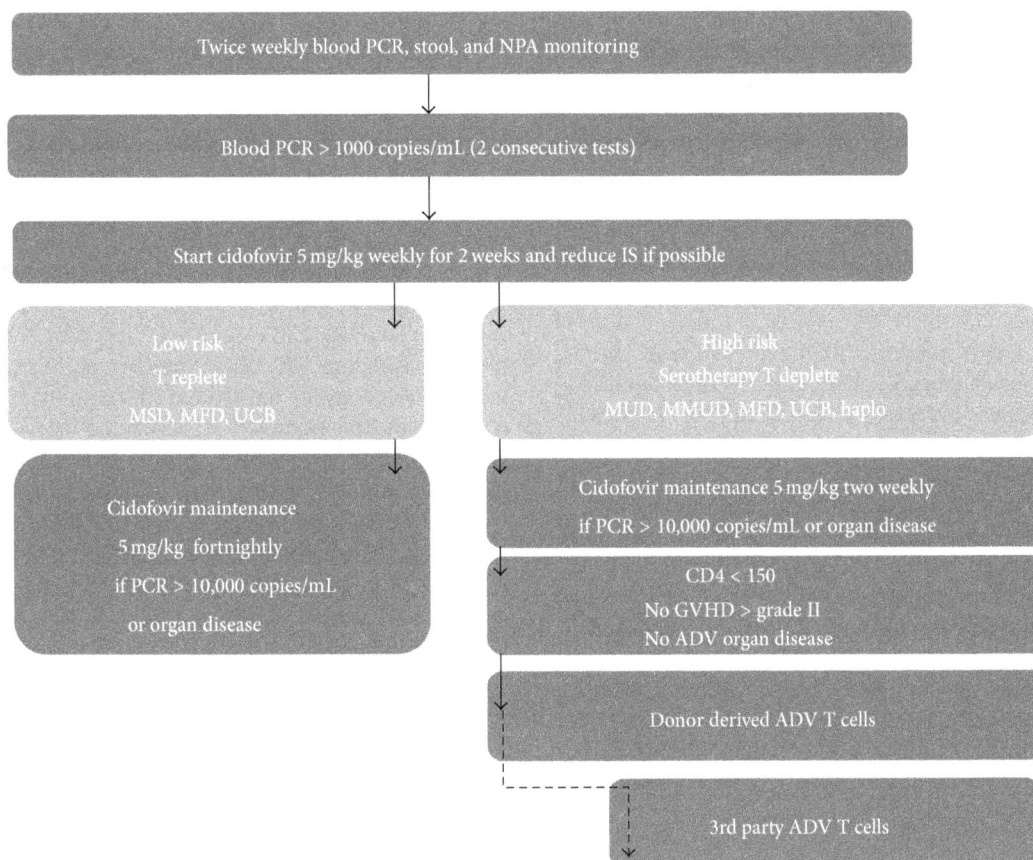

Abbreviations:

MSD: matched sibling donor

MFD: matched family donor

UCB: umbilical cord blood

MUD: matched unrelated donor

MMUD: mismatched unrelated donor

Haplo: haploidentical

GVHD: Graft versus Host Disease

FIGURE 2: Algorithm for the management of ADV reactivation in children after allogeneic stem cell transplantation.

Ribavirin is a nucleoside analogue for which *in vitro* anti-ADV activity has been reported but it differs against different subtypes. It is active on most ADV isolates from species A, B, and D and in all isolates from species C [49]. There is anecdotal evidence of successful treatment of ADV in immunocompromised patients but larger studies have not been as supportive [43, 50] (reviewed in [15]). There is no provable role for ganciclovir or for immunoglobulin therapy in immunocompromised patients [14, 15].

More recently a new oral therapy has been trialled for the treatment of ADV infections in immunocompromised patients. CMX001 (hexadecyloxypropyl cidofovir) is an orally bioavailable lipid conjugate of cidofovir with good oral bioavailability and can achieve higher intracellular levels of active drug compared with cidofovir; it may also have a better safety profile [51]. The drug was trialled in 13 immunocompromised patients and nearly two-thirds had a ≥10-fold drop in viral load after 1 week of therapy [51]. CMX001 is currently being studied in a randomised, placebo-controlled, Phase 2

trial for the preemptive treatment of adenovirus disease versus placebo in 48 paediatric and adult haematopoietic cell transplant recipients (ADV Halt Trial, NCT01241344).

7.2. Withdrawal of Immunosuppression. Chakrabarti et al. reported on the success of pre-emptive reduction or withdrawal of immunosuppressive therapy at first detection of adenovirus. In a group of 76 adult allograft recipients, 15 developed adenovirus disease/infection. Twelve patients had immunosuppression withdrawn or reduced and 9 had resolution of infection, whereas all 3 patients in whom immunosuppression had to be continued succumbed to adenovirus disease [34]. Similarly in paediatric transplant recipients withdrawal of immunosuppression together with early antiviral therapy led to the resolution of adenoviraemia in 19/26 (86%) patients [33]. Hence in the posttransplant setting we would recommend the following algorithm for the treatment of ADV (see Figure 2).

7.3. Adoptive Immunotherapy. It is clear that recovery from ADV infection requires cellular immune reconstitution after allogeneic HSCT. Adoptive immunotherapy using both unmanipulated T cells and virus-specific T cells has therefore been evaluated as approaches to reconstitute antiviral immunity.

Unmanipulated donor lymphocyte infusions (DLI) containing virus-specific T cells have been trialled in patients with EBV infections which resulted in clearance of infection but increased the risk of GHVD due to high frequency of alloreactive cells [52]. In 1995 Walter et al. infused clones of CMV-specific CD8+ cytotoxic T lymphocytes from donors into 14 recipients of allogeneic bone marrow in an attempt to reconstitute cellular immunity against CMV. All 14 patients had reconstituted CMV immunity by days 42 to 49 after marrow transplantation. The transferred CD8+ clones persisted for at least 8 weeks after completion of T-cell therapy [53].

Hromas et al. reported the first successful treatment of adenovirus infection with DLI. The patient developed severe ADV-associated haemorrhagic cystitis after a T cell depleted graft and did not respond to antiviral drugs or immunoglobulin. After infusion of 1×10^6/kg CD3+ cells on day +61 the patient improved over a period of 5 weeks without developing GVHD. This successful treatment supported the rationale for the adoptive transfer of adenovirus-specific CTL [54]. Earlier studies on adoptive immunotherapy have been summarised in recent reviews [47, 55–58].

8. Generation of T Cells Against ADV

In order to increase antiviral efficacy and to reduce the risk of alloreactivity, techniques were developed to isolate only ADV-specific T cells to be given to patients. Smith et al. in 1996 used donor peripheral blood dendritic cells as antigen-presenting cells to manufacture cytotoxic T cells (CTLs) that recognise ADV. Dendritic cells (DCs) from donors were infected with either wild-type adenovirus serotype 5 (Ad) or Ad5 strain *dl312*, an Ad5 mutant with the E1A region deleted resulting in a virus defective in early and late viral gene transcription. The adenovirus-specific T cells were subsequently expanded using virion-pulsed irradiated DCs [17]. The majority of the CTLs were CD4+ T cells and were directed against the input virion proteins. They demonstrated cross-reactivity but were unable to kill target cells in a standard 4–6-hour assay (requiring 18 hours to kill) and could not be adequately expanded into CTL lines [59].

Following on from this, in 2004 Leen and her group developed a protocol to reactivate ADV-specific memory T cells from donors' PBMCs using clinical-grade ADV vector. PBMCs from 6 healthy ADV-seropositive volunteers were stimulated with autologous dendritic cells (DCs) transduced with Ad5f35 (replication-defective ADV vector). CD4+ and CD8+ ADV-specific T cells were isolated and expanded with autologous EBV-transformed lymphoblastoid cell lines (LCLs) and showed ADV specific killing [59]. Because the generation of DCs to act as stimulator cells requires a large volume of blood, a second protocol using Ad5f35GFP-transduced PBMCs as both stimulators and responders was used. Expansion was again carried out with LCLs, and the

resultant expanded T cells had specific reactivity against both ADV and EBV. These CTL lines generated using Ad5f35 vector were able to recognise and kill autologous cells infected with wild-type adenovirus isolates from different serotypes and groups including Ad2, Ad4, Ad7, and Ad11 [59].

In 2006 Leen et al. reported on the prophylactic clinical use of trispecific (EBV, CMV, and ADV) CTLs on 11 adult and paediatric patients after haematopoietic stem cell transplant. Donor PBMCs transduced with a recombinant adenoviral vector encoding the CMV antigen pp65 (Ad5f35pp65) were used to reactivate CMV- and ADV-specific T cells. Subsequent stimulation with EBV-transformed LCLs transduced with the same vector reactivated EBV-specific T cells whilst maintaining the expansion of activated ADV- and CMV-specific T cells (Figure 3(c)). Fifteen donor CTL lines were generated and all showed cytolytic activity against all three viruses [62, 63]. Eleven patients received from 5×10^6 to 1×10^8 cells/m^2 at 35 to 150 days after HSCT. CMV- and EBV-specific CTLs consistently expanded in all individuals treated within 4 weeks of administration, whereas ADV-specific CTLs expanded only in those with active or recent infection. All patients with preinfusion viral infection/reactivation had reduction in viral titre and resolution of disease symptoms, contemporaneous with expansion of virus-specific T cells detected in peripheral blood [62].

In order to increase the frequency of adenovirus-specific T cells within their CTL lines, Leen and her group removed competition from the immunodominant CMV antigen and manufactured bivirus-specific CTL lines directed only to EBV and adenovirus [64]. Twenty CTL lines were made, of which 13 were administered to paediatric stem cell transplant recipients: 7 unrelated and 6 haploidentical transplants. The frequency of adenovirus hexon-specific T cells in the bivirus CTL was significantly higher than in the trivirus CTL study (median ADV cells 308 spot forming colonies/10^5 CTL [range 46–350] compared to 86 SFC/10^5 CTL [46–350] in bivirus product) [62, 64]. Each patient received from 5×10^6 to 1.35×10^8 cells/m^2 at 40 to 150 days after HSCT. There were no toxicities related to CTL therapy and no subject developed de novo GVHD after cell infusion. None of the 13 patients developed EBV-associated lymphoproliferative disease, and 2 of the subjects had resolution of their adenoviral disease [64]. More recently in a multicentre study, banked third-party virus-specific T cells (VSTs) were administered to 50 patients with severe, refractory CMV, ADV, or EBV infections [65]. Thirty-two virus-specific lines were generated from individuals with common HLA polymorphisms immune to EBV, CMV, or ADV, of which 18 lines were administered to 50 post-HSCT patients with severe, refractory illness due to infection with one of these viruses. The virus specific T cells were generated by transduction of PBMC with clinical-grade Ad5f35pp65 vector followed by stimulation with EBV-transformed LCL that had been transduced with the same chimeric vector. The VSTs were then cryopreserved until required. Patients were excluded from the study if they had received T-cell serotherapy within 28 days of proposed administration date. The cumulative rates of complete or partial responses at 6 weeks after infusion were 74% for the

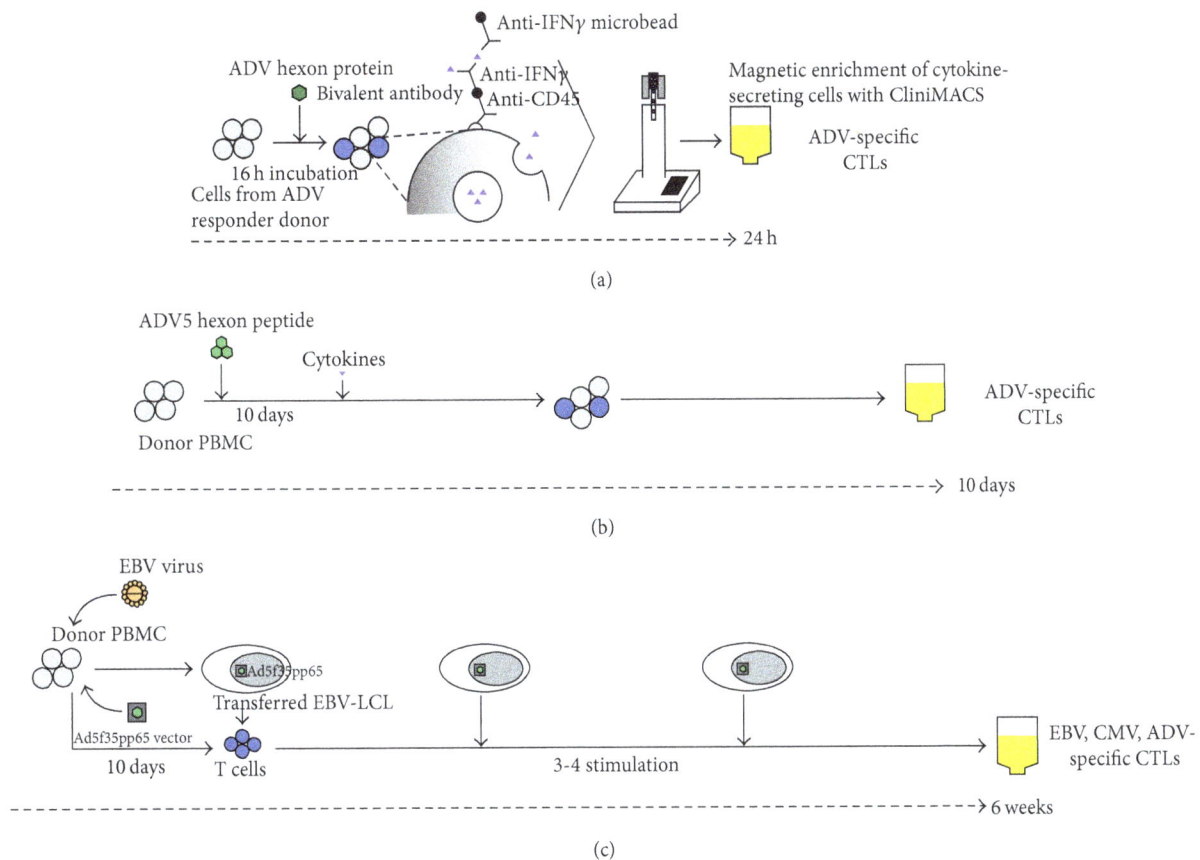

FIGURE 3: Protocols for generating virus-specific T cells. (a) Donor identified as ADV responder by IFN-γ secretion assay (Miltenyi Biotec, Bergisch Gladbach, Germany). Peripheral blood mononuclear cells (PBMC) isolated and incubated overnight with ADV Hexon protein. Responding cells captured with IFN-γ reagent, anti-IFN-γ microbead and magnetically enriched with CliniMACS (Miltenyi Biotec) [60]. (b) Donor PBMC incubated over 10 days with ADV5 hexon peptide and cytokines. Expanded cells isolated and infused into patients after QA/QC testing [61]. (c) EBV-transformed B cell lines (EBV-LCLs) generated from donor PBMCs by infecting with EBV virus. Donor PBMCs are transfected with Ad5f35pp65 vector (replication-competent adenovirus-negative) and later restimulated several times by EBV-LCLs that have been transduced with the same vector [62].

entire group. No immediate infusion-related adverse events were noted, 2 patients developed de novo GVHD (grade 1). Six out of eight patients who did not have line available and continued with standard therapy died of their viral disease. This approach of using "off-the-shelf" third-party VSTs is promising as it appears to remove some of the barriers to the wider application of cell therapy in viral reactivations post-transplant. It avoids the lengthy time and cost of producing individual lines, and does not appear to cause GVHD from alloreactivity of the third-party cells [65].

Once it has been established that ADV-specific T cells can be expanded in vitro and that they are effective and protective in vivo, the next challenge was to overcome logistics of manufacturing these products. The protocol described above of activating donor PBMCs with autologous monocytes transduced with the Ad5f3pp65 vector followed by restimulation with Ad5f35pp65-transduced EBV-LCL takes in total 10–14 weeks. This implies that products have to be manufactured in advance if they were to be made immediately available for acutely ill patients; and comes with it cost implications. Different cell selection and culture practices were therefore explored to develop more rapid and cost-effective strategies for production of CTLs.

9. Cytokine Based Selection of Antigen-Specific T Cells from Donor Peripheral Blood Mononuclear Cells

In 2004 Feuchtinger et al. described a clinical-grade strategy to isolate and expand donor derived human ADV-specific T lymphocytes using the Miltenyi Biotec (Bergisch Gladbach, Germany) interferon-γ (IFN-γ) secretion assay. PBMCs were isolated from suitable donors and stimulated with type C adenoviral antigen (BioWhittaker, Verviers, Belgium) for 16 hours. T cells with antigen-specific secretion of IFN-γ were detected on the following day and these cytokine-secreting cells were magnetically enriched using CliniMACS device (Miltenyi Biotech). A mean number of 3.4×10^6 cells were obtained with a mean purity of 85% ADV-specific T cells. These isolated cells were then expanded ex vivo in a median of 18 days (range 7–29 days) to greater than 10^8 total cells using

IL-2 and autologous feeder cell stimulation. The generated T cells showed ADV-specific IFN-γ release and specific killing of ADV-infected cells. Alloreactive proliferation of the generated lines in mixed lymphocyte cultures was significantly reduced when compared to unmanipulated PBMCs [66].

The above method of generating ADV-specific T cells was adopted clinically in 2006 by Feuchtinger's group for nine children with systemic ADV infection after HSCT for mainly leukaemia or lymphoma. These children underwent myeloablative conditioning regimen with T-cell depletion for HSCT and had ADV viraemia not controlled by antivirals. T-cell transfer was performed if a sufficient ADV-specific T-cell response was detected in the donor (>0.01% of T cells). A mean of 14×10^3/kg (range 1.2–50×10^3/kg) T cells were infused at a median of +77 days after transplant (range +40–+378). T-cell infusion was well tolerated in all nine patients, except for one case with aggravation of preexisting skin GVHD that was seen at days 10 to 14. Five out of six evaluable patients had significant decrease in viral DNA in peripheral blood and stool with an *in vivo* expansion of specific T cells. Those without a specific T-cell response after adoptive T-cell transfer had either increasing or unchanged viral DNA load in peripheral blood. Three patients in whom followup was possible had sustained ADV-specific T-cell response detected 4 to 6 months after T-cell transfer. Efficacy was independent of T-cell dose transferred, suggesting efficient *in vivo* expansion. Four patients died of whom 3 died from adenovirus-associated, preexisting multiorgan failure. Three out of 4 patients who died did not have specific T-cell response after immunotherapy [67].

Chatziandreou et al. also reported on the successful isolation of ADV-specific T cells using a similar protocol [69]. Using the Miltenyi IFN-γ secretion and capture assay with adenovirus lysate, ADV-specific T cells were isolated, expanded, and restimulated over 2 weeks. The numbers of eluted virus-specific cells from six ADV-positive donors ranged from 1 to 7×10^5 cells, with the majority being CD4+ cells. After a 2-week culture period, a 1.5 to 2 log expansion was seen with cell numbers averaging at 1×10^7 cells. This would enable infusions of up to 10^5 ADV-specific cells/kg for most adults and larger amounts of paediatric patients. This approach offers the advantage of a short 14-day culture period, allowing for generation of cells in response to first detection of virus during routine screening. It is therefore less labour intensive and has a more favourable cost: benefit profile [69]. Using a similar IFN-γ capture protocol, five patients have been treated at Great Ormond Street Hospital with ADV-specific T cells either from the original donor ($n = 3$) or third-party haploidentical parents ($n = 2$) [60]. All 5 children had undergone either *in vivo* or *ex vivo* T cell depletion as part of their conditioning regimen and had peak ADV loads in blood ranging from 5.6×10^4/mL to 22×10^6/mL before cell infusion. IFN-γ secreting ADV-specific T cells in the donations were enriched to between 19 and 64% after 24 hours and infused directly without *ex vivo* expansion (Figure 3(a)), with 4 children receiving 10^4 T cells/kg and 1 child receiving 10^5 T cells/kg at an average of 80 days after the original stem cell graft. Three patients cleared

ADV in blood after a single infusion of 10^4/kg and had demonstrable ADV-specific T cells in circulation detected by IFN-γ secretion assay. No acute, infusion-related toxicities were observed. Three patients died: one due to bystander GVHD after cell infusion even though viraemia had resolved [70], the other two failed to clear virus and died at days 175 and 56, respectively [60].

10. Peptide Expanded T Cells

More recently in order to generate CTLs from a greater majority of healthy donors in a short period of time, Comoli et al. used a pool of five 30 mer peptides derived from HAdV5 hexon protein, to generate 21 T-cell lines with limited alloreactivity starting from median of 20×10^6 donor PMBC and expanded to 75×10^6 cells at the end of 26 days. This would have been sufficient for infusion aimed at 0.5×10^6 cells/kg [71]. In 2010 Aïssi-Rothe et al. used clinical-grade PepTivator-ADV5 Hexon (Miltenyi Biotec, Germany) and 6 hr incubation time to generate IFN-γ secreting ADV-specific T cells which were expanded over a median of 2-week period with IL2 and irradiated autologous feeder cells (Figure 3(b)). Up to 85×10^6 ADV T cells were generated with a mean of 1.7 log expansion and a reduction of 1.3 log in alloreactivity [61].

11. Stimulation with Viral DNA Plasmids

In 2011 the Baylor group took an alternative approach to rapidly select virus-specific T cells. Instead of using adenovectors to stimulate T cells, dendritic cells nucleofected with DNA plasmids encoding LMP2, EBNA1, and BZLF1 (EBV), hexon and penton (ADV), and pp65 and IE1 (CMV) were used as antigen-presenting cells. Secondly, EBV-LCLs were removed and replaced by gas permeable culture device (G-Rex) that promotes expansion and survival of large cell numbers after a single stimulation. Activated T-cells were cultured in the presence of IL-4 (1,000 u/mL) and IL-7 (10 ng/mL). This approach reduced the time of manufacturing from 10 weeks to 10 days, as well as the cost of production by >90% [72]. Using this method, 22 trivirus and 14 bivirus CTL lines were produced with a 1.5 log expansion from 15×10^6 starting PBMCs. 10 patients with viral reactivation (either single or dual) were treated between day 27 and 52 months after HSCT, with each patient receiving 0.5 to 2×10^7 cells/m^2. Complete virological responses associated with increased frequency of virus specific T cells were seen in 80%. One patient developed stage 2 skin GVHD after infusion but no other toxicities were observed [68]. Similarly this approach was used to develop a single preparation of polyclonal (CD4+ and CD8+) CTLs that is specific for 7 viruses (EBV, CMV, adenovirus, BK, human herpes virus 6, respiratory syncytial virus, and influenza) [73].

12. Isolation Protocols Using T-Cell Activation Markers

Apart from using IFN-γ production as a way to capture antigen-specific T cells, alternative isolation strategies based on

TABLE 2: Clinical trials using virus-specific cytotoxic T cells in the HSCT setting.

Reference number (centre)	Virus specificity	Expansion protocol	Antigen used	Infused number and type of cells	Patients treated	Clinical results
[62] (Texas)	EBV, CMV, ADV	Donor PBMCs infected with vector and restimulated, repetitively, with irradiated EBV-LCLs transduced with same vector over 10–12 weeks	Clinical-grade Ad5f35pp65 vector	Median 5×10^7 polyclonal cells/m² infused at 35–150 d after HSCT (median 62 d)	11 infused (children and adults; 10 prophylactically, 1 treated for ADV infection)	3/3 cleared CMV and 3/3 cleared EBV infection/PTLD without antivirals; 3 patients with infection and 1 with disease cleared ADV after-CTL. No GVHD
[67] (Tuebingen)	ADV	IFN-γ selection after 16 h stimulation Cytokine-secreting cells magnetically enriched	Adenoviral antigen type C (nonclinical grade)	1.2–50×10^3/kg ADV-reactive polyclonal T cells infused	9 children with ADV infection	5 out of 6 with ADV responded 1 died at 30 days from ADV infection 5 deaths (3 due to ADV infection)
[64] (Texas)	EBV + ADV	PBMCs infected with vector Responder cells restimulated weekly with irradiated autologous LCL transduced with the same vector IL-2 being added twice weekly from day 14. CTLs cryopreserved after 3 or 4 simulations	Ad5f35^{null} vector MOI 200 vp/cell	20 CTL lines with EBV and ADV specificity produced, 13 lines infused Dose of 5×10^6 to 1.35×10^8 cells/m² at 40 to 150 days after HSCT (median 77 days)	13 children [(M)MUD or haplo] 2 with active ADV disease; 11 prophylactic	No toxicities or GVHD, monitored for 3 months. Only detected increases in ADV-sp T cells in peripheral blood in those with active ADV infection (2 out of 13)
[60] (London)	ADV	PBMCs stimulated for 16 hrs with ADV-hexon antigen Cytokine-secreting cells selected using anti-IFN-γ microbeads and Miltenyi Mini-MACS column within 24 h	Commercially available purified ADV-hexon antigen (Binding Site, UK)	3 received γ-captured cells from original stem cell donor Cells (10^4–10^5/kg) received on average 80 d after original graft (range 34–122)	5 patients treated (3 with original donor; 2 third-party haploidentical donor)	Blood viraemia resolved in 3 IFN-γ secreting ADV-specific T cells present in 4 patients 3 died—1 of bystander GVHD after clearing virus
[65] (Texas)	ADV, CMV, EBV	Banked 3rd party PMBCs transduced with vector and stimulated with EBV-LCL transduced with same vector	Ad5f35pp65 vector	32 virus-specific lines from individuals with common HLA polymorphisms immune to EBV, CMV, or ADV Each patient received up to 2×10^7 cells/m²	18 lines administered to 50 patients with severe viral illness with one of the viruses	Cumulative rates of complete or partial responses at 6 weeks were 74% for the whole group 2 de novo GVHD (grade 1).
[68] (Texas)	ADV, CMV, EBV	Donor PBMCs stimulated with nucleofacted DCs and cultured over 2-3 weeks with IL4 and IL7.	DCs nucleofacted with range of EBV, CMV, and ADV viral antigens	22 trivirus and 14 bivirus CTL lines. Each patient received 0.5–2×10^7 cells/m²	10 patients with viral reactivation treated between day 27 and month 52 after HSCT	Viral clearance and increased frequency of VSTs in 80% 1 stage 2 skin GVHD

other T-cell activation markers have been investigated. Khanna et al. generated antigen-specific T cells lines for ADV, EBV, CMV, A fumigatus, and C albicans based on magnetic cell separation of CD154+ T cells after 16 hours of stimulation with antigens, followed by expansion in presence of IL2, IL7, and IL15 over 14 days. Purity of the product was between 8 to 15%, with a higher frequency of virus-specific T cells compared to fungus-specific T cells [74]. Leibold et al. compared the specificity, expansion/differentiation potential, and Th1 response against CMV and ADV after isolation of antigen specific T cells based on IFN-γ release or expression of activation markers (CD137 ND CD154). Isolation of T cells based on expression markers is feasible and less time consuming, but it resulted in smaller proportion of Th1 cells compared to IFN-γ capture which may correspond to less effector function *in vivo* [75].

Because CD4+ T cells are critical in human ADV infection, Haveman et al. explored the possibility to selectively expand and isolate ADV-specific CD4+ T cells. PBMCs were stimulated with 15 mer pan-DR binding CD4+ T cell epitopes of ADV serotype 5 peptides using artificial APCs, composed of liposomes harbouring ADV peptide/HLA class-II complexes [76]. The resultant T-cell lines after 7-day culture period produced mainly proinflammatory cytokines (TNF-α, IFN-γ, MDC, RANTES, and MIP-1α), expressed perforin and granzyme B, had specific ADV-killing, and were not alloreactive [76].

Table 2 summarises recent clinical trials on the use of virus-specific T cells.

13. Financial Implications

The economic burden of viral reactivation has been assessed recently at one of the main Paediatric transplant centres in the UK. By calculating the cost of antiviral drugs and excess inpatient hospital stay, viral reactivation costs an estimate of £22500 per patient (compared to £800 per day for routine inpatient costs following HSCT) [36]. On the other hand, although generating virus-specific T cells can be a costly operation, it could result in less patients with ADV infection requiring prolonged hospital stay and/or ICU admissions. Advances are being made in cell production techniques to reduce production time and generation of single CTL product with specificity against multiple viruses will be more cost effective.

14. Summary

It is undeniable that adenovirus can cause significant morbidity and mortality in immunocompromised children. Current antiviral therapy with cidofovir is not always successful, although current available data on the new drug CMX001 seems promising. Ultimately clearance of adenovirus requires reconstitution of T-cell immunity which is often delayed after haematopoietic stem cell transplant, especially in T-cell depleted grafts. Major advances have been made over the past decade in adoptive transfer of virus-specific T cells. However there is still ground to be covered to move T-cell

immunotherapy from specialist centres to standard-of-care therapy available to all transplant recipients.

Acknowledgments

Winnie Ip is supported by the Technology Strategy Board (TSB), a business-led executive nondepartmental UK government public body which is providing funding support for a clinical trial of adenovirus-specific T cells jointly with Cellmedia Ltd. Waseem Qasim receives support from Great Ormond Street Hospital Children's Charity and the National Institute of Health Research via Biomedical Research Councils.

References

[1] W. P. Rowe, R. J. Huebner, L. K. Gilmore et al., "Isolation of a cytopathogenic agent from human adenoids undergoing spontaneous degeneration in tissue culture," *Proceedings of the Society for Experimental Biology and Medicine*, vol. 84, no. 3, pp. 570–573, 1953.

[2] T. Walls, A. G. Shankar, and D. Shingadia, "Adenovirus: an increasingly important pathogen in paediatric bone marrow transplant patients," *The Lancet Infectious Diseases*, vol. 3, no. 2, pp. 79–86, 2003.

[3] A. Heim, "Advances in the management of disseminated adenovirus disease in stem cell transplant recipients: impact of adenovirus load (DNAemia) testing," *Expert Review of Anti-Infective Therapy*, vol. 9, no. 11, pp. 943–945, 2011.

[4] T. Lion, R. Baumgartinger, F. Watzinger et al., "Molecular monitoring of adenovirus in peripheral blood after allogeneic bone marrow transplantation permits early diagnosis of disseminated disease," *Blood*, vol. 102, no. 3, pp. 1114–1120, 2003.

[5] T. Kojaoghlanian, P. Flomenberg, and M. S. Horwitz, "The impact of adenovirus infection on the immunocompromised host," *Reviews in Medical Virology*, vol. 13, no. 3, pp. 155–171, 2003.

[6] C. M. Robinson, G. Singh, J. Y. Lee et al., "Molecular evolution of human adenoviruses," *Scientific Reports*, vol. 3, p. 1812, 2013.

[7] J. C. Hierholzer, "Adenoviruses in the immunocompromised host," *Clinical Microbiology Reviews*, vol. 5, no. 3, pp. 262–274, 1992.

[8] L. Lenaerts, E. De Clercq, and L. Naesens, "Clinical features and treatment of adenovirus infections," *Reviews in Medical Virology*, vol. 18, no. 6, pp. 357–374, 2008.

[9] C. I. A. Toogood, J. Crompton, and R. T. Hay, "Antipeptide antisera define neutralizing epitopes on the adenovirus hexon," *Journal of General Virology*, vol. 73, no. 6, pp. 1429–1435, 1992.

[10] H. Gahéry-Ségard, F. Farace, D. Godfrin et al., "Immune response to recombinant capsid proteins of adenovirus in humans: antifiber and anti-penton base antibodies have a synergistic effect on neutralizing activity," *Journal of Virology*, vol. 72, no. 3, pp. 2388–2397, 1998.

[11] S. M. Sumida, D. M. Truitt, A. A. C. Lemckert et al., "Neutralizing antibodies to adenovirus serotype 5 vaccine vectors are directed primarily against the adenovirus hexon protein," *Journal of Immunology*, vol. 174, no. 11, pp. 7179–7185, 2005.

[12] S. M. Sumida, D. M. Truitt, M. G. Kishko et al., "Neutralizing antibodies and CD8$^+$ T lymphocytes both contribute to immunity to adenovirus serotype 5 vaccine vectors," *Journal of Virology*, vol. 78, no. 6, pp. 2666–2673, 2004.

[13] B. Heemskerk, A. C. Lankester, T. Van Vreeswijk et al., "Immune reconstitution and clearance of human adenovirus viremia in pediatric stem-cell recipients," *Journal of Infectious Diseases*, vol. 191, no. 4, pp. 520–530, 2005.

[14] F. Legrand, D. Berrebi, N. Houhou et al., "Early diagnosis of adenovirus infection and treatment with cidofovir after bone marrow transplantation in children," *Bone Marrow Transplantation*, vol. 27, no. 6, pp. 621–626, 2001.

[15] P. Ljungman, "Treatment of adenovirus infections in the immunocompromised host," *European Journal of Clinical Microbiology and Infectious Diseases*, vol. 23, no. 8, pp. 583–588, 2004.

[16] P. Flomenberg, V. Piaskowski, R. L. Truitt, and J. T. Casper, "Characterization of human proliferative T cell responses to adenovirus," *Journal of Infectious Diseases*, vol. 171, no. 5, pp. 1090–1096, 1995.

[17] C. A. Smith, L. S. Woodruff, G. R. Kitchingman, and C. M. Rooney, "Adenovirus-pulsed dendritic cells stimulate human virus-specific T-cell responses in vitro," *Journal of Virology*, vol. 70, no. 10, pp. 6733–6740, 1996.

[18] C. A. Smith, L. S. Woodruff, C. Rooney, and G. R. Kitchingman, "Extensive cross-reactivity of adenovirus-specific cytotoxic T cells," *Human Gene Therapy*, vol. 9, no. 10, pp. 1419–1427, 1998.

[19] B. Heemskerk, L. A. Veltrop-Duits, T. Van Vreeswijk et al., "Extensive cross-reactivity of CD4+ adenovirus-specific T cells: implications for immunotherapy and gene therapy," *Journal of Virology*, vol. 77, no. 11, pp. 6562–6566, 2003.

[20] M. Olive, L. Eisenlohr, N. Flomenberg, S. Hsu, and P. Flomenberg, "The adenovirus capsid protein hexon contains a highly conserved human CD4+ T-cell epitope," *Human Gene Therapy*, vol. 13, no. 10, pp. 1167–1178, 2002.

[21] A. M. Leen, U. Sili, E. F. Vanin et al., "Conserved CTL epitopes on the adenovirus hexon protein expand subgroup cross-reactive and subgroup-specific CD8+ T cells," *Blood*, vol. 104, no. 8, pp. 2432–2440, 2004.

[22] J. Tang, M. Olive, R. Pulmanausahakul et al., "Human CD8+ cytotoxic T cell responses to adenovirus capsid proteins," *Virology*, vol. 350, no. 2, pp. 312–322, 2006.

[23] J. Tang, M. Olive, K. Champagne et al., "Adenovirus hexon T-cell epitope is recognized by most adults and is restricted by HLA DP4, the most common class II allele," *Gene Therapy*, vol. 11, no. 18, pp. 1408–1415, 2004.

[24] A. M. Leen, A. Christin, M. Khalil et al., "Identification of hexon-specific CD4 and CD8 T-cell epitopes for vaccine and immunotherapy," *Journal of Virology*, vol. 82, no. 1, pp. 546–554, 2008.

[25] M. L. Zandvliet, J. H. F. Falkenburg, E. van Liempt et al., "Combined CD8+ and CD4+ adenovirus hexon-specific T cells associated with viral clearance after stem cell transplantation as treatment for adenovirus infection," *Haematologica*, vol. 95, no. 11, pp. 1943–1951, 2010.

[26] G. A. Hale, H. E. Heslop, R. A. Krance et al., "Adenovirus infection after pediatric bone marrow transplantation," *Bone Marrow Transplantation*, vol. 23, no. 3, pp. 277–282, 1999.

[27] D. R. Carrigan, "Adenovirus infections in immunocompromised patients," *American Journal of Medicine*, vol. 102, no. 3A, pp. 71–74, 1997.

[28] A. F. Shields, R. C. Hackman, and K. H. Fife, "Adenovirus infections in patients undergoing bone marrow transplantation," *The New England Journal of Medicine*, vol. 312, no. 9, pp. 529–533, 1985.

[29] P. Flomenberg, J. Babbitt, W. R. Drobyski et al., "Increasing incidence of adenovirus disease in bone marrow transplant recipients," *Journal of Infectious Diseases*, vol. 169, no. 4, pp. 775–781, 1994.

[30] D. S. Howard, G. L. Phillips II, D. E. Reece et al., "Adenovirus infections in hematopoietic stem cell transplant recipients," *Clinical Infectious Diseases*, vol. 29, no. 6, pp. 1494–1501, 1999.

[31] A. Baldwin, H. Kingman, M. Darville et al., "Outcome and clinical course of 100 patients with adenovirus infection following bone marrow transplantation," *Bone Marrow Transplantation*, vol. 26, no. 12, pp. 1333–1338, 2000.

[32] V. Runde, S. Ross, R. Trenschel et al., "Adenoviral infection after allogeneic stem cell transplantation (SCT): report on 130 patients from a single SCT unit involved in a prospective multi center surveillance study," *Bone Marrow Transplantation*, vol. 28, no. 1, pp. 51–57, 2001.

[33] B. Kampmann, D. Cubitt, T. Walls et al., "Improved outcome for children with disseminated adenoviral infection following allogeneic stem cell transplantation," *British Journal of Haematology*, vol. 130, no. 4, pp. 595–603, 2005.

[34] S. Chakrabarti, V. Mautner, H. Osman et al., "Adenovirus infections following allogeneic stem cell transplantation: incidence and outcome in relation to graft manipulation, immunosuppression, and immune recovery," *Blood*, vol. 100, no. 5, pp. 1619–1627, 2002.

[35] T. Feuchtinger, J. Lücke, K. Hamprecht et al., "Detection of adenovirus-specific T cells in children with adenovirus infection after allogeneic stem cell transplantation," *British Journal of Haematology*, vol. 128, no. 4, pp. 503–509, 2005.

[36] P. Hiwarkar, H. B. Gaspar, K. Gilmour et al., "Impact of viral reactivations in the era of pre-emptive antiviral drug therapy following allogeneic haematopoietic SCT in paediatric recipients," *Bone Marrow Transplant*, vol. 48, no. 6, pp. 803–808, 2013.

[37] F. M. Munoz, P. A. Piedra, and G. J. Demmler, "Disseminated adenovirus disease in immunocompromised and immunocompetent children," *Clinical Infectious Diseases*, vol. 27, no. 5, pp. 1194–1200, 1998.

[38] T. Feuchtinger, C. Richard, M. Pfeiffer et al., "Adenoviral infections after transplantation of positive selected stem cells from haploidentical donors in children: an update," *Klinische Padiatrie*, vol. 217, no. 6, pp. 339–344, 2005.

[39] V. Erard, M.-L. Huang, J. Ferrenberg et al., "Quantitative real-time polymerase chain reaction for detection of adenovirus after T cell-replete hematopoietic cell transplantation: viral load as a marker for invasive disease," *Clinical Infectious Diseases*, vol. 45, no. 8, pp. 958–965, 2007.

[40] M. W. Schilham, E. C. Claas, W. Van Zaane et al., "High levels of adenovirus DNA in serum correlate with fatal outcome of adenovirus infection in children after allogeneic stem-cell transplantation," *Clinical Infectious Diseases*, vol. 35, no. 5, pp. 526–532, 2002.

[41] R. S. Sellar and K. S. Peggs, "Management of multidrug-resistant viruses in the immunocompromised host," *British Journal of Haematology*, vol. 156, no. 5, pp. 559–572, 2012.

[42] J. A. Hoffman, A. J. Shah, L. A. Ross, and N. Kapoor, "Adenoviral infections and a prospective trial of cidofovir in pediatric hematopoietic stem cell transplantation," *Biology of Blood and Marrow Transplantation*, vol. 7, no. 7, pp. 388–394, 2001.

[43] P. Bordigoni, A.-S. Carret, V. Venard, F. Witz, and A. L. Faou, "Treatment of adenovirus infections in patients undergoing allogeneic hematopoietic stem cell transplantation," *Clinical Infectious Diseases*, vol. 32, no. 9, pp. 1290–1297, 2001.

[44] P. Ljungman, P. Ribaud, M. Eyrich et al., "Cidofovir for adenovirus infections after allogeneic hematopoietic stem cell transplantation: a survey by the Infectious Diseases Working Party of the European Group for Blood and Marrow Transplantation," *Bone Marrow Transplantation*, vol. 31, no. 6, pp. 481–486, 2003.

[45] U. Yusuf, G. A. Hale, J. Carr et al., "Cidofovir for the treatment of adenoviral infection in pediatric hematopoietic stem cell transplant patients," *Transplantation*, vol. 81, no. 10, pp. 1398–1404, 2006.

[46] D. Neofytos, A. Ojha, B. Mookerjee et al., "Treatment of adenovirus disease in stem cell transplant recipients with cidofovir," *Biology of Blood and Marrow Transplantation*, vol. 13, no. 1, pp. 74–81, 2007.

[47] C. A. Lindemans, A. M. Leen, and J. J. Boelens, "How I treat adenovirus in hematopoietic stem cell transplant recipients," *Blood*, vol. 116, no. 25, pp. 5476–5485, 2010.

[48] S. A. Lacy, M. J. M. Hitchcock, W. A. Lee, P. Tellier, and K. C. Cundy, "Effect of oral probenecid coadministration on the chronic toxicity and pharmacokinetics of intravenous cidofovir in cynomolgus monkeys," *Toxicological Sciences*, vol. 44, no. 2, pp. 97–106, 1998.

[49] F. Morfin, S. Dupuis-Girod, E. Frobert et al., "Differential susceptibility of adenovirus clinical isolates to cidofovir and ribavirin is not related to species alone," *Antiviral Therapy*, vol. 14, no. 1, pp. 55–61, 2009.

[50] A. C. Lankester, B. Heemskerk, E. C. J. Claas et al., "Effect of ribavirin on the plasma viral DNA load in patients with disseminating adenovirus infection," *Clinical Infectious Diseases*, vol. 38, no. 11, pp. 1521–1525, 2004.

[51] D. F. Florescu, S. A. Pergam, M. N. Neely et al., "Safety and efficacy of CMX001 as salvage therapy for severe adenovirus infections in immunocompromised patients," *Biology of Blood and Marrow Transplantation*, vol. 18, no. 5, pp. 731–738, 2012.

[52] E. B. Papadopoulos, M. Ladanyi, D. Emanuel et al., "Infusions of donor leukocytes to treat Epstein-Barr virus-associated lymphoproliferative disorders after allogeneic bone marrow transplantation," *The New England Journal of Medicine*, vol. 330, no. 17, pp. 1185–1191, 1994.

[53] E. A. Walter, P. D. Greenberg, M. J. Gilbert et al., "Reconstitution of cellular immunity against cytomegalovirus in recipients of allogeneic bone marrow by transfer of T-cell clones from the donor," *The New England Journal of Medicine*, vol. 333, no. 16, pp. 1038–1044, 1995.

[54] R. Hromas, K. Cornetta, E. Srour, C. Blanke, and E. R. Broun, "Donor leukocyte infusion as therapy of life-threatening adenoviral infections after T-cell-depleted bone marrow transplantation," *Blood*, vol. 84, no. 5, pp. 1689–1690, 1994.

[55] C. M. Bollard, I. Kuehnle, A. Leen, C. M. Rooney, and H. E. Heslop, "Adoptive immunotherapy for posttransplantation viral infections," *Biology of Blood and Marrow Transplantation*, vol. 10, no. 3, pp. 143–155, 2004.

[56] A. M. Leen and C. M. Rooney, "Adenovirus as an emerging pathogen in immunocompromised patients," *British Journal of Haematology*, vol. 128, no. 2, pp. 135–144, 2005.

[57] A. M. Leen, G. D. Myers, C. M. Bollard et al., "T-cell immunotherapy for adenoviral infections of stem-cell transplant recipients," *Annals of the New York Academy of Sciences*, vol. 1062, pp. 104–115, 2005.

[58] A. M. Leen, T. Tripic, and C. M. Rooney, "Challenges of T cell therapies for virus-associated diseases after hematopoietic stem cell transplantation," *Expert Opinion on Biological Therapy*, vol. 10, no. 3, pp. 337–351, 2010.

[59] A. M. Leen, U. Sili, B. Savoldo et al., "Fiber-modified adenoviruses generate subgroup cross-reactive, adenovirus-specific cytotoxic T lymphocytes for therapeutic applications," *Blood*, vol. 103, no. 3, pp. 1011–1019, 2004.

[60] W. Qasim, K. Gilmour, H. Zhan et al., "Interferon-gamma capture T cell therapy for persistent Adenoviraemia following allogeneic haematopoietic stem cell transplantation," *British Journal of Haematology*, vol. 161, no. 3, pp. 449–452, 2013.

[61] L. Aïssi-Rothe, V. Decot, V. Venard et al., "Rapid generation of full clinical-grade human antiadenovirus cytotoxic t cells for adoptive immunotherapy," *Journal of Immunotherapy*, vol. 33, no. 4, pp. 414–424, 2010.

[62] A. M. Leen, G. D. Myers, U. Sili et al., "Monoculture-derived T lymphocytes specific for multiple viruses expand and produce clinically relevant effects in immunocompromised individuals," *Nature Medicine*, vol. 12, no. 10, pp. 1160–1166, 2006.

[63] Y. Fujita, C. M. Rooney, and H. E. Heslop, "Adoptive cellular immunotherapy for viral diseases," *Bone Marrow Transplantation*, vol. 41, no. 2, pp. 193–198, 2008.

[64] A. M. Leen, A. Christin, G. D. Myers et al., "Cytotoxic T lymphocyte therapy with donor T cells prevents and treats adenovirus and Epstein-Barr virus infections after haploidentical and matched unrelated stem cell transplantation," *Blood*, vol. 114, no. 19, pp. 4283–4292, 2009.

[65] A. M. Leen, C. M. Bollard, A. M. Mendizabal et al., "Multicenter study of banked third-party virus-specific T cells to treat severe viral infections after hematopoietic stem cell transplantation," *Blood*, vol. 121, no. 26, pp. 5113–5123, 2013.

[66] T. Feuchtinger, P. Lang, K. Hamprecht et al., "Isolation and expansion of human adenovirus-specific $CD4^+$ and $CD8^+$ T cells according to IFN-γ secretion for adjuvant immunotherapy," *Experimental Hematology*, vol. 32, no. 3, pp. 282–289, 2004.

[67] T. Feuchtinger, S. Matthes-Martin, C. Richard et al., "Safe adoptive transfer of virus-specific T-cell immunity for the treatment of systemic adenovirus infection after allogeneic stem cell transplantation," *British Journal of Haematology*, vol. 134, no. 1, pp. 64–76, 2006.

[68] U. Gerdemann, U. L. Katari, A. Papadopoulou et al., "Safety and clinical efficacy of rapidly-generated trivirus-directed T cells as treatment for Adenovirus, EBV and CMV infections after allogeneic hematopoietic stem cell transplant," *Molecular Therapy*, 2013.

[69] I. Chatziandreou, K. C. Gilmour, A.-M. McNicol et al., "Capture and generation of adenovirus specific T cells for adoptive immunotherapy," *British Journal of Haematology*, vol. 136, no. 1, pp. 117–126, 2007.

[70] W. Qasim, S. Derniame, K. Gilmour et al., "Third-party virus-specific T cells eradicate adenoviraemia but trigger bystander graft-versus-host disease," *British Journal of Haematology*, vol. 154, no. 1, pp. 150–153, 2011.

[71] P. Comoli, M. W. Schilham, S. Basso et al., "T-cell lines specific for peptides of adenovirus hexon protein and devoid of alloreactivity against recipient cells can be obtained from HLA-haploidentical donors," *Journal of Immunotherapy*, vol. 31, no. 6, pp. 529–536, 2008.

[72] U. Gerdemann, J. F. Vera, C. M. Rooney, and A. M. Leen, "Generation of multivirus-specific T cells to prevent/treat viral infections after allogeneic hematopoietic stem cell transplant," *Journal of Visualized Experiments*, no. 51, 2011.

[73] U. Gerdemann, J. M. Keirnan, U. L. Katari et al., "Rapidly generated multivirus-specific cytotoxic T lymphocytes for the

prophylaxis and treatment of viral infections," *Molecular Therapy*, vol. 20, no. 8, pp. 1622–1632, 2012.

[74] N. Khanna, C. Stuehler, B. Conrad et al., "Generation of a multipathogen-specific T-cell product for adoptive immunotherapy based on activation-dependent expression of CD154," *Blood*, vol. 118, no. 4, pp. 1121–1131, 2011.

[75] J. Leibold, J. Feucht, A. Halder et al., "Induction of Thelper1-driven antiviral T-cell lines for adoptive immunotherapy is determined by differential expression of IFN-gamma and T-cell activation markers," *Journal of Immunotherapy*, vol. 35, no. 9, pp. 661–669, 2012.

[76] L. M. Haveman, M. Bierings, M. R. Klein et al., "Selection of perforin expressing CD4$^+$ adenovirus-specific T-cells with artificial antigen presenting cells," *Clinical Immunology*, vol. 146, no. 3, pp. 228–239, 2013.

17

Aromatic Amines Exert Contrasting Effects on the Anticoagulant Effect of Acetaldehyde upon APTT

La'Teese Hall, Sarah J. Murrey, and Arthur S. Brecher

Department of Chemistry, Bowling Green State University, Bowling Green, OH 43403, USA

Correspondence should be addressed to Arthur S. Brecher; artbrec@bgsu.edu

Academic Editor: Bashir A. Lwaleed

The pharmacological effects of amphetamine, procaine, procainamide, DOPA, isoproterenol, and atenolol upon activated partial thromboplastin time in the absence and presence of acetaldehyde have been investigated. In the absence of acetaldehyde, amphetamine and isoproterenol exhibit a procoagulant effect upon activated partial thromboplastin time, whereas atenolol and procaine display anticoagulant effects upon activated partial thromboplastin time. DOPA and procainamide do not alter activated partial thromboplastin time. Premixtures of procaine with acetaldehyde produce an additive anticoagulant effect on activated partial thromboplastin time, suggesting independent action of these compounds upon clotting factors. Premixtures of amphetamine with acetaldehyde, as well as atenolol with acetaldehyde, generate a detoxication of the anticoagulant effect of acetaldehyde upon activated partial thromboplastin time. A similar statistically significant decrease in activated partial thromboplastin time is seen when procainamide is premixed with acetaldehyde for 20 minutes at room temperature. Premixtures of DOPA and isoproterenol with acetaldehyde do not affect an alteration in activated partial thromboplastin time relative to acetaldehyde alone. Hence, a selective interaction of atenolol, procaine, and amphetamine with acetaldehyde to produce detoxication of the acetaldehyde is suggested, undoubtedly due to the presence of amino, hydroxyl, or amide groups in these drugs.

1. Introduction

The physiological and pharmacological effects of alcohol upon brain and CNS function have been the subject of many studies. Ethanol is readily metabolized in the body to CO_2 and H_2O by well-established enzymatic pathways (reviewed in [1]). Acetaldehyde (AcH), the primary metabolite in ethanol metabolism, is a highly reactive molecule which reacts readily with nucleophiles [2–4]. Among these compounds are amines, amides, imidazoles, thiols, and hydroxyls which are found in proteins, nucleic acids, select carbohydrates, and lipids. In an earlier communication, it was reported that highly reactive biogenic amine hormones, such as dopamine, epinephrine, serotonin, norepinephrine, and histamine, each of which contain primary or secondary amines, or hydroxyl groups, appear to readily react with AcH at room temperature (RT) and to "detoxify" the AcH, as evidenced by their capacity to reduce the anticoagulant effect of AcH on activated partial thromboplastin time (APTT) upon preincubation of the amines with AcH at room

temperature (RT) [5]. It was further suggested that covalent interaction of the AcH with the biogenic amines would also "neutralize" their hormonal influences. As a consequence of these earlier investigations a new study of the effect of drugs with neurological impacts upon AcH, as followed by APTT, was initiated. In the study presented herein, the effects of amphetamine, procaine, procainamide, atenolol, and isoproterenol upon AcH are explored and compared with that of DOPA, the biological precursor to catecholamines and melanin. The ability of AcH-exposed drugs to prolong coagulation times, as a measure of pharmacological function, was investigated.

2. Materials and Methods

Procainamide, lot #54F-0048, procaine-HCl, lot #125K0697, isoproterenol, D-amphetamine, L-DOPA, lot #077K1844, and 5-atenolol, lot #044K3485, were purchased from Sigma-Aldrich Corporation, St. Louis, MD. APTT reagent, lot #2006-02-02/527313A, 0.025 $\underline{M}$ CaCl$_2$, lot #05-17-2004/5006872, Ci-Trol coagulation control, Level I, lots #2009-02-05/508114, 2006-01-19/538162/245, and 2010-06-07/548137/255, were obtained from Dade Behring, Marburg. Assess TM Level I plasma lot #N1106614 was obtained from Instrumentation Laboratory Company, Lexington, MA. Brockman I aluminum oxide, lot #0791DY, was purchased from Aldrich Chemical Company, Milwaukee, WI. Acetaldehyde (AcH), 99%, batch #00339MB, was secured from Sigma-Aldrich and passed through short columns of aluminum oxide in order to remove oxidation products. It was subsequently stored under N$_2$ at −20°C until further use.

APTT assays were carried out as originally described elsewhere [6]. A fibrosystem fibrometer precision coagulation timer, model 5, Becton, Dickinson and Company, Cockeysville, MD, was employed to assay the APTTs.

3. Methods

3.1. Effect of Amphetamine Concentration on APTT. To 90 μL of reconstituted plasma was added 10 μL of ISB or 10 μL of $10^{-1}, 10^{-2}$, or 10^{-3} $\underline{M}$ amphetamine. The solutions were mixed in fibrometer cups and stored for 20 min at RT. Subsequently, 100 μL of APTT reagent at 37°C was added thereto and the mixtures were incubated at 37°C for an additional five min, after which time 100 μL of 0.025 $\underline{M}$ CaCl$_2$ at 37°C was delivered in order to initiate the clotting reaction.

3.2. Effect of Amphetamine and AcH upon APTT. To 90 μL of reconstituted plasma was added 20 μL of ISB to serve as a control. To a second 90 μL aliquot of plasma were added 10 μL of ISB and 10 μL of 0.1 $\underline{M}$ amphetamine to give a final concentration of 4.5×10^{-2} $\underline{M}$ amphetamine in plasma. To a third aliquot of plasma were added 10 μL of 447 m$\underline{M}$ AcH and 10 μL ISB, to give an AcH concentration of 20.3 m$\underline{M}$ in plasma. Lastly, to a fourth aliquot of 90 μL of plasma was added 20 μL of a mixture of equal volumes of amphetamine and 447 m$\underline{M}$ AcH (which was stored for five min at RT). Each sample was mixed and stored for 20 min at RT, after which time 100 μL of APTT reagent at 37°C was added thereto. The mixture was subsequently stored at 37°C for five min prior to initiation of clotting upon addition of 100 μL of 0.025 m$\underline{M}$ CaCl$_2$ at 37°C.

3.3. Effect of Isoproterenol Concentration on APTT. To fibrometer cups containing 90 μL of reconstituted Level I human plasma were added 10 μL of ISB and 10 μL of 10^{-1} $\underline{M}$, 10^{-2} $\underline{M}$, or 10^{-3} $\underline{M}$ isoproterenol in ISB. The solutions were mixed, stoppered, and stored for 20 min at RT. Subsequently, 100 μL APTT reagent was added thereto at 37°C and the mixture was further stored at 37°C for five min. Lastly, 0.025 $\underline{M}$ CaCl$_2$ (100 μL) at 37°C was added to initiate clotting.

3.4. Effect of Isoproterenol and AcH upon APTT. To 90 μL aliquots of plasma in fibrometer cups was added 20 μL ISB or three alternative mixtures: (1) 10 μL ISB + 10 μL 10^{-1} $\underline{M}$ isoproterenol; (2) 10 μL ISB + 10 μL 223.5 m$\underline{M}$ AcH; and (3) 20 μL of a 1 : 1 mixture of 10^{-1} $\underline{M}$ isoproterenol and 223.5 m$\underline{M}$ AcH. The solutions were mixed, stoppered, and stored at RT for 20 min, after which time 100 μL of APTT reagent at 37°C was added thereto. After further storage at 37°C for five min, 100 μL of 0.025 $\underline{M}$ CaCl$_2$ at 37°C was added in order to initiate clotting.

3.5. Effect of Atenolol and AcH upon APTT. To six 90 μL aliquots of Level I plasma in fibrometer cups was added either 20 μL ISB (1° control); 10 μL ISB and 10 μL of 0.075 $\underline{M}$ atenolol (in 30% ethanol); 10 μL ISB and 10 μL of 223 m$\underline{M}$ AcH; 10 μL of 0.075 $\underline{M}$ atenolol, followed five minutes later by 10 μL of 223 m$\underline{M}$ AcH; 10 μL of 223 m$\underline{M}$ AcH, followed five minutes later by 10 μL of 0.075 $\underline{M}$ atenolol; or 20 μL of a 1 : 1 mixture of atenolol: AcH which had been stored at RT for five min. Upon standing at RT for five min, 100 μL of APTT reagent was added thereto and the mixture was incubated at 37°C for an additional five min. Subsequently, clotting was initiated by addition of 100 μL of 0.025 $\underline{M}$ CaCl$_2$ at 37°C. In separate experiments, the effect of atenolol-treated plasma was compared to control plasma containing approximately 1% ethanol.

3.6. Effect of Procainamide, Procaine, DOPA, and AcH upon APTT. To six fibrometer cups were added 90 μL of plasma and each of the following: (1) 20 μL ISB; (2) 10 μL ISB and 10 μL of 0.05 $\underline{M}$ procainamide (to a final concentration of 4.5 m$\underline{M}$ in plasma); (3) 10 μL ISB and 10 μL of 223.5 $\underline{M}$ AcH (to a final concentration of 20.3 m$\underline{M}$ in plasma); (4) ten μL of procainamide, followed ten minutes later by 10 μL of AcH; (5) ten μL of AcH, followed ten minutes later by 10 μL of procainamide; (6) 20 μL aliquot of a 1 : 1 mixture of procainamide and AcH which had been previously stored and stoppered at RT for ten min. After standing at RT for ten min, 100 μL of APTT reagent at 37°C was added thereto, and the cups were incubated at 37°C for five min. Subsequently, clotting was initiated upon addition of 100 μL of 0.025 $\underline{M}$ CaCl$_2$. Four additional fibrometer cups contained a control stored at RT for 20 min, as well as plasma-procainamide, plasma-AcH, and plasma/procainamide-AcH premixtures stored for 20 min at RT. In an analogous manner, the effects of procaine and DOPA upon AcH were studied utilizing 9.1 m$\underline{M}$ procaine in plasma and 0.9 m$\underline{M}$ DOPA in plasma (due to solubility limitations).

3.7. Statistical Analyses. The data were analyzed by application of student's t-test. P values ≤ 0.05 were assumed to be statistically significant. In all groups of experiments, n = 4, 5, 6, 7, or 10, as indicated above in Methods section.

4. Results

The neurohormone, DOPA, and the neurotropic drugs, isoproterenol, atenolol, amphetamine, procaine, and procainamide each contain the benzene ring and various structural modifications. Each one presents a diverse picture relating to its effect upon APTT and its influence on the anticoagulant effect of AcH as a consequence of the presence/absence of functional groups which may interact with AcH. In essence, it was observed that amphetamine and isoproterenol exhibit a procoagulant effect upon APTT whereas atenolol and procaine display an anticoagulant effect upon APTT. Procainamide and DOPA have no statistical effect upon APTT under the conditions employed. AcH prolongs the APTT. Premixtures of amphetamine, atenolol, procaine, and procainamide with AcH exhibit a "detoxication" of the anticoagulant effect of AcH, that is, reduction in the anticoagulant activity of AcH. Successive additions of atenolol and AcH to plasma produce an additive anticoagulant effect, as does procaine. Successive additions of procainamide and AcH to plasma do not exhibit an additive anticoagulant effect with a 10-min exposure to plasma.

4.1. Effect of Atenolol and Acetaldehyde upon APTT.

Atenolol additions to plasma to concentrations of 10^{-2} $\underline{M}$ and 5×10^{-3} $\underline{M}$ produced APTTs of 53.6 ± 0.8 sec ($n = 4$; $P = 0$) and 41.3 ± 0.1 sec ($n = 4$; $P = 0$) relative to their respective controls of 39.7 ± 0.6 and 37.8 ± 0.3 sec ($n = 4$) (Figure 1). At concentrations of 1×10^{-3} $\underline{M}$ and 1×10^{-4} $\underline{M}$, a slight procoagulant effect was observed with $P = 0.07$, approaching significance for the former concentration and a statistically significant $P = 0.01$ for the latter concentration. In studies involving both atenolol and acetaldehyde, it was noted that 7.5×10^{-3} $\underline{M}$ atenolol in plasma and 20.3 m $\underline{M}$ acetaldehyde in plasma each prolonged APTT, with values of 42.6 ± 0.7 ($P = 0.002$) and 42.8 ± 0.9 sec ($P = 0.002$), respectively, relative to a control of 34.0 ± 0.4 sec ($n = 4$) (Figure 2). Preincubation time of plasma with the drug was 5 min at RT. Hence, atenolol and acetaldehyde each exhibited anticoagulant effects. When atenolol was added initially to plasma for five min at RT and acetaldehyde was subsequently added for an additional five min prior to concluding the APTT, a value of 54.5 ± 0.8 sec ($P = 0$) was obtained. The atenolol and AcH effects on plasma were additive. When the order of addition of the reagents to plasma was reversed, an APTT of 59.0 ± 1.8 sec ($P = 0$) was noted. However, when atenolol and acetaldehyde were mixed and preincubated at RT for five min prior to addition to plasma for an additional five min at RT before concluding the APTT, an APTT of 45.9 ± 2.4 sec ($P = 0$) was observed. The drop in APTT from 54.5″ to 45.9″ suggested that atenolol partially inactivated the effect of acetaldehyde by exerting a detoxifying effect. The increase in APTT by the addition of acetaldehyde to plasma prior to addition of atenolol reflected the effect of increased exposure time of plasma to acetaldehyde.

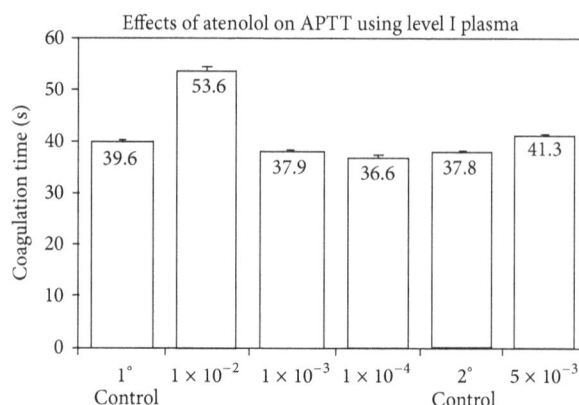

FIGURE 1: Effects of atenolol upon APTT using Level I plasma ($n = 4$; $P = 0$ for 1×10^{-2} $\underline{M}$ and 5×10^{-3} $\underline{M}$ atenolol) ($n = 4$; $P = 0.07$ for 1×10^{-3} $\underline{M}$ atenolol and $P = 0.01$ for 1×10^{-4} $\underline{M}$ atenolol).

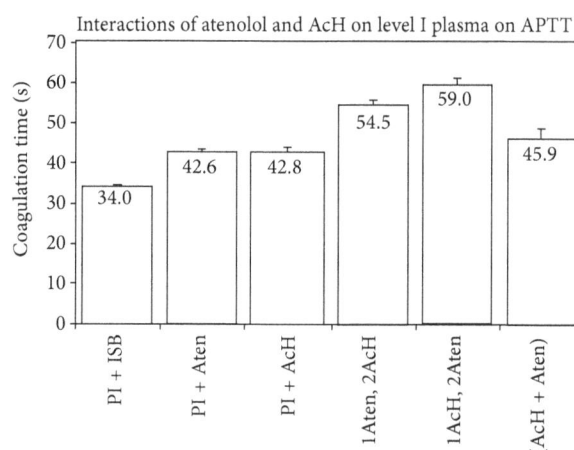

FIGURE 2: Interactions of atenolol and AcH on Level I plasma on APTT ($n = 4$; $P = 0.002$ for atenolol and for AcH; $P = 0$ for 1 Aten/2 AcH and for 1 AcH/2 Aten; $P = 0.02$ for the AcH and Aten premixture).

4.2. Effect of Amphetamine and Acetaldehyde.

Figure 3 indicates that 0.01 $\underline{M}$ D-amphetamine exerted a statistically significant procoagulant effect upon APTT upon preincubation with plasma for 20 min at RT, with an APTT of 24.3 ± 0.8 sec ($P \leq 0.02$) relative to a control of 28.4 ± 1.1 sec ($n = 5$). At 10^{-3} and 10^{-4} $\underline{M}$ levels of amphetamine, there was no significant difference between control and experimental values. In an examination of the interactive effect of amphetamine and acetaldehyde upon the APTT reaction, it was observed that 0.01 $\underline{M}$ amphetamine, upon exposure to plasma for 20 min at RT, exhibited an APTT of 26.4 ± 0.8 sec relative to a control plasma of 29.5 ± 0.9 sec, whereas 40.6 m$\underline{M}$ acetaldehyde under the same conditions affected an APTT of 48.5 ± 2.2 sec (Figure 4). A premixture of acetaldehyde and amphetamine, standing at RT for 20 min prior to incubation with plasma for 20 min, resulted in an APTT of 35.4 ± 1.6 sec ($n = 10$, $P \leq 0.01$) corresponding to a decrease of 13.1 sec in clotting time and a detoxication of the acetaldehyde by amphetamine.

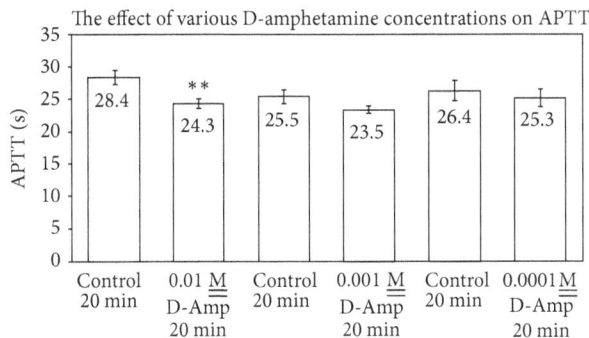

FIGURE 3: Effect of various D-amphetamine concentrations on APTT ($n = 5$; $P \leq 0.02$ for 0.01 $\underline{M}$ D-Amp) ($n = 10$; $P \leq 0.01$ for the 20 min D-Amp-AcH mixture). ∗∗ indicate that $P \leq 0.05$ relative to the control APTTs.

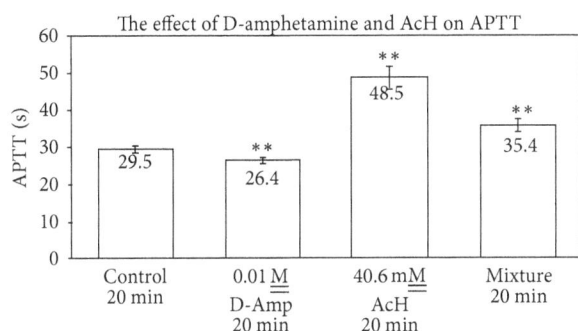

FIGURE 4: The effect of D-amphetamine and AcH on APTT ($n = 10$; $P \leq 0.01$ for the D-Amp-AcH mixture).

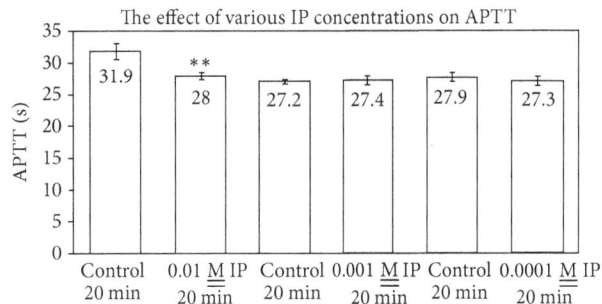

FIGURE 5: Effect of various isoproterenol concentrations upon APTT ($n = 4$; $P = 0.03$ for 0.01 $\underline{M}$ IP).

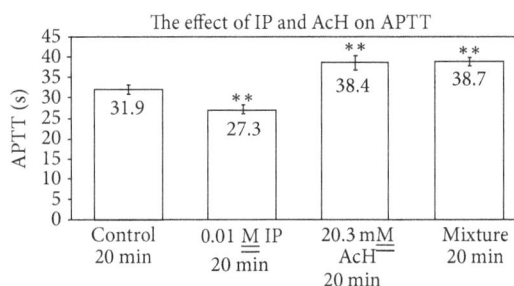

FIGURE 6: Effect of isoproterenol and acetaldehyde on APTT ($n = 6$; $P = 0.01$).

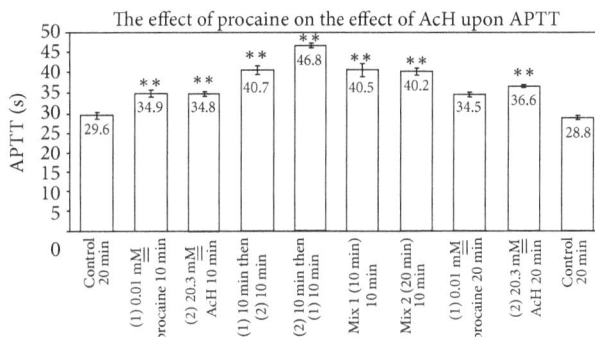

FIGURE 7: Effect of procaine and acetaldehyde upon APTT ($n = 6$; $P = 0.001$).

4.3. Effect of Isoproterenol and Acetaldehyde upon APTT.

As indicated in Figure 5, 1×10^{-2} $\underline{M}$ isoproterenol exerts a small but statistically significant procoagulant effect upon APTT since its clotting time is 28.0 ± 0.6 sec relative to the control of 31.9 ± 1.3 sec ($n = 4$, $P = 0.03$). At concentrations of isoproterenol at 10^{-3} and 10^{-4} $\underline{M}$, no statistical difference is seen as compared to controls. The data in Figure 6 show that a premixture of isoproterenol and acetaldehyde exhibits essentially identical APTTs as acetaldehyde alone, with values of 38.7 ± 1.1 sec and 38.4 ± 1.8 sec, relative to the control of 31.9 ± 1.1 sec. In this series ($n = 6$, $P = 0.01$), the isoproterenol exhibited a procoagulant effect of 27.3 ± 1.1 sec. Hence, isoproterenol did not apparently react with acetaldehyde or affect its toxicity on APTT.

4.4. Effect of Procaine and Acetaldehyde upon APTT.

Figure 7 shows that 0.01 $\underline{M}$ procaine and 20.3 m$\underline{M}$ acetaldehyde each prolong APTT, relative to control APTT of 29.6 ± 0.8 sec, with APTTs of 34.9 ± 0.9 and 34.8 ± 0.5 sec, respectively ($P = 0.001$, resp.), when preincubation times of procaine or acetaldehyde are for 10 min at RT, indicating anticoagulant effects ($n = 6$). When procaine and acetaldehyde at the same concentrations are preincubated with plasma for 20 min at RT, the respective APTTs are 34.5 ± 0.6 sec and 36.6 ± 0.3 sec, relative to a control of 28.8 ± 0.5 sec ($P = 0.0001$, resp.).

The increase in the anticoagulant effect of acetaldehyde with longer preincubation times with plasma has been previously reported [6]. Premixtures of procaine with acetaldehyde, upon storage for 10 or 20 min at RT before addition to plasma for an additional 10 min at RT before assay for APTT, resulted in APTTs of 40.5 ± 1.6 sec and 40.2 ± 0.9 sec, respectively ($P = 0.0001$, resp.). These essentially reflect an additive effect of each drug upon the components of the coagulation cascade. When procaine is added to plasma first for a ten-minute preincubation, followed by acetaldehyde second for an additional ten minutes, an APTT of 40.7 ± 1.0 sec is noted. When the order of addition to plasma is reversed, an APTT of 46.8 ± 0.6 sec is obtained, reflecting an increase in clotting

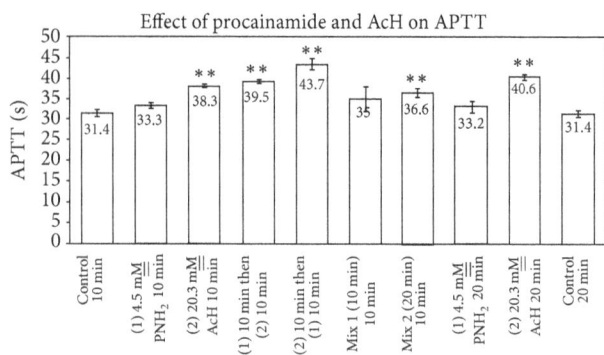

FIGURE 8: Effect of procainamide and acetaldehyde upon APTT (n = 6; P = 0.0001 for AcH; for 1 procainamide, 2 AcH; and for 1 AcH, 2 procainamide; P = 0.0035 for the 20 min premix of procainamide with AcH and is n.s. (0.3) for the 10 min premix).

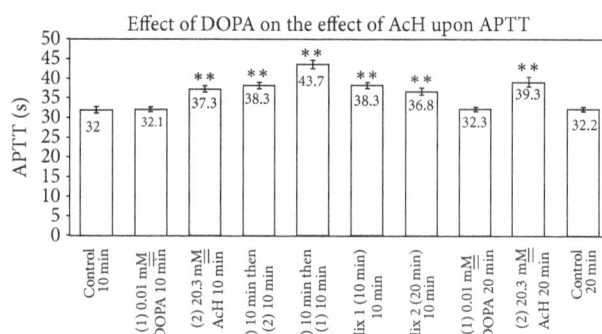

FIGURE 9: Effect of DOPA and acetaldehyde upon APTT (n = 7; $P \leq 0.05$ relative to the controls).

time as a consequence of prolonged exposure of plasma to acetaldehyde.

4.5. Effect of Procainamide and Acetaldehyde upon APTT.

Procainamide, 4.5 mM, and acetaldehyde, 20.3 mM, each prolonged APTT, relative to the control of 31.4 ± 0.9 sec, with APTTs of 33.3 ± 0.6 sec and 38.3 ± 0.4 sec, respectively, when preincubated with plasma at RT for ten min (n = 6, P = 0.0001 for acetaldehyde). Whereas the acetaldehyde-containing plasma gave a statistically significant difference from the control, the procainamide value was not statistically different (P = 0.1) (Figure 8). When incubations of procainamide and acetaldehyde with plasma were extended to 20 min at RT, APTTs of 33.2 ± 1.4 sec and 40.6 ± 0.7 sec, respectively, relative to a control of 31.4 ± 0.8 sec were obtained. Acetaldehyde, again, affected a greater prolongation of clotting time in 20 min as compared to 10 min. The procainamide-containing plasma did not statistically significantly alter APTT in 20 min as compared to its control plasma. Whereas 20.5 mM acetaldehyde added to plasma produced APTTs of 38.3 ± 0.4 and 40.6 ± 0.7 sec (P = 0.0001 in both cases) in 10 and 20 min, respectively, 10- and 20-min premixtures of procainamide with acetaldehyde generated APTTs of 35 ± 3.2 and 36.6 ± 1.1 sec, respectively. The latter (20 min) values exhibited statistical differences between acetaldehyde alone and the acetaldehyde-procainamide premixture suggesting a detoxication of acetaldehyde by procainamide as a consequence of interaction. When procainamide was preincubated with plasma for ten min at RT after which acetaldehyde was subsequently added thereto, an APTT of 39.5 ± 0.4 sec was seen. When the order of addition of the compounds was reversed, an APTT of 43.7 ± 1.4 sec was noted. The increase in APTT was a reflection of the increased time of exposure of plasma to acetaldehyde.

4.6. Effect of DOPA and Acetaldehyde on APTT.

Figure 9 shows that 0.01 M DOPA does not significantly affect APTT after preincubation for 10 or 20 min (n = 7) (P = 0.92, n.s.). Whereas 20.3 mM acetaldehyde significantly prolongs

APTT upon preincubation with plasma for 10 min (P = 0.0001) as well as 20 min (P = 0.0002), premixtures of acetaldehyde with DOPA for 10 min or 20 min do not differ statistically from acetaldehyde alone in their APTT values. Preincubation of acetaldehyde alone with plasma gives a higher APTT after 20 min contact as compared to 10 min contact (39.3 sec relative to 37.3 sec), confirming all previous time course studies. Similarly, order of addition of reagents affected APTT since addition, first, of acetaldehyde to plasma with a 10-min contact time, followed by addition of DOPA thereto, gave an elevated APTT relative to the reverse order of addition (43.7 sec. relative to 37.3 sec) once again suggesting that longer contact times for interaction of acetaldehyde with plasma give greater prolongation of clotting times. Interestingly, however, it was observed that a 20-min premixture presented an APTT of 36.8 ± 1.0 sec whereas the APTT obtained when acetaldehyde was preincubated with plasma for 10 min prior to a second 10 min preincubation with added DOPA was 43.7 ± 1.0 sec, inferring that an interaction between acetaldehyde and DOPA has occurred in the 20-min preincubation time.

5. Discussion

The comparisons and contrasts between the structures as well as physiological and pharmacological effects of aromatic drugs such as amphetamine, isoproterenol, atenolol, procaine, and procainamide relative to the naturally occurring DOPA are marked. Furthermore, their response to interaction with AcH, the primary metabolite in alcohol metabolism, adds to the fascinating diversity in physiological and pharmacological responses. The comparison of these compounds with results obtained in earlier studies on such biogenic amine hormones as dopamine, epinephrine, norepinephrine, serotonin, and histamine also bears notice [5].

In contrast to the biogenic amines listed above (DA, E, NE, 5-HT, and H), all of the compounds in the current study, with the exception of the naturally occurring DOPA, namely, amphetamine, isoproterenol, atenolol, procaine, and procainamide, are drugs. Each is aromatic and each bears a broad resemblance to E, NE, and DA in that they contain the benzene ring. DOPA, procainamide, procaine, and amphetamine contain the primary amine group. Procaine, procainamide, and isoproterenol contain 2° N's, whereas atenolol, isoproterenol, and DOPA also contain hydroxyl groups (which should be capable of reacting with aldehydic functional groups). Procainamide, lastly, also contains a 1° amide group. Hence, many groups are susceptible to reactivity with AcH. Whereas each drug contains nucleophiles and rings, they differ amongst themselves in their ability to affect the APTT reaction. Accordingly, amphetamine and isoproterenol exhibit a procoagulant effect upon addition to plasma, whereas atenolol and procaine have an anticoagulant effect upon APTT. Procainamide and naturally occurring DOPA do not affect the APTT under the conditions employed. It should be noted that DA, the metabolic product of DOPA by decarboxylation, has a modest procoagulant effect upon APTT, as do EP and 5-H [5]. NE and histamine, however, do not statistically affect APTT [5].

Notwithstanding the similarities and diversities of the drugs studied herein with regard to nucleophilic properties and aromaticity, the difference in pharmacological effect upon APTT, relative to interactions of the drugs with AcH, is striking. Amphetamine, which exhibited a small, but statistically significant, procoagulant effect upon APTT, had a profound "detoxifying" effect upon APTT as a consequence of premixing the drug for 20 min at RT with AcH prior to addition to plasma (Figures 3 and 4). Essentially, the major anticoagulant effect of AcH upon APTT was markedly reduced by premixing with amphetamine. Atenolol, which exhibits an anticoagulant effect upon APTT, similarly statistically reduces the anticipated APTT when premixtures thereof with AcH are added to plasma. Individually, Aten and AcH each prolong APTT (Figure 2). Premixtures thereof are far less than additive in their APTT effect suggesting an interaction of the two, leading to a partial detoxication. When Aten is added to plasma prior to AcH, an APTT is recorded which is less than that when AcH is added first and Aten second. This is in agreement with earlier published results from this laboratory signifying that AcH affects a time-dependent increasing anticoagulant effect upon clotting time (PT). Although AcH reacts instantaneously with nucleophiles [2, 3], some reactions are reversible while others are irreversible [7, 8]. Presumably, this would explain increases and some slight ultimate decreases in coagulation times over extended periods of time, as tertiary structures of some proteins/enzymes are altered. Of further note is the fact that successive addition of Aten and AcH to plasma lends an additive effect upon APTT, suggesting that each of these components reacts at different sites on proteins, resulting in anticoagulant effects, when they do not react with one another. Whereas procainamide alone has no significant anticoagulant effect on APTT, successive additions of procainamide and AcH to plasma for 10 min at RT result in an anticoagulant effect corresponding to that of AcH alone and statistically significant (Figure 8). Upon premixing procainamide and AcH for 10 min prior to addition to plasma, there is no statistically significant reduction in the anticoagulant activity. However, when the premixture stands at RT for 20 min, a statistical drop in anticoagulant activity is observed, that is, a partial detoxication of the anticoagulant activity. This suggests that a slow reaction between AcH

and procainamide, perhaps of a reversible nature, may be occurring. Of course, a reversible dissociation of AcH from the protein, with time, may also be occurring.

Procaine differs from procainamide in that the former exhibits an anticoagulant effect upon APTT, while successive additions of procaine and AcH to plasma produce an additive effect upon APTT, reflecting independent action of each compound upon protein components of the coagulation scheme (Figure 7). Interestingly, premixtures of procaine and AcH for 10 min, as well as 20 min, are reflected by an additive effect upon the APTT. This may be a reflection of the difference in reactivity of procaine, with an ester link, and procainamide, with an amide (2° amine) link.

Isoproterenol and DOPA, with their procoagulant and nonstatistical effects upon APTT, appear also to exert no statistical effect upon APTT when premixed with AcH (Figures 6 and 9). In the case of isoproterenol, AcH alone and AcH-IP mixtures show identical APTTs (Figure 6). In the DOPA experiments, successive additions behave as though DOPA was ineffective in influencing APTT in the presence of AcH. Similarly, 10-min and 20-min mixtures of AcH with DOPA behaved as if DOPA were absent (Figure 9). These data differ markedly from those with dopamine, which has a slight procoagulant effect and which decreases the anticoagulant effect of AcH when added successively to plasma as a premix with AcH [5]. The aromatic amines, epi, norepi, 5-HT, and histamine, each lower the anticoagulant effect of AcH upon plasma when preincubated with AcH at RT [5].

Clinically, the drugs exhibit powerful effects. Amphetamines, as well as methamphetamine (MDMA) and cocaine, are linked with increased blood pressure, cardiac arrhythmias, stroke, TIAs, infarctions, and hemorrhages [9, 10]. Amphetamines promote neurotransmission by blocking presynaptic uptake of catecholamines, thereby elevating their presence at the synapses, with the consequential saturation of postsynaptic receptors [10]. MDMA inhibits mitochondrial ALDH2 and cytosolic ALDH1 [11]. Long term serotonergic neurotoxicity of MDMA in rats is extended by ethanol as a result of the increased presence of acetaldehyde which inhibits ALDH1 and ALDH2 [12].

Isoproterenol, which is a β_1-β_2 adrenergic agonist, causes cardiac hypertrophy and myocardial infarction in mice and rats [13–20]. Galindo et al. [13] observed the modification of 865 genes by isoproterenol. Notably, however, caffeic acid lowers the extent of membrane damage by isoproterenol in male albino Wistar rats. Sesamol, neferine, and vitamin A protect rodents from damages by isoproterenol. Rats on an ethanol diet exhibit higher survival rates as a consequence of isoproterenol-induced MI. The alcoholic rats exhibited higher levels of ADH and ALDH [20].

The β-adrenergic blocker, atenolol, has antihypertensive, antianginal, and antiarrhythmic properties [21–27]. The antiarrhythmic effect is seen on administration of atenolol to rats with epinephrine-induced arrhythmia [26]. The combined application of ethanol and atenolol generates a reduced arrhythmic response in comparison to individual administration. Atenolol has been applicable for the treatment of ethanol-withdrawal syndrome [28, 29]. It also lowers the rate of reinfarction after an initial MI [23] thereby lowering mortality rates.

DOPA and dopamine are integrally related since DOPA is a metabolic product of tyrosine and dopamine is a sequential metabolic product of DOPA. Both are catecholamines and are precursors to norepinephrine and epinephrine. Together with 5-HT, they comprise biogenic amine hormones which decrease the anticoagulant effect of AcH upon APTT [5]. The most likely scenario involved is the formation of Schiff bases as well as hemiacetals and acetals between the AcH and the amines and hydroxyl moieties of these hormones, thereby detoxifying the AcH [5]. Johnson [30] noted in animal studies that lower levels of 5-HT are seen with an increase in alcoholic drinking. This may be reflected in the interaction of AcH with 5-HT to form Schiff bases. Sato et al. [31] have reported that patients treated with antiparkinsonism drugs who were on DOPA and dopamine agonists had elevated PTs. Among the most interesting developments in recent years is the report by Sandler et al. that 1-methyl-6,7-dihydroxy-1,2,3,4-tetrahydroisoquinoline, also known as salsolinol, was seen in the urine of parkinsonism patients under treatment with L-DOPA [32]. Further studies with rats and humans have led to the observation of salsolinol in rat adrenals and in the urine of alcoholics [33]. Salsolinol was reported to be a condensation product of dopamine and AcH [34]. N-Methyl salsolinol, a metabolic product of salsolinol, induced apoptosis in neurons [35] as a neurotoxin [36]. Hence, DOPA and dopamine engage both Parkinson's disease and AcH, although DOPA is not an agent utilizable for alcoholism [37].

Unlike the afore discussed metabolites and drugs, procaine and procainamide have not been explored for their interactions with alcoholism or acetaldehyde to any major extent. However, some effects of paraldehyde have been briefly studied in earlier years [38–40]. Interactions of biogenic amine hormones with AcH, as well as metabolic studies on their catabolic products, remain an ongoing field of interest.

Conflict of Interests

The authors declare that there is no conflict of interests regarding the publication of this paper.

Acknowledgment

The authors express their deep appreciation to Professor Robert Harr, Chairperson of the Medical Technology Program at BGSU, for his generous contribution of plasma and APTT reagents which were used during this investigation.

References

[1] A. S. Brecher, "The effect of acetaldehyde on plasma," in *Comprehensive Handbook of Alcohol Related Pathology*, V. R. Preedy and R. Watson, Eds., pp. 1223–1244, Academic Press, Elsevier Science, London, UK, 2005.

[2] H. Fraenkel-Conrat and H. S. Olcott, "Reaction of formaldehyde with proteins. VI. Crosslinking of amino groups with phenol, imidazole, or indole groups," *The Journal of Biological Chemistry*, vol. 174, pp. 827–843, 1948.

[3] H. Fraenkel-Conrat and H. S. Olcott, "The reaction of formaldehyde with proteins. V. Cross-linking between amino and primary amide or guanidyl groups," *Journal of the American Chemical Society*, vol. 70, no. 8, pp. 2673–2684, 1948.

[4] S. Ratner and H. T. Clarke, "The action of formaldehyde upon cysteine," *Journal of the American Chemical Society*, vol. 59, no. 1, pp. 200–206, 1937.

[5] S. J. Murrey and A. S. Brecher, "Interaction of biogenic amine hormones with acetaldehyde," *Digestive Diseases and Sciences*, vol. 55, no. 1, pp. 21–27, 2010.

[6] A. S. Brecher and M. T. Adamu, "Short- and long-term effects of acetaldehyde on plasma," *Alcohol*, vol. 26, no. 1, pp. 49–53, 2002.

[7] D. J. Tuma, T. Hoffman, and M. F. Sorrell, "The chemistry of acetaldehyde-protein adducts," *Alcohol and Alcoholism*, vol. 1, pp. 271–276, 1991.

[8] M. F. Sorrell, D. J. Tuma, and A. J. Barak, "Evidence that acetaldehyde irreversibly impairs glycoprotein metabolism in liver slices," *Gastroenterology*, vol. 73, no. 5, pp. 1138–1141, 1977.

[9] T. P. Enevoldson, "Recreational drugs and their neurological consequences," *Journal of Neurology, Neurosurgery & Psychiatry*, vol. 75, supplement 111, pp. iii9–iii15, 2004.

[10] K. Esse, M. Fossati-Bellani, A. Traylor, and S. Martin-Schild, "Epidemic of illicit drug use, mechanisms of action/addiction and stroke as a health hazard," *Brain and Behavior*, vol. 1, no. 1, pp. 44–54, 2011.

[11] V. V. Upreti, N. D. Eddington, K.-H. Moon, B.-J. Song, and I. J. Lee, "Drug interaction between ethanol and 3,4-methylenedioxymethamphetamine ("ecstasy")," *Toxicology Letters*, vol. 188, no. 2, pp. 167–172, 2009.

[12] M. Izco, L. Orio, E. O'Shea, and M. I. Colado, "Binge ethanol administration enhances the MDMA-induced long-term 5-HT neurotoxicity in rat brain," *Psychopharmacology*, vol. 189, no. 4, pp. 459–470, 2007.

[13] C. L. Galindo, M. A. Skinner, M. Errami et al., "Transcriptional profile of isoproterenol-induced cardiomyopathy and comparison to exercise-induced cardiac hypertrophy and human cardiac failure," *BMC Physiology*, vol. 9, no. 1, article no. 23, 2009.

[14] L. C. Heather, A. F. Catchpole, D. J. Stuckey, M. A. Cole, C. A. Carr, and K. Clarke, "Isoproterenol induces *in vivo* functional and metabolic abnormalities; similar to those found in the infarcted rat heart," *Journal of Physiology and Pharmacology*, vol. 60, no. 3, pp. 31–39, 2009.

[15] X. Li, R. Zhou, P. Zheng et al., "Cardioprotective effect of matrine on isoproterenol-induced cardiotoxicity in rats," *Journal of Pharmacy and Pharmacology*, vol. 62, no. 4, pp. 514–520, 2010.

[16] K. S. Kumaran and P. S. M. Prince, "Preventive effect of caffeic acid on lysosomal dysfunction in isoproterenol-induced myocardial infarcted rats," *Journal of Biochemical and Molecular Toxicology*, vol. 24, no. 2, pp. 115–122, 2010.

[17] L. Vennila and K. V. Pugalendi, "Efficacy of sesamol on plasma and tissue lipids in isoproterenol-induced cardiotoxicity in Wistar rats," *Archives of Pharmacal Research*, vol. 35, no. 8, pp. 1465–1470, 2012.

[18] G. Lalitha, P. Poornima, A. Archanah, and V. V. Padma, "Protective effect of neferine against isoproterenol-induced cardiac toxicity," *Cardiovascular Toxicology*, vol. 13, no. 2, pp. 168–179, 2013.

[19] H. Pipaliya and J. Vaghasiya, "Cardio protective effect of vitamin A against isoproterenol-induced myocardial infarction," *Journal*

of Nutritional Science and Vitaminology, vol. 58, no. 6, pp. 402–407, 2012.

[20] A. Remla, P. V. G. Menon, P. A. Kurup, and S. Kumari, "Effect of ethanol administration on metabolism of lipids in heart and aorta in isoproterenol induced myocardial infarction in rats," *Indian Journal of Experimental Biology*, vol. 29, no. 3, pp. 244–248, 1991.

[21] L. D. Gottlieb, R. I. Horwitz, M. L. Kraus, S. R. Segal, and C. M. Viscoli, "Randomized controlled trial in alcohol relapse prevention: role of atenolol, alcohol craving, and treatment adherence," *Journal of Substance Abuse Treatment*, vol. 11, no. 3, pp. 253–258, 1994.

[22] M. Klapholz, "β-blocker use for the stages of heart failure," *Mayo Clinic Proceedings*, vol. 84, no. 8, pp. 718–729, 2009.

[23] V. Hinstridge and T. M. Speight, "An overview of therapeutic interventions in myocardial infarction. Emphasis on secondary prevention," *Drugs*, vol. 42, no. 2, pp. 8–20, 1991.

[24] M. E. Pedersen and J. R. Cockcroft, "The vasodilatory beta-blockers," *Current Hypertension Reports*, vol. 9, no. 4, pp. 269–277, 2007.

[25] M. A. A. Saad, A. M. Abbas, V. Boshra, M. Elkhateeb, and I. A. El Aal, "Effect of Angiotensin II Type 1 receptor blocker, Candesartan, and β₁ adrenoceptor blocker, Atenolol, on brain damage in ischemic stroke," *Acta Physiologica Hungarica*, vol. 97, no. 2, pp. 159–171, 2010.

[26] B. Filipek, J. Krupinska, T. Librowski, K. Zebala, I. Piasecka, and W. Peikoszewski, "The effect of ethanol on the antiarrhythmic action of atenolol," *Polish Journal of Pharmacology and Pharmacy*, vol. 41, no. 3, pp. 207–211, 1989.

[27] H. Douard, B. Mora, and J.-P. Broustet, "Comparison of the anti-anginal efficacy of nicardipine and nifedipine in patients receiving atenolol: a randomized, double-blind, crossover study," *International Journal of Cardiology*, vol. 22, no. 3, pp. 357–363, 1989.

[28] L. D. Gottlieb, "The role of beta blockers in alcohol withdrawal syndrome," *Postgraduate Medicine*, no. 169–174, 1988.

[29] R. I. Horwitz, L. D. Gottlieb, and M. L. Kraus, "The efficacy of atenolol in the outpatient management of the alcohol withdrawal syndrome. Results of a randomized clinical trial," *Archives of Internal Medicine*, vol. 149, no. 5, pp. 1089–1093, 1989.

[30] B. A. Johnson, "The role of serotonergic agents as treatments for alcoholism," *Drugs of Today*, vol. 39, no. 9, pp. 665–672, 2003.

[31] Y. Sato, M. Kaji, N. Metoki, H. Yoshida, and K. Satoh, "Coagulation-fibrinolysis abnormalities in patients receiving antiparkinsonian agents," *Journal of the Neurological Sciences*, vol. 212, no. 1-2, pp. 55–58, 2003.

[32] M. Sandler, S. B. Carter, K. R. Hunter, and G. M. Stern, "Tetrahydroisoquinoline alkaloids: in vivo metabolites of L-dopa in man," *Nature*, vol. 241, no. 5390, pp. 439–443, 1973.

[33] M. Hirst, D. R. Evans, C. W. Gowdey, and M. A. Adams, "The influences of ethanol and other factors on the excretion of urinary salsolinol in social drinkers," *Pharmacology Biochemistry and Behavior*, vol. 22, no. 6, pp. 993–1000, 1985.

[34] J. Adachi, Y. Mizoi, T. Fukunaga, M. Kogame, I. Ninomiya, and T. Naito, "Effect of acetaldehyde on urinary salsolinol in healthy man after ethanol intake," *Alcohol*, vol. 3, no. 3, pp. 215–220, 1986.

[35] M. Naoi, W. Maruyama, and G. M. Nagy, "Dopamine-derived salsolinol derivatives as endogenous monoamine oxidase inhibitors: occurrence, metabolism, and function in human brains," *NeuroToxicology*, vol. 25, no. 1-2, pp. 193–204, 2004.

[36] W. Maruyama, G. Sobue, K. Matsubara, Y. Hashizume, P. Dostert, and M. Naoi, "A dopaminergic neurotoxin, 1(R)2(N)-dimethyl-6,7-dihydroxy-1,2,34-tetrahydroisoquinoline, N-methyl (R) salsolinol and its oxidation product, 1,2(N)-dimethyl-6,7-dihydroxyisquinolinium ion, accumulate in the nigro-straiatal system of the human brain," *Neuroscience Letters*, vol. 223, pp. 61–64, 1997.

[37] P. Batel, "The treatment of alcoholism in France," *Drug and Alcohol Dependence*, vol. 39, supplement 1, pp. S15–S21, 1995.

[38] R. C. Elliott and J. P. Quilliam, "Some actions of centrally active and other drugs on the transmission of single nerve impulses through the isolated superior cervical ganglion preparation of the rabbit," *British Journal of Pharmacology and Chemotherapy*, vol. 23, pp. 222–240, 1964.

[39] D. A. Brown and J. P. Quilliam, "The effects of some centrally acting drugs on ganglionic transmission in the cat," *The British Journal of Pharmacology and Chemotherapy*, vol. 23, pp. 241–256, 1964.

[40] D. A. Brown and J. P. Quillian, "Observations on the mode of action of some central depressant drugs on transmission through the cat superior cervical ganglion," *British Journal of Pharmacology*, vol. 23, pp. 257–272, 1964.

18

Thrombin-Accelerated Quick Clotting Serum Tubes: An Evaluation with 22 Common Biochemical Analytes

Wai-Yoong Ng and Chin-Pin Yeo

Department of Pathology, Clinical Biochemistry Laboratories, Singapore General Hospital, Outram Road, Singapore 169608

Correspondence should be addressed to Wai-Yoong Ng; ng.wai.yoong@sgh.com.sg

Academic Editor: Frits R. Rosendaal

Clot activator serum tubes have significantly improved turnaround times for result reporting compared to plain tubes. With increasing workload and service performance expectations confronting clinical laboratories with high-volume testing and with particular emphasis on critical analytes, attention has focussed on preanalytical variables that can be improved. We carried out a field study on the test performance of BD vacutainer rapid serum tubes (RSTs) compared to current institutional issued BD vacutainer serum separator tubes (SSTs) in its test result comparability, clotting time, and stability on serum storage. Data from the study population ($n = 160$) of patients attending outpatient clinics and healthy subjects showed that results for renal, liver, lipids, cardiac, thyroid, and prostate biochemical markers were comparable between RSTs and SSTs. Clotting times of the RSTs were verified to be quick with a median time of 2.05 min. Analyte stability on serum storage at $4°C$ showed no statistically significant deterioration except for bicarbonate, electrolytes, and albumin over a period of 4 days. In conclusion, RSTs offered savings in the time required for the clotting process of serum specimens. This should translate to further trimming of the whole process from blood collection to result reporting without too much sacrifice on test accuracy and performance compared to the current widely used SSTs in most clinical laboratories.

1. Introduction

The performance of laboratory services is often expected to demonstrate delivery of accurate test results in the shortest possible time. To meet service targets, turnaround times are constantly under scrutiny for further improvement. What is perhaps less understood are the various influences that determine the prompt delivery of results from the journey of the blood specimen which begins at the blood collection point and continues to testing and result reporting. Studies have indicated that much of the delay is due to factors at the preanalytical phase including specimen delivery efficiencies [1, 2]. A key factor is the clotting time of blood collected for serum testing, and current blood collection tubes (with clot activator and gel separation) require a recommended 30-min standing time for clotting. Hence, at times, specimens reaching the laboratory through a fast delivery service (example, for STAT specimens) may not have clotted completely to allow immediate testing.

To mitigate the clotting time issue, some laboratories are using plasma specimens for STAT testing. However, it is known that plasma is not exactly an adequate substitute for serum [3, 4]. Plasma has its own set of areas for concern, for example, problem of adequate mixing of blood with anticoagulants, difference in result values for some analytes when measured in serum or plasma, especially potassium and lactate dehydrogenase, thus requiring changes in reference intervals [5]. With its inherent known limitations particularly in the more recent reports of issues with cardiac markers, plasma may not be the specimen of choice [6–9].

The Becton Dickinson BD vacutainer rapid serum tube (RST BD 368774) has a 5-min clotting time which is advantageous for any immediate processing in the high-volume clinical laboratory. Commercially available in 2010 with supporting data on its use on various popular instrument platforms, more recent studies have shown that RSTs can replace plasma gel tubes [10]. The RSTs were shown to produce equivalent Troponin-T results compared to SSTs

[11, 12] and give less false-positive Troponin-I and Troponin-T results compared to plasma gel tubes [13, 14]. Manufacturer's white papers have supporting data that RSTs showed same results as current serum tubes or plasma tubes except for some analytes, for example, total protein, hence, a suitable alternative to the use of plasma gel tubes in the STAT environment.

As RSTs were recently introduced in our region, we carried out a field study on its quick clotting performance and tests accuracies of routine chemistries often requested by the emergency department and outpatient clinics. The RSTs were compared with the current SSTs (serum separation tube BD 367986) on test results for general biochemical indices such as renal, liver, lipids, cardiac markers, and thyroid function. A subset of archived samples (at 4°C) was further evaluated for analyte stability by retesting for the same analytes each day for up to 5 days.

2. Methods and Materials

Blood specimens were collected from adult healthy subjects ($n = 85$) and patients ($n = 75$) for routine chemistries—renal panel, liver panel, lipid panel, cardiac markers, thyroid hormones, and prostate specific antigen. Patients were randomly selected at the outpatient clinics for participation. Both blood specimens in RSTs and current institutional issued SSTs were obtained from the participants in no particular order with only the order of draw (for various specimen type) adhered to for those patients with various other tests requested. Blood tubes were mixed with 5 inversions as a standard protocol before dispatched to the clinical laboratories for testing.

To determine the clotting time, an empirical visual approach was taken to manually time the clotting process for some RST and SST ($n = 30$). Tube pairs (RST, SST) were placed side by side with occasional tilting of the tubes to check on the clot process. Once a firm clot (>50% no flow) was shown, the timer (on a stop watch) was stopped.

2.1. Workflow and Analyte Testing. Following accessioning of requested tests, the workflow for patient samples followed the usual process through the central lab automation system where specimen tubes are placed through the automated routing process of centrifugation, aliquoting, testing in linked analyzers, and finally archived in the specimen stockyard. For healthy subject specimens, they were manually processed for centrifugation and testing.

RST and SST specimen tubes for patients processed through the central lab automation system were analyzed on the automation-line-connected Beckman Coulter DxC 800 analyzers for the renal panel (urea, creatinine, bicarbonate, sodium, potassium, chloride, and glucose), liver panel (total protein, albumin, total bilirubin, alkaline phosphatase ALP, alanine aminotransferase ALT, and aspartate aminotransferase AST), and lipid panel (total cholesterol, HDL-cholesterol, triglycerides) and DxI 800 for thyroid hormones (thyroid stimulating hormone TSH, free thyroxine fT4). Sera from healthy subjects for the same analytes (renal, liver, and lipids) were analyzed on the Roche MODULAR

EVO analyzer. Thyroid hormones for both subject populations were analyzed on the DxI 800. The cardiac markers (Troponin-T, creatine kinase-MB CK-MB, and N-terminal brain natriuretic peptide NT-proBNP) and prostate-specific antigen (PSA) were analyzed on a Roche cobas6000 analyzer.

2.2. Stability Study. Paired blood specimens collected in RSTs and SSTs ($n = 31$) that were tested for renal, liver, and lipid panels, cardiac markers and thyroid hormones were archived at 4°C (D1). The samples were re-tested for the same analytes each day (D2–D5) for the next 4 days. Storage of the study samples was in the same cold room as other routine blood specimens.

2.3. Data Analysis. Results were analyzed using Passing-Bablok and Bland-Altman plots for association and differences. Tube comparison results analyzed by the Student's t-test were applied for each analyte. Analysis of variance (ANOVA) procedure for group mean differences against the initial first day D1 over the next 4 days' (D2–D5) results for serum stability at different days of storage was performed. Differences are considered statistically significant at a P value of <0.05.

This study has institutional ethics approval (CIRB2011/855/B) with informed consent from all participants.

3. Results and Discussion

All study analytes from the healthy subjects were readily tested; however, not all of these analytes were requested for the outpatients, hence, the unequal number of tests for each analyte (85–129 results). Subjects' demographics gave the following: 70 males, 90 females of average age 43 years (range 20–77). There were 85 healthy subjects and 75 patients. A summary of the tests and instrument platform associated is shown in Table 1.

Visual review of the clotting process clearly verified a much shorter clot formation in the RSTs at less than 5 min compared to SSTs. Of the 30 RSTs and SSTs observed, clots formed almost immediately for the RSTs. The RSTs gave an overall mean clotting time of 2.07 min (range 1–4 min, median 2.05 min). Blood in SSTs did not clot at 5 min and most required at least 15 min to show signs of clotting.

Most parallel test results for RSTs and SSTs agreed very well. Means of the RSTs were in close agreement with that of the control (SST) tube for all 22 analytes (Table 2). No statistical significant differences in results were indicated for the RSTs compared to SSTs. It is noted that absolute differences were small, for example, potassium −0.5 to +0.5 mmol/L although translated in percent difference would be large. As shown in the table, results for renal and liver panels that are universally requested were similarly observed on both types of blood collection tubes. Results for cardiac markers were also of similar mean values between the two tubes.

Graphical illustrations of the select analytes chosen for their high workload, requirement of short turnaround time, and panic value reporting especially in the accident and emergency setting (Figure 1), showed strong correlations

TABLE 1: Tests associated with instrument platforms.

	Group	Principle	Instruments for health, patients
Urea, creatinine Bicarbonate, glucose	Renal	Chemistry	MOD, DxC800
Sodium, potassium, chloride	Electrolyte	Electrochemistry	MOD, DxC800
Total protein, albumin Total Bilirubin, ALP, ALT, AST	Liver	Chemistry	MOD, DxC800
Cholesterol, HDL, triglycerides	Lipid	Chemistry	MOD, DxC800
TSH, free T4	Thyroid	Immunoassay	DxI800
Troponin T, CK-MB, NT-proBNP	Cardiac	Immunoassay	cobas6000
PSA	Prostate	Immunoassay	cobas6000

Beckman Coulter: DxC800, DxI800.
Roche Diagnostics: MODULAR EVO, cobas6000.

TABLE 2: Summary statistics for RST results compared with control (SST) tubes.

Analyte	Units	n	RST mean	Range	SST mean	Range	Diff mean	95% CI range	t-test P value
Urea	mmol/L	106	4.8	2.2, 17.5	4.9	2.3, 17.4	0.0	−0.6, 0.7	0.90
Creatinine	μmol/L	127	81.9	46, 370	82.7	40, 371	−0.7	−12, 9	0.89
Bicarbonate	mmol/L	104	24.9	15.4, 29.9	25.0	19.0, 29.9	−0.1	−5.8, 3.8	0.71
Glucose	mmol/L	97	5.4	2.9, 20.2	5.4	2.3, 20.3	0.0	−0.3, 0.6	0.94
Sodium	mmol/L	106	140.1	132, 146	140.3	133, 148	−0.2	−4, 4	0.52
Potassium	mmol/L	108	4.2	3.4, 5.1	4.2	3.3, 5.1	0.0	−0.5, 0.5	0.70
Chloride	mmol/L	106	103.7	99, 110	103.7	98, 109	0.0	−4, 3	1.00
Total protein	g/L	107	71.9	55, 85	71.6	55, 84	0.3	−3, 4	0.69
Albumin	g/L	127	39.1	24, 49	38.8	24, 48	0.3	−2, 2	0.52
Total Bilirubin	μmol/L	110	11.2	4.0, 33.0	11.4	4.4, 34.0	−0.2	−19, 4	0.80
ALP	U/L	108	66.3	28, 338	66.4	35, 331	−0.2	−13, 7	0.97
ALT	U/L	129	25.7	4, 374	25.6	4, 375	−0.2	−5, 7	0.95
AST	U/L	121	25.3	8, 465	25.6	10, 451	−0.3	−5, 14	0.96
Cholesterol	mmol/L	93	5.21	3.23, 9.39	5.18	3.17, 9.11	0.03	−0.32, 0.36	0.84
HDL	mmol/L	93	1.47	0.10, 2.72	1.48	0.66, 2.75	−0.01	−0.95, 0.20	0.86
Triglycerides	mmol/L	93	1.18	0.41, 4.83	1.16	0.41, 4.70	0.02	−0.12, 0.13	0.88
TSH	mU/L	98	2.125	0.015, 43.4	2.040	0.015, 39.9	0.085	−0.406, 3.50	0.88
fT4	pmol/L	98	11.7	4.0, 19.5	11.7	4.4, 19.4	−0.04	−3.3, 2.4	0.88
Troponin-T	μg/L	86	0.003	0.003, 0.01	0.003	0.003, 0.01	−0.0002	−0.013, 0	0.44
CK-MB	μg/L	86	1.86	0.71, 5.65	1.89	0.78, 5.71	−0.03	−0.19, 0.24	0.85
NT-proBNP	pg/mL	85	44.4	5.0, 229	44.1	5.0, 228	0.33	−2.6, 7.71	0.95
PSA	μg/L	87	0.33	0.003, 4.60	0.34	0.003, 4.50	0.00	−0.06, 0.10	0.97

Diff: absolute difference (RST − SST).
95% CI: minimum, maximum.
Range: minimum, maximum.

between RSTs and SSTs as evidenced by near equivalent slopes as determined with Passing-Bablok regression fits. Most of the tests gave a slope of 1.00 and zero y-intercepts as summarised in Table 3. Selected analytes also displayed these tight fittings with Spearman's correlations ranging from 0.91 to 1.00. Bland-Altman difference plots showed low mean biases in general (Figure 2, Table 3). In the case for Troponin-T, none of the results were reported as positive (>0.03 μg/L), and the few results ($n = 8$) that were >0.003 μg/L (lowest detectable level) still gave a Passing-Bablok slope of 1.00.

TABLE 3: Summary of Passing-Bablok regression and Bland-Altman bias between RST and SST.

Analyte	Sample size	Passing-Bablok		Correl rs	mBias%	95% CI bias		95% limitAgrmt	
		Slope	Constant			Min.	Max.	Min.	Max.
Urea	106	1.00	0.00	0.99	−0.7	−1.5	−0.0	−8.2	6.7
Creatinine	127	0.98	0.55	0.99	−0.9	−1.7	−0.1	−9.7	8.0
Bicarbonate	104	1.00	0.00	0.86	−0.5	−1.6	0.5	−11.1	10.0
Glucose	97	1.00	0.00	0.99	0.8	0.1	1.5	−6.2	7.7
Sodium	106	1.00	0.00	0.82	−0.2	−0.4	0.0	−2.2	1.8
Potassium	108	1.00	0.00	0.91	0.3	−0.3	1.0	−6.2	6.9
Chloride	106	1.00	0.00	0.83	0.0	−0.2	0.2	−2.4	2.4
Total protein	107	1.00	0.00	0.95	0.4	0.0	0.7	−3.0	3.7
Albumin	127	1.00	0.00	0.98	0.7	0.4	1.0	−2.7	4.0
Total Bilirubin	110	1.00	0.00	0.94	−1.5	−4.4	1.3	−31.4	28.4
ALP	108	1.00	0.00	0.99	−0.6	−1.4	0.2	−8.9	7.8
ALT	129	1.00	0.00	0.98	−2.1	−3.9	−0.3	−22.3	18.2
AST	121	1.00	0.00	0.96					
Cholesterol	93	0.99	0.04	0.99	0.6	0.2	1.1	−3.4	4.7
HDL	93	1.02	−0.03	0.99	−2.0	−5.6	1.6	−36.3	32.2
Triglycerides	93	1.00	0.02	1.00	1.5	1.0	2.0	−3.5	6.5
TSH	98	1.06	−0.01	0.99	2.8	1.1	4.4	−13.3	18.8
fT4	98	0.96	0.48	0.84	−0.3	−1.8	1.3	−15.5	15.0
Troponin-T	86	1.00	0.00	0.88	0.0	0	0	0	0
CK-MB	86	1.00	−0.03	1.00	−1.7	−2.5	−1.0	−8.6	5.1
NT-proBNP	85	1.01	−0.16	1.00	0.9	−0.7	2.4	−13.3	15.0
PSA	87	0.98	0.00	0.97	−2.1	−4.9	0.8	−28.3	24.1

Passing Bablok: slope, constant.
Correl: Spearman's correlation coefficient: rs
mBias%: Bland-Altman mean Bias with 95% confidence interval and 95% limits of agreement.

Stability studies of archived specimens showed that serum in RSTs has the same stability as in SSTs at 4°C, tested up to 5 days for the renal, liver, and lipid panels, cardiac markers, and thyroid hormones except for bicarbonate whose levels differ substantially each day and would have clinical impact (Table 4). The mean values for bicarbonate decrease daily with large differences between days with statistical significance shown immediately on the next day D2, averaging −25.6% to 7.2% and corresponding medians of −25.8% to 1.1%. For the electrolytes sodium, potassium, and chloride, differences between days were less than 12%, averaging 0.7% to 6.2% with corresponding median values of 0% to 6.8%. Though statistically significant at D3 and D4, the differences have little clinical impact. This is also shown with albumin, another analyte that showed some incremental increase on storage but of little clinical impact.

Although insufficient serum was available to test for all analytes on the fifth day of storage (D5; only 8 cases have results), similar group means were obtained and included in the ANOVA computation (data not shown). The result trending of the analytes was similar to D2–D4, that is, all ANOVA tested analytes showed no statistical significant difference except for bicarbonate, sodium, potassium, chloride, and albumin.

Turnaround times for test results depend on how fast the test can be performed, how fast the blood sample reaches the laboratory, how fast the laboratory processes the specimen, and how fast the results are reported. Hence, there are potential areas for improvement at the preanalytical, analytical, and postanalytical phases. There have been various studies on the preanalytical phase with blood collection tubes being one of the improvement areas [1, 2, 15]. For a fast turnaround for tests from the emergency department and outpatient clinics, use of plasma tubes is one answer to the limitation of a 30-minute clotting time imposed by the standard blood collection tubes with serum separator and clot activator.

In addition, RSTs have also been shown to give comparable results for reproductive hormones (e.g., follicle stimulating hormone, luteinizing hormone, human chorionic gonadotropin, and estradiol) and similarly for cardiac markers and thyroid hormones, on other instrument platforms—Siemens ADVIA Centaur, Beckman Access II,

TABLE 4: Stability of serum in RSTs over 4 days indicated by repeat testing.

Analyte	Units	Range*	D1 **n = 31	D2 **n = 31	D3 **n = 27	D4 **n = 18	ANOVA
Urea	mmol/L	2.3, 75	4.24 (0.21)	4.17 (0.20)	4.13 (0.19)	4.07 (0.22)	NS
Creatinine	μmol/L	47, 108	72.0 (2.80)	75.2 (2.91)	76.7 (3.03)	75.5 (2.88)	NS
Bicarbonate	mmol/L	22.0, 28.5	25.3 (0.31)	18.8 (0.39)	16.9 (0.25)	16.9 (0.30)	d2, d3, d4
Glucose	mmol/L	3.5, 9.0	4.97 (0.19)	5.06 (0.19)	5.16 (0.22)	5.21 (0.31)	NS
Sodium	mmol/L	135, 144	140 (0.40)	143 (0.49)	147 (0.53)	148 (0.78)	d3, d4
Potassium	mmol/L	3.4, 5.0	4.1 (0.05)	4.2 (0.05)	4.4 (0.07)	4.4 (0.08)	d3, d4
Chloride	mmol/L	101, 107	104 (0.32)	105 (0.40)	107 (0.37)	109 (0.51)	d3, d4
Total Protein	g/L	60, 80	71.0 (0.74)	72.2 (0.74)	73.6 (0.97)	73.4 (1.14)	NS
Albumin	g/L	34, 44	38.8 (0.45)	39.1 (0.49)	40.7 (0.53)	41.4 (0.63)	d3, d4
Total Bilirubin	μmol/L	4.4, 23.5	9.69 (0.89)	8.95 (0.81)	8.79 (0.79)	8.26 (1.05)	NS
ALP	U/L	39, 331	73.4 (10.7)	75.9 (11.3)	81.8 (12.9)	95.8 (19.6)	NS
ALT	U/L	7, 36	16.4 (1.22)	16.1 (1.12)	15.3 (1.24)	16.0 (1.60)	NS
AST	U/L	10, 26	15.6 (0.71)	16.2 (0.70)	16.7 (0.85)	18.1 (1.11)	NS
Cholesterol	mmol/L	3.17, 6.27	4.84 (0.14)	4.91 (0.14)	4.99 (0.16)	4.89 (0.20)	NS
HDL	mmol/L	0.79, 2.75	1.47 (0.06)	1.46 (0.06)	1.51 (0.07)	1.52 (0.10)	NS
Triglycerides	mmol/L	0.42, 2.88	1.18 (0.10)	1.22 (0.10)	1.26 (0.11)	1.33 (0.16)	NS
TSH	mU/L	0.487, 6.20	1.889 (0.21)	1.893 (0.21)	2.010 (0.24)	2.360 (0.34)	NS
fT4	pmol/L	8.7, 14.6	11.3 (0.24)	10.9 (0.24)	11.1 (0.26)	11.2 (0.36)	NS
CK-MB	μg/L	0.88, 4.82	1.80 (0.15)	1.88 (0.14)	1.65 (0.14)	1.61 (0.21)	NS
NT-proBNP	pg/mL	5.0, 100.6	35.9 (4.98)	37.3 (4.97)	37.9 (5.28)	47.5 (7.00)	NS

*Range: minimum, maximum.
**D1: day 1, D2: day 2, D3: day 3, D4: day 4.
Result: mean (SD).
d2, d3, d4: $P < 0.05$.
Note: same stability shown on SST tubes.

Abbott AxSYM, and Ortho Clinical Vitros eCi (data not shown).

It should, however, be clearly made known that as thrombin is used to accelerate clotting, the endogenous pathways involving thrombin would be affected with these tubes. Those patients for coagulation studies are likely to be affected and should not have their blood collected with the RSTs. Similarly, RSTs are not recommended for patients on heparin therapy, thrombin inhibitor therapy, or with deficiency in the clotting factors as latent clotting has been observed on patients on high dose heparin treatment resulting with APTT > 150 sec [10]. In our study, none of the 75 outpatients recruited for this study had coordered coagulation tests on the day of study participation that would suggest any recent high dose heparin therapy typically administered in an inpatient setting. It would, however, be prudent to confine the use of RSTs which are primarily suited for fast turnaround needs, to subjects without recent history of coagulation treatment, for example, cardiac surgery.

4. Conclusions

This present study has observed concordance of common analytes on evaluation of serum from the standard blood collection tubes and the quick clotting tubes. The new RSTs have also been reported to give very similar results as SSTs [10, 16]. With quick clotting, RSTs potentially allow time gains in terms of reduced turnaround times and circumvent the use of plasma specimens to achieve service performance improvements. As observed in other studies, the rapid clotting tubes, RSTs, could bridge the concern of short turnaround service performance for many healthcare institutions that have converted to the use of plasma instead of serum.

A notable aspect of our study depicts hospital-based clinical practice conditions for the collection of blood specimens and real situation tests' performance. In summary, RSTs gave comparable test results as current serum separator tubes for some of the most common biochemical analytes ordered in the emergency and outpatient setting. This tube development would be helpful to achieve short turnaround times for serum specimens needing STAT reporting.

Disclosure

The authors have no conflict of interests regarding the publication of this study. Becton Dickinson and Company, Singapore, played no role in the design, data analysis, or in

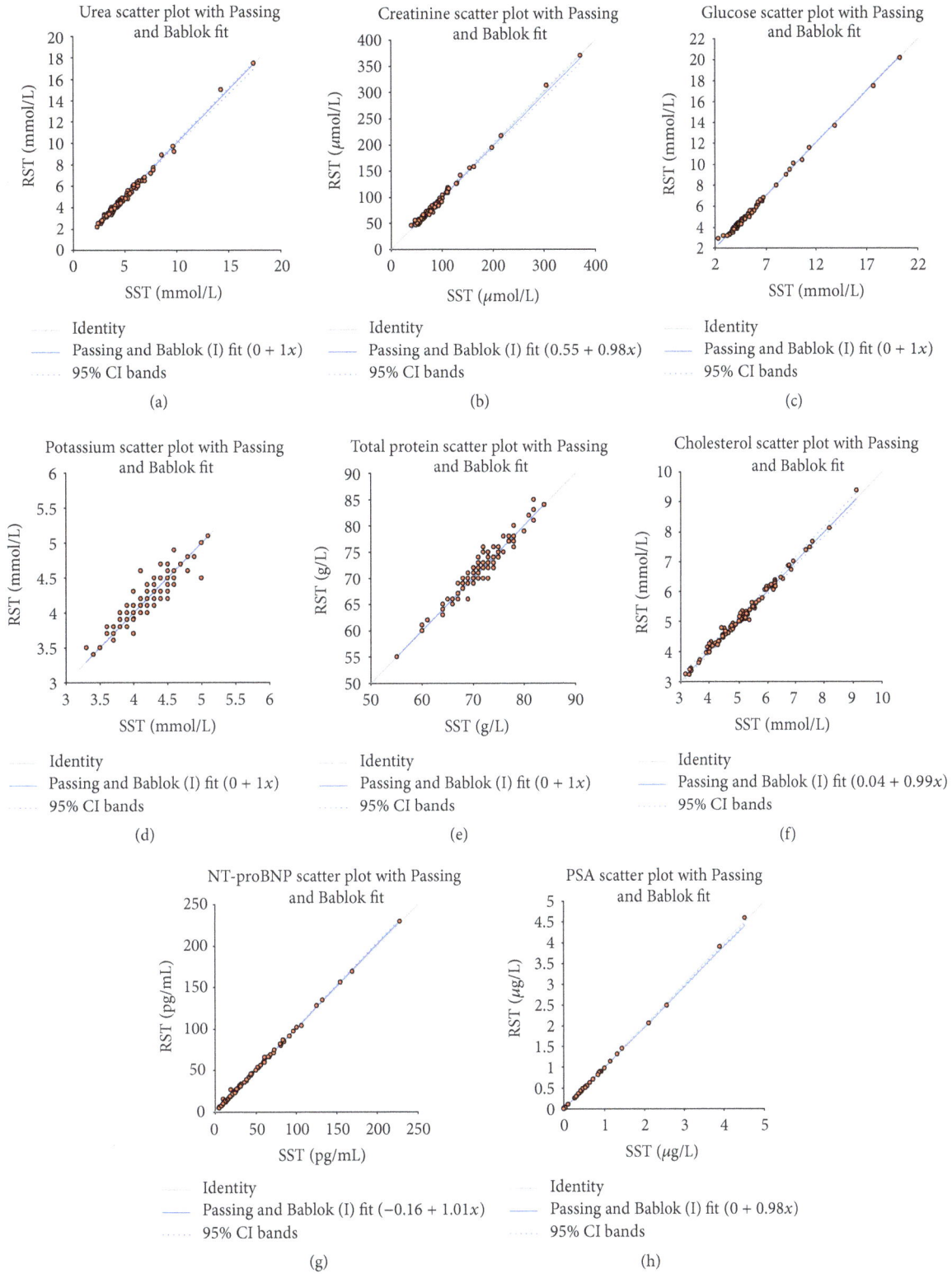

FIGURE 1: Comparison of results for RST and SST for the select analytes. Select analytes: Passing-Bablok regression analysis. (a) urea, (b) creatinine, (c) glucose, (d) potassium, (e) total protein, (f) cholesterol, (g) NT-proBNP, and (h) PSA.

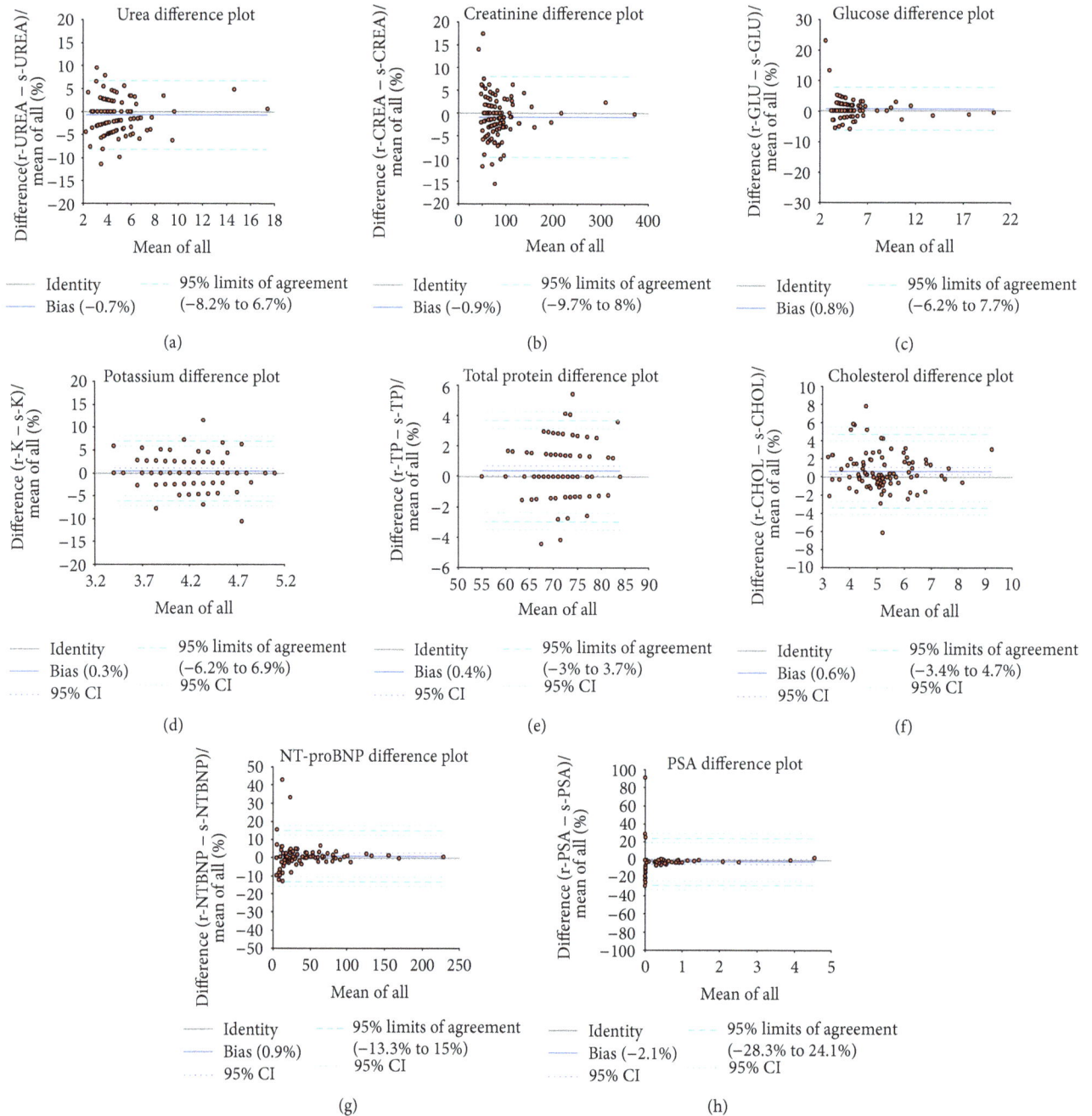

FIGURE 2: Bland-Altman difference plots for select analytes. Select analytes: (a) urea, (b) creatinine, (c) glucose, (d) potassium, (e) total protein, (f) cholesterol, (g) NT-proBNP, and (h) PSA.

the writing of the report aside from providing the rapid serum tubes for the study.

Acknowledgments

The authors wish to thank Chiu Yuet Wah, James Low Pak Wai, Chiong Sieu Ping, and Tiong Chiau Chiae for their contributions to the study. The authors thank Becton Dickinson and Company, Singapore, for the supply of rapid serum tubes used in the study.

References

[1] P. G. Manor, "Turnaround times in the laboratory: a review of the literature," *Clinical Laboratory Science*, vol. 12, no. 2, pp. 85–89, 1999.

[2] H. J. Chung, W. Lee, S. Chun, H. I. Park, and W. K. Min, "Analysis of turnaround time by subdividing three phases for outpatient chemistry specimens," *Annals of Clinical and Laboratory Science*, vol. 39, no. 2, pp. 144–149, 2009.

[3] R. R. Miles, R. F. Roberts, A. R. Putnam, and W. L. Roberts, "Comparison of serum and heparinized plasma samples for

measurement of chemistry analytes," *Clinical Chemistry*, vol. 50, no. 9, pp. 1704–1706, 2004.

[4] B. L. Boyanton Jr. and K. E. Blick, "Stability studies of twenty-four analytes in human plasma and serum," *Clinical Chemistry*, vol. 48, no. 12, pp. 2242–2247, 2002.

[5] T. K. Er, L. Y. Tsai, Y. J. Jong, and B. H. Chen, "Selected analyte values in serum versus heparinized plasma using the SYNCHRON LX PRO assay methods/instrument," *Laboratory Medicine*, vol. 37, no. 12, pp. 731–732, 2006.

[6] H. Stiegler, Y. Fischer, J. F. Vazquez-Jimenez et al., "Lower cardiac tropinin T and I results in heparin-plasma than in serum," *Clinical Chemistry*, vol. 46, no. 9, pp. 1338–1344, 2000.

[7] M. Panteghini, "Performance of today's cardiac troponin assays and tomorrow's," *Clinical Chemistry*, vol. 48, no. 6, pp. 809–810, 2002.

[8] M. Panteghini and F. Pagani, "On the comparison of serum and plasma samples in troponin assays," *Clinical Chemistry*, vol. 49, no. 5, pp. 835–836, 2003.

[9] R. Dominici, I. Infusino, C. Valente, I. Moraschinelli, and C. Franzini, "Plasma or serum samples: measurements of cardiac troponin T and of other analytes compared," *Clinical Chemistry and Laboratory Medicine*, vol. 42, no. 8, pp. 945–951, 2004.

[10] G. Dimeski, P. P. Masci, M. Trabi, M. F. Lavin, and J. de Jersey, "Evaluation of the Becton-Dickinson rapid serum tube: does it provide a suitable alternative to lithium heparin plasma tubes?" *Clinical Chemistry and Laboratory Medicine*, vol. 48, no. 5, pp. 651–657, 2010.

[11] J. Huyakorn, J. Chance, J. Berube, M. Alsberge, P. Harper, and D. L. Uettwiller-Geiger, "Evaluation of the BD Vacutainer rapid serum tubes for cardiac marker assays on three instrument platforms," *Pathology*, vol. 41, supplement 1, p. 70, 2009.

[12] C. Koch, A. Wockenfus, A. Saenger, A. Jaffe, and B. Karon B, "Validation of the BD rapid serum tubes for STAT troponin-T testing on the Roche c411," *Clinical Chemistry*, vol. 57, supplement 10, p. A100, 2011.

[13] F. G. Strathmann, M. M. Ka, P. M. Rainey, and G. S. Baird, "Use of the BD vacutainer rapid serum tube reduces false-positive results for selected Beckman Coulter Unicel DxI immunoassays," *American Journal of Clinical Pathology*, vol. 136, no. 2, pp. 325–329, 2011.

[14] C. D. Koch, A. M. Wockenfus, A. K. Saenger, A. S. Jaffe, and B. S. Karon, "BD rapid serum tubes reduce false positive plasma troponin T results on the Roche Cobas e411 analyzer," *Clinical Biochemistry*, vol. 45, no. 10-11, pp. 842–844, 2012.

[15] R. Prusa, J. Doupovcova, D. Warunek, and A. K. Stankovic, "Improving laboratory efficiencies through significant time reduction in the preanalytical phase," *Clinical Chemistry and Laboratory Medicine*, vol. 48, no. 2, pp. 293–296, 2010.

[16] K. Middleton, V. Parvu, S. Church, A. Mouser, and R. Rosa, "Comparison of the BD Vacutainer rapid serum tube with a range of commercially available serum separator tubes for clotting time," *Biochemia Medica*, vol. 21, no. 2, p. A6, 2011, (1st EFCC-BD European Conference on Preanalytical Phase).

19

Persistent Polyclonal B Cell Lymphocytosis B Cells Can Be Activated through CD40-CD154 Interaction

Emmanuelle Dugas-Bourdages,[1] Sonia Néron,[2,3] Annie Roy,[2] André Darveau,[3] and Robert Delage[1]

[1]Centre Universitaire d'Hématologie et d'Oncologie de Québec, CHU de Québec, Hôpital de l'Enfant-Jésus, 1401 18ième rue, Québec, QC, Canada G1J 1Z4

[2]Héma-Québec, Recherche et Développement, 1070 avenue des Sciences-de-la-Vie, Québec, QC, Canada G1V 5C3

[3]Département de Biochimie, de Microbiologie et de Bio-Informatique, Pavillon Alexandre-Vachon, 1045 avenue de la Médecine, Bureau 3428, Université Laval, Québec, QC, Canada G1V 0A6

Correspondence should be addressed to Robert Delage; robert.delage@fmed.ulaval.ca

Academic Editor: Emili Montserrat

Persistent polyclonal B cell lymphocytosis (PPBL) is a rare disorder, diagnosed primarily in adult female smokers and characterized by an expansion of CD19$^+$CD27$^+$IgM$^+$ memory B cells, by the presence of binucleated lymphocytes, and by a moderate elevation of serum IgM. The clinical course is usually benign, but it is not known whether or not PPBL might be part of a process leading to the emergence of a malignant proliferative disorder. In this study we sought to investigate the functional response of B cells from patients with PPBL by use of an optimal memory B cell culture model based on the CD40-CD154 interaction. We found that the proliferation of PPBL B cells was almost as important as that of B cells from normal controls, resulting in high immunoglobulin secretion with *in vitro* isotypic switching. We conclude that the CD40-CD154 activation pathway is functional in the memory B cell population of PPBL patients, suggesting that the disorder may be due to either a dysfunction of other cells in the microenvironment or a possible defect in another B cell activation pathway.

1. Introduction

Persistent polyclonal B cell lymphocytosis (PPBL) is a rare and presumably nonmalignant lymphoproliferative disorder diagnosed predominantly in women [1, 2], although a few men have also been diagnosed with this condition [3–5]. Clinical symptoms are nonspecific except for mild fatigue in most individuals with this disorder [1, 6]. Patients, usually cigarette smokers, present with elevated polyclonal serum IgM and a persistent polyclonal lymphocytosis of memory B cell origin as evidenced, on flow cytometry, by a population of CD27$^+$IgM$^+$IgD$^+$ cells with normal κ/λ ratio [7–11] representing more than 70% of their total B lymphocytes [12]. The blood smear in these patients is characterized by the presence of mostly atypical lymphocytes with abundant cytoplasm and mature nuclei. Binuclearity can be observed in 1–9% of their

lymphocytes [13]. Patients predominantly express the HLA-DR7 phenotype, while this particular allele usually occurs in only 26% of the normal Caucasian population [14].

The clinical course is usually benign, but we have previously described the case of one individual who developed a diffuse large-B-cell lymphoma (DLBCL) 19 years after a diagnosis of PPBL [15]. Overall, a small proportion of patients with PPBL has been reported in the literature to have developed a malignant disease [16–18]. Although the pathophysiology of this disorder remains largely unknown, a familial link is one of its constant features, suggesting the existence of an underlying genetic defect [19]. Despite the apparent polyclonal nature of the B cell proliferation, the frequency of rearrangements between the *bcl-2* and Ig heavy chain genes is 100-fold greater than that observed in normal

B cells, and multiple *bcl-2/Ig* gene rearrangements have been observed in all PPBL patients [20]. An isochromosome 3q+ (i3)(q10) has also been described in a varying proportion of the B cell population [3, 18]. Such genetic aberrations were always restricted to the B cells, indicating the presence of a distinct clonal cytogenetic population in PPBL patients [3]. This confirms that some B cells in this disorder are distinct from their normal counterparts. However, sparse information is as yet available on the functional properties of B cells in PPBL.

It has been shown that PPBL B cells are memory cells presenting the $CD27^+IgM^+IgD^+$ immunotype [11, 21] with a large repertoire diversity [11, 22] and that they could originate from the B cell populations of the splenic marginal zone [23]. Marginal zone $CD27^+IgM^+IgD^+$ B cells likely are memory cells that can be generated independently from a germinal center reaction and T cell help, while also being able to respond to the CD40-CD154 interaction [24, 25]. The binding of CD40 to CD154 expressed on activated T cells plays a central role in B cell activation, proliferation, and immunoglobulin isotype switching [26]. B lymphocytes from healthy controls grow perfectly well in a culture system based on this interaction in the presence of IL-4 [26, 27]. However, we have previously shown that PPBL B lymphocytes were unable to proliferate following *in vitro* CD40-CD154 interaction. These observations were suggestive of a possible defect in the CD40 pathway, although CD40 expression, sequencing, and tyrosine phosphorylation appeared to be normal [28]. Others have reported later that the circulating $CD19^+CD27^+$ memory B cells from normal individuals were unresponsive to high-level CD40-CD154 interaction [29]. Finally, it has been shown that a reduced-intensity CD40-CD154 interaction in the presence of IL-2, IL-4, and IL-10 results in the proliferation, expansion, and immunoglobulin secretion of normal memory $CD19^+CD27^+$ B cells [30, 31].

Since PPBL B cells share the CD27 expression of normal memory B cells, we have designed a study to investigate the response of B lymphocytes from patients with PPBL in cultures with low-intensity CD40-CD154 interaction and to further characterize these cells, especially their isotype switching and immunoglobulin secretion.

2. Patients and Methods

2.1. Patients and Healthy Controls. This study was conducted on six female patients (8010, 8011, 8013, 8030, 8031, and 8032) ranging from 47 to 69 years. All individuals were asked to answer a questionnaire inquiring about their habits and health status. PPBL patients were initially diagnosed and followed at St-Sacrement and later at Enfant-Jésus hospitals of the CHU de Québec. Diagnostic criteria were (a) a persistent $CD19^+/CD5^-$ B cell lymphocytosis of at least 6 months' duration with a normal κ/λ ratio; (b) a polyclonal increase in the serum IgM concentration; (c) the presence on the blood smear of binucleated lymphocytes as previously described [11, 28]; and (d) the presence of multiple bcl-2/Ig gene rearrangements in peripheral blood lymphocytes. Blood was collected from all patients after informed consent was

obtained. This study has been approved by the Research Ethics Board of the CHU de Québec. Peripheral blood mononuclear cells (PBMCs) were obtained from healthy individuals following routine platelet collection by recovering the cells from leukoreduction chambers, as described previously [32]. Consequently, comparison against samples obtained from healthy individuals participating in Héma-Québec's study was approved by Héma-Québec's Research Ethic Committee and all these samples were obtained following each individual's informed consent.

2.2. Isolation of Human Peripheral B Cells from PPBL Samples. PBMCs were isolated from peripheral blood by Ficoll-paque density gradient centrifugation (Amersham Pharmacia Biotech, Baie d'Urfé, Canada), suspended in freezing medium (Roswell Park Memorial Institute (RPMI) medium (Gibco-BRL, Burlington, Ont, Canada)), supplemented with 20% fetal bovine serum supplemented with 5% DMSO (FBS; Hyclone, Logan, UT, USA), and kept frozen in liquid nitrogen. B cells, from patients or from healthy controls, were purified by negative selection from thawed PBMCs cryopreserved for 3 months or less, using the StemSep CD19 mixture according to the manufacturer's instructions (Stem Cell Technologies, Vancouver, Canada) [30]. Purified human B cells were 95% or more $CD19^+$ as determined by flow cytometry.

2.3. In Vitro Stimulation of Human B Cells with $CD154^+$ Adherent Cells. L4.5 cells originate from a genetically modified L929 cell line (CCL-1, American Type Culture Collection, Manassas, VA) and express about $21,000 \pm 4000$ CD154 molecules per cell [30, 33]. Purified B cells from PPBL patients and controls ($\sim2.5 \times 10^5$ cells/mL) were seeded in Primaria plates (BD Biosciences, Mountain View, CA) in the presence of gamma-irradiated (75 Gy/7500 rad) L4.5 cells in a ratio of either 3 or 25 B cells per L4.5 cell, corresponding to high and low stimulations, respectively [30]. B cells were cultured in Iscove's modified Dulbecco's medium (IMDM) supplemented with 10% ultralow IgG FBS containing $10\,\mu g/mL$ insulin, $5.5\,\mu g/mL$ transferrin, $6.7\,ng/mL$ sodium selenite (all from Invitrogen, Burlington, ON, Canada), and a mixture of cytokines, namely, $5\,ng/mL$ IL-2 ($\sim50\,U/mL$), $40\,ng/mL$ IL-10 ($\sim20\,U/mL$) (both from PeproTech, Rocky Hill, NJ, USA), and $3.5\,ng/mL$ IL-4 ($100\,U/mL$) (R&D Systems, Minneapolis, MN, USA). Three separate culture experiments were performed, each consisting of cells purified from 1 healthy control and 2 patients. Cell counts and viability were evaluated in triplicate by Trypan blue dye exclusion. Cultured B cells were always ≥95% $CD19^+$ and, unless otherwise specified, viability was >90%.

2.4. Flow Cytometry Analysis. Allophycocyanin-conjugated anti-CD27 and anti-IgG, PerCP-cyanin 5.5-conjugated anti-CD19, and PE-conjugated anti-IgD and their conjugated isotype controls were all from BD Biosciences. Polyvalent goat IgG FITC-anti-IgM antibodies were from The Jackson Laboratory (Mississauga, Ontario, Canada). All stainings were performed using $1\,\mu g$ of each Ab for 1×10^6 cells. Cells were

TABLE 1: Clinical data of PPBL patients.

Characteristics	Patients					
	8010	8011	8013	8030	8031	8032
Age (years)	50	47	59	69	56	49
Lymphocytosis ($\times 10^9$/L)	6,4	2,5	3,9	2,8	4,4	2,4
Lymphocytosis (% total leukocytosis)	58,4	32,1	36,5	42,5	56,6	48,7
B cells/μL	5250	1550	910	1200	2240	760
Serum IgM (g/L)	12,1	7,8	3,8	9,6	9,5	7,3
Number of *BCL-2/Ig* rearrangements[a]	3	5	3	7	5	5
HLA	A 2, 9 B 14, 44 Dr 2, 5	A 9, 30 B 13, 14 Dr 5, 13	A 9, 39 B 14, 35 Dr 5, 13	A 1, 3 B 7, 57 Dr 7, 14	ND	A 11, 29 B 35, 44 Dr 7, 14
Cigarette smoking[b]	Yes	Stopped × 7 years	Yes	Stopped × 3 years	Yes	Stopped × 5 years

[a] *BCL-2/Ig* gene rearrangement was determined as previously described by Delage et al., 2001 [19].
[b] Information was reported on day of blood collection.

fixed with 2% paraformaldehyde. Isotype-matched control Ab staining was >95% double-negative cells. Regions containing dead cells were delineated using 7-amino-actinomycin D staining, following manufacturer's instructions (BD Biosciences). Analyses were done by gating ≥10,000 cells with a FACSCalibur Flow cytometer and the CellQuest Pro software (BD Biosciences). Data were subsequently analyzed with FCS Express II software (De Novo Software, Thornhill, ON, Canada).

2.5. Ig-Secretion Rate. The IgG and IgM secretion rates were determined on either day 13 or 14. Briefly stated, cells were harvested, washed with PBS, and seeded at $1\text{-}2 \times 10^6$ cells/mL in bare IMDM medium. Supernatants were collected after 18 to 22 hours and IgG and IgM concentrations were determined by standard enzyme-linked immunoadsorbent assay (ELISA), as previously described [29]. When indicated, IgG and IgM contents were also determined by ELISA in culture supernatants.

3. Results

3.1. Patient Profiles. The six patients studied were all female and displayed the clinical features associated with PPBL (Table 1). As described earlier [19], these were a higher than normal circulating lymphocyte count ($n = 2,4$ to $6,4 \times 10^9$/L), due to an increased number of B cells, and a polyclonal increase in their serum IgM ($n = 3,8$ to $12,1$ g/L). Their κ/λ ratio was consistent with a polyclonal origin of the lymphoproliferation in all cases (data not shown). A *Bcl2/Ig* gene rearrangement was present in everyone (Table 1). All patients were cigarette smokers, either presently or previously.

3.2. Phenotypic Characterization of Peripheral B Cells from Patients. Flow cytometry was done on purified B cells from

each of the six patients to evaluate CD19, CD27, IgD, and IgM expression (Figure 1). As previously reported [11], 73% ± 13% (mean ± SD; range of 58% to 87%) of the CD19+ B cell populations were characterized by CD27 positivity and 90% ± 6% (mean ± SD; range of 81% to 96%) expressed IgD and IgM. All B cells from PPBL patients also expressed CD40 (data not shown). Such high frequency of CD27+IgM+IgD+ B cell subset in the purified CD19+ cells was as expected and in agreement with the clinical data of our PPBL patients.

3.3. PPBL B Cells Respond to Low CD40 Stimulation. B cells from PPBL patients and healthy individuals were submitted to culture with high (3 B cells per L4.5 cell) and low (25 B cells per L4.5 cell) stimulation conditions and their proliferation was monitored for 13 to 14 days (Figure 2). As previously observed, the response of PPBL B cells to a high CD154 interaction was still 6- to 30-fold lower than that of control B cells, presumably due to their high frequency of CD27+IgM+IgD+ cells. Conversely, all PPBL B cell samples responded to the low stimulation conditions, with an expansion factor of anywhere between 3 and 20 times higher than that observed in the high CD40-CD154 interaction experiments. However, the response of PPBL B cells to a low CD40 interaction was lower than that of control B cells, which contained a normal ratio of naive CD27− and memory CD27+ B cells (data not shown). It is likely that the degree of proliferation of the dominant CD27+IgM+IgD+ B cell subpopulation observed in our patients is much lower than the otherwise more prominent CD27− B cell subpopulations of our controls [11].

3.4. Evolution of PPBL B Cells following Long-Term CD40 Stimulation. The phenotypes of PPBL B cells following low CD40 stimulation were monitored for CD19, CD27, IgM, and IgD expression on days 9 and 14. Phenotypic profiles for one representative PPBL sample and an example of control B cells are presented below (Figure 3(a)). The frequencies for

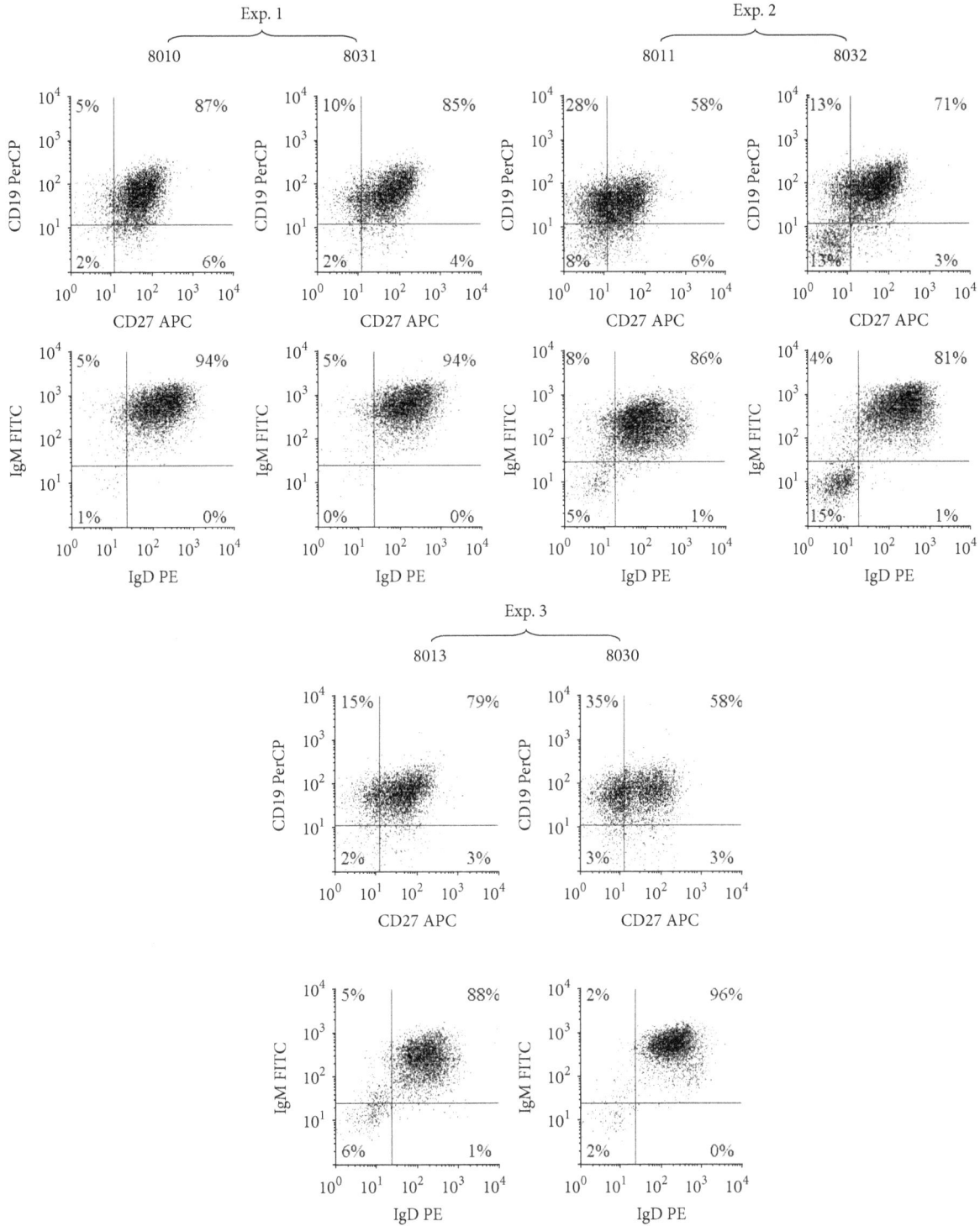

FIGURE 1: Phenotypes of B cells isolated from the blood samples of six patients with persistent polyclonal B cell lymphocytosis. Flow cytometry analysis of CD19, CD27, IgD, and IgM expression was done on purified peripheral B cells. More than 95% of purified cells were CD19$^+$CD40+ cells for all these patient samples. All analyses were done as described in methods.

CD19$^+$CD27$^-$, CD19$^+$CD27$^+$, IgM$^-$IgD$^-$, and IgM$^+$IgD$^-$ cells are shown as the mean values for all PPBL samples (n = 6) and the three controls (Figure 3(b)). Phenotypic evolution of the CD19$^+$ B cells, similar in all PPBL samples, differed from that of control B cells by showing a higher frequency of CD27$^+$ and IgM$^+$IgD$^-$ cells (Figures 3(a) and 3(b)). In all samples, two main phenotypes, corresponding to CD19$^+$CD27$^-$ and CD19$^+$CD27$^+$ cells, were observed during days 9 through 14. Based upon CD27 expression, the evolution of B cells from PPBL patients, following low CD40 stimulation, appeared

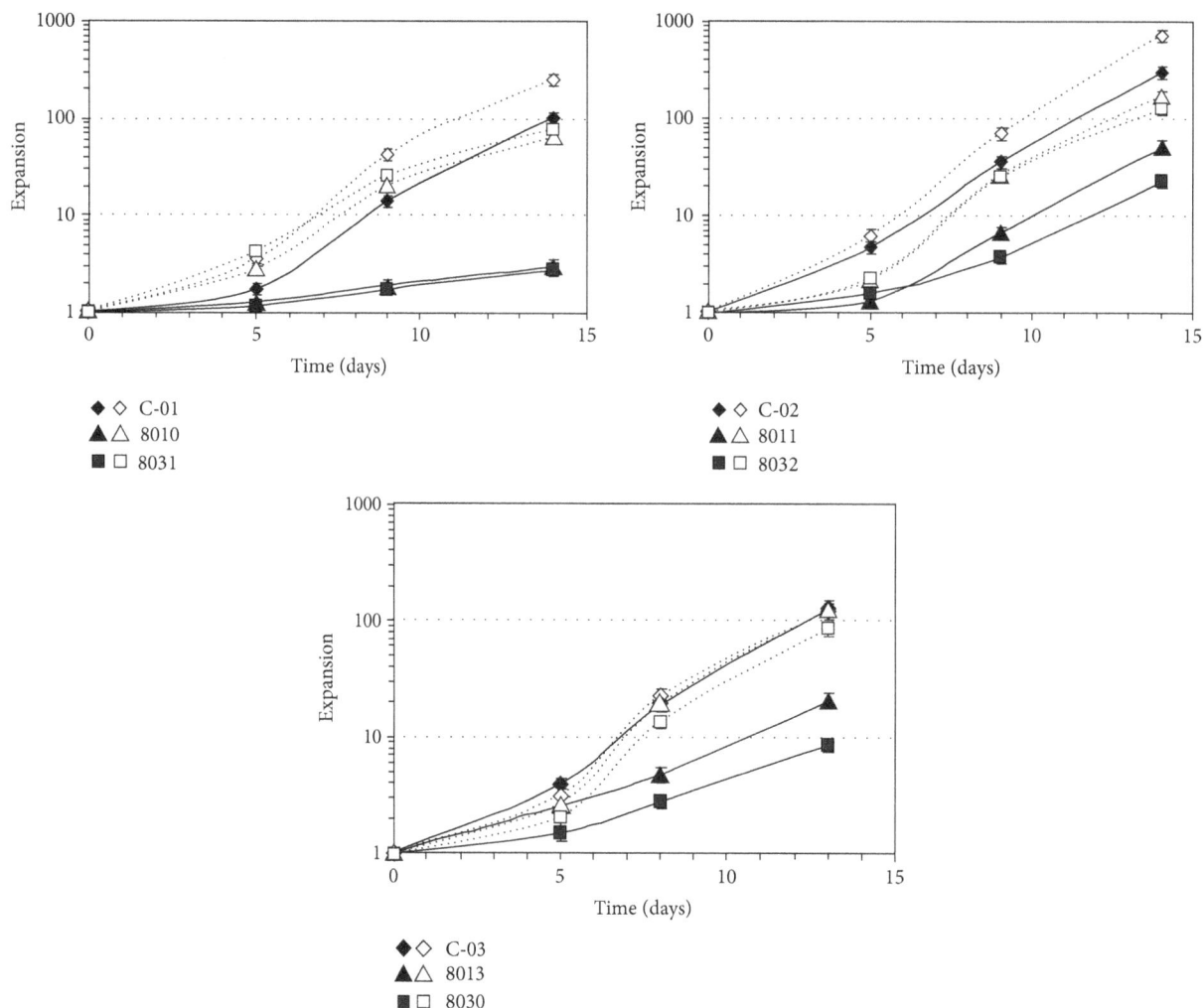

FIGURE 2: PPBL B cells proliferate following low CD154 interaction. Purified B cells isolated from samples obtained from healthy individuals (C-01, C-02, and C-03) and from patients with PPBL (8010, 8011, 8013, 8030, 8031, and 8032) were activated *in vitro* using a low level (open symbols; dashed line) or a high level (filled symbols; plain line) of CD154 interaction in the presence of cytokines, as indicated in methods. Expansion factors were evaluated using viable cell counts performed in triplicate at the indicated times. Error bars can be smaller than symbols.

similar to that of B cells from healthy controls. At rest, 81 to 96% of PPBL B cells were $IgD^{lo}IgM^+$ (Figure 1), a phenotype similar to that of normal marginal zone B cells [11, 34]. Following CD40 stimulation, surface IgD almost vanished in all PPBL B cell samples (Figures 3(a) and 3(b)). Additionally, the frequency of total IgM^+ B cells decreased in controls, from 88 to 95% (day 0) to less than 10% of $CD19^+$ cells (day 14), while remaining at 57% ± 15% in PPBL samples. Overall, these results indicate that the response of PPBL B cells to CD40 stimulation leads to phenotype changes that are quite similar to those observed in normal B cell populations but that remains biased towards growth of IgM^+ B cell subsets.

3.5. PPBL B Cells Are Able to Switch to and to Secrete IgG. Based on the above results, flow cytometry analyses of CD40-activated PPBL B cells were performed in order to monitor their expression of IgG (Figure 4(a)). It was thus found that a heightened proportion of IgM^-IgD^- B cells correlated quite

precisely with the emergence of IgG^+ B cells. Furthermore, high IgG secretion rates, similar to those observed in control B cells, were observed in CD40-activated B cells from the six PPBL patient samples (Figure 4(b)). Conversely, IgM secretion rates within PPBL B cells were higher than those seen in control B cells, in concordance with the higher proportion of IgM^+ cells. In addition, the capacity of PPBL B cells to switch isotypes and to secrete IgG suggests that their *in vitro* response to CD40 is similar to that of normal B cells. Another proof of the *in vitro* isotype switching capacity of PPBL B cells is in the observed difference between IgM/IgG ratios at days 5 and 14 for cultures in a low interaction CD40-CD154 medium. On day 5, the IgM/IgG ratio of PPBL B cells varied between 6 and 205, whereas at the end of the cultures (day 14), the IgM/IgG ratio was nearly or completely reversed in favour of IgG (0,4 to 3,5) (Figure 5). These observations are in agreement with the reported isotype switching capacity of normal $CD27^+IgD^+IgM^+$ human B cells [35].

(a)

(b)

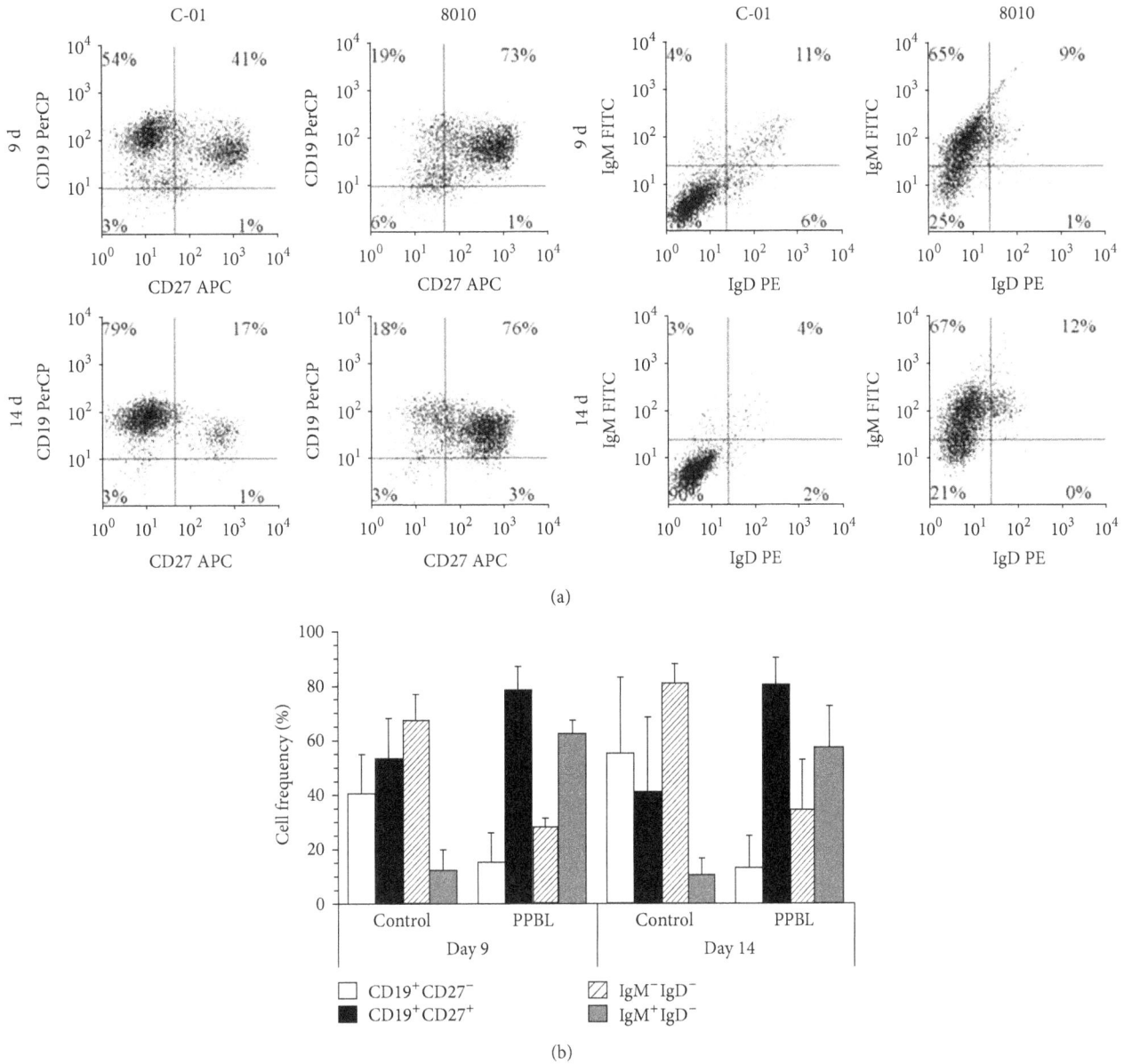

FIGURE 3: Phenotypes of PPBL B cells following low CD154 interaction. CD19, CD27, IgD, and IgM expressions were evaluated by flow cytometry on B cells receiving a low level of CD154 interaction (shown in Figure 2), at days 8 to 9 (9 d) or 13 to 14 (14 d), as indicated. (a) Phenotypic profiles are shown for one control (C-01) and one PPBL sample (8010). (b) The frequencies of cells in the three control samples and the 6 PPBL samples are shown for the main subsets of CD19$^+$CD27$^-$, CD19$^+$CD27$^+$, IgM$^-$IgD$^-$, and IgM$^+$IgD$^-$ cells, as illustrated in. (a) Data is presented as mean ± SD.

4. Discussion

The importance of a functional CD40 molecule in B cell development, proliferation, and immunoglobulin production is well illustrated by the X-linked hyper-IgM syndrome, which is the outcome of an inadequate interaction between CD40 on B lymphocytes and its ligand, CD154, presented by activated T cells [36, 37]. This deficiency affects the interaction between activated CD4$^+$ T cells and all other cell types expressing CD40, namely, B cells, dendritic cells, monocytes/macrophages, platelets, and activated endothelial and epithelial cells. This inherited condition is characterized by a defective class-switch recombination, resulting in normal or increased levels of serum IgM associated with deficiencies of IgG, IgA, and IgE. Moreover, the lymphoid organs of affected individuals are devoid of germinal centres and they are unable to develop memory B cells in response to T-dependent antigens [38]. The characteristics associated with this disorder are partially reminiscent of those observed in patients affected with persistent polyclonal B cell lympho-proliferation. Indeed, patients with PPBL showed elevated serum IgM and polyclonal B cell proliferation. Consequently,

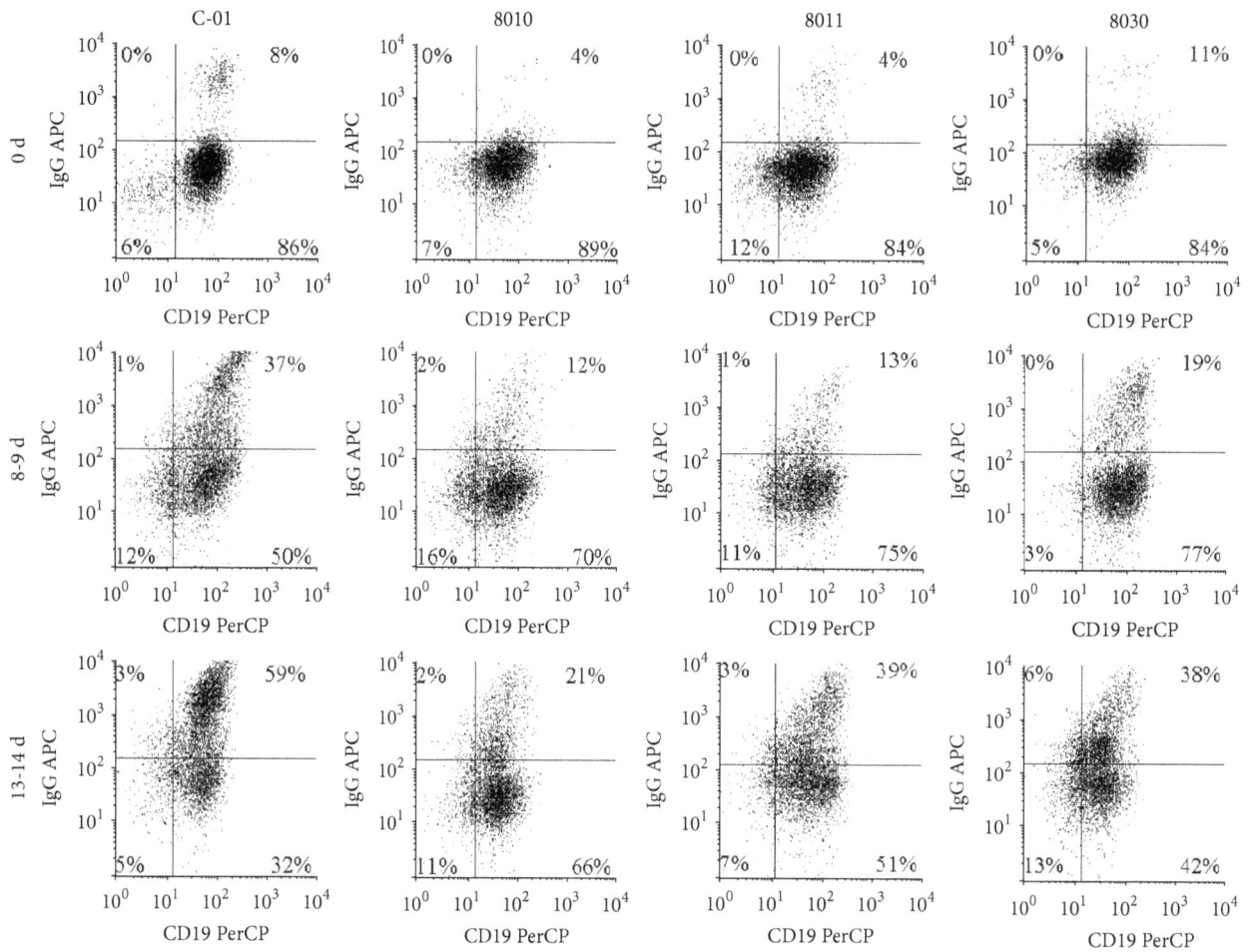

(a)

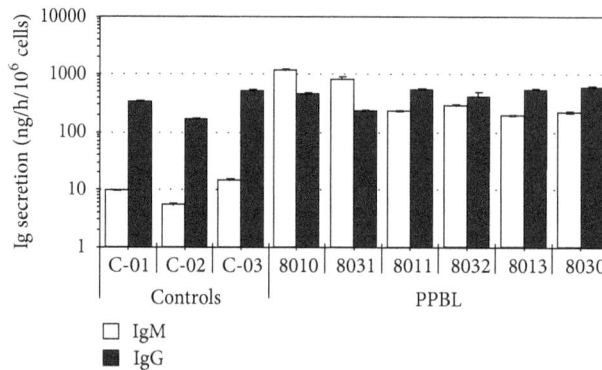

(b)

FIGURE 4: PPBL B cells can morph into IgG secreting cells following long-term CD154 stimulation. B cells stimulated with a low level of CD154 interaction (Figure 2) were analyzed for their ability to express and secrete IgG. (a) The proportion of IgG+ within CD19+ cells before (0 d) and after exposure to a low level of CD154 interaction (8 d and 13 d for 8030 and 9 d and 14 d for 8010 and 8011) was determined by flow cytometry. These phenotypes are representative of the six analyzed samples. (b) IgG and IgM secretion rates were determined at the end of the culture periods on all samples (patients and healthy controls).

we asked ourselves whether or not there was a similar pathophysiology between these two disorders, specifically, a defect in the CD40-CD154 signaling pathway. Although many cases of hyper-IgM syndrome are related to genetic abnormalities affecting CD154 and preventing its interaction with its receptor [39–41], a subset of patients has been described in whom the disorder rather stems from the presence of defects in the CD40-induced B cell activation

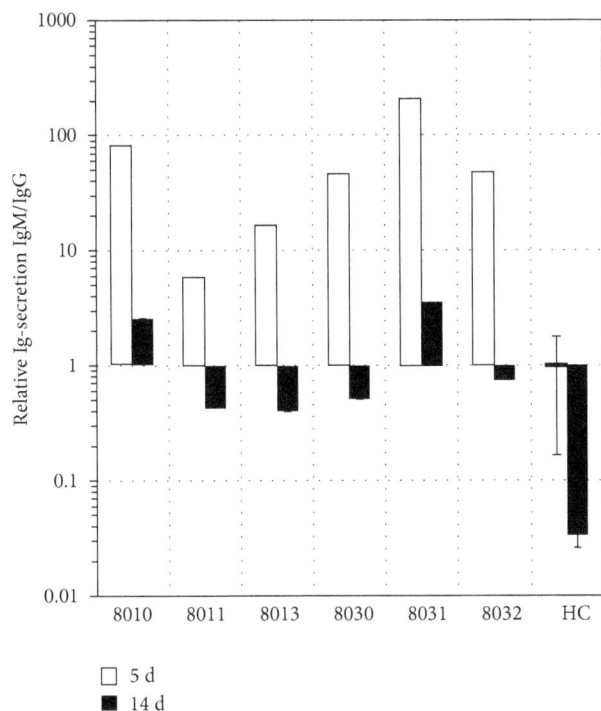

FIGURE 5: Isotype switching during culture of PPBL B cells with low CD154 interaction. The IgG and IgM secretion ratios of PPBL CD19$^+$ cells stimulated with a low level of CD154 interaction were determined by ELISA in supernatant collected after 5 days (5 d) and evaluated on day 14 (14 d), for all patient samples. Four healthy controls submitted to identical culture conditions (HC) were analyzed similarly and data is presented as the mean ± SD.

pathway [42, 43]. When B lymphocytes isolated from this subset of hyper-IgM syndrome patients are stimulated in vitro in the CD40-dependent cell culture system in the presence of an intact ligand, they are still unable to proliferate and undergo immunoglobulin isotype switching. Likewise, we had already demonstrated that B lymphocytes isolated from PPBL patients did not respond to the expansion signal delivered through CD40 when the level of interaction between CD40 and CD154 was high, indicating a possible defect in the CD40 signaling pathway, despite normal expression, sequencing, and tyrosine phosphorylation of CD40 [28]. It was later demonstrated that PPBL B cells were in essence memory B cells harbouring the CD27$^+$IgM$^+$IgD$^+$ immunotype [11, 21]. The peripheral CD19$^+$CD27$^+$ memory B cells from normal individuals were then reported to be unresponsive to high-level CD40 stimulation [29]. However, it has been shown recently that a reduced intensity of CD40-CD154 interaction in the presence of IL-2, IL-4, and IL-10 results in the proliferation, expansion, and immunoglobulin secretion of normal memory CD19$^+$CD27$^+$IgM$^+$ B cells [30]. We thus performed a culture of PPBL B cells in the low-interaction CD40-CD154 medium and obtained a proliferation of the CD19$^+$CD27$^+$IgM$^+$ B cells that was 6 to 20 times higher than that observed with the high CD154 interaction medium. We demonstrated that these lymphocytes were capable of proliferating in vitro in the presence of precise and optimal

culture conditions, that is, a low level of interaction between CD40 and CD154 (3 cells expressing the CD154 ligand for 25 B lymphocytes) in the presence of IL-2, 4, and 10. We can now confirm that PPBL patients did not demonstrate any defect in the CD40-induced signaling pathway.

The following interesting observation was made: the CD19$^+$IgG$^+$ cell population, encompassing globally less than 5% of the cell population at the beginning of the culture in PPBL patients, increased beyond 25% on day 14. Meanwhile, we observed the emergence of a CD19$^+$CD27$^-$ cell population and the disappearance of surface IgD as in normal controls. Such downregulation of IgD is traditionally observed in B cell subsets following their activation within germinal center [44] and is usually associated with further secretion of immunoglobulin. Similarly, when cultured under proper condition, B cells from patients with PPBL showed a heightened proportion of IgM$^-$IgD$^-$ B cells along with an emergence of IgG$^+$ B cells and high immunoglobulin secretion. By dosing immunoglobulin secretion from cultured controls and patients' B cells, we observed a much larger immunoglobulin secretion rate in the low interaction culture system than in the high interaction CD40-CD154 medium. Those results were expected in controls, since we already knew that a low level interaction medium promotes differentiation and secretion of memory B cells whereas a high interaction medium preferentially stimulates proliferation of normal B cells [30]. In the low-level CD40-CD154 interaction medium, we observed much larger IgG and IgM secretion rate from PPBL B cells than from healthy control B cells. We believe that this is attributable to the IgM-rich B lymphocyte subpopulations seen in large quantities, relative to controls, in PPBL patient. It is also possible that PPBL B cells were able to differentiate faster than those from controls.

The high proportion of IgM$^+$IgD$^+$ B cell population and increased IgM levels in PPBL patients suggest a difficulty in normally completing isotype switching. On day 14, immunoglobulin isotype analysis showed higher IgG than IgM levels. These results strongly demonstrate the capacity of in vitro isotype switching of PPBL B cells. We also observed that IgG preferential secretion occurred in the low-level CD40-CD154 medium, thus reinforcing the in vitro isotype switching hypothesis.

5. Conclusion

In summary, we have shown throughout this study that PPBL B cells could proliferate in a CD40-CD154 culture system under proper conditions and that proliferation also results in IgM and IgG secretion, all of which indicating an adequate CD40 signaling pathway. Moreover, this report provides the first evidence of in vitro immunoglobulin isotype switching of CD19$^+$CD27$^+$IgM$^+$ B cells from PPBL, while denoting that this capacity may be impaired in vivo [45]. These results also indicate that these same CD19$^+$CD27$^+$IgM$^+$ B cells are not as abnormal as we initially believed and thus that PPBL may arise, as recently proposed, from a deregulation of the microenvironment [46] or from a defect in a different B cell activation pathway, resulting in extensive proliferation.

Conflict of Interests

There is no conflict of interests for all authors.

Authors' Contribution

Emmanuelle Dugas-Bourdages performed research, analyzed data, and wrote the paper. Sonia Néron designed research, analyzed data, and wrote the paper. Annie Roy performed research. André Darveau designed research, analyzed data, and wrote the paper. Robert Delage designed research, analyzed data, and wrote the paper.

Acknowledgments

This work was supported by a studentship grant to Emmanuelle Dugas-Bourdages from the Leukemia & Lymphoma Society of Canada. The authors are grateful to Dr. Pierre F. Leblond and Phillipe Richer for their help in editing the paper.

References

[1] D. S. Gordon, B. M. Jones, S. W. Browning, T. J. Spira, and D. N. Lawrence, "Persistent polyclonal lymphocytosis of B lymphocytes," *The New England Journal of Medicine*, vol. 307, no. 4, pp. 232–236, 1982.

[2] H. Mossafa, H. Malaure, M. Maynadie et al., "Persistent polyclonal B lymphocytosis with binucleated lymphocytes: a study of 25 cases. Groupe Francais d'Hematologie Cellulaire," *The British Journal of Haematology*, vol. 104, no. 3, pp. 486–493, 1999.

[3] E. Callet-Bauchu, N. Renard, S. Gazzo et al., "Distribution of the cytogenetic abnormality +i(3)(q10) in persistent polyclonal B-cell lymphocytosis: a FICTION study in three cases," *British Journal of Haematology*, vol. 99, no. 3, pp. 531–536, 1997.

[4] E. Cornet, J. F. Lesesve, H. Mossafa et al., "Long-term follow-up of 111 patients with persistent polyclonal B-cell lymphocytosis with binucleated lymphocytes," *Leukemia*, vol. 23, no. 2, pp. 419–422, 2009.

[5] X. Troussard, H. Mossafa, G. Flandrin et al., "Identity between hairy B-cell lymphoproliferative disorder and persistent polyclonal B lymphocytosis?" *Blood*, vol. 90, no. 5, pp. 2110–2113, 1997.

[6] P. Feugier, A. K. De March, J. F. Lesesve et al., "Intravascular bone marrow accumulation in persistent polyclonal lymphocytosis: a misleading feature for B-cell neoplasm," *Modern Pathology*, vol. 17, no. 9, pp. 1087–1096, 2004.

[7] K. C. Carstairs, W. H. Francombe, J. G. Scott, and E. W. Gelfand, "Persistent polyclonal lymphocytosis of B lymphocytes, induced by cigarette smoking?" *The Lancet*, vol. 325, no. 8437, p. 1094, 1985.

[8] P. Casassus, P. Lortholary, H. Komarover, F. Lejeune, and J. Hors, "Cigarette smoking-related persistent polyclonal B lymphocytosis. A premalignant state," *Archives of Pathology and Laboratory Medicine*, vol. 111, no. 11, article 1081, 1987.

[9] M. A. Chan, S. H. Benedict, K. C. Carstairs, W. H. Francombe, and E. W. Gelfand, "Expansion of B lymphocytes with an unusual immunoglobulin rearrangement associated with atypical lymphocytosis and cigarette smoking," *The American Journal of Respiratory Cell and Molecular Biology*, vol. 2, no. 6, pp. 549–552, 1990.

[10] A. Delannoy, D. Djian, G. Wallef et al., "Cigarette smoking and chronic polyclonal B-cell lymphocytosis," *Nouvelle Revue Francaise d'Hematologie*, vol. 35, no. 2, pp. 141–144, 1993.

[11] M. M. Loembe, S. Néron, R. Delage, and A. Darveau, "Analysis of expressed V_H genes in persistent polyclonal B cell lymphocytosis reveals absence of selection in $CD27^+IgM^+IgD^+$ memory B cells," *European Journal of Immunology*, vol. 32, pp. 3678–3688, 2002.

[12] R. Küppers, U. Klein, M.-L. Hansmann, and K. Rajewsky, "Cellular origin of human B-cell lymphomas," *The New England Journal of Medicine*, vol. 341, no. 20, pp. 1520–1529, 1999.

[13] X. Troussard, H. Mossafa, F. Valensi et al., "Polyclonal lymphocytosis with binucleated peripheral lymphocytes. Morphological, immunological, cytogenetic and molecular analysis in 15 cases," *Presse Medicale*, vol. 26, no. 19, pp. 895–899, 1997.

[14] S. Agrawal, E. Matutes, J. Voke, M. J. S. Dyer, T. Khokhar, and D. Catovsky, "Persistent polyclonal B-cell lymphocytosis," *Leukemia Research*, vol. 18, no. 10, pp. 791–795, 1994.

[15] J. Roy, C. Ryckman, V. Bernier, R. Whittom, and R. Delage, "Large cell lymphoma complicating persistent polyclonal B cell lymphocytosis," *Leukemia*, vol. 12, no. 7, pp. 1026–1030, 1998.

[16] E. Lawlor, M. Murray, D. S. O'Briain et al., "Persistent polyclonal B lymphocytosis with Epstein-Barr virus antibodies and subsequent malignant pulmonary blastoma," *Journal of Clinical Pathology*, vol. 44, no. 4, pp. 341–342, 1991.

[17] M. Schmidt-Hieber, T. Burmeister, A. Weimann et al., "Combined automated cell and flow cytometric analysis enables recognition of persistent polyclonal B-cell lymphocytosis (PPBL), a study of 25 patients," *Annals of Hematology*, vol. 87, no. 10, pp. 829–836, 2008.

[18] X. Troussard, E. Cornet, J. F. Lesesve, C. Kourel, and H. Mossafa, "Polyclonal B-cell lymphocytosis with binucleated lymphocytes (PPBL)," *OncoTargets and Therapy*, vol. 1, pp. 59–66, 2008.

[19] R. Delage, L. Jacques, M. Massinga-Loembe et al., "Persistent polyclonal B-cell lymphocytosis: further evidence for a genetic disorder associated with B-cell abnormalities," *British Journal of Haematology*, vol. 114, no. 3, pp. 666–670, 2001.

[20] R. Delage, J. Roy, L. Jacques, V. Bernier, J.-M. Delàge, and A. Darveau, "Multiple bcl-2/Ig gene rearrangements in persistent polyclonal B-cell lymphocytosis," *British Journal of Haematology*, vol. 97, no. 3, pp. 589–595, 1997.

[21] A. Himmelmann, O. Gautschi, M. Nawrath, U. Bolliger, J. Fehr, and R. A. Stahel, "Persistent polyclonal B-cell lymphocytosis is an expansion of functional IgD^+CD27^+ memory B cells," *British Journal of Haematology*, vol. 114, no. 2, pp. 400–405, 2001.

[22] I. Salcedo, A. Campos-Caro, A. Sampalo, E. Reales, and J. A. Brieva, "Persistent polyclonal B lymphocytosis: an expansion of cells showing IgVH gene mutations and phenotypic features of normal lymphocytes from the CD27+ marginal zone B-cell compartment," *British Journal of Haematology*, vol. 116, no. 3, pp. 662–666, 2002.

[23] I. Del Giudice, S. A. Pileri, M. Rossi et al., "Histopathological and molecular features of persistent polyclonal B-cell lymphocytosis (PPBL) with progressive splenomegaly," *British Journal of Haematology*, vol. 144, no. 5, pp. 726–731, 2009.

[24] J.-C. Weill, S. Weller, and C.-A. Reynaud, "Human marginal zone B cells," *Annual Review of Immunology*, vol. 27, pp. 267–285, 2009.

[25] S. G. Tangye and K. L. Good, "Human IgM^+CD27^+ B cells: memory B cells or "memory" B cells?" *The Journal of Immunology*, vol. 179, no. 1, pp. 13–19, 2007.

[26] G. Van Kooten and J. Banchereau, "CD40-CD40 ligand," *Journal of Leukocyte Biology*, vol. 67, no. 1, pp. 2–17, 2000.

[27] J. Banchereau, P. de Paoli, A. Vallé, E. Garcia, and F. Rousset, "Long-term human B cell lines dependent on interleukin-4 and antibody to CD40," *Science*, vol. 251, no. 4989, pp. 70–72, 1991.

[28] M. M. Loembé, J. Lamoureux, N. Deslauriers, A. Darveau, and R. Delage, "Lack of CD40-dependent B-cell proliferation in B lymphocytes isolated from patients with persistent polyclonal B-cell lymphocytosis," *British Journal of Haematology*, vol. 113, no. 3, pp. 699–705, 2001.

[29] J. F. Fecteau and S. Néron, "CD40 stimulation of human peripheral B lymphocytes: distinct response from naïve and memory cells," *Journal of Immunology*, vol. 171, no. 9, pp. 4621–4629, 2003.

[30] S. Néron, C. Racine, A. Roy, and M. Guérin, "Differential responses of human B-lymphocyte subpopulations to graded levels of CD40-CD154 interaction," *Immunology*, vol. 116, no. 4, pp. 454–463, 2005.

[31] J. F. Fecteau, A. Roy, and S. Néron, "Peripheral blood CD27+ IgG+ B cells rapidly proliferate and differentiate into immunoglobulin-secreting cells after exposure to low CD154 interaction," *Immunology*, vol. 128, no. 1, pp. e353–e365, 2009.

[32] S. Néron, L. Thibault, N. Dussault et al., "Characterization of mononuclear cells remaining in the leukoreduction system chambers of apheresis instruments after routine platelet collection: a new source of viable human blood cells," *Transfusion*, vol. 47, no. 6, pp. 1042–1049, 2007.

[33] S. Néron, A. Pelletier, M.-C. Chevrier, G. Monier, R. Lemieux, and A. Darveau, "Induction of LFA-1 independent human B cell proliferation and differentiation by binding of CD40 with its ligand," *Immunological Investigations*, vol. 25, no. 1-2, pp. 79–89, 1996.

[34] S. Weller, M. C. Braun, B. K. Tan et al., "Human blood IgM "memory" B cells are circulating splenic marginal zone B cells harboring a prediversified immunoglobulin repertoire," *Blood*, vol. 104, no. 12, pp. 3647–3654, 2004.

[35] C. Werner-Favre, F. Bovia, P. Schneider et al., "IgG subclass switch capacity is low in switched and in IgM-only, but high in IgD+IgM+, post-germinal center (CD27+) human B cells," *European Journal Immunology*, vol. 31, pp. 243–249, 2001.

[36] V. Lougaris, R. Badolato, S. Ferrari, and A. Plebani, "Hyper immunoglobulin M syndrome due to CD40 deficiency: clinical, molecular, and immunological features," *Immunological Reviews*, vol. 203, pp. 48–66, 2005.

[37] N. S. Longo, P. L. Lugar, S. Yavuz et al., "Analysis of somatic hypermutation in X-linked hyper-IgM syndrome shows specific deficiencies in mutational targeting," *Blood*, vol. 113, no. 16, pp. 3706–3715, 2009.

[38] L. A. Vogel and R. J. Noelle, "CD40 and its crucial role as a member of the TNFR family," *Seminars in Immunology*, vol. 10, no. 6, pp. 435–442, 1998.

[39] R. C. Allen, R. J. Armitage, M. E. Conley et al., "CD40 ligand gene defects responsible for X-linked hyper-IgM syndrome," *Science*, vol. 259, no. 5097, pp. 990–993, 1993.

[40] J. P. DiSanto, J. Y. Bonnefoy, J. F. Gauchat, A. Fischer, and G. de Saint Basile, "CD40 ligand mutations in x-linked immunodeficiency with hyper-IgM," *Nature*, vol. 361, no. 6412, pp. 541–543, 1993.

[41] U. Korthauer, D. Graf, H. W. Mages et al., "Defective expression of T-cell CD40 ligand causes X-linked immunodeficiency with hyper-IgM," *Nature*, vol. 361, no. 6412, pp. 539–541, 1993.

[42] M. E. Conley, M. Larché, V. R. Bonagura et al., "Hyper IgM syndrome associated with defective CD40-mediated B cell activation," *Journal of Clinical Investigation*, vol. 94, no. 4, pp. 1404–1409, 1994.

[43] A. Durandy, C. Hivroz, F. Mazerolles et al., "Abnormal CD40-mediated activation pathway in B lymphocytes from patients with hyper-IgM syndrome and normal CD40 ligand expression," *The Journal of Immunology*, vol. 158, no. 6, pp. 2576–2584, 1997.

[44] V. Pascual, Y.-J. Liu, A. Magalski, O. de Bouteiller, J. Banchereau, and J. D. Capra, "Analysis of somatic mutation in five B cell subsets of human tonsil," *The Journal of Experimental Medicine*, vol. 180, no. 1, pp. 329–339, 1994.

[45] K. Hafraoui, M. Moutschen, J. Smet, F. Mascart, N. Schaaf-Lafontaine, and G. Fillet, "Selective defect of anti-pneumococcal IgG in a patient with persistent polyclonal B cell lymphocytosis," *European Journal of Internal Medicine*, vol. 20, no. 3, pp. e62–e65, 2009.

[46] M. A. Berkowska, C. Grosserichter-Wagener, H. J. Adriaansen et al., "Persistent polyclonal B-cell lymphocytosis: extensively proliferated CD27+IgM+IgD+ memory B cells with a distinctive immunophenotype," *Leukemia*, vol. 28, pp. 1560–1564, 2014.

20

Prevalence and Specificity of RBC Alloantibodies in Indian Patients Attending a Tertiary Care Hospital

Shamsuz Zaman, Rahul Chaurasia, Kabita Chatterjee, and Rakesh Mohan Thapliyal

Department of Transfusion Medicine, All India Institute of Medical Sciences, New Delhi 110029, India

Correspondence should be addressed to Shamsuz Zaman; rxhope@gmail.com

Academic Editor: Meral Beksac

Background. Red blood cell (RBC) alloimmunization results from genetic disparity of RBC antigens between donor and recipients. Data about alloimmunization rate in general patient population is scarce especially from resource limited countries. We undertook this study to determine prevalence and specificity of RBC alloantibodies in patients admitted in various clinical specialties at a tertiary care hospital in North India. *Methods.* Antibody screening was carried out in 11,235 patients on automated QWALYS 3 platform (Diagast, Loos, France). Antibody identification was carried out with an 11-cell identification panel (ID-Diapanel, Diamed GmbH, Switzerland). *Results.* The overall incidence of RBC alloimmunization in transfused patients was 1.4% (157/11235), with anti-E being the most common specificity (36.3%), followed by anti-D (16%), anti-c (6.4%), anti-c + E (6.4%), anti-C + D (5.1%), and anti-K (4.5%). The highest incidence of alloimmunization was observed in hematology/oncology patients (1.9%), whereas in other specialties the range was 0.7–1%. *Conclusion.* As alloimmunization complicates the transfusion outcomes, authors recommend pretransfusion antibody screening and issue of Rh and Kell matched blood to patients who warrant high transfusion requirements in future.

1. Introduction

Red blood cell (RBC) transfusion is a lifesaving therapy for complications of anemia and treatment of the symptoms and signs of hypoxia. However, the risk of RBC alloimmunization is always a concern for patients receiving RBC transfusions [1]. Alloimmunization occurs because of red cells antigenic differences between donor and recipient or between mother and fetus. As no two humans, except identical twins, have the same genetic makeup, blood transfusion exposes the patient to numerous "foreign" antigens. These foreign antigens are potential immunogens which can lead to development of antibodies in the recipient within days, weeks, or months after a transfusion [2].

Alloantibodies may cause hemolytic disease of new born (HDN), hemolytic transfusion reaction (HTR, acute, or delayed), or decrease in the survival of transfused RBCs. Presence of alloantibodies in patients leads to difficulty in finding compatible RBC units and, thus, delay in issuing compatible blood [3]. The prevalence of clinically significant alloantibodies has been reported from less than 0.3% to

up to 60% of samples depending on the study populations and the test method sensitivity [4, 5]. Not uncommonly, autoantibodies can also be found along with alloantibodies which have been reported to be as high as 28% [6]. The concomitant presence of auto- and alloantibodies may further complicate serological workup and add to difficulty in obtaining a suitable crossmatch-compatible blood and may result in further decrement in posttransfusion survival of RBCs [7, 8]. Theoretically, risk of alloimmunization can be significantly decreased by typing the donors' and patients' clinically significant antigens. This extended matching would be an ultimate solution, although the associated costs and logistics will raise serious concerns especially in resource limited countries [3]. Moreover, due to different distribution of blood groups in patient and general population, managing inventory in the face of extended-crossmatching will further pose serious challenges [9].

Previously performed studies have largely concentrated on multiply transfused patient populations or antenatal women [10–14]. Data about relative frequency of RBC alloantibodies in the general patient population receiving occasional RBC transfusions has not been studied extensively. In the current study, we analyzed the prevalence and specificity of RBC alloantibodies in patient population from various clinical specialties by employing automated QWALYS 3 system (Diagast, Loos, France) for antibody screening. Antibody screen-positive samples were further analyzed for their antibody specificity.

2. Material and Methods

Data of antibody screening between years 2012 and 2013 were retrieved from case records at Department of Transfusion Medicine, All India Institute of Medical Sciences, New Delhi, and assessed for the presence of alloantibodies. During the study period all patients for whom routine transfusion requests were received or any incompatibility was reported were included in the study. All cases underwent antibody screening and if found positive were subjected to antibody characterization/identification. All antenatal women and patients with only autoantibodies were excluded from the study. All cardiac surgery, neurosurgery, and trauma patients were also excluded as these specialties are not catered by our transfusion facility.

2.1. Serological Workup. Blood grouping and antibody screening were performed on QWALYS 3 (fully automated system, Diagast, Loos, France) based on Erythrocyte Magnetization Technology. This system uses ABD-Lys and Hemascreen for blood grouping and antibody screening, respectively. The detailed principle and methodology of the system are excellently reviewed by Schoenfeld et al. [15]. Briefly, the system utilizes magnetic hemagglutination and avoids steps of centrifugation and washing. All serum samples positive on automated antibody screen were referred to immunohematology laboratory where antibody identification was performed manually using commercial 11-red cell panel (ID-DiaPanel, BioRad, Switzerland). An autocontrol using the patient's cell and serum was tested in parallel with each screen to exclude presence of autoantibodies.

2.2. Blood Transfusion Protocol. Patients with a negative antibody screen received a transfusion of ABO and Rh(D)-compatible RBCs by an immediate spin crossmatch technique. For alloimmunized patients, antigen-negative, crossmatch-compatible RBCs were transfused. The treating clinicians were informed regarding the presence and nature of alloantibody.

2.3. Statistical Analysis. The analysis and data management were performed using SPSS software version 16 (SPSS, Inc., Chicago, IL, USA).

3. Results

In total, 11235 patients (6573 males and 4662 females, mean age 32.37 years, and range 1–83 years) from various clinical specialties who received packed RBCs were included in the study. Demographic details, ABO and Rh distribution are shown in Table 1. The antibody screen was positive in 215 patients. On further characterization 157 (73%) patients were

TABLE 1: Demographic profile of study population.

	Total patients $n = 11235$	Alloimmunized patients $n = 157$
Gender		
Male	6573	57
Female	4662	100
Age group (years)		
<10	2427	9
11–20	2168	37
21–30	1831	32
31–40	1393	30
41–50	1180	21
51–60	1292	19
>60	944	9
ABO group distribution		
O	3449	56
A	2764	25
B	3910	52
AB	1112	24
Rh group distribution		
Rh D positive	10392	115
Rh D negative	843	42

found to have alloantibodies and 58 (27%) patients with only autoantibodies were excluded from study. Concomitant presence of autoantibodies was found in 9 patients (0.08%). The overall prevalence of RBC alloimmunization was 1.4%. Females had a higher alloimmunization rate of 2.1% versus 0.9% in males; difference was clinically significant ($P < 0.05$). Distribution of patients according to clinical specialties is given in Table 2. The highest number of alloimmunized patients belonged to hematology/oncology group ($n = 118$) with prevalence rate of 1.9%, whereas in other specialties the alloimmunization rate was between 0.7 and 1.0%. A total of 13 different alloantibodies either singly or in combination were identified in 157 patients. Antibodies to the Rh blood group system were the most frequent being present in 120 (76.4%) patients. 19 patients (12.1%) showed presence of multiple alloantibodies. The prevalence of autoantibodies along with alloantibodies was found to be 5.7% ($n = 9$) of total alloimmunized patients. In 12 (7.6%) instances, specificity of antibodies could not be determined. The specificities of alloantibodies identified are shown in Table 3.

4. Discussion

RBC alloimmunization results from the antigenic disparity of red cells between donor and recipient or between mother and fetus. Current standard pretransfusion testing protocols require detection and identification of clinically significant antibodies reacting in antihuman globulin (AHG) phase after incubation at 37°C.

In present study, the overall alloimmunization rate was 1.4% which was low when compared with a study done by

TABLE 2: Distribution of patients according to clinical specialties.

Specialty	Total number of patients	Mean age	Alloimmunized patients	Auto- + alloantibody	Sex M/F
Hematology/oncology	6282	41.6 ± 17.6	118 (1.9%)	7	46/72
Gynecology	964	39.8 ± 18.8	8 (0.8%)	0	0/8
Orthopedics	1575	43.75 ± 14.1	11 (0.7%)	0	5/6
Nephrology/urology	923	33.6 ± 11.7	8 (0.9%)	0	3/5
Gastroenterology/gastrosurgery	908	35.5 ± 12.0	6 (0.7%)	0	1/5
Others	583	30.1 ± 11.2	6 (1%)	2	1/5
Total	11235		157 (1.4%)	9 (0.08%)	

TABLE 3: Specificities of alloantibodies.

Antibody(ies)	Number of patients	Percentage
Alloantibodies		
Anti-c	10	6.4
Anti-C	3	1.9
Anti-c and anti-E	10	6.4
Anti-C + D	8	5.1
Anti-C + D + E	1	0.6
Anti-D	25	16.0
Anti-e	1	0.6
Anti-E	57	36.3
Anti-Fy^a	1	0.6
Anti-Jk^a	3	1.9
Anti-K	7	4.5
Anti-Kp^a	1	0.6
Anti-Le^a	4	2.5
Anti-Lu^a	1	0.6
Anti-M	4	2.5
Auto- + alloantibodies		
Auto- + alloanti-c	2	1.3
Auto- + alloanti-E	3	1.9
Auto- + alloanti-K	3	1.9
Auto- + alloanti-S	1	0.6
Not determined	12	7.6
Total	157	≈100%

Thakral et al. who reported prevalence of 3.4% [16]. This difference could be due to varied study populations. In a similar study in Tehran, prevalence of alloimmunization reported was 0.97% which was comparable to our study [17]. Female patients had higher rate of alloimmunization than male in our study (2.1 versus 0.9%, $P < 0.05$). A systematic review by Verduin et al. also showed that women have slightly higher rate of alloimmunization than men although they categorically state that, based solely on sex difference, results do not justify recommending additional matching for women [18]. The high prevalence of alloimmunization in hematology/oncology (n = 118, 1.9%) could be due to high incidences of RBC antigenic exposures in this group. In other specialties alloimmunization rate ranged from 0.7 to 1.0%. In a similar study, Schonewille also reported that

occasionally transfused patients have alloimmunization rate ranging between 1 and 3% [19]. The most prevalent antibodies in our study were against E (36.3%), D (16.0%), and c (6.4%) and c + E (6.4%), C + D (5.1%), and K (4.5%) antigens. Al-Joudi et al. also reported anti-E as the most common antibody [20]. Study by Thakral et al. also showed 22.2% prevalence of anti-E; however, the most common alloantibody detected by them was anti-c (38.8%) [16]. The differences in antibody specificity could be attributed to the difference in the study population at both centers. In our study of 34 patients with anti-D (either singly or in combination) majority (n = 22) were multiparous females who might have formed anti-D due to previous pregnancies or transfusions. The rest of the 12 patients were transfusion dependent due to underlying medical/oncologic conditions and might have received Rh(D)-incompatible transfusions leading to the formation of anti-D in these patients. The underlying clinical conditions of these 12 multiply transfused patients were thalassemia (n-6), aplastic anemia (n-3), carcinoma (n-2), and AIHA (n-1). A study by Schonewille et al. evaluated alloimmunization in myeloproliferative and lymphoproliferative diseases and reported 4 (7.8%) patients who formed anti-D antibody [1]. Sadeghian et al. studied the development of alloimmunization among Iranian transfusion-dependent thalassemia patients and found that 8 out of 9 alloimmunized patients formed anti-D in the course of the disease with marked preponderance in female patients [21].

Most of the studies done outside India report incidence of anti-K as high as 23% [17, 22, 23]. Low prevalence of anti-K in our study (4.5%) could be due to low frequency of Kell antigen in Indian population (1.97%) as compared to frequency of 8.8% in Caucasian population [24]. Nineteen (12.1%) alloimmunized patients showed presence of multiple antibodies. Al-Joudi et al. also reported multiple antibodies in 23.1% of patients [20]. Since pretransfusion antibody screening in patients' samples is not a routine practice in India, these patients might have received antigen-mismatched blood leading to formation of multiple alloantibodies. Unfortunately, the records of previous transfusions received elsewhere were not available to us. Nine patients (5.7%) had coexisting autoantibodies along with alloantibodies. Ahrens et al. had reported increased risk of autoantibody formation in face of concomitant alloimmunization [6]. We were not able to determine the specificity of antibody(ies) in 12 (7.6%) patients. This may be due to lack of indigenous red cell panels [25]. Salamat et al. also emphasized that red cell panels sourced from local population would be better for detection of antibodies as cell panels from nonindigenous populations may miss certain antibodies against antigens in local population [26]. The frequency of RBC alloantibodies varies considerably depending upon numerous factors, for example, demographics, number of transfusions, pregnancy, genetic constitution, immune competence, disease factors, time and frequency of screening, and sensitivity of the methodology [8, 27]. Although the patients from other specialties were not exempt from the risk of alloantibody formation, we found the highest proportion of alloimmunized patients in hematology/oncology group. The issue of routine antibody screening of all patients requiring transfusion, that too, in resource limited countries is highly debatable [28]. Thus, for prevention of alloimmunization, authors recommend the transfusion of Rh and Kell antigen-matched blood to those patients whose natural history of disease dictates high transfusion requirements in future.

Conflict of Interests

The authors declare that there is no conflict of interests regarding the publication of this paper.

References

[1] H. Schonewille, H. L. Haak, and A. M. van Zijl, "Alloimmunization after blood transfusion in patients with hematologic and oncologic diseases," *Transfusion*, vol. 39, no. 7, pp. 763–771, 1999.

[2] P. W. Jenner and P. V. Holland, *Clinical Practice of Transfusion Medicine*, Edited by: L. D. Petz, S. N. Swisher, S. Kleinman, R. K. Spence, R. G. Strauss, Churchill Livingston, New York, NY, USA, 1996.

[3] S. Zalpuri, J. J. Zwaginga, S. le Cessie, J. Elshuis, H. Schonewille, and J. G. van der Bom, "Red-blood-cell alloimmunization and number of red-blood-cell transfusions," *Vox Sanguinis*, vol. 102, no. 2, pp. 144–149, 2012.

[4] H. Schonewille, L. M. G. Van De Watering, and A. Brand, "Additional red blood cell alloantibodies after blood transfusions in a nonhematologic alloimmunized patient cohort: is it time to take precautionary measures?" *Transfusion*, vol. 46, no. 4, pp. 630–635, 2006.

[5] R. H. Walker, D.-T. Lin, and M. B. Hartrick, "Alloimmunization following blood transfusion," *Archives of Pathology and Laboratory Medicine*, vol. 113, no. 3, pp. 254–261, 1989.

[6] N. Ahrens, A. Pruss, A. Kähne, H. Kiesewetter, and A. Salama, "Coexistence of autoantibodies and alloantibodies to red blood cells due to blood transfusion," *Transfusion*, vol. 47, no. 5, pp. 813–816, 2007.

[7] R. M. Leger and G. Garratty, "Evaluation of methods for detecting alloantibodies underlying warm autoantibodies," *Transfusion*, vol. 39, no. 1, pp. 11–16, 1999.

[8] A. Gharehbaghian, B. Ghezelbash, S. Aghazade, and M. T. Hojjati, "Evaluation of alloimmunization rate and necessity of blood type and screening test among patients candidate for elective surgery," *International Journal of Hematology-Oncology and Stem Cell Research*, vol. 8, no. 1, pp. 1–4, 2014.

[9] C. Tayou Tagny, V. Fongué Fongué, and D. Mbanya, "The erythrocyte phenotype in ABO and Rh blood groups in blood donors and blood recipients in a hospital setting of Cameroon: adapting supply to demand," *Revue Medicale de Bruxelles*, vol. 30, no. 3, pp. 159–162, 2009.

[10] J. Varghese, M. P. Chacko, M. Rajaiah, and D. Daniel, "Red cell alloimmunization among antenatal women attending a tertiary care hospital in south India," *Indian Journal of Medical Research*, vol. 138, no. 2013, pp. 68–71, 2013.

[11] K. J. Moise Jr., "Non-anti-D antibodies in red-cell alloimmunization," *European Journal of Obstetrics & Gynecology and Reproductive Biology*, vol. 92, no. 1, pp. 75–81, 2000.

[12] S. Pahuja, M. Pujani, S. K. Gupta, J. Chandra, and M. Jain, "Alloimmunization and red cell autoimmunization in multitransfused thalassemics of Indian origin," *Hematology*, vol. 15, no. 3, pp. 174–177, 2010.

[13] R. Gupta, D. K. Singh, B. Singh, and U. Rusia, "Alloimmunization to red cells in thalassemics: emerging problem and future strategies," *Transfusion and Apheresis Science*, vol. 45, no. 2, pp. 167–170, 2011.

[14] R. Sood, R. N. Makroo, V. Riana, and N. L. Rosamma, "Detection of alloimmunization to ensure safer transfusion practice," *Asian Journal of Transfusion Science*, vol. 7, no. 2, pp. 135–139, 2013.

[15] H. Schoenfeld, K. Bulling, C. V. Heymann et al., "Evaluation of immunohematologic routine methods using the new erythrocyte-magnetized technology on the QWALYS 2 system," *Transfusion*, vol. 49, no. 7, pp. 1347–1352, 2009.

[16] B. Thakral, K. Saluja, R. R. Sharma, and N. Marwaha, "Red cell alloimmunization in a transfused patient population: a study from a tertiary care hospital in north India," *Hematology*, vol. 13, no. 5, pp. 313–318, 2008.

[17] K. Reyhaneh, G. Ahmad, K. Gharib, V. Vida, K. Raheleh, and T. N. Mehdi, "Frequency & specificity of RBC alloantibodies in patients due for surgery in Iran," *The Indian Journal of Medical Research*, vol. 138, pp. 252–256, 2013.

[18] E. P. Verduin, A. Brand, and H. Schonewille, "Is female sex a risk factor for red blood cell alloimmunization after transfusion? A systematic review," *Transfusion Medicine Reviews*, vol. 26, no. 4, pp. 342.e5–353.e5, 2012.

[19] H. Schonewille, *Red Blood Cell Alloimmunization after Blood Transfusion*, Leiden University Press, 2008.

[20] F. Al-Joudi, A. B. Ali, M. B. Ramli, S. Ahmed, and M. Ismail, "Prevalence and specificities of red cell alloantibodies among blood recipients in the Malaysian State of Kelantan," *Asian Journal of Transfusion Science*, vol. 5, no. 1, pp. 42–45, 2011.

[21] M. H. Sadeghian, M. R. Keramati, Z. Badiei et al., "Alloimmunization among transfusion-dependent thalassemia patients," *Asian Journal of Transfusion Science*, vol. 3, no. 2, pp. 95–98, 2009.

[22] R. Ameen, O. Al-Eyaadi, S. Al-Shemmari, R. Chowdhury, and A. Al-Bashir, "Frequency of red blood cell alloantibody in Kuwaiti population," *Medical Principles and Practice*, vol. 14, no. 4, pp. 230–234, 2005.

[23] N. M. Heddle, R. L. Soutar, P. L. O'Hoski et al., "A prospective study to determine the frequency and clinical significance of alloimmunization post-transfusion," *British Journal of Haematology*, vol. 91, no. 4, pp. 1000–1005, 1995.

[24] N. Agarwal, R. M. Thapliyal, and K. Chatterjee, "Blood group phenotype frequencies in blood donors from a tertiary care hospital in North India," *Blood Research*, vol. 48, no. 1, pp. 51–54, 2013.

[25] R. Chaudhary and N. Agarwal, "Safety of type and screen method compared to conventional antiglobulin crossmatch procedures for compatibility testing in Indian setting," *Asian Journal of Transfusion Science*, vol. 5, no. 2, pp. 157–159, 2011.

[26] N. Salamat, F. A. Bhatti, M. Yaqub, M. Hafeez, and A. Hussain, "Indigenous development of antibody screening cell panels at Armed Forces Institute of Transfusion (AFIT)," *Journal of the Pakistan Medical Association*, vol. 55, no. 10, pp. 439–443, 2005.

[27] E. H. Estey and F. R. Appelbaum, *Leukemia and Related Disorders: Integrated Treatment Approaches*, Humana Press, New York, NY, USA, 2012.

[28] A. Treml and K. E. King, "Red blood cell alloimmunization: lessons from sickle cell disease," *Transfusion*, vol. 53, no. 4, pp. 692–695, 2013.

Absence of Association between *CCR5* rs333 Polymorphism and Childhood Acute Lymphoblastic Leukemia

Carlos Eduardo Coral de Oliveira,[1] **Marla Karine Amarante,**[2] **Aparecida de Lourdes Perim,**[2] **Patricia Midori Murobushi Ozawa,**[1] **Carlos Hiroki,**[1] **Glauco Akelinghton Freire Vitiello,**[1] **Roberta Losi Guembarovski,**[1] **and Maria Angelica Ehara Watanabe**[1]

[1] *Laboratory of Study and Application of DNA Polymorphisms, Department of Pathological Sciences, Biological Sciences Center, State University of Londrina, Rodovia Celso Garcia Cid, (PR 445), Km 380, 86051-970 Londrina, PR, Brazil*
[2] *Laboratory of Hematology, Department of Pathology, Clinical and Toxicological Analysis, Health Sciences Center, State University of Londrina, Londrina, PR, Brazil*

Correspondence should be addressed to Maria Angelica Ehara Watanabe; maewatuel@gmail.com

Academic Editor: Helen A. Papadaki

Acute lymphoblastic leukemia (ALL) is a malignant disorder that originates from one single hematopoietic precursor committed to B- or T-cell lineage. Ordinarily, these cells express CCR5 chemokine receptor, which directs the immune response to a cellular pattern and is involved in cancer pathobiology. The genetic rs333 polymorphism of CCR5 (Δ32), results in a diminished receptor expression, thus leading to impaired cell trafficking. The objective of the present study was to investigate the effect of *CCR5* chemokine receptor rs333 polymorphism in the pathogenesis of ALL. The genotype distribution was studied in 79 patients and compared with 80 control subjects, in a childhood population of Southern Brazil. Genotyping was performed using DNA samples amplified by polymerase chain reaction with sequence-specific primers (PCR-SSP). The homozygous (Δ32/Δ32) deletion was not observed in any subject involved in the study. Heterozygous genotype was not associated with ALL risk (OR 0.7%; 95% CI 0.21–2.32; $P > 0.05$), nor recurrence status of ALL (OR 0.86; 95% CI 0.13–5.48; $P > 0.05$). This work demonstrated, for the first time, no significant differences in the frequency of the CCR5/Δ32 genotype between ALL and control groups, indicating no effect of this genetic variant on the ALL susceptibility and recurrence risk.

1. Introduction

Leukemia is the most common childhood cancer, although overall incidence is rare. Within this population, acute lymphoblastic leukemia (ALL) occurs approximately five times more frequently than acute myelogenous leukemia (AML) and accounts for approximately 78% of all childhood leukemia diagnoses [1]. In Brazil, the National Cancer Institute (INCA) estimated 9,370 new cases of leukemia in 2014, with the highest age incidence of 1–4 years [2].

The specific biological and molecular mechanisms that account for the aggressiveness and poor therapy response of some ALL cases remain to be elucidated. Once chemokines and their receptors have been discovered as essential and selective mediators in leukocyte migration to inflammatory sites and to secondary lymphoid organs, it is reasonable that they also play a critical role in tumor initiation, promotion, and progression [3, 4]. Moreover, updated research indicates that cancer cells subvert the normal chemokine system, and these molecules and their receptors become important constituents of the tumor microenvironment with very different ways to exert tumor-promoting roles [5].

The CC chemokine receptor 5 (CCR5) belongs to the trimeric guanine nucleotide-binding-protein-coupled seven-transmembrane receptor superfamily, which comprises the largest superfamily of human proteins [6]. It exerts its activity via G protein and binds to the chemokines RANTES (CCL5), MIP-1α (CCL3), and MIP-1β (CCL4) [7]. This receptor is involved in the chemotaxis of leucocytes to inflammation sites [8] and plays important function in the recruitment of macrophages, T cells, and monocytes [9].

The importance of CCR5 for immune response is dependent on the type of stimuli; moreover, in some cases, compensating mechanisms override the absence of CCR5 expression and function. Noteworthy, CCR5 may exert a far more important role in the immune response than in immune cells traffic regulation [10].

It has been shown that CCR5 expression in stromal cells as well as hematopoietic cells contributes to tumor metastasis. For instance, CCR5 is involved in chondrosarcomas metastasization [11] and oral cancer cells migration [12]. Its expression correlates with multiple myeloma cell growth, bone marrow homing, and osteolysis [13].

Aster and colleagues [14] showed that T-cell ALL is a disease primarily caused by aberrant activation of the NOTCH1 signaling pathway. In this context, expression and function of important chemokine receptors, such as CCR5 and CCR9, are partially controlled by the oncogenic NOTCH1 isoform in T-cell ALL, regulating blast malignant properties and localization of extramedullary infiltrations [15].

Additionally, CCR5 has been related to play a key role in metastasis of aggressive NK-cells leukemia to the liver of patients, contributing to hepatosplenomegaly and hepatic failure [16, 17]. Also, Davies et al. [18] showed that the G allele of rs1799987 polymorphism in *CCR5* was associated with more favorable minimal residual disease status than the A allele when comparing "best" and "worst" risk groups of B-cell ALL, adjusted for prognostic features. Considering the lower activity of *CCR5* promoter in the presence of this polymorphism [19], this evidence indicated that both acquired and host genetics influence response to cancer therapy. Thus, it is plausible that CCR5 might play a role in ALL pathogenesis and prognosis.

It is known that the polymorphism rs333 in *CCR5*, a common 32-base pair deletion (Δ32), causes truncation and loss of this receptor on lymphoid cell surface, with complete retention in the endoplasmic reticulum within homozygous or diminished expression in heterozygous genotype [20]. The *CCR5* studies have demonstrated the importance of Δ32 mutation, particularly in the susceptibility to HIV infection [21], since CCR5 is a coreceptor in the primary stage of infection that is essential for the AIDS onset [22].

Our research group has reported polymorphic allelic variants related to the immune system and tumor development in different cancer types. Nevertheless, there are no data relating *CCR5*/Δ32 polymorphism to ALL population. In this context, the present work analyzed rs333 polymorphism of *CCR5* in ALL patients from the southern region of Brazil.

2. Materials and Methods

2.1. Human Subjects. Following approval from the Human Ethics Committee of the State University of Londrina,

Paraná, Brazil (CAAE number 171231134.0000.5231), inclusion of the individuals to the study was conditioned by an obtained written informed consent form from parents regarding the use of their children and adolescents blood samples. Seventy-nine ALL patients were enrolled and diagnostic criteria were based on the guidelines proposed by Hematology Department of the University Hospital of Londrina. Recurrence risk status of ALL patients was evaluated through the GBTLI Protocol (Brazilian Group of Childhood Leukemia Treatment Protocol-99) which is based on the Cancer Therapy Evaluation Program, proposed by the National Cancer Institute, and takes into account age at diagnosis, leukocyte count, immunophenotyping, involvement of tissues other than bone marrow, and responsiveness to treatment. The control group is comprised of 80 healthy individuals free of neoplasia, matched by age and gender.

2.2. Genomic DNA Extraction. Genomic DNA was extracted from whole blood by Biopur Mini Spin Plus Kit (Biometrix Diagnostica, Curitiba, Brazil), according to the manufacturer's instructions. DNA was eluted in 50 μL of milliQ water and quantified by NanoDrop 2000c spectrophotometer (Thermo Fisher Scientific Inc., Wilmington, USA) at a wavelength of 260/280 nm. Final preparation was stored at −20°C and used as templates in polymerase chain reactions (PCR).

2.3. Optimization of PCR for CCR5. The method of genotyping (rs333) was optimized in the Laboratory of Study and Application of DNA Polymorphisms of the State University of Londrina using genomic DNA and specific primers for *CCR5*: *Primer sense*: 5′ ACC AGA TCT CAA AAA GAA 3′ and *Primer antisense*: 5′ CAT GAT GGT GAA GAT AAG CCT CA 3′ (GenBank accession AF009962). Genotyping of CCR5 was determined by PCR-SSP. The samples were amplified using 1.25 units of Taq polymerase (Invitrogen, Carlsbad, USA) in a Mastercycler Gradient Thermal Cycler (Eppendorf, Hamburg, Germany). PCR conditions were: denaturation step at 94°C for 5 min, 35 cycles of 1 min at 94°C, 1 min at 58°C and 1 min at 72°C, and 10 min of elongation at 72°C. PCR products (225 bp or 193 bp) were analyzed on polyacrylamide gel (10%), stained with silver nitrate (AgNO₃).

2.4. Statistical Analysis. Contingency tables and Fisher's exact test were used to calculate differences in genotype distributions and allele frequencies. $P < 0.05$ was considered to indicate a statistically significant difference. Goodness of fit of Hardy-Weinberg equilibrium was tested by calculating the expected frequencies of each genotype and comparing them with the observed value using a chi-square test.

3. Results

The distribution of *CCR5* alleles in both ALL and control groups was in accordance with the assumption of Hardy-Weinberg equilibrium ($P > 0,05$). The mean age of controls and ALL patients was 10.8 years ± 5.65 and 8.7 years ± 6.20, respectively, all of whom were predominantly from Caucasoid population, due to European colonization.

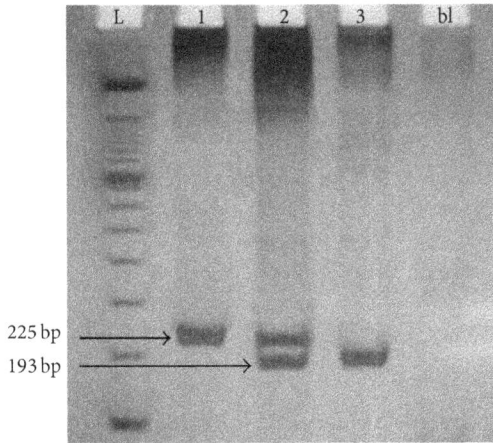

FIGURE 1: *CCR5* genotype profile. The PCR products were detected using silver staining method after polyacrylamide gel electrophoresis. *Lane* L: DNA Ladder 100 bp; *lane* 1: CCR5 wild-type homozygous genotype (CCR5/CCR5, 225 bp); *lane* 2: heterozygous genotype (CCR5/Δ32, 225 bp, and 193 bp); and *lane* 3: variant allele homozygous genotype (Δ32/Δ32, 193 bp); bl represents blank reaction (without DNA).

TABLE 1: Genotype distribution of *CCR5* rs333 polymorphism and recurrence risk status analysis in ALL and control groups.

| | Genotypes | | OR | 95% CI | P^* |
	CCR5/CCR5	CCR5/Δ32			
Control (80)	73 (91.25%)	7 (8.75%)	0.7	0.21–2.32	0.76
ALL (79)	74 (92.5%)	5 (7.5%)			
High risk (50)	47 (94%)	3 (6%)	0.86	0.13–5.48	1.00
Low risk (29)	27 (93.1%)	2 (6.9%)			

*Fisher's exact test, $P > 0.05$. OR: odds ratio; CI: confidence interval.

The patients and controls were matched for sex and gender, although there was a modest higher frequency of males in ALL group (53.16%) than in controls (48.75%). Fifty (63.29%) ALL patients were classified in high recurrence risk group and 29 (36.71%) in low recurrence risk group. The possible observed genotypes for *CCR5* rs333 polymorphism are shown in Figure 1.

Genotyping results did not show any homozygous individuals for Δ32 deletion in both groups. The heterozygous CCR5/Δ32 genotypes were observed in 8.75% ($n = 7$) of controls and 7.5% ($n = 5$) of ALL patients. To determine if there was a statistically significant increased risk of ALL development related to the *CCR5* genotypes, we conducted logistic regression analysis (Table 1), which showed that individuals with one copy of Δ32 variant allele did not exhibit ALL-associated risk. No statistical difference was observed when allelic frequency of Δ32 at rs333 in ALL patients was associated with control subjects (OR = 0.71; 95%CI = 0.22–2.30; $P = 0.77$).

In addition, we compared the *CCR5* genotype distribution in ALL patients classified in high risk or low risk, according to recurrence status. From five (7.5%) ALL Δ32 carriers, three were classified as high-risk patients. However,

association study between both recurrence statuses did not reach statistical significance.

The *CCR5* genotypes distribution in ALL patients and controls was stratified by gender. Subgroup analyses revealed that the effect of gender was not significantly different among *CCR5* genotypes (female ALL versus female control, OR = 0.52; 95%CI = 0.09–3.07, and male ALL versus male control, OR = 0.97; 95%CI = 0.18–5.14).

4. Discussion

Chemokines and their receptors are key regulators of immune activities and in parallel could play conflicting roles in malignancy. While most combinations of these receptors and chemokines are active in cancer, many findings in the field have emphasized the chemokine CCL5 and its cognate receptor CCR5 [23].

The gene variants of the chemokine and chemokine receptor genes associated with inflammation may be involved in cancer initiation and progression [24]. Considering the remarkable difference in CCR5/Δ32 allele frequency among worldwide populations, we aimed to survey the genetic variations in *CCR5* in ALL patients and control individuals.

The patients' age in this study was the expected for ALL, which is frequent in children and younger patients. Moreover, as previously mentioned, both sample groups were composed predominantly of Caucasian individuals from Southern Brazil. However, due to high degree of miscegenation of Brazilian population and the demand to use genetic markers for correct characterization of individuals [25, 26] in our country, these data have not been explored in relation to the variants analyzed.

Chemokines and chemokine receptors are among factors that may influence ALL progression and localization [15]. A 32-base pair nucleic acid deletion in *CCR5* exists and causes a frameshift mutation in the amino acids comprising the second extracellular loop. This deletion leads to premature truncation of the protein, disabling its ability to translocate to the membrane, impairing expression and ligand binding at the cell surface, and causing membrane receptor deficiency that may influence leukocyte trafficking [27].

Based on this, we hypothesized that the ability of CCR5 to bind its ligands and signal recruitment of pathogenic T cells into target tissues may be impaired, thus imparting ALL protection. Although there were no differences in the frequency of CCR5/CCR5 and CCR5/Δ32 genotypes between patient and control groups, the variant genotype had no effect on the ALL susceptibility.

These results corroborated with studies in different disorders, such as leishmaniasis, breast, laryngeal, thyroid, and brain carcinoma, which also identified no differences in the frequency of these alleles among healthy subjects and patients of Southern Brazilian population [28–30] and worldwide [31–33].

Intensive multiagent chemotherapy regimens and introduction of risk-stratified therapy have substantially improved cure rates for children with ALL. Current risk allocation schemas are imperfect, as some children are classified as lower-risk and treated with less intensive therapy relapse, while others deemed higher-risk are probably overtreated [34]. In this context, genetic polymorphisms in chemokine receptors could predict outcome and be considered an independent risk factor to stratify and allocate therapy in ALL.

More than half of the patients with ALL were classified in higher-risk group, according to the clinical and laboratory findings at diagnosis, as defined by GBTLI LLA-99 protocol [2]. When the genotype data were analyzed for stratified group of ALL, the results indicated that the presence of Δ32 did not influence this clinical parameter. Similarly, a recent study conducted by our research group has not found association among tumor suppressor *TP53* and chemokine *CXCL12* polymorphisms and ALL recurrence risk status [35].

5. Conclusion

The comprehension about cellular and molecular mechanisms of ALL is critically important for the development of new approaches to hematological neoplasia treatment. Although any association of rs333 polymorphism of *CCR5* was verified, we believe that the current research must lead to a better definition of the host-tumor relationship particularly with respect to immunologic response and interrelation of CCR5 and ALL development. Given the sample size of the present case-control association study, strong conclusions are not possible; however, future investigation involving much larger cases may determine the absence of clinical implications for CCR5/Δ32 alleles in relation to ALL pathogenesis.

Conflict of Interests

The authors declare that there is no conflict of interests regarding the publication of this paper.

Acknowledgments

The authors would like to acknowledge the volunteers who made this study possible, the University Hospital of Londrina, and Londrina Cancer Institute, PR, Brazil, for their collaboration. This study was supported by Conselho Nacional de Desenvolvimento Científico e Tecnológico (CNPq), Coordenação de Aperfeiçoamento de Pessoal de Nível Superior (CAPES), Fundação Araucária do Paraná, Secretaria da Ciência, Tecnologia e Ensino Superior (SETI), Fundo Estadual para a Infância e Adolescência (FIA/PR) e Secretaria da Família e Desenvolvimento Social (SEDS), and Coordination of Undergraduate Studies of Londrina State University (PROPPG-UEL).

References

[1] M. Belson, B. Kingsley, and A. Holmes, "Risk factors for acute leukemia in children: a review," *Environmental Health Perspectives*, vol. 115, no. 1, pp. 138–145, 2007.

[2] INCA, *Estimate 2014: Cancer Incidence in Brazil*, INCA, Rio de Janeiro, Brazil, 2013.

[3] F. Balkwill, "Cancer and the chemokine network," *Nature Reviews Cancer*, vol. 4, no. 7, pp. 540–550, 2004.

[4] J. Vandercappellen, J. Van Damme, and S. Struyf, "The role of CXC chemokines and their receptors in cancer," *Cancer Letters*, vol. 267, no. 2, pp. 226–244, 2008.

[5] D. Aldinucci and A. Colombatti, "The inflammatory chemokine CCL5 and cancer progression," *Mediators of Inflammation*, vol. 2014, Article ID 292376, 12 pages, 2014.

[6] C. J. Raport, J. Gosling, V. L. Schweickart, P. W. Gray, and I. F. Charo, "Molecular cloning and functional characterization of a novel human CC chemokine receptor (CCR5) for RANTES, MIP-1β, and MIP-1α," *Journal of Biological Chemistry*, vol. 271, no. 29, pp. 17161–17166, 1996.

[7] M. Samson, O. Labbe, C. Mollereau, G. Vassart, and M. Parmentier, "Molecular cloning and functional expression of a new human CC-chemokine receptor gene," *Biochemistry*, vol. 35, no. 11, pp. 3362–3367, 1996.

[8] P. Proost, A. Wuyts, and J. van Damme, "The role of chemokines in inflammation," *Clinical and Experimental Medicine*, vol. 26, no. 4, pp. 211–223, 1996.

[9] P. Spagnolo, E. A. Renzoni, A. U. Wells et al., "C-C chemokine receptor 5 gene variants in relation to lung disease in sarcoidosis," *American Journal of Respiratory and Critical Care Medicine*, vol. 172, no. 6, pp. 721–728, 2005.

[10] E.-M. Weiss, A. Schmidt, D. Vobis et al., "Foxp3-mediated suppression of cd95l expression confers resistance to activation-induced cell death in regulatory T cells," *Journal of Immunology*, vol. 187, no. 4, pp. 1684–1691, 2011.

[11] C.-H. Tang, A. Yamamoto, Y.-T. Lin, Y.-C. Fong, and T.-W. Tan, "Involvement of matrix metalloproteinase-3 in CCL5/CCR5 pathway of chondrosarcomas metastasis," *Biochemical Pharmacology*, vol. 79, no. 2, pp. 209–217, 2010.

[12] J.-Y. Chuang, W.-H. Yang, H.-T. Chen et al., "CCL5/CCR5 axis promotes the motility of human oral cancer cells," *Journal of Cellular Physiology*, vol. 220, no. 2, pp. 418–426, 2009.

[13] E. Menu, E. De Leenheer, H. De Raeve et al., "Role of CCR1 and CCR5 in homing and growth of multiple myeloma and in the development of osteolytic lesions: a study in the 5TMM model," *Clinical and Experimental Metastasis*, vol. 23, no. 5-6, pp. 291–300, 2006.

[14] J. C. Aster, W. S. Pear, and S. C. Blacklow, "Notch signaling in leukemia," *Annual Review of Pathology: Mechanisms of Disease*, vol. 3, pp. 587–613, 2008.

[15] L. Mirandola, M. Chiriva-Internati, D. Montagna et al., "Notch1 regulates chemotaxis and proliferation by controlling the CC-chemokine receptors 5 and 9 in T cell acute lymphoblastic leukaemia," *Journal of Pathology*, vol. 226, no. 5, pp. 713–722, 2012.

[16] H. Makishima, T. Ito, N. Asano et al., "Significance of chemokine receptor expression in aggressive NK cell leukemia," *Leukemia*, vol. 19, no. 7, pp. 1169–1174, 2005.

[17] H. Makishima, T. Ito, K. Momose et al., "Chemokine system and tissue infiltration in aggressive NK-cell leukemia," *Leukemia research*, vol. 31, no. 9, pp. 1237–1245, 2007.

[18] S. M. Davies, M. J. Borowitz, G. L. Rosner et al., "Pharmacogenetics of minimal residual disease response in children with B-precursor acute lymphoblastic leukemia: a report from the children's oncology group," *Blood*, vol. 111, no. 6, pp. 2984–2990, 2008.

[19] D. H. McDermott, P. A. Zimmerman, F. Guignard, C. A. Kleeberger, S. F. Leitman, and P. M. Murphy, "CCR5 promoter polymorphism and HIV-1 disease progression," *The Lancet*, vol. 352, no. 9131, pp. 866–870, 1998.

[20] M. Chelli and M. Alizon, "Determinants of the trans-dominant negative effect of truncated forms of the CCR5 chemokine receptor," *Journal of Biological Chemistry*, vol. 276, no. 50, pp. 46975–46982, 2001.

[21] E. M. V. Reiche, M. A. E. Watanabe, A. M. Bonametti et al., "Frequency of CCR5-Δ32 deletion in human immunodeficiency virus type 1 (HIV-1) in healthy blood donors, HIV-1-exposed seronegative and HIV-1-seropositive individuals of southern Brazilian population," *International Journal of Molecular Medicine*, vol. 22, no. 5, pp. 669–675, 2008.

[22] A. P. Galvani and J. Novembre, "The evolutionary history of the CCR5-Delta32 HIV-resistance mutation," *Microbes and Infection*, vol. 7, no. 2, pp. 302–309, 2005.

[23] P. Weitzenfeld and A. Ben-Baruch, "The chemokine system, and its CCR5 and CXCR4 receptors, as potential targets for personalized therapy in cancer," *Cancer Letters*, 2013.

[24] C. Kucukgergin, F. K. Isman, S. Dasdemir et al., "The role of chemokine and chemokine receptor gene variants on the susceptibility and clinicopathological characteristics of bladder cancer," *Gene*, vol. 511, no. 1, pp. 7–11, 2012.

[25] V. R. Arruda, C. E. Grignolli, M. S. Gonçalves et al., "Prevalence of homozygosity for the deleted alleles of glutathione S-transferase mu (GSTM1) and theta (GSTT1) among distinct ethnic groups from Brazil: relevance to enviromental carcinogenesis?" *Clinical Genetics*, vol. 54, no. 3, pp. 210–214, 1998.

[26] F. C. Parra, R. C. Amado, J. R. Lambertucci et al., "Color and genomic ancestry in Brazilians," *Proceedings of the National Academy of Sciences of the United States of America*, vol. 100, no. 1, pp. 177–182, 2003.

[27] J. S. Maier-Moore, C. A. Cañas, G. Tobón et al., "The CCR5 delta 32 polymorphism (rs333) is not associated with Sjogren's syndrome or type 1 diabetes in colombians," *Clinical Immunology*, vol. 148, no. 2, pp. 206–208, 2013.

[28] S. M. Muxel, S. D. Borelli, M. K. Amarante et al., "Association study of CCR5 delta 32 polymorphism among the HLA-DRB1 Caucasian population in northern Paraná, Brazil," *Journal of Clinical Laboratory Analysis*, vol. 22, no. 4, pp. 229–233, 2008.

[29] K. Brajão de Oliveira, E. M. Vissoci Reiche, H. Kaminami Morimoto et al., "Analysis of the CC chemokine receptor 5 delta32 polymorphism in a Brazilian population with cutaneous leishmaniasis," *Journal of Cutaneous Pathology*, vol. 34, no. 1, pp. 27–32, 2007.

[30] M. N. Aoki, A. C. D. S. do Amaral Herrera, M. K. Amarante, J. L. do Val Carneiro, M. H. P. Fungaro, and M. A. E. Watanabe, "CCR5 and p53 codon 72 gene polymorphisms: implications in breast cancer development," *International Journal of Molecular Medicine*, vol. 23, no. 3, pp. 429–435, 2009.

[31] N. Degerli, E. Yilmaz, and F. Bardakci, "The Δ32 allele distribution of the CCR5 gene and its relationship with certain cancers in a Turkish population," *Clinical Biochemistry*, vol. 38, no. 3, pp. 248–252, 2005.

[32] K. Guleria, S. Sharma, M. Manjari et al., "p.R72P, PIN3 Ins16bp polymorphisms of TP53 and CCR5?32 in north Indian breast cancer patients," *Asian Pacific Journal of Cancer Prevention*, vol. 13, no. 7, pp. 3305–3311, 2012.

[33] A. Zafiropoulos, N. Crikas, A. M. Passam, and D. A. Spandidos, "Significant involvement of CCR2-64I and CXCL12-3a in the development of sporadic breast cancer," *Journal of Medical Genetics*, vol. 41, no. 5, p. e59, 2004.

[34] D. T. Teachey and S. P. Hunger, "Predicting relapse risk in childhood acute lymphoblastic leukaemia," *British Journal of Haematology*, vol. 162, no. 5, pp. 606–620, 2013.

[35] A. de Lourdes Perim, R. L. Guembarovski, J. M. Oda et al., "CXCL12 and TP53 genetic polymorphisms as markers of susceptibility in a Brazilian children population with acute lymphoblastic leukemia (ALL)," *Molecular Biology Reports*, vol. 40, no. 7, pp. 4591–4596, 2013.

22

Hypertransfusion Therapy in Sickle Cell Disease in Nigeria

Ademola Samson Adewoyin and Jude Chike Obieche

Department of Haematology and Blood Transfusion, University of Benin Teaching Hospital, PMB 1111, Benin City, Edo State, Nigeria

Correspondence should be addressed to Ademola Samson Adewoyin; drademola@yahoo.com

Academic Editor: Peter Bader

Introduction. Hypertransfusion refers to chronic blood transfusion therapy aimed at ameliorating disease complications in various haemopathies particularly the haemoglobinopathies. In sickle cell disease, hypertransfusion is aimed at maintaining patient's haemoglobin level at 10 to 11 g/dL using haemoglobin AA blood and its resultant dilutional effect on sickle haemoglobin is sustained by intermittent long-term transfusions. *Aim and Objective*. This paper highlights hypertransfusion and its privileged position as a secondary measure in prevention and treatment of sickle cell disease, especially in the Nigerian context. *Materials and Methods*. Relevant literatures were searched on PubMed, Google Scholar and standard texts in haematology and transfusion medicine. Keywords used in the search are hypertransfusion, sickle cell disease, chronic transfusion, and Nigeria. Literatures gathered were reviewed, summarized, and presented in this paper. *Result*. Immense clinical benefit is associated with hypertransfusion therapy including prevention of stroke and amelioration of severe sickle cell disease especially in transplant ineligible patients. Careful patient selections, appropriate blood component, and prevention of transfusion hazards as well as oversight function of an experienced haematologist are pertinent to a successful hypertransfusion therapy. *Conclusion*. Improved knowledge of the benefits and practice of hypertransfusion will effectively translate into improved health status even among Nigerian sickle cell disease patients.

1. Introduction

Sickle cell disease (SCD) is the commonest monogenetic disease worldwide and its greatest burden is found in Sub-Saharan Africa especially Nigeria [1, 2]. In most parts of West Africa, the prevalence of sickle cell trait ranges between 10 and 40% of the population [3]. However, in some areas in Uganda, prevalence has been reported to be as high as 45% while in Nigeria about 20 to 30% of the population are trait carriers [4, 5]. A recent survey in South-south Nigeria revealed that about 2.39% of the population is affected by sickle cell disease [6]. In Africa, significant morbidity and mortality are still associated with the disease, hence the need for effective and definite control measures [7, 8].

Care and treatment of SCD patients require expertise commitment, as well as a wide array of therapeutic and prophylactic measures including adequate analgesia, anticoagulation as indicated, transfusion of requisite blood components when necessary, haemopoietic stem cell transplantation, oxygen therapy when needed, routine prophylactic medications (antimalarial, multivitamins supplements, low dose aspirin, and antioxidants), hydroxyurea therapy, adequate hydration, and immunization against infectious pathogens especially in early childhood. Moreover, care of SCD patients requires a multispecialist team including haematologists, orthopedic surgeons, plastic surgeons, urologists, nephrologists, specialist nurses, counselors, and medical social workers [9].

Carrier detection and genetic counseling have been recommended by World Health Organization for the control of SCD [10]. In Nigeria, efforts at public education on sickle cell disease and its prevention as well as carrier detection with genetic counseling have not made sufficient far reaching improvements in sickle cell disease control. There is still a palpable dearth of public knowledge about sickle cell disease [11–14]. Studies have also shown the option of selective abortion following prenatal diagnosis to be unacceptable to a significant proportion of persons [15, 16]. At the primary prevention level, there are currently no functional nationwide neonatal screening policies or programs for early detection and optimal treatment. Though it is expected that a country like Nigeria with very high prevalence of sickle cell trait should have a nationwide program at all levels of care for control and care of sickle cell disease, available evidence suggests that effective control of SCD in Nigeria is still largely infantile.

Apart from premarital counseling and continuous medical education, a number of other strategies including chronic transfusion have been scientifically proven to reduce complications and improve quality of life in SCD patients. This work therefore is aimed at collecting and summarizing available information on the practice and utilization of hypertransfusion in the care of SCD patients in Nigeria.

2. Hypertransfusion Therapy in Sickle Cell Disease

Hypertransfusion refers to a chronic blood transfusion regimen with therapeutic intention of reducing sickle haemoglobin levels over a long period of time [17, 18]. Generally, blood transfusion in medicine entails safe transfer and infusion of blood components into an individual to meet specific physiological needs. Such needs include improving haemoglobin level for better tissue oxygenation, replacement of deficient coagulation factors, and platelet transfusions [19, 20]. Transfusion modalities in SCD include top up (simple), exchange, and chronic blood transfusions. The different transfusion plans have specific benefits in various clinical scenarios in SCD.

Traditionally, transfusion in sickle cell disease was carried out only in emergencies until the early 1980s when the benefits of chronic transfusion began to gain clinical appreciation [21]. Approach to hypertransfusion may be the conservative transfusion therapy aimed at maintaining haemoglobin level around 10 to 11 g/dL with about 50% reduction in haemoglobin S level or the aggressive approach aimed at reducing sickle haemoglobin level below 30% [22]. The goal of hypertransfusion in sickle cell disease is to reduce the level of circulating haemoglobin S below a target level for prevention and treatment of disease complications associated with sickle haemoglobinopathies. Red cell transfusion also serves to correct the attendant anaemia in SCD, suppress endogenous erythropoiesis, and reduce haemolysis. Hypertransfusion has been found to effectively mitigate the complications of sickle cell anaemia in some randomized studies [23–28]. It is well-established that there is a high correlation between disease manifestations and level of circulating haemoglobin S [29]. The bulk of the disease burden is due to high percentage of sickle haemoglobin within the red cells and the plasma sickle haemoglobin levels.

As a rule, transfusion therapy in sickle cell disease is carried out with haemoglobin AA blood. Besides reducing the level of circulating haemoglobin S, exogenous supply of haemoglobin AA red cells also suppresses endogenous erythropoiesis, thereby suppressing intrinsic sickle haemoglobin

levels. The primary event in sickle cell disease pathogenesis is deoxyhaemoglobin precipitation. Normal red cells contain about 200–300 million soluble haemoglobin A molecules. However, red cells in sickle cell disease contain high level (80–90%) of the less soluble sickle haemoglobin which crystallizes out of solution under low oxygen tension. Under conditions of low oxygen tension (PaO_2 less than 35–40 mmHg), haemoglobin S molecules undergo nucleation with progressive polymerization of haemoglobin molecules and eventual crystallization into tactoids with seven double strands which cross-links. This gives rise to the crescent shape appearance of the sickled red cells on blood cytology. With reoxygenation, the polymers dissolve. However, with repeated deoxygenation and reoxygenation in different vascular beds, the red cells permanently acquire a sickle shape. This is termed irreversible sickle red cells (ISCs) when seen on peripheral blood smear. Again, the percentage of ISCs has been shown to correlate directly with severity of haemolysis and inversely with frequency and severity of vasoocclusive crisis [30–32].

At the molecular level, there is substitution of valine for glutamate at position 6 of the beta sickle haemoglobin chain due to the single base change from adenine to thymidine. The resultant HbS exposes a hydrophobic patch under low oxygen tension and interactions between these patches lead to nucleation and eventual polymerization [30]. ISCs are less deformable and more prone to fragmentation which results in intravascular haemolysis. High circulating level of sickle haemoglobin causes significant pathology in sickle cell disease. When released, tetrameric haemoglobin dissociates into dimers with molecular weight of 34 kDA. Free haemoglobin, being an avid scavenger of nitric oxide (NO), leads to reduction in NO bioavailability. Lysis of red cells releases the arginase-1 which breaks down arginine, a metabolic substrate required in biosynthesis of NO. This further contributes to reduction in NO synthesis and further depletion of plasma NO levels. Vasospasm in sickle cell disease results from marked depletion of NO, a potent vasodilator. Defect in ornithine pathway favors alternate pathways with increased production of prolines and polyamines. These byproducts induce smooth muscle proliferation; the resultant proliferative vasculopathy produces disease complications such as pulmonary hypertension, retinopathy, cerebrovascular disease, and chronic leg ulcers. Some other disease manifestations such as bone pain crisis and osteonecrosis are associated with heightened blood viscosity and microvascular occlusion by the irreversibly sickled red cells. Deformable sickle cells are known to express CD36 and very late antigen 4 (VLA4). CD36 and VLA4 interact with vascular endothelium via thrombospondin and VCAM-1, respectively, leading to vasoocclusion with subsequent ischaemic injury and organ infarctions [22, 29]. In line with the current understanding of the pathophysiology of SCD, disease manifestations and complications can therefore be averted by treatment protocols aimed at reducing the circulating ISCs, plasma sickle haemoglobin levels, and therapeutic suppression of the disordered host erythropoiesis in these patients. Thus, hypertransfusion is currently indicated in treatment of SCD as further discussed below.

2.1. Clear Indications for Use of
Hypertransfusion Therapy [33–41]

(i) Prevention of first stroke (cerebrovascular disease).

(ii) Prevention of repeat stroke.

(iii) Transcranial Doppler (TCD) ultrasonography with cerebral blood flow > 2 m/sec (highly predictive of stroke).

(iv) Delayed growth and development in children.

(v) Frequent acute chest syndrome unresponsive to hydroxyurea.

(vi) Frequent severe bone pain crisis requiring three or more hospital admissions per annum and unresponsive to hydroxyurea therapy.

(vii) Severe SCD lacking HLA-matching donor.

(viii) Sickle chronic lung disease.

(ix) Chronic vital organ failure.

(x) Pregnant women with bad obstetric history and frequent bone pains.

2.2. Relative Indications [25, 40, 42]

(i) Sickle cell leg ulcers (to improve tissue oxygenation and wound healing and reduce vasculopathy).

2.3. Controversial Indications [35, 40]

(i) Recurrent sickle cell priapism.

(ii) Preparation for infusion of contrast media.

(iii) "Silent" cerebral infarct and/or neurocognitive damage.

2.4. Inappropriate Indications [35]

(i) Steady state (compensated anaemia).

(ii) Uncomplicated pain episodes.

(iii) Infections.

(iv) Minor surgery that does not require general anaesthesia.

(v) Aseptic necrosis of the hip or shoulder (unless indicated for surgery).

(vi) Uncomplicated pregnancy.

2.5. Relative Contraindications [36]

(i) Multiple red cell alloantibodies.

(ii) Poor venous access.

2.6. Suggested Guidelines on Hypertransfusion

(i) Decision to initiate a chronic hypertransfusion regimen in a patient should be individualized. Benefit to

risk should be carefully assessed and a clear indication must be present.

(ii) Decision to hypertransfuse should be communicated to the patient and relatives in clear terms (stating the benefits and potential adverse effects) and informed consent should be obtained.

(iii) Design a clearly written therapeutic plan and all clinical staff must be duly communicated.

(iv) Blood bank must be duly informed and necessary pretransfusion services commenced.

(v) Prehypertransfusion laboratory work-up should include: blood type with extended red cell phenotyping, antibody screening for unexpected antibodies if indicated, serum ferritin levels, screening for hepatitis A, B, and C, retroviral disease status, liver function test, electrocardiogram/echocardiography, and possibly audiologic/ophthalmologic examinations [35, 43].

(vi) Therapeutic goals such as the final (posttransfusion) haematocrit and the target sickle haemoglobin level should be set before each transfusion episode.

(vii) On the average, most patients will require 2-3 units every 4–6 weeks. As such, transfusion requirement should be established in each individual patient and monitored as changes may occur with time [44].

(viii) Rapid transfusion should be avoided to prevent hyperviscosity. Overtransfusion or supertransfusion (where haemoglobin level is raised above 11 g/dL) should be avoided [29].

(ix) Transfusion requirement will vary from patient to patient depending on quality of the donor unit, associated morbidities, and biologic variables in the patients.

(x) The aim is to keep the haematocrit below 35% to prevent hyperviscosity [29, 33, 45]. Increased viscosity may precipitate hypertransfusion syndrome if haematocrit is elevated too rapidly or haematocrit is greater than 35% [29].

(xi) If the pretransfusion haematocrit is >35%, chances are that hyperviscosity may be contributing to acute complications like acute chest syndrome, stroke, and chronic complications like chronic pain syndrome, osteonecrosis, and ocular disease [26]. Such patients should have one or two units removed, followed by repeated exchange transfusions until desired sickle haemoglobin reduction is achieved [29].

(xii) The patient should report to the outpatient clinic or day-care unit at least 24 hours before each planned transfusion for a full blood count, reticulocyte count, and initial sickle haemoglobin level.

(xiii) Formula for estimation of required transfusion volume and its dilutional effect of transfusion on HbS levels are as follows [29, 34]:

(a) simple red cell transfusions: PRBCV (mL) = $[(\mathrm{HCT}_d - \mathrm{HCT}_i)/\mathrm{HCT}_{rp}] \times \mathrm{TBV}$,

(b) dilutional effects of transfusion on Hb S levels:
$Hb\ S_f(\%) = \{1 - [(PRBCV \times HCT_{rp})/(TBV \times HCT_i) + (PRBCV \times HCT_{rp})]\} \times Hb\ S_i$,

(c) manual partial exchange transfusion: exchange volume (mL) $= [(HCT_d - HCT_i) \times TBV]/[HCT_{rp} - \{(HCT_i + HCT_d)/2\}]$,

(d) automated exchange transfusion: red cell volume (mL) $= HCT_i \times TBV$, where

PRBCV: packed red blood cell volume,

HCT_d: desired haematocrit,

HCT_i: initial haematocrit,

TBV: estimated total blood volume in mL (children 80 mL/kg, adults 65–70 mL/kg),

$Hb\ S_f$: final Hb S levels,

HCT_{rp}: haematocrit of replacement cells (usually 0.7 to 0.8),

$Hb\ S_i$: initial Hb S levels.

(xiv) Patient should be immunized for hepatitis B and C. Booster doses should be given annually to maintain good antibody levels [41].

(xv) Monitor for iron overload and commence s/c desferrioxamine infusion when serum ferritin > 1000 ug/L or >20 units of red cell concentrate has been administered [36]. Oral iron chelators like deferasirox (exjade, asunra) are locally available.

(xvi) Overall, the managing physician should ensure that the right blood and the right amount are administered to the right patient at the right time in the right place.

2.7. Potential Hazards of Hypertransfusion. The art of blood transfusion is not without potential hazards to its recipients. Awareness of complications associated with blood transfusion and hypertransfusion (in particular) helps to position the clinician with strategies to keep these untoward effects to the barest minimum. Hazards of blood transfusion are vast and may be categorized as acute or chronic, immunologic or nonimmunologic. They may also be categorized as early (arising within 24 hours of commencement), delayed (up to 4 weeks), or long-term. Early complications include allergic reactions, anaphylaxis, febrile nonhaemolytic transfusion reaction (FNHTR), acute haemolysis, volume overload, hypothermia, metabolic derangements including hyperkalaemia, hypocalcaemia, and acid-base disturbances, transfusion related acute lung injury, thrombophlebitis, citrate toxicity, bacterial contamination, air embolism, and clotting abnormalities. Late complications include delayed haemolysis, alloimmunization, transfusion associated graft versus host disease, iron overload, transfusion transmissible infections, post transfusion purpura, and transfusion associated immune-modulation. Suffice to say, red cell alloimmunization and iron overload are peculiar complications of chronic blood transfusion in SCD.

Generally, the most frequent transfusion hazard is febrile nonhaemolytic transfusion reaction [46, 47]. Usually, this is caused by exposure of an alloimmunized recipient to foreign antigens on donor leucocytes and platelets leading to

the release of pyrogens such as IL-1 and TNF-alpha. Also, leakage of cytokines from inflammatory cells in the stored blood has been proposed to cause FNHTR. Risk of FNHTR is higher with multiply transfused patients and in multiparous women. FNHTR usually begins within thirty minutes to one hour of transfusion and manifest with fever, chills, headache, or itching. Treatment is to discontinue transfusion, exclude other causes of fever such as bacterial contamination and haemolytic reaction, underlying disease in the patient, and administer antipyretics and antihistamine. Leucodepleted red cell, premedication with antipyretic, and slow speed of transfusion are preferable in subsequent transfusions.

Acute haemolysis (AHTR) is the most dangerous transfusion reaction. It is usually due to incompatible blood components from clerical errors. Transfusion of incompatible units leads to immune response and activation of complement cascade leading to intravascular haemolysis. Also massive release of inflammatory cytokines (cytokine storm) and anaphylatoxins leads to hypotension and acute renal failure. Severe intravascular haemolysis can trigger disseminated intravascular coagulopathy and fatality may ensue. Acute haemolytic transfusion reaction (AHTR) is an emergency. Usually, AHTR begins within few minutes of starting the transfusion. Conscious patients complain of pain or heat at the infusion site, restlessness (akathisia), and loin pain. Fever develops with associated chills and rigor, tachycardia, hypotension/shock, and bleeding tendencies. Hypotension and oozing from venipuncture sites may be the only signs in an unconscious patient.

In event of a suspected AHTR, transfusion should be stopped immediately. Then, maintain plasma volume with crystalloids and manage complications that may arise. Haemovigilance unit should be notified immediately. Investigation of AHTR includes checks for haemolysis (visual examination of patient's plasma and urine, spherocytosis on blood film, increased serum bilirubin, and LDH levels), checking the compatibility form, blood label and patient's identity, repeat blood grouping of recipient pre- and posttransfusion blood sample and on donor's blood unit, repeat cross-matching of donor blood against recipient's pre- and posttransfusion samples, direct antiglobulin test on pre- and posttransfusion samples, run coagulation profile, D-dimer to rule out DIC, and finally electrolyte/urea/creatinine to rule out acute renal failure [48].

Urticarias are due to allergens (usually plasma proteins) in the donor blood to which the recipient has been previously sensitized. Patient develops rashes and pruritus within minutes of transfusion. Treatment is to slow the transfusion rate and administer antihistamine. if patient is unresponsive to antihistamines, discontinue transfusion. Anaphylaxis is a form of severe allergy, quite rare, and is associated with immunoglobulin-A deficient recipients. Infusion of immunoglobulin-A containing blood component into the recipient triggers the formation of IgA/anti-IgA aggregates with the activation of alternate complement pathway. Release of anaphylatoxins (C5a and C3a) mediates anaphylaxis. Transfusion should be stopped immediately and patient is given adrenaline, chlorpheniramine/promethazine, and hydrocortisone. Hypothermia, metabolic derangements (hyperkalaemia, hypocalcaemia, and acid-base imbalance), citrate toxicity, and clotting abnormalities are associated with large volume transfusions and are unlikely in hypertransfusion therapy. Thrombophlebitis may occur as in any condition warranting insertion of a peripheral or central venous catheter. Peripheral line should be changed every 3-4 days and removed when not in use.

Delayed haemolysis is an immunological reaction that occurs in alloimmunized individuals with low (undetectable) antibody titre which is often missed during compatibility testing. Implicated antibodies include non-D Rh (E, C, and c), kell, duffy, and kidd antibodies [49, 50]. On reexposure to the antigen, a secondary (anamnestic) immune response ensues with massive antibody production, manifesting about 5 to 10 days later with fever, jaundice, and declining haemoglobin levels (incongruent with expected haemoglobin rise). Usually, it is less severe than AHTR and the haemolysis is extravascular. Antibody screening and identification are important. Least incompatible blood is indicated for subsequent transfusions.

Transfusion associated graft versus host disease (GvHD) is associated with immune-compromised recipients. It results from immune attack of recipient tissues by immune-competent donor T lymphocytes. Blood components for immune-compromised persons should be irradiated (25 Gy) before use.

With proper donor selection blood screening for pathogens, the risk of transfusion transmissible infection (TTI) is negligible. However, in developing nations such as Nigeria, TTIs still pose a major challenge. International standards such as predonation questionnaire and ELISA based TTI screening are yet to become a routine in many blood banking facilities. In addition, there is poor haemovigilance reporting; as such there is little or no data for monitoring and evaluation of transfusion services.

Alloimmunization to donor red cell antigens and iron overload from repeated transfusions poses a serious challenge to effective hypertransfusion therapy. One unit of red cell concentrate contains about 200–250 mg of iron. Daily physiological loss of iron (through desquamation of skin and mucous membrane) is only about 1 mg. As such, the repeated transfusions and heightened haemolysis in sickle cell disease create a positive iron balance, leading to transfusion siderosis over time. Excess iron in the body will get deposited in virtually every organ in the body, most especially the heart, liver, skin, and endocrine organs and gonads. That would lead to heart failure, diabetes mellitus, skin pigmentation, and gonadal failure. It is advised that iron status of such patients should be monitored every 6 months. Iron chelation therapy should be commenced early when liver iron store exceeds 7 mg/g in adults or 4 mg/g in children [36, 51]. Another useful indicator is to begin iron chelation after cumulative transfusion of 120 mL/kg of red cell concentrate which equates to transfusions in excess of 20 to 30 units of red cells [36]. Serum ferritin levels greater than 1000 ng/mL can be used in steady state but can be quite unreliable. Serum ferritin is an acute phase reactant and is falsely elevated in inflammations, liver disease, and high vitamin C stores. Compared with standard

transfusion therapy, erythrocytapheresis greatly reduces the risk of iron overload but the cost is more.

Recipient alloimmunization is another serious problem that occurs with multiple transfusions. It reduces the chances of a successful transfusion at subsequent times. As a rule, patients being planned for hypertransfusion should have an extended red cell typing to identify other clinically significant blood group antigens including Rh, kell, kidd, and duffy [42, 43, 52]. As much as possible, a group of identical blood units should be transfused. For patients already alloimmunized, antigen negative or the least incompatible blood unit should be transfused. Studies show that 18 to 36% of multiply transfused sickle cell anaemia patients become alloimmunized [53, 54]. Some studies have reported a lower incidence of alloimmunisation with a closer donor-recipient matching for minor red cell antigens and race [54, 55]. However, a recent study of 182 patients with SCD who received antigen matched (phenotype matching for Rh-D, C, E, and K antigen) and racially matched blood revealed a significant alloimmunization rate of 58% and 15% for those received chronic transfusions and episodic transfusions, respectively [56]. Findings from this study suggest that little benefit may be associated with racial and phenotypic red cell matching possibly due to Rh variants that are not detected by red cell phenotyping [56]. Genotypic matching of red cell concentrate may, however, be more beneficial. Further research is required to clarify these positions. Chronic blood transfusion has been associated with hypersplenism and splenomegaly, which may result in increased transfusion requirements over time [57].

3. Current Practice, Challenges, and Prospects of Hypertransfusion in Nigeria

Predating this paper, I found sparse local data on the prevalence and pattern of blood use in Nigerian SCD population. Barbara Otaigbe recently reported a high rate of blood use among paediatric SCD patients in south-south Nigeria and noted the commonest indication for simple transfusions to be severe anaemia [58]. However, no report was made on the use of hypertransfusion in the study [58]. However, in a recent report by Oniyangi et al., chronic transfusion therapy was used in prevention of recurrent stroke among some SCD children in Abuja and it showed some beneficial effects [59].

Furthermore, there is dearth of scientific data on the level of awareness, knowledge, and practice of hypertransfusion in SCD among Nigerian general duty doctors and specialists alike. As such, its current challenges may include poor awareness, poor knowledge, and lack of technical expertise among health care givers. Insufficient supply of blood and blood components due to inefficient blood banking services even at tertiary health care levels is a major challenge in our blood banks [60, 61]. Also, the financial burden of the therapy to the patient, the family, and the society at large is quite heavy as most of the blood supply is commercially driven or at best family replacement donations [60, 61]. Procurement of blood from commercial vendors further increases the risk of transfusion acquired infections and cost of transfusion services which has to be borne by the patient and caregivers.

Recently, Ejeliogu et al. reported that HIV transmission is still transmissible through blood transfusion in Nigerian patients with SCD especially commercially sourced units transfused in peripheral hospitals [62]. In another recent report, Lagunju et al. reported a low acceptance rate of chronic transfusion therapy among caregivers of SCD children in Ibadan [63]. Major reasons for decline included its high cost, unavailability of blood, and the need to regularly seek for donors. The mean cost of chronic blood transfusion (excluding chelation therapy) was found to be 3,276 US Dollars (SD = 1,168) per annum [63].

Moreover, the cost of instituting iron chelation therapy adds to the overall cost of hypertransfusion therapy. Invariably, hypertransfusion therapy may cost beyond the reach of most eligible Nigerian SCD patients. The option of erythrocytapheresis is relatively inaccessible and unaffordable. Thus, the practice of hypertransfusion in Nigeria may be bewildered by suboptimal transfusion services and complications such as monitoring and treatment of iron overload. It behooves us to say that its successful use in the Nigerian context cannot be disconnected from general improvements in our national transfusion service. As well, specialized supports including financial aids, trained professionals, and comprehensive sickle cell centers/clinics should be dedicated to treatment of SCD. Better government commitment to the treatment and prevention of sickle cell disease is necessary to expedite proper healthcare delivery to affected persons.

4. Conclusion

Hypertransfusion is an effective disease modifying strategy in the management of SCD patients. Despite its applicability, there is still little data on its utilization in Nigeria. The reason for the scarcity of information on this treatment modality could be nonusage of the strategy, low acceptance rate, and/or poor attitude to documentation and analysis of such data.

Considering the potential benefits of chronic blood transfusion on quality of life and overall survival in sickle cell disease, we advocate that selected Nigerian patients with adequate resources should be offered hypertransfusion following proper patient education and informed decision on its potential benefits, complications, and cost of therapy. Apheresis for red cell exchange should be provided, accessed, and used when indicated.

Other disease modifying strategies in management of sickle cell disease such as haemopoietic stem cell transplantation are either not readily available or not affordable in developing countries. Therefore, this paper serves as a wake-up call to physicians in Nigeria to practice and promote judicious use of hypertransfusion therapy.

The term hypertransfusion is not exclusive to treatment of SCD alone. There are other clinical indications that may warrant a chronic transfusion regimen, conditions such as major thalassaemia, refractory myelodysplastic syndrome, and aplastic anaemia. However, the strategic therapeutic choice for hypertransfusion in SCD is freshly donated (less than 24 hours), sickle negative, leucodepleted, phenotypically matched, cytomegalovirus negative, and perhaps a minority and racially matched red cell concentrate.

Further efforts should be directed at educating professionals involved in sickle cell disease management at all levels of healthcare to boost their technical knowledge and expertise. Amongst the few disease-modifying interventions that are currently available in SCD care, only haemopoietic stem cell transplantation (HSCT) is potentially curative. However, because of its potential toxicities, HSCT tends to be employed more readily in patients with severe sickle cell disease aged less than 16 years and having a matched sibling donor [64]. Gene therapy offers great hope of cure theoretically but effective vector for stem cell gene transfer is yet to be designed [65]. Hydroxyurea therapy has also been shown to significantly improve outcome in SCD [66–68]. Still yet, hypertransfusion remains a cornerstone strategy especially in those that are unresponsive to hydroxyurea or when hydroxyurea is contraindicated. With effective practice of hypertransfusion, patients with severe sickle cell disease can live a near normal life, with significant reduction of disease morbidity and mortality.

Conflict of Interests

The authors declare that there is no conflict of interests regarding the publication of this paper.

References

[1] D. J. Weatherall and J. B. Clegg, "Inherited haemoglobin disorders: an increasing global health problem," *Bulletin of the World Health Organization*, vol. 79, no. 8, pp. 704–712, 2001.

[2] B. Modell and M. Darlison, "Global epidemiology of haemoglobin disorders and derived service indicators," *Bulletin of the World Health Organization*, vol. 86, no. 6, pp. 480–487, 2008.

[3] WHO Regional Office for Africa, "Sickle cell disease prevention and control," November 2013, http://www.afro.who.int/en/nigeria/nigeria-publications/1775-sickle%20cell%20disease.html.

[4] G. R. Serjeant and B. E. Sergent, "The epidemiology of sickle cell disorder: a challenge for Africa," *Archives of Ibadan Medicine*, vol. 2, no. 2, pp. 4–52, 2001.

[5] A. L. Okwi, W. Byarugaba, C. M. Ndugwa, A. Parkes, M. Ocaido, and J. K. Tumwine, "An up-date on the prevalence of sickle cell trait in Eastern and Western Uganda," *BMC Blood Disorders*, vol. 10, article 5, 2010.

[6] B. Nwogoh, A. S. Adewoyin, O. E. Iheanacho, and G. N. Bazuaye, "Prevalence of haemoglobin variants in Benin City, Nigeria," *Annals of Biomedical Sciences*, vol. 11, no. 2, pp. 60–64, 2012.

[7] S. D. Grosse, I. Odame, H. K. Atrash, D. D. Amendah, F. B. Piel, and T. N. Williams, "Sickle cell disease in Africa: a neglected cause of early childhood mortality," *American Journal of Preventive Medicine*, vol. 41, no. 6, supplement 4, pp. S398–S405, 2011.

[8] J. Makani, T. N. Williams, and K. Marsh, "Sickle cell disease in Africa: burden and research priorities," *Annals of Tropical Medicine and Parasitology*, vol. 101, no. 1, pp. 3–14, 2007.

[9] M. Brozovic and S. Davies, "Management of sickle cell disease," *Postgraduate Medical Journal*, vol. 63, no. 742, pp. 605–609, 1987.

[10] "Sickle Cell Anaemia. Agenda item 11.4," in *Proceedings of the 59th World Health Assembly*, Geneva, Switzerland, May 2006, http://www.who.int/gb/ebwha/pdf_files/WHA59-REC1/WHA59_2006_REC1-en.pdf.

[11] F. A. Olatona, K. A. Odeyemi, A. T. Onajole, and M. C. Asuzu, "Effects of health education on knowledge and attitude of youth corps members to sickle cell disease and its screening in Lagos State," *Journal of Community Medicine & Health Education*, vol. 2, no. 7, article 163, 2012.

[12] R. S. Owolabi, P. Alabi, D. Olusoji, S. Ajayi, T. Otu, and A. Ogundiran, "Knowledge and attitudes of secondary school students in Federal Capital Territory, Abuja, Nigeria towards sickle cell disease," *Nigerian Journal of Medicine*, vol. 20, no. 4, pp. 479–485, 2011.

[13] S. Abubakar, U. M. Lawan, M. S. Mijinyawa, S. I. Adeleke, and H. Sabiu, "Perceptions about sickle cell disease and its prevention among undergraduates of tertiary institutions in Kano State, Nigeria," *Nigerian Journal of Clinical Medicine*, vol. 3, no. 1, 2010.

[14] G. N. Bazuaye and E. E. Olayemi, "Knowledge and attitude of senior secondary school students in Benin City Nigeria to sickle cell disease," *World Journal of Medical Sciences*, vol. 4, no. 1, pp. 46–49, 2009.

[15] D. A. Adekanle and A. S. Adeyemi, "Prevention of Sickle cell disease by prenatal diagnosis-opinion of female health workers in Osogbo, South-Western Nigeria," *Ibom Medical Journal*, vol. 2, no. 1, pp. 20–22, 1997.

[16] M. A. Durosinmi, A. I. Odebiyi, I. A. Adediran, N. O. Akinola, D. E. Adegorioye, and M. A. Okunade, "Acceptability of prenatal diagnosis of sickle cell anaemia (SCA) by female patients and parents of SCA patients in Nigeria," *Social Science & Medicine*, vol. 41, no. 3, pp. 433–436, 1995.

[17] N. Win, "Blood transfusion therapy for Haemoglobinopathies," in *Practical Management of Haemoglobinopathies*, I. E. Okpala, Ed., pp. 99–106, Blackwell Publishing, 2004.

[18] G. R. Serjeant, "Chronic transfusion programmes in sickle cell disease: problem or panacea?" *British Journal of Haematology*, vol. 97, no. 2, pp. 253–255, 1997.

[19] M. F. Murphy, T. B. Wallington, P. Kelsey et al., "Guidelines for the clinical use of red cell transfusions," *British Journal of Haematology*, vol. 113, no. 1, pp. 24–31, 2001.

[20] G. Liumbruno, F. Bennardello, A. Lattanzio, P. Piccoli, and G. Rossetti, "Recommendations for the transfusion of red blood cells," *Blood Transfusion*, vol. 7, no. 1, pp. 49–64, 2009.

[21] J. Pendergrast, "Transfusion of Patients with Thalassemia and Sickle Cell Disease," https://www.lhsc.on.ca/lab/bldbank/assets/LLSGSymposium11/Pendergrast%202011%5B1%5D.pdf.

[22] K. Natarajan, "Disorders of haemoglobin structure: sickle cell anaemia and related abnormalities," in *Williams Haematology*, M. A. Lichtman, Ed., vol. 47, pp. 667–700, McGraw-Hill, 2006.

[23] S. Charache, "The treatment of sickle cell anemia," *Archives of Internal Medicine*, vol. 133, no. 4, pp. 698–705, 1974.

[24] M. J. Telen, "Principles and problems of transfusion in sickle cell disease," *Seminars in Hematology*, vol. 38, no. 4, pp. 315–323, 2001.

[25] M. Koshy, L. Burd, D. Wallace, A. Moawad, and J. Baron, "Prophylactic red-cell transfusions in pregnant patients with sickle cell disease. A randomized cooperative study," *The New England Journal of Medicine*, vol. 319, no. 22, pp. 1447–1452, 1988.

[26] S. Laulan, J. F. Bernard, and P. Boivin, "Systematic blood transfusions in adult homozygous sicle-cell anaemia," *Presse Medicale*, vol. 19, no. 17, pp. 785–789, 1990.

[27] A. R. Cohen, M. B. Martin, J. H. Silber, H. C. Kim, K. Ohene-Frempong, and E. Schwartz, "A modified transfusion program for prevention of stroke in sickle cell disease," *Blood*, vol. 79, no. 7, pp. 1657–1661, 1992.

[28] M. T. Lee, S. Piomelli, S. Granger et al., "Stroke prevention Trial in Sickle Cell Anaemia (STOP): extended Follow up and final results," *Blood*, vol. 108, no. 3, pp. 847–852, 2006.

[29] W. F. Rosse, M. Narla, L. D. Petz, and M. H. Steinberg, "New views of sickle cell disease pathophysiology and treatment," in *American Society of Haematology Education Book*, vol. 2000, pp. 2–17, 2000.

[30] D. C. Rees, T. N. Williams, and M. T. Gladwin, "Sickle-cell disease," *The Lancet*, vol. 376, no. 9757, pp. 2018–2031, 2010.

[31] G. R. Serjeant, B. E. Serjeant, and P. F. Milner, "The irreversibly sickled cell; a determinant of haemolysis in sickle cell anaemia," *British Journal of Haematology*, vol. 17, no. 6, pp. 527–533, 1969.

[32] W. M. Lande, D. L. Andrews, M. R. Clark et al., "The incidence of painful crisis in homozygous sickle cell disease: correlation with red cell deformability," *Blood*, vol. 72, no. 6, 1988.

[33] Z. Y. Aliyu, A. R. Tumblin, and G. J. Kato, "Current therapy of sickle cell disease," *Haematologica*, vol. 91, no. 1, pp. 7–10, 2006.

[34] A. S. Wayne, S. V. Kevy, and D. G. Nathan, "Transfusion management of sickle cell disease," *Blood*, vol. 81, no. 5, pp. 1109–1123, 1993.

[35] M. H. Steinberg, "Management of sickle cell disease," *The New England Journal of Medicine*, vol. 340, no. 13, pp. 1021–1030, 1999.

[36] E. P. Vinchinsky, "Transfusion therapy in sickle cell disease," http://sickle.bwh.harvard.edu/transfusion.html.

[37] R. Adams, V. McKie, F. Nichols et al., "The use of transcranial ultrasonography to predict stroke in sickle cell disease," *The New England Journal of Medicine*, vol. 326, no. 9, pp. 605–610, 1992.

[38] R. J. Adams, V. C. McKie, L. Hsu et al., "Prevention of a first stroke by transfusions in children with sickle cell anemia and abnormal results on transcranial Doppler ultrasonography," *The New England Journal of Medicine*, vol. 339, pp. 5–11, 1998.

[39] S. T. Miller, E. Wright, M. Abboud et al., "Impact of chronic transfusion on incidence of pain and acute chest syndrome during the Stroke Prevention Trial (STOP) in sickle-cell anemia," *Journal of Pediatrics*, vol. 139, no. 6, pp. 785–789, 2001.

[40] Z. R. Rogers, "Review: clinical transfusion management in sickle cell disease," *Immunohematology*, vol. 22, no. 3, pp. 126–131, 2006.

[41] Sickle Cell Disease in Childhood, *Standards and Guidelines for Cliinical Care*, NHS Sickle Cell and Thalassaemia Screening Programme, London, UK, 2nd edition, 2010.

[42] H. H. Al-Saeed and A. H. Al-Salem, "Principles of blood transfusion in sickle cell anemia," *Saudi Medical Journal*, vol. 23, no. 12, pp. 1443–1448, 2002.

[43] Sickle cell society, Standards for the clinical care of adults with sickle cell disease in the United Kingdom, Chapter 6: Blood transfusion 2008.

[44] W. H. Zinkham, A. J. Seidler, and T. S. Kickler, "Variable degrees of suppression of hemoglobin S synthesis in subjects with hemoglobin SS disease on a long-term transfusion regimen," *Journal of Pediatrics*, vol. 124, no. 2, pp. 215–219, 1994.

[45] H. Qureshi, *Red Cell Transfusion in Sickle Cell Disease*, University Hospital of Leicester NHS Trust, 2010.

[46] B. A. Gwalam, M. M. Bowdo, A. I. Dutse, and A. Kaliya-Gwarzo, "Patterns of acute blood transfusion reactions in Kano, north-western Nigeria," *Nigerian Journal of Basic and Clinical Sciences*, vol. 9, pp. 27–32, 2012.

[47] O. P. Arewa, N. O. Akinola, and L. Salawu, "Blood transfusion reactions: evaluation of 462 transfusions at a tertiary hospital in Nigeria," *African Journal of Medicine and Medical Sciences*, vol. 38, no. 2, pp. 143–148, 2009.

[48] J. O. Adewuyi, "Blood group serology," in *Companion to Practical Haematology*, vol. 10, pp. 74–84, 2007.

[49] L. A. M. Bashawri, "Red cell alloimmunization in sickle-cell anaemia patients," *Eastern Mediterranean Health Journal*, vol. 13, no. 5, pp. 1181–1189, 2007.

[50] K. Yazdanbakhsh, R. E. Ware, and F. Noizat-Pirenne, "Red blood cell alloimmunization in sickle cell disease: pathophysiology, risk factors, and transfusion management," *Blood*, vol. 120, no. 3, pp. 528–537, 2012.

[51] Mid-Atlantic Sickle Cell Disease Consortium (MASCC) Guidelines, "Chronic transfusion in children with sickle cell disease," Sickle cell disease in children and adolescents: diagnosis, guidelines for comprehensive care and protocols for management of acute and chronic complications, 2001.

[52] I. A. Shulman, "Prophylactic phenotype matching of donors for the transfusion of nonalloimmunized patients with sickle cell disease," *Immunohematology*, vol. 22, no. 3, pp. 101–102, 2006.

[53] E. P. Vichinsky, A. Earles, R. A. Johnson, M. S. Hoag, A. Williams, and B. Lubin, "Alloimmunization in sickle cell anemia and transfusion of racially unmatched blood," *The New England Journal of Medicine*, vol. 322, no. 23, pp. 1617–1621, 1990.

[54] D. R. Ambruso, J. H. Githens, R. Alcorn et al., "Experience with donors matched for minor blood group antigens in patients with sickle cell anemia who are receiving chronic transfusion therapy," *Transfusion*, vol. 27, no. 1, pp. 94–98, 1987.

[55] E. P. Vichinsky, N. L. C. Luban, E. Wright et al., "Prospective RBC phenotype matching ina stroke-Prevention trial in sickle cell anemia: a multicenter transfusion trial," *Transfusion*, vol. 41, no. 9, pp. 1086–1092, 2001.

[56] S. T. Chou, T. Jackson, S. Vege, K. Smith-Whitley, D. F. Friedman, and C. M. Westhoff, "High prevalence of red blood cell alloimmunization in sickle cell disease despite transfusion from Rh-matched minority donors," *Blood*, vol. 122, no. 6, pp. 1062–1071, 2013.

[57] A. R. Cohen, G. R. Buchanan, M. Martin, and K. Ohene-Frempong, "Increased blood requirements during long-term transfusion therapy for sickle cell disease," *Journal of Pediatrics*, vol. 118, no. 3, pp. 405–407, 1991.

[58] B. Otaigbe, "Prevalence of blood transfusion in sickle cell anaemia patients in South-South Nigeria: a two-year experience," *International Journal of Medicine and Medical Science Research*, vol. 1, no. 1, pp. 13–18, 2013.

[59] O. Oniyangi, P. Ahmed, O. T. Otuneye et al., "Strokes in children with sickle cell disease at the National Hospital, Abuja, Nigeria," *Nigerian Journal of Paediatrics*, vol. 40, no. 2, pp. 158–164, 2013.

[60] A. O. Emeribe, A. O. Ejele, E. E. Attai, and E. A. Usanga, "Blood donation and patterns of use in southeastern Nigeria," *Transfusion*, vol. 33, no. 4, pp. 330–332, 1993.

[61] S. G. Ahmed, U. A. Ibrahim, and A. W. Hassan, "Adequacy and pattern of blood donations in North-eastern Nigeria: the implications for blood safety," *Annals of Tropical Medicine and Parasitology*, vol. 101, no. 8, pp. 725–731, 2007.

[62] E. U. Ejeliogu, S. N. Okolo, S. D. Pam et al., "Is human immunodeficiency virus still transmissible through blood transfusion in children with Sickle cell anaemia in Jos, Nigeria?" *British Journal of Medicine and Medical Research*, vol. 4, no. 21, pp. 3912–3923, 2014.

[63] A. I. Lagunju, B. J. Brown, and O. O. Sodeinde, "Chronic Blood transfusion for primary and secondary stroke prevention in Nigerian children with Sickle cell disease: a five year appraisal," *Pediatric Blood and Cancer*, vol. 60, no. 12, pp. 1940–1945, 2013.

[64] K. W. Chan, "Haemopoeitic stem cell transplantation for sickle cell disease: more options and many unanswered questions," *Journal of Blood Disorders & Transfusion*, vol. 4, p. e106, 2013.

[65] M. J. Stuart and R. L. Nagel, "Sickle-cell disease," *The Lancet*, vol. 364, no. 9442, pp. 1343–1360, 2004.

[66] M. H. Steinberg, "Hydroxyurea treatment for sickle cell disease." *TheScientificWorldJournal*, vol. 2, pp. 1706–1728, 2002.

[67] R. E. Ware and B. Aygun, "Advances in the use of hydroxyurea," *Hematology*, pp. 62–69, 2009.

[68] S. C. Davies and A. Gilmore, "The role of hydroxyurea in the management of sickle cell disease," *Blood Reviews*, vol. 17, no. 2, pp. 99–109, 2003.

23

Imatinib Mesylate Effectiveness in Chronic Myeloid Leukemia with Additional Cytogenetic Abnormalities at Diagnosis among Black Africans

Tolo Diebkilé Aïssata,[1] Duni Sawadogo,[2] Clotaire Nanho,[1] Boidy Kouakou,[1] N'dogomo Meité,[1] N'Dhatz Emeuraude,[1] Ayémou Roméo,[1] Sekongo Yassongui Mamadou,[1] Paul Kouéhion,[1] Konan Mozart,[1] Gustave Koffi,[1] and Ibrahima Sanogo[1]

[1] *Department of Clinical Hematology, Yopougon Teaching Hospital, P.O. Box 632, Abidjan 21, Cote d'Ivoire*
[2] *Department of Biological Hematology, Yopougon Teaching Hospital, P.O. Box 632, Abidjan 21, Cote d'Ivoire*

Correspondence should be addressed to Tolo Diebkilé Aïssata; aissata_tolo@yahoo.fr

Academic Editor: Giuseppe G. Saglio

Imatinib mesylate provides good results in the treatment of CML in general. But what about the results of this treatment in CML associated with additional cytogenetic abnormalities at diagnosis among black Africans? For this, we retrospectively studied 27 cases of CML associated with additional cytogenetic abnormalities, diagnosed in the department of clinical hematology of the University Hospital of Yopougon in Côte d'Ivoire, from May 2005 to October 2011. The age of patients ranged from 13 to 68 years, with a mean age of 38 years and a sex ratio of 2. Patients were severely symptomatic with a high Sokal score of 67%. CML in chronic phase accounted for 67%. The prevalence of additional cytogenetic abnormalities was 29.7%. There were variants of the Philadelphia chromosome (18.5%), trisomy 8 (14.8%), complex cytogenetic abnormalities (18.5%), second Philadelphia chromosome (14.8%), and minor cytogenetic abnormalities (44.4%). Complete hematologic remission was achieved in 59%, with 52% of major cytogenetic remission. The outcome was fatal in 37% of patients. Death was related in 40% to hematologic toxicity and in 30% to acutisation. The median survival was 40 months.

1. Introduction

Chronic myeloid leukemia (CML) is characterized by the predominant proliferation of cells of grainy line and by the existence of a cytogenetic abnormality that is the translocation t (9; 22) (q34; q11) with BCR/ABL rearrangement.

If CML develops inexorably towards the acute transformation, the time necessary for this transformation is variable. Twenty five percent of patients will survive more than 5 years, 5% over 10 years. For others, the acute transformation occurs immediately or very soon after the diagnosis of the disease.

This difference in overall survival may be partly explained by the Sokal score but also by the existence or not of additional cytogenetic abnormalities at diagnosis. Major additional cytogenetic abnormalities at diagnosis have a negative impact on survival and mean progression to the accelerated or blast phase [1–4].

Currently, the first-line treatment of this CML is based on imatinib mesylate. Imatinib mesylate or STI-571 or Glivec was discovered right in 1988 as a highly potent and selective inhibitor of ABL tyrosine kinases. This drug has become the first-line treatment of Ivorian patients with CML and with low income, since GIPAP (Glivec International Patient Assistance Program) kindly provides Côte d'Ivoire with it. Some resistance to this treatment may be associated with additional cytogenetic abnormalities [1, 5].

The aim of our study was to determine the effectiveness of imatinib mesylate in the CML with additional cytogenetic abnormalities. The study was approved by an ethics committee and was carried out in accordance with the Declaration

Kaplan-Meier graphe de survie cum. pour colonne 1
Variable censure : ⟨sans⟩

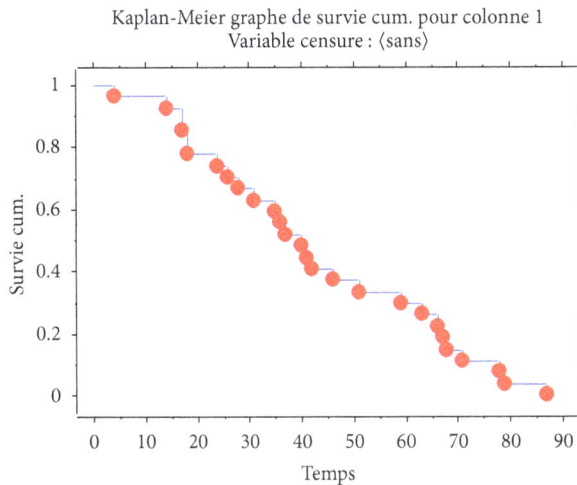

FIGURE 1: Curve of overall survival in CML patients with additional cytogenetic abnormalities.

of Helsinki. A written consent was signed before inclusion in the protocol.

2. Patients and Methods

Our study was carried out in the department of clinical hematology of the University Hospital of Yopougon in Abidjan, Côte d'Ivoire. It was retrospective and descriptive. It involved records of in-patients or out-patients from May 2005 to October 2011. All in-patients or out-patients with CML diagnosed by blood count, myelogram, and cytogenetic or molecular biology with additional chromosomal abnormality and treated by imatinib mesylate were included. Twenty-seven CML patients with additional cytogenetic abnormalities treated by imatinib mesylate were retained.

Each medical record was exploited through a personal survey form with collection of epidemiological data (age, sex), clinical data (lymphadenopathy, splenomegaly, hepatomegaly, performance status, bone pain, and fever), biological data (white blood cell count, platelet count, hemoglobin count, blood blasts rates, blood promyelocytes rates, and the result of cytogenetic or molecular biology), evolutional data (Sokal classification, evolutionary stages, and death), treatment data (hematologic remission, cytogenetic remission, molecular remission, and overall survival).

Complete hematologic remission corresponds to the normalization of blood counts with disappearance of clinical signs of disease.

Complete cytogeneticremission corresponds to the absence of the Philadelphia chromosome at the cytogenetic examination (0% Ph + metaphases). It may be partial (1–35% Ph + metaphases) or minor (35%–95% Ph + metaphases) or minimal (96%–100% Ph + metaphases).

The major molecular response corresponds to the disappearance of BCR/ABL transcript.

Patients were seen again for clinical examination, blood count, and biochemical tests once a week for 4 weeks, then every 3 months. Cytogenetic response was assessed every 6 months during the first year, then once a year.

TABLE 1: Epidemiological, clinical, and biological features of patients.

Variables	Numbers (%)
Age (years) mean age 38 years (13–68)	
11–30	13 (48)
31–50	9 (33)
51–70	5 (19)
Sex	
Male	18 (67)
Female	9 (33)
Socioeconomic level	
Low	10 (37)
Average	17 (63)
Reason for consultation	
Hyperleukocytosis	17 (63)
Hyperleukocytosis + splenomegaly	10 (37)
Performance status	
0 and 1	0 (0)
2 and 3	13 (48)
4	14 (52)
Bone pains	
Presence	13 (48)
Fever	
Presence	20 (74)
Hepatomegaly	
Presence	13 (48)
Lymphadenopathy	
Presence	6 (22)
Splenomegaly	
0 cm	0 (0)
1–9 cm	7 (26)
≥10 cm	7 (26)
Hemogram (median values and extremes)	
White Blood Cells (10^9/L)	341.2 (140–650)
Hemoglobin (g/dL)	8.5 (5.7–12.4)
Platelets (10^9/L)	340 (57–1992)
Polynuclear basophiles (%)	5 (0–9)
Blasts (%)	7 (0–16)
Promyelocytes (%)	8 (0–18)
Sokal score	
Low	0 (0)
Intermediate	9 (33)
High	18 (67)

Imatinib mesylate was administered at a dose of 400 mg/day in chronic phase and 600 mg/day in accelerated phase, doses that were adjusted according to tolerance and response. The box of the drug was delivered to the patient in the hospital under medical supervision. The delivery of the second box was preceded by the handing over by the patient of the first empty box and so on. Doses were reduced for neutropenia and thrombocytopenia of grade 3 or 4.

TABLE 2: List of additional cytogenetic anomalies at diagnosis of the 27 patients in the study.

No patient	Cytogenetic abnormalities
1	47,XX, +8, t (9;22) (q34;11) [100]
2	47,XY, +8, t (9;22) (q34;11) [1]
3	47,XX, +8, t (9;22) (q34;11) [1]
4	47,XX, +8, t (9;22) (q34;11) [1]
5	46,XY, t (9;22) (q34;q11), add (1) (p36.3) [12]
6	46,XY, t (9;22) (q34;q11), add (2) (p25) [6]
7	46,XX, del (7) (q22;q31), t (9;22) (q34;q11) [100]
8	46,XY, del (7) (q31), t (9;22) (q34;q11) [2]
9	46,XY, del (12) (p12), t (9;22) (q34;q11) [12]
10	46,XY, del (3) (p12p14), t (9;22) (q34;q11) [5]
11	46,XX, del (1) (q12) add (1) (q44), t (9;22) (q34;11) [3]
12	46,XX, t (9;22) (q34;q11), add (13) (p11), add (20) (p13) [23]
13	46,XY, t (9;22) (q34;q11) t (16;20) (q23;q12) [3]
14	46,XX, dup (14) (q22;q32), t (9;22) (q34;q11) [5]
15	46,XX, t (4;11) (q13;p12), t (9;22) (q34;q11) [11]
16	46,XX, inv (12), t (9;22) (q34;11) [100]
17	47,XY, del (13) (q21), t (9;10;22) (q34;p14;q11) + mar 1 [3]
18	46,XY, t (1;3;9;22) (p35;p22;q34;q11) [20]
19	46,XY, t (2;9;22) (q37;q34;q11) [100]
20	46,XY, t (6;9;22) (q22; q34;q11) [3]
21	46,XY, t (3; 9; 22) (q27; q34; q11), der (21) t (21;?) p (12;?) [15]
22	47,XY, der (22), t (9;22) (q34;q11) [100]
23	45-46,XY, t (9;22) (q34;q11), der (12), t(12;14), (q10;q10), add (13), (p11.2), -14, -mar
24	46,XY, t (3; 13) (p25; q14), t(9; 22) (q34; q11) [28]/52, idem, +6,+7,+8,+19,+21, +der(22), t(9;22) (q34;q11)
25	46,XY, del (2) (p22), der (9), t(9;22) (q34;q11), der (22), t(9;22) (q34;q11), +mar 1, +mar 2 [20]
26	46,XY, t (9;22) (q34;q11), der (9), der (22q) [7]/47,XY, idem, der (22) [11]
27	45,XY, -17, t (9;22) (q34;q11), add(19) (q13.4), -mar [19]/45,XY, -17, t (9;22) (q34;q11), add(19) (q13.4) [11]

The assessment of the socioeconomic level was done according to indirect criteria which were occupation, number of children, and type of housing.

Data were analyzed using Epi-Info version 6.04b. The calculation of overall survival was performed according to the Kaplan-Meier method with the existence in the record of a date of inclusion (date of entry) and a point date (date of death or latest news) mentioned in day, month, year (Figure 1).

3. Results

From May 2005 to October 2011 the diagnosis of CML was made in 91 patients. Among these 91 patients, 27 were carriers of additional cytogenetic abnormalities, that is, 29.7% (Table 2). The epidemiological, clinical, and biological features of those patients are summarized in Table 1. The age ranged from 13 to 68 years with an average of 38 years. The sex ratio was 2.

4. Discussion

The mean age of our patients was 38 years with extremes of 13 and 68 years. Our lower average age also reported by other

authors [6] could be related to the pyramid of ages of the African people.

The sex ratio was 2. So there were two times more additional cytogenetic abnormalities in men than in women. This male predominance was also noted by Luatti et al. [1] who in his study found 86% of men with an additional cytogenetic abnormality against 59% of men who did not have any with a $P = 0.02$.

The socioeconomic level of our study population was low or medium. It is this socio-economic class which is taken into account by the GYPAP program, and it is this group that consults in public hospitals, the more affluent preferring private clinics.

Clinically, the reason for consultation was made by leukocytosis, associated or not with splenomegaly in 100% of cases.

Generally, our patients were severely symptomatic with a performance status ≥ 2 in 100%, splenomegaly in 100%, fever in 74%, hepatomegaly in 48%, bone pains in 48% and lymphadenopathy in 22%. Splenomegaly was relatively large, ≥ 10 cm in 74%, probably due to the long period of consultation. Our patients were characterized by the long period of consultation in clinical hematology because most of them would first consult traditional healers, then a general

TABLE 3: Therapeutic and evolutionary features.

Variables	Numbers (%)
Evolutionary phase	
Chronic phase	18 (67)
Accelerated phase	9 (33)
Hematologic remission	
Complete	16 (59)
Partial	11 (41)
Cytogenetic or molecular remission	
Major cytogenetic response (Ph+ ≤ 35%)	14 (52)
Complete cytogenetic response (Ph+ 0%)	7 (26)
Partial cytogenetic response (Ph+ 1%–35%)	7 (26)
Minor cytogenetic response (Ph+ 36%–95%)	8 (30)
Minimal cytogenetic response (Ph+ 96%–100%)	4 (15)
Complete molecular response	1 (3)
Outcome	
Alive	17 (63)
Dead	10 (37)
Causes of death	
Acutisation	3 (30)
Hematologic toxicity	4 (40)
Pulmonary tuberculosis	1 (10)
Epilepsy	1 (10)
Unspecified	1 (10)
Adverse effects grade 3 and 4	
Hematologic toxicity	
Anemia	10 (37)
Leukopenia	9 (33)
Thrombocytopenia	8 (29)
Duration of follow-up (median and extreme values in months)	37 (4–87)

practitioner. And the time between the date of entry and the date of treatment with imatinib was long for three reasons

(i) Most of the time patients do not have funds available for biological and radiology assessment; the waiting period before parents accept to help them can often be long.

(ii) Cytogenetics is not performed in Côte d'Ivoire; therefore, the sample has to be sent to France.

(iii) The patient must be enrolled on GIPAP program and must wait till the imatinib is send to him.

All the long delays (consultation and treatment) contribute to alter the condition of the patient, to increase the volume of his spleen, his white blood cell count and the Sokal score, and favor the transition to the accelerate phase of the disease.

These symptoms were mainly found in patients with the accelerated phase of the disease (33%) and/or with a high Sokal score (67%), whereas in the study by Koffi et al. [6]

that takes into account all cases of CML diagnosed in our department, there were 59% of performance status quoted at 0 to 1 and 10% who had no splenomegaly.

However, according to Luatti et al. [1], there is no significant difference concerning the size of the spleen in patients with CML with or without additional cytogenetic abnormalities ($P = 0.10$), just as there is no significant difference concerning the Sokal score ($P = 0.66$).

Biologically, the median of white blood cell count was 314.2×10^9/L, that of platelet count 340×10^9/L; those of polynuclear basophiles, blasts, and promyelocytes were respectively, 5%, 7%, and 8%. Concerning these parameters, according to Luatti et al. [1], there are no significant differences between the two groups of patients with CML with or without additional cytogenetic abnormalities, except for the rate of blasts in the peripheral blood. The median rate of blasts in the peripheral blood was 2.5% versus 1% ($P = 0.03$).

However, our median rate of white blood cells was higher, and our median hemoglobin rate was lower than the values reported by Braziel et al. [7] The difference in platelets was not significant.

In our study, we found 29.7% of additional cytogenetic abnormalities. There were 5 cases of variants of Philadelphia chromosome (no. 17 to 21), 5 cases of complex cytogenetic abnormalities (no. 23 to 27), that is, 18.5% each, 4 cases of trisomy 8 (no. 1 to 4), 4 cases of second philadelphia chromosome (22, 24 to 26), that is, 14.8% each and 12 cases of minor cytogenetic abnormalities (no. 5 to 16), that is, 44.4%. Our overall rate of additional cytogenetic abnormalities is relatively high compared to that reported in the literature which is, 5 to 18% [1, 2, 4, 7–10]. For some there was no statistically significant difference between the future and the type of additional cytogenetic abnormalities [2, 11], for others, the difference was significant [4, 12]. In fact, according Fabarius [4], the PFS was 90% versus 50%, and the overall survival to 92% versus 53%, respectively, in those without and with major additional cytogenetic abnormalities with $P < 0.001$.

The median survival was 40 months. Regarding the survival median that was 40 months, it should be noted that 14 patients had less than 40 months of survival, deaths having occurred precociously due to hematologic toxicity particularly. Three patients were enrolled in 2011.

On the therapeutic level, we obtained 59% of complete hematologic response (CHR) and 41% of partial hematologic response (PHR). Our results are below those of Koffi et al. [6] who had 76% of CHR and 24% of PHR. As for Luatti et al. [1], they achieved 100% of CHR in patients with additional cytogenetic abnormalities. Our low rate of CHR could be related to the Sokal score (33% of intermediate score and 67% of high score). But it should be noted that in the study of Luatti et al. [1], there were 29% of intermediate Sokal score and 38% of high Sokal score in patients with additional cytogenetic abnormalities.

Concerning the cytogenetic and molecular response, only one patient (3%) achieved a major molecular response. He was carrying a trisomy 8. There was major cytogenetic response (52%), complete cytogenetic response (26%), partial cytogenetic response (26%), minor cytogenetic response (30%), minimal cytogenetic response (15%).

The outcome was fatal in 37%, and the causes of death were dominated by hematologic toxicity (40%), followed by acutisation (30%). In one patient (10%), acutisation occurred at the interruption of the treatment against medical advice.

Normally, patients during treatment with imatinib are reviewed once a week for 4 weeks, then every 3 months for a complete blood count and biochemical tests.

Unfortunately, this control rate is not respected by patients, and they return only in case of complications (anemia, neutropenia, thrombocytopenia, fever, etc.). In addition, they often do not have the means to finance a good hematologic resuscitation (transfusions, antibiotics, etc.). This explains the death by hematologic toxicity (Table 3).

Acknowledgments

The authors are grateful to Novartis for providing imatinib mesylate, the Max Foundation and Axios International for facilitating the delivery of the drugs, and Pasteur Cerba of Paris (France) for cytogenetic analysis.

References

[1] S. Luatti, F. Castagnetti, G. Marzocchi et al., "Additional chromosomal abnormalities in Philadelphia-positive clone: adverse prognostic impact on frontline imatinib therapy: a GIMEMA Working Party on CML analysis," *Blood*, vol. 120, no. 4, pp. 761–767, 2012.

[2] H. H. Hsiao, Y. C. Liu, H. J. Tsai et al., "Additional chromosome abnormalities in chronic myeloid leukemia," *Kaohsiung Journal of Medical Sciences*, vol. 27, no. 2, pp. 49–54, 2011.

[3] N. Meggysi, A. Kozma, G. Halm et al., "Additional chromosome abnormalities, BCR-ABL tyrosine kinase domain mutations and clinical outcome in Hungarian tyrosine kinase inhibitor-resistant chronic myelogenous leukemia patients," *Acta Haematol*, vol. 127, no. 1, pp. 34–42, 2012.

[4] A. Fabarius, A. Leitner, A. Hochhaus et al., "Impact of additional cytogenetic aberrations at diagnosis on prognosis of CML: long-term observation of 1151 patients from the randomized CML Study IV," *Blood*, vol. 118, no. 26, pp. 6760–6768, 2011.

[5] S. Marktel, D. Marin, N. Foot et al., "Chronic myeloid leukemia in chronic phase responding to imatinib: the occurrence of additional cytogenetic abnormalities predicts disease progression," *Haematologica*, vol. 88, no. 3, pp. 260–267, 2003.

[6] K. G. Koffi, D. C. Nanho, E. N'Dathz et al., "The effect of imatinib mesylate for newly diagnosed Philadelphia chromosome-positive, chronic-phase myeloid leukemia in sub-saharan african patients: the experience of côte d'ivoire," *Advances in Hematology*, vol. 2010, Article ID 268921, 6 pages, 2010.

[7] R. M. Braziel, T. M. Launder, B. J. Druker et al., "Hematopathologic and cytogenetic findings in imatinib mesylate-treated chronic myelogenous leukemia patients: 14 Months' experience," *Blood*, vol. 100, no. 2, pp. 435–441, 2002.

[8] U. Bacher, T. Haferlach, W. Hiddemann, S. Schnittger, W. Kern, and C. Schoch, "Additional clonal abnormalities in Philadelphia-positive ALL and CML demonstrate a different cytogenetic pattern at diagnosis and follow different pathways at progression," *Cancer Genetics and Cytogenetics*, vol. 157, no. 1, pp. 53–61, 2005.

[9] A. Zaccaria, N. Testoni, A. M. Valenti et al., "Chromosome abnormalities additional to the Philadelphia chromosome at the diagnosis of chronic myelogenous leukemia: pathogenetic and prognostic implications," *Cancer Genetics and Cytogenetics*, vol. 199, no. 2, pp. 76–80, 2010.

[10] C. Belli, M. F. Alú, G. Alfonso, M. Bianchini, and I. Larripa, "Novel variant Ph translocation t(9;22;11) (q34;q11.2;p15)inv(9)(p13q34) in chronic myeloid leukemia involving a one-step mechanism," *Cytogenetic and Genome Research*, vol. 132, no. 4, pp. 304–308, 2011.

[11] M. Holzerová, E. Faber, J. Veselovská et al., "Imatinib mesylate efficacy in 72 previously treated Philadelphia-positive chronic myeloid leukemia patients with and without additional chromosomal changes: single-center results," *Cancer Genetics and Cytogenetics*, vol. 191, no. 1, pp. 1–9, 2009.

[12] X. Y. Su, N. Wong, Q. Cao et al., "Chromosomal aberrations during progression of chronic myeloid leukemia identified by cytogenetic and molecular cytogenetic tools: implication of 1q12-21," *Cancer Genetics and Cytogenetics*, vol. 108, no. 1, pp. 6–12, 1999.

24

The Genetic Architecture of Multiple Myeloma

Steven M. Prideaux, Emma Conway O'Brien, and Timothy J. Chevassut

Brighton and Sussex Medical School, Sussex University, Falmer, Brighton BN1 9PS, UK

Correspondence should be addressed to Timothy J. Chevassut; t.chevassut@bsms.ac.uk

Academic Editor: Gösta Gahrton

Multiple myeloma is a malignant proliferation of monoclonal plasma cells leading to clinical features that include hypercalcaemia, renal dysfunction, anaemia, and bone disease (frequently referred to by the acronym CRAB) which represent evidence of end organ failure. Recent evidence has revealed myeloma to be a highly heterogeneous disease composed of multiple molecularly-defined subtypes each with varying clinicopathological features and disease outcomes. The major division within myeloma is between hyperdiploid and nonhyperdiploid subtypes. In this division, hyperdiploid myeloma is characterised by trisomies of certain odd numbered chromosomes, namely, 3, 5, 7, 9, 11, 15, 19, and 21 whereas nonhyperdiploid myeloma is characterised by translocations of the immunoglobulin heavy chain alleles at chromosome 14q32 with various partner chromosomes, the most important of which being 4, 6, 11, 16, and 20. Hyperdiploid and nonhyperdiploid changes appear to represent early or even initiating mutagenic events that are subsequently followed by secondary aberrations including copy number abnormalities, additional translocations, mutations, and epigenetic modifications which lead to plasma cell immortalisation and disease progression. The following review provides a comprehensive coverage of the genetic and epigenetic events contributing to the initiation and progression of multiple myeloma and where possible these abnormalities have been linked to disease prognosis.

1. Overview of Myeloma Genetics

Myeloma is a genetically complex disease which develops via a multistep process whereby plasma cells are driven towards malignancy through the accumulation of genetic "hits" over time. This multistep process permits myeloma to have various recognisable clinical phases, distinguished by biological parameters, along its development (Table 1). The earliest of these phases is termed monoclonal gammopathy of undetermined significance (MGUS) and is an indolent, asymptomatic, premalignancy phase characterized by a small clonal population of plasma cells within the bone marrow of <10% [1]. MGUS has a prevalence of >5% in adults aged over 70 and a progression risk to myeloma quantified at 1% per year [2, 3]. Following MGUS is smouldering multiple myeloma (SMM), another asymptomatic phase distinguished from MGUS by a greater intramedullary tumour cell content of >10% and an average risk of progression to myeloma of 10% per year for the first five years [4]. Next, myeloma itself is recognised, whereby malignant clones cause clinically relevant end-organ damage including the features of CRAB. The final phase is plasma cell leukemia (PCL), an aggressive disease end-point characterised by the existence of extramedullary clones and rapid progression to death. The basic premise of this disease progression is that the accumulation of genetic "hits" across different cellular pathways drives malignant change through deregulation to the intrinsic biology of the plasma cell. With advancements in molecular biology, many of these disrupted genes and pathways have now been characterised and the current challenge is therefore how to correctly interpret these molecular findings and develop them into clinically useful advances.

1.1. Myeloma Intraclonal Heterogeneity. Alongside aiding the characterisation of genes and pathways disrupted in myeloma, molecular studies have also revealed that intraclonal heterogeneity is a common feature of the malignancy [5, 6]. This heterogeneity adds an extra layer of complexity to myeloma progression as it is apparent that genetic "hits" are not acquired in a linear fashion but rather through nonlinear branching pathways synonymous to Darwin's evolution of

TABLE 1: Diagnostic criteria for myeloma of undetermined significance (MGUS), smouldering multiple myeloma (SMM), myeloma, and plasma cell leukemia (PCL). Reproduced from international myeloma working group, 2003 [37].

MGUS	SMM	Myeloma	PCL
Serum M-protein <30 g/L		M-protein in serum and/or urine.* No specific concentration required	Presence of ≥20% circulating plasma cells
Bone marrow clonal plasma cells <10%. **If done**—low level of plasma cell infiltration in a trephine biopsy	Serum M-protein ≥30 g/L **AND/OR** Bone marrow clonal plasma cells ≥10%	Confirmed clonal plasma cells in bone marrow	Absolute level of >2.0 × 10^9/L
Absence of end-organ disease and symptoms	Absence of end-organ disease and symptoms	Presence of myeloma-related organ or tissue impairment (ROTI)**	

*1-2% of patients have no detectable M-protein in serum or urine but do have myeloma-related organ or tissue impairment (ROTI) and increased intramedullary plasma cells; this is termed nonsecretory myeloma. **ROTI: corrected serum calcium >0.25 mmol/L above the upper limit of normal or >2.75 mmol/L, creatinine >173 mmol/L, Hb 2 g/dL below the lower limit of normal or <10 g/dL, lytic bone lesions or osteoporosis with compression fractures (may be clarified by CT or MRI), symptomatic hyperviscosity, amyloidosis, recurrent bacterial infections (>2 episodes in 12 months).

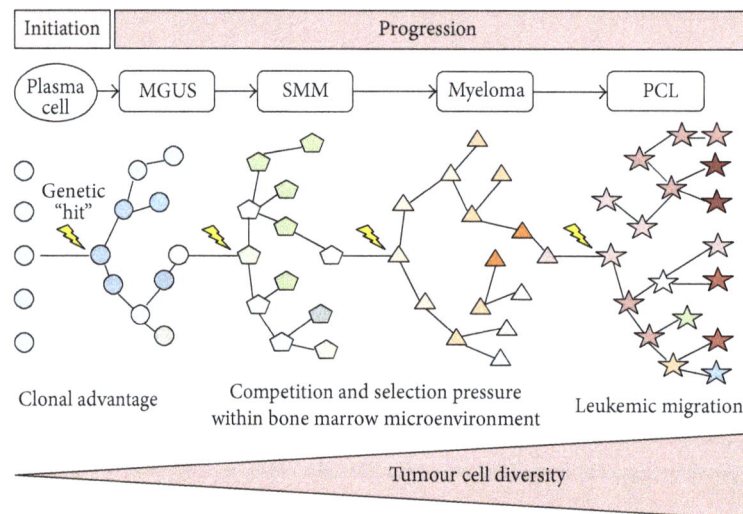

FIGURE 1: *Initiation and progression of myeloma.* A postgerminal centre B cell receives a genetic "hit" which immortalizes the cell and initiates transition to the indolent phase of monoclonal gammopathy of undetermined significance (MGUS). MGUS clones may then transition through the other disease phases of smouldering multiple myeloma (SMM), myeloma, and plasma cell leukemia (PCL) as genetic "hits", which confer a survival advantage and are acquired over time. Clonal evolution develops through branching pathways whereby numerous ecosystems composed of multiple subclones exist at each disease phase, as represented by the differing shapes. At the end of this process, proliferative clones no longer become confined to the bone marrow and expand rapidly as a leukemic phase. At each disease phase, the precursor clones are present only at a low level as they have been outcompeted by more advantageous clones. It should be noted that the above figure represents an oversimplification of myeloma initiation and progression, as the process is highly complex with multiple pathways possible at any one time (adapted from Morgan et al., 2012 [8]).

the species [7, 8]. A model of myeloma development through branching pathways is represented in Figure 1. This model however is designed as an oversimplification and should be viewed as a gross overview of disease progression as the process is highly complex with multiple progression pathways possible [8]. This analogy to Darwin's work explains that plasma cell clones acquire genetic lesions randomly and that these aberrations are then selected out based on their survival advantage. Consideration of intraclonal heterogeneity is important for disease understanding, as it is likely that the findings from many genomic studies represent the genetic

aberrations in the predominant clonal population at the time of sampling and that these results may not be applicable to all subclonal populations. This has particular therapeutic relevance, as the genes and pathways deregulated in the predominant clonal population are unlikely to be uniform across the many subclones allowing drug resistance and relapse to occur through the evolution and progression of these minority populations.

1.2. Nonhyperdiploid and Hyperdiploid Myeloma. Along the progression from MGUS to PCL, genetic aberrations can

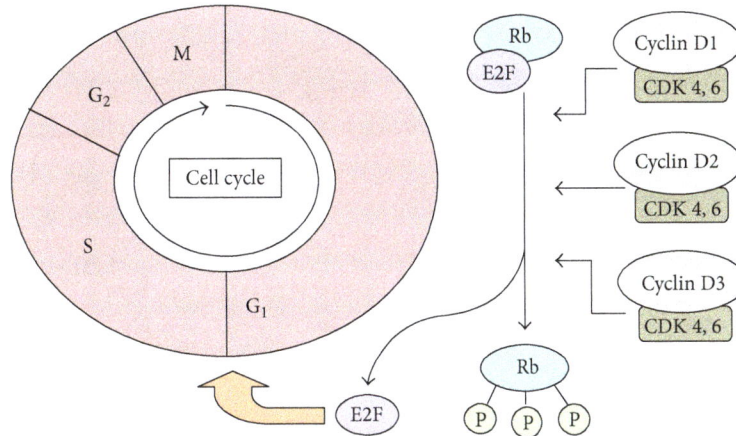

FIGURE 2: *Overexpression of cyclin D genes influence cell cycle progression at the G$_1$/S transition point in myeloma.* Increased cyclin D gene expression through hyperdiploid or nonhyperdiploid events in myeloma facilitates activation of a cyclin-dependent kinase (CDK 4 or 6). The respective CDK then phosphorylates Rb (retinoblastoma protein), which subsequently resides from its role inhibiting E2F transcription factors allowing these to facilitate cell cycle progression at the G$_1$/S transition. G$_1$: Gap-1 phase; S: synthesis phase; G2: Gap-2 phase; M: mitosis; P: phosphate group.

be classified as primary events, contributing to plasma cell immortalisation, or secondary events, contributing to disease progression. This classification facilitates the division of myeloma into two broad groups, nonhyperdiploidy myeloma and hyperdiploidy myeloma, based on one of two genetic aberrations observed in the primary phase [9, 10], a distinction originally suggested by Smadja et al., supported by the work of others, who put forward the idea of myeloma representing two closely related diseases [11–13]. Non-hyperdiploidy myeloma involves the translocation (*t*) of immunoglobulin heavy chain alleles (IGH@) at 14q32 with various partner chromosomes including 4, 6, 11, 16, and 20. These primary translocations occur due to aberrant class switch recombination (CSR) in lymph node germinal centres and act to juxtapose the partner chromosome oncogenes under the influence of the IGH@ enhancer region. Hyper-diploidy myeloma is generally associated with better survival and involves trisomies of the odd numbered chromosomes 3, 5, 7, 9, 11, 15, 19, and 21 coupled to a low prevalence of IGH@ translocations [14, 15]. Either directly, or indirectly, one consequence of hyperdiploid and nonhyperdiploid events is to result in deregulation of the G$_1$/S cell cycle transition point via the overexpression of cyclin D genes, an event shown to be a key early molecular abnormality in myeloma (Figure 2) [16]. For completion, it should be stated that exceptions to the hyperdiploidy and nonhyperdiploidy divisions do exist and that cases with primary translocations and multiple trisomies are detected in a minority.

1.3. Secondary Genetic Events and the Bone Marrow Microenvironment. Secondary genetic events drive disease progression and are generally found at higher frequencies in SMM, myeloma, and PCL. These secondary events cooperate with primary events to produce the malignant phenotype of myeloma and include secondary translocations, copy number variations (CNV), loss of heterozygosity (LOH), acquired mutations, and epigenetic modifications. Coupled to the development of these secondary events, clonal cells require a specialised relationship with bone marrow stromal cells for growth and survival. Studies have shown that this microenvironment interaction is highly complex, involving positive and negative interactions between the many cell types mediated through a variety of adhesion molecules, receptors, and cytokines [17, 18]. Furthermore, the derangement of these stromal-clone interactions has been shown to have important consequences in facilitating plasma cell homing to the bone marrow [18], promoting plasma cell immortalisation, and helping spread to secondary bone marrow sites [19, 20]. This stromal-clone relationship is relatively poorly understood at present but represents an area where investigation is ongoing and treatments are likely to be developed [21, 22].

1.4. Inherited Variation. Several studies have demonstrated that the majority of, if not all, myeloma cases pass through the MGUS phase [23, 24]. Therefore, in order to gain a fuller understanding of the disease, it is important to consider the genetic and environmental factors influencing transition to this indolent phase. From familial studies on index cases of myeloma, it is apparent that inherited genetic variation can predispose to the development of MGUS as these families have a two- to four-fold increased risk of developing the premalignant condition [25]. By investigating these families further, molecular epidemiology studies identified three genetic loci with associated gene pairs (2p: *DNMT3A* and *DTNB*, 3p: *ULK4* and *TRAK1*, 7p: *DNAH11* and *CDCA7L*) which incur a modest but increased risk of developing myeloma [26]. The complete functional role of these gene pairs is currently unknown, although deregulation of the proto-oncogene *MYC* encoding a transcription factor which regulates genes involved in DNA replication, cell proliferation, and apoptosis, has been implicated [26]. From these initial studies, it is likely that more susceptibility loci will

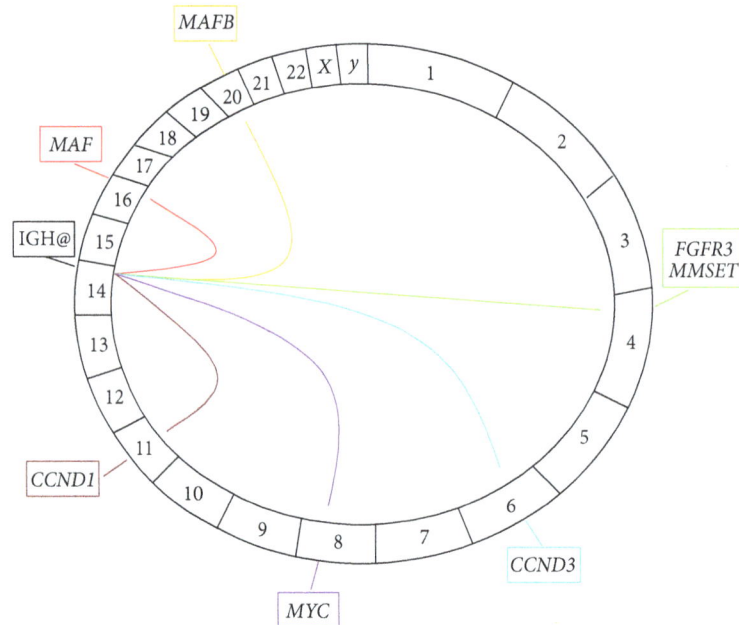

FIGURE 3: *The key chromosomal translocations in myeloma*. A Circos plot, with the chromosomes arranged in a clockwise direction, demonstrating the key translocations in myeloma. The translocations are represented as lines emerging from the immunoglobulin heavy chain (IGH@) locus on chromosome 14 to their respective partner chromosomes. The genes involved in each translocation are represented in boxes outside the plot. All translocations represent primary events except $t(8;14)$ involving *MYC* which is a secondary translocation.

be identified in the future and that these may be correlated to specific myeloma subtypes. The reliable identification of those at risk of developing myeloma would be an important advancement as it may facilitate comprehensive disease monitoring and early disease detection. Furthermore, it could be postulated that future targeted therapies or gene knockdown interventions may be developed against these susceptibility loci to restrict progression to myeloma altogether.

2. Chromosomal Translocations in Myeloma

Chromosomal translocations account for 40–50% of primary events in myeloma and strongly influence disease phenotype [9]. Secondary translocations, not associated with aberrant CSR, occur later in disease and are likely to represent progression events. The key primary and secondary translocations occurring in myeloma are highlighted in Figure 3.

2.1. $t(4;14)$ in Myeloma. The $t(4;14)$ is observed in 15% of myeloma cases and has been associated with an adverse prognosis in a variety of clinical settings such as those receiving high dose therapy with autologous stem cell transplant (ASCT) [27–30]. Pathologically, $t(4;14)$ results in the overexpression of two genes, *FGFR3* and *MMSET*, by juxtaposition next to the IGH@ enhancers [31]. The upregulation of *FGFR3* results in the ectopic expression of the FGFR3 tyrosine kinase receptor, an aberration with a currently unclear role in myelomagenesis. Interestingly, the pathogenic role of *FGFR3* is somewhat in question, as approximately 30% of $t(4;14)$ tumours are imbalanced and lack *FGFR3* expression due to loss of the derivative 14 chromosome [28, 32]. Furthermore, in

these 30% lacking *FGFR3* expression, the adverse prognosis of $t(4;14)$ remains [28], lending support for the role of the second gene *MMSET*. *MMSET* is overexpressed in all $t(4;14)$ tumours and encodes a chromatin-remodelling factor with histone methyltransferase (HMT) activity [27]. As for *FGFR3*, the exact role *MMSET* plays in pathogenesis is unclear although epigenetic regulation and a role in DNA repair have been suggested [33, 34]. In keeping with the unifying event of cyclin D deregulation, $t(4;14)$ with *MMSET* and/or *FGFR3* overexpression have been shown to upregulate *CCND2*, and in some instances *CCND1*, through an unknown mechanism [9]. It is interesting to note that despite the poor prognosis associated with $t(4;14)$ a clear survival advantage in these tumours has recently been demonstrated through early treatment with the proteasome inhibitor bortezomib [35, 36], with a suggestion that prolonged bortezomib treatment can overcome the adverse prognosis altogether [35, 36]. This point demonstrates that future myeloma prognostication is likely to be determined by the success of therapeutically targeting high-risk lesions through a personalised approach.

2.2. $t(6;14)$ and $t(11;14)$ in Myeloma. The $t(6;14)$ is a rare translocation present in 2% of myeloma patients which results in the direct upregulation of the *CCND3* gene via juxtaposition to the IGH@ enhancers [27, 38]. $t(11;14)$ is more common, occurring in approximately 17% of myeloma patients and also directly upregulates a cyclin D gene in the form *CCND1* [27, 39]. Gene expression studies have shown that the overexpression of *CCND3* and *CCND1* results in a clustering of downstream gene expression suggesting that activation of these two genes results in the deregulation of common downstream transcriptional events [27]. Due to the seeming importance of cyclin D gene deregulation in myeloma, cyclin D inhibitors with a variety of specificities have shown promise targeting myeloma *in vitro* [40, 41], with many of these inhibitors now entering early human trials. Unlike $t(4; 14)$, the overall prognostic impact of these two translocations is neutral [42], although $t(11; 14)$ patients do show considerable heterogeneity and in some instances the translocation may manifest with an aggressive phenotype such as PCL.

2.3. t(14; 16) and t(14; 20) in Myeloma. The $t(14; 16)$ and $t(14; 20)$ both result in increased expression of a *MAF* family oncogene and combined are identified in 5–10% of presenting myeloma cases [27]. Specifically, $t(14; 16)$ results in overexpression of the *MAF* gene splice variant *c-MAF*, a transcription factor which upregulates a number of genes including *CCND2* by binding directly to its promoter [43]. $t(14; 16)$ has been associated with a poor prognosis in a number of clinical series [29, 44], although this concept has recently been challenged by retrospective multivariate analysis on 1003 newly diagnosed myeloma patients which showed $t(14; 16)$ not to be prognostic [45]. $t(14; 20)$ is the rarest translocation involving the IGH@ and results in upregulation of the *MAF* gene paralog *MAFB*. Microarray studies have demonstrated that *MAFB* overexpression results in a very similar gene expression profile (GEP) to that seen with *c-MAF* [27], suggesting that common downstream targets, including *CCND2*, are deregulated by each. Interestingly, $t(14; 20)$ is associated with a poor prognosis when present in myeloma but correlates to long-term stable disease when found in MGUS and SMM [46]. This suggests that the translocation alone is not responsible for the poor prognosis but that additional genetic events are required.

2.4. Secondary Translocations in Myeloma. As opposed to primary translocations, secondary translocations are CSR-independent events occurring later in disease. Furthermore, although the most frequent secondary translocation is $t(8; 14)$, they do not always involve the IGH@ at 14q32 with approximately 40% linking different partner genes [47]. The gene typically deregulated by secondary translocations is *MYC*, the overexpression of which is linked directly to late disease stages and indirectly to a poor prognosis via a strong correlation to high levels of serum β_2-microglobulin (Sβ_2M) [48], an established indicator of a poor prognosis [49]. The frequency of *MYC* overexpression from secondary translocations supports its role as a progression event, as it is infrequently witnessed in MGUS but seen in 15% of myelomas and 50% of advanced disease [48, 50]. In opposition to this, a mouse model has previously demonstrated that the sporadic activation of a *MYC* transgene in germinal centre B cells of MGUS-prone mice results in the universal development of myeloma [51], whereas as previously discussed, an association also exists between *MYC* deregulation and certain genetic loci linked with myeloma susceptibility [26]. From these conflicting findings, it appears that *MYC* may play a role in both early and late disease phases and that further studies are required to elucidate an exact role for the gene.

3. Copy Number Variations in Myeloma

Copy number variations result from gains and losses of DNA and are common events in myeloma. These gains and losses can be both focal or of an entire chromosome/chromosome arm. In general, losses of DNA contribute to malignancy through loss of tumour suppressor genes, whereas gains are pathogenic through oncogene overexpression/activation.

3.1. Hyperdiploidy. Hyperdiploidy involves trisomies of the odd numbered chromosomes and is an event witnessed in approximately 50% of myeloma cases [14]. More common in elderly patients and associated with a high incidence of bone disease, hyperdiploidy confers a relatively favourable prognosis in the majority of cases [14], a factor held particularly true in instances where amplification 5q31.3 is concurrently present [52]. The underlying mechanism to generate hyperdiploidy is unknown, although one hypothesis, based on what is suggested to occur in hyperdiploid acute lymphoblastic leukemia, is that a single catastrophic mitosis results in the gain of whole chromosomes rather than their serial accumulation over time [53]. Along with the underlying mechanism, the consequence of hyperdiploidy towards myelomagenesis is poorly understood. However, alongside the known dysfunction of cyclin D genes, recent GEP studies have demonstrated that a high proportion of protein biosynthesis genes, specifically ribosomal protein genes representing end-points in MYC, NF-κB, and MAPK signalling pathways, are also concurrently overexpressed in hyperdiploid tumours [54, 55]. One explanation for this is that these genes are overexpressed due to rapid cell proliferation. This however is unlikely, as myeloma has a distinctively low proliferation rate. Instead, it is proposed that the overexpression is driven by gene copy number increases, with hyperdiploid cells then possessing more ribosomes and translational initiation factors to promote myelomagenesis through the overexpression of cellular growth genes [54].

3.2. Gain of 1q. Gain of the chromosome 1q arm (+1q) is an event observed in 35–40% of presenting myeloma cases and one which is frequently observed along with loss of 1p [56–59]. +1q is associated with a poor prognosis in patients treated both intensively and nonintensively and is an observation which remains when other adverse cytogenetic lesions which frequently coexist are removed [57, 60, 61]. Despite this knowledge, the relevant genes on 1q are not fully explored. One region of the chromosome arm which has been identified as a frequently minimally amplified region; however, 1q21 does contain many candidate oncogenes in the form of *CKS1B, ANP32E, BCL-9*, and *PDZK1* [57, 60, 62]. The importance of this region is supported by the demonstration of a strong association between +1q21 and an adverse prognosis using both fluorescence *in situ* hybridization (FISH) and GEP techniques [56, 57, 61]. Of these genes, *ANP32E*, a protein phosphatise 2A inhibitor with a role in chromatin remodelling and transcriptional regulation, is of particular interest as it has been shown to be independently associated with shortened survival [57]. These findings support the importance of +1q in myeloma pathogenesis and suggest that patients in this group may benefit from specific inhibitors of the candidate genes and pathways identified.

3.3. Loss of 1p.

Whole arm deletion or interstitial deletions of the 1p chromosome arm are observed in approximately 30% of myeloma patients and are associated with a poor prognosis in a range of treatment settings [57, 63, 64]. Molecular genetics has revealed that two regions of 1p, 1p12, and 1p32.3 are particularly important in myeloma pathogenesis when deleted. 1p12 may be hemi- or homozygously deleted and contains the candidate tumour suppressor gene *FAM46C* [5]. The function of *FAM46C* is unknown, although recent sequencing and homology studies have shown that its expression is correlated to both that of ribosomal proteins and eukaryotic initiation/elongation factors involved in protein translation [5]. *FAM46C* is considered a gene of significance as it has been shown to be frequently mutated in myeloma whilst also being independently correlated to a poor prognosis [5, 57, 58, 63]. 1p32.3 may also be hemi- and homozygously deleted and contains the two target genes, *FAF1* and *CDKN2C*. *CDKN2C* is a cyclin-dependent kinase 4 inhibitor involved in negative regulation of the cell cycle, whereas *FAF1* encodes a protein involved in initiation and/or enhancement of apoptosis through the Fas pathway. Homozygous deletion of 1p32.3 is associated with a poor prognosis in those receiving ASCT whereas in those receiving nonintensive treatment its prognostic impact is neutral [63]. Significant evidence points to *CDKN2C* as being the influential gene lost through homozygous 1p32.3 deletion [63, 65], although as *CDKN2C* and *FAF1* lie in such close proximity, the vast majority of deletions lose both genes and therefore the importance of *FAF1* relative to *CDKN2C* is difficult to delineate.

3.4. Loss of Chromosome 13/13q.

Chromosome 13 deletion is observed in approximately 50% of myeloma cases and is commonly associated with nonhyperdiploid tumours [66–68]. In approximately 85% of cases, deletion of chromosome 13 constitutes a monosomy or loss of the q arm, whereas in the remaining 15% various interstitial deletions occur [66, 69]. With this, the identification of key genes contributing to myeloma pathogenesis is challenging as often a level of gene function remains from the residual allele(s). Despite this, molecular studies have shown that the tumour suppressor gene *RB1* is significantly underexpressed in del(13/13q) and may therefore result in inferior negative cell cycle regulation [57]. To establish the prognostic impact of del(13/13q) is challenging due to its frequent association with other high-risk lesions, such as that of *t*(4; 14) where it is concurrently present in approximately 90% of cases [59]. When del(13/13q) is detected via conventional cytogenetics a link to poor survival exists [70, 71]. However, when detected via FISH, and in the absence of coexisting high-risk lesions, its significance towards survival is lost [42, 72]. This finding suggests that the historical link between del(13/13q) and a poor prognosis is therefore a surrogate of its association with high-risk lesions. One caveat to this statement however is that few long term follow-up studies comparing patient outcomes with or without these high-risk lesions have been completed whereas

several long-term studies comparing the presence or absence of del(13/13q) do exist. In one of these studies, conducted by Gahrton et al. [73], a 96-month followup of 357 myeloma patients treated with either autologous transplantation or tandem autologous/reduced intensity conditioning allogenic transplantation (auto/RICallo) showed that whilst del(13/13q) acted as a poor prognostic marker for those receiving autologous transplantation this factor was apparently overcome for patients with del(13/13q) receiving auto/RICallo. This therefore suggests that del(13/13q) may have value as a poor prognostic marker for long-term outcomes in those receiving autologous transplantation.

3.5. Loss of 17p.

The majority of chromosome 17 deletions are hemizygous and of the whole p arm, a genetic event observed in approximately 10% of new myeloma cases with this frequency increasing in later disease stages [29, 74]. The relevant gene deregulated in del(17p) is thought to be the tumour suppressor gene *TP53*, as GEP has shown that myeloma samples with monoallelic 17p deletions express significantly less *TP53* compared to nondeleted samples [57]. Furthermore, in cases without del(17p) the rate of *TP53* mutation is <1%, whereas in cases with del(17p) this rises to 25–37% [75]; a finding providing some evidence that monoallelic 17p deletion contributes to disruption of the remaining allele. The *TP53* gene has been mapped to 17p13 and is known to function as a transcriptional regulator influencing cell cycle arrest, DNA repair, and apoptosis in response to DNA damage. In myeloma, del(17p) is the most important molecular finding for prognostication as it linked to an aggressive disease phenotype, a greater degree of extramedullary disease, and shortened survival [29, 42, 76]. It is hypothesised that PCL is largely a consequence of *TP53* dysfunction, as the majority of these cases have abnormalities in the gene [74]. Furthermore, most, if not all, human myeloma cell lines which survive in laboratory cell culture have *TP53* deficiency, further suggesting its importance in extramedullary disease. Despite the consensus that *TP53* is the relevant gene disrupted in del(17p); however, it should be stated that no direct biological evidence exists to support this hypothesis and that further exploration of the genetic consequences of the deletion is required.

3.6. Other Chromosomal Losses.

Many other chromosomal deletions, focal copy number losses, and regions of LOH are seen in myeloma, and as with the deletions of 1p, 13/13q, and 17p, the relatively high frequencies of these events in regions containing tumour suppressor genes suggest they are "driver" lesions contributing to myelomagenesis. Chromosome 11q deletion is observed in 7% of myeloma cases and harbours the tumour suppressor genes *BIRC2* and *BIRC3* [57]. del(14q) is a common event found in 38% of cases and includes the tumour suppressor gene *TRAF3* [57]. 16q deletion is another common event, seen in 35% of myeloma cases, and contains the tumour suppressor genes *CYLD* and *WWOX* [57]. All of these genes, except *WWOX* which is implicated in apoptosis [77], are involved in the NF-κB pathway and demonstrate that activation of this signalling

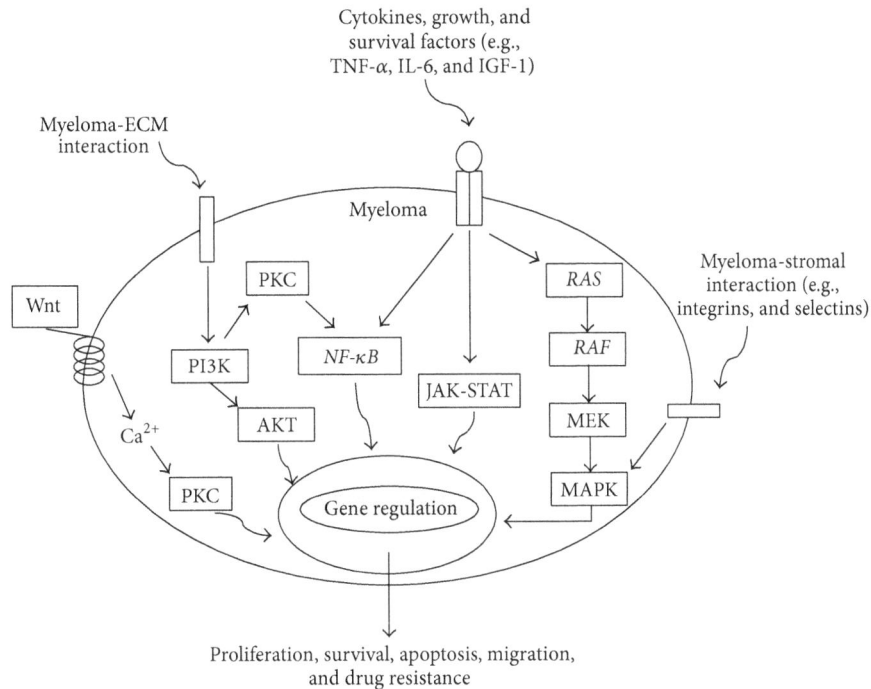

FIGURE 4: *Signalling pathways involved in myeloma pathogenesis.* The various pathways involved in myeloma pathogenesis may be stimulated via exogenous factors, such as Wnt proteins, myeloma-stromal interactions, cytokines, growth and survival factors, and myeloma-extracellular matrix (ECM) interactions, or the pathways may be aberrantly activated endogenously through genetic abnormalities such as activating mutations in *RAS*, *RAF*, and *NF-κB* genes.

pathway is important in myeloma pathogenesis [57, 78, 79]. del(12p) is another lesion of interest in myeloma, as a recent single-nucleotide polymorphism (SNP) assay found it to be an independent adverse prognostic marker in 192 newly diagnosed patients [52]; a finding however not repeated in other studies [57]. Two further common chromosomal arm deletions frequently witnessed in myeloma are del(6q) and del(8p), observed 33% and 19–24% of cases, respectively [57, 80–82]. The relevance of del(6q) towards survival is as yet not clear. For del(8p) however, it has been shown that this aberration acts as an independently poor prognostic factor for both progression free survival (PFS) and overall survival (OS) [80, 81]. Furthermore, it has been shown that the tumour necrosis factor-related apoptosis-inducing ligand (TRALI) receptor gene is located on 8p, and that during del(8p) a consequential downregulation of TRALI occurs [83]. As TRALI is associated with TNF-induced apoptosis, it is proposed that with reduced receptor expression in del(8p) the sensitivity of tumour cells to TRAIL-medicated apoptosis may be decreased providing an advantage for the immune escape of malignant clones from surveillance by natural killer cells and cytotoxic T lymphocytes [84].

4. Deregulation of Myeloma Cellular Pathways and Processes

A range of signalling pathways are deregulated in myeloma and contribute towards pathogenesis through associations with proliferation, survival, apoptosis, migration, and drug

resistance (Figure 4) [85]. Other cellular processes such as DNA repair, RNA editing, protein homeostasis, and cell differentiation may also contribute towards myelomagenesis through aberrant functioning.

4.1. NF-κB. NF-κB comprises a family of structurally related transcription factors which are upregulated during cellular stress to mediate gene responses. Salient to cancer, aberrant activation of NF-κB contributes to cell survival, proliferation and adhesion pathways. In myeloma, the NF-κB pathway is constitutively active in at least 50% of cases and is likely to represent a "driver" event due to its differing activation frequency between MGUS and later disease phases [78, 79]. Interestingly, NF-κB may be upregulated in both plasma cells and surrounding bone marrow stromal cells. In these supporting cells, NF-κB stimulates the release of key cytokines such as IL-6, BAFF and APRIL resulting in paracrine stimulation and critical survival signals to malignant clones [86, 87]. Activation of NF-κB within myeloma cells occurs through a range of mechanisms, including the inactivation of pathway suppressors through gene deletions and/or mutations, and pathway hyperactivity due to translocations and copy number gains [78, 79]. Furthermore, a recent whole genome sequencing (WGS) and whole exome sequencing (WES) study expanded the possible mechanisms through which the pathway may be activated by demonstrating 14 novel mutations/rearrangements affecting 11 NF-κB pathway genes [5]. The frequency with which NF-κB is deregulated in myeloma supports its importance in pathogenesis, although the prognostic impact for many of the implicated genes are yet to be fully elucidated. As the pathway involves the proteasome, inhibitors of this protein complex have been developed, with evidence suggesting that tumours "addicted" to the NF-κB pathway are particularly sensitive to these drugs [79]. Any adverse prognosis of NF-κB activation may therefore be potentially therapeutically ameliorated in the future.

4.2. Cell Proliferation. Of the pathways highlighted in Figure 4, three of them, the MAPK pathway, the JAK-STAT pathway, and the PI3K pathway, are particularly implicated in myelomagenesis through influences on cell proliferation.

4.2.1. The Mitogen Activated Protein Kinase (MAPK) Pathway. The MAPK pathway is a highly conserved cellular signalling cascade involved in cell differentiation, proliferation, and survival. The pathway may be stimulated via a range of inflammatory cytokines, such as TNF-a, IL-6, and IGF-1, which in turn activate the downstream kinase cascades RAS, RAF, MEK, and MAPK ultimately influencing gene expression. Two dominant oncogenes in the MAPK pathway, deregulated in many cancers, are *NRAS* and *KRAS*. These genes are frequently mutated in myeloma with a combined prevalence of 20–35% [88]. *RAS* mutations are likely to represent progression events as they are rarely found in MGUS but occur more frequently in later disease [89]. Additionally, *RAS* mutations are a poor prognostic marker, frequently being associated to a more aggressive disease phenotype and shortened survival times [88]. Recently however, it has been suggested that *KRAS*, and not *NRAS*, is the more influential gene impacting on prognosis [88], a finding which may have important consequences if genetic lesions are used to define risk. Due to the importance of *RAS* mutations and the MAPK pathway across many cancers, therapeutic inhibitors within this area are a key focus of research.

Showing further importance of the MAPK pathway, a recent study by Chapman et al. identified that seven out of 161 (4%) myeloma patients harboured a previously unobserved mutation in the *BRAF* gene [5]. *BRAF* encodes a serine/threonine-protein kinase in which activating mutations are known to be important in many cancers including melanoma and hairy cell leukemia [90]. This has particular clinical relevance, as myeloma patients with *BRAF* mutations may benefit from newly developed BRAF inhibitors, drugs which in some instances have shown marked clinical activity [91]. The premise to perform genome analysis for *BRAF* mutations on 161 samples arose from an original WGS/WES study on 38 myeloma samples which revealed the mutation in one patient [5]. This highlights the advantage of WGS/WES, in that the technique can be used as a screening tool to identify unknown genetic aberrations across the whole genome/exome, a benefit which may prove paramount in identifying novel therapeutic targets and disease biomarkers.

4.2.2. The JAK-STAT Pathway. The JAK-STAT pathway is constitutively activated in 50% of myeloma samples as well as a proportion of surrounding bone marrow stromal cells [92, 93]. The principal method thought to induce JAK-STAT activation is through autocrine and paracrine stimulation with IL-6, a cytokine shown to be important in myelomagenesis through the regulation of growth and survival [94, 95]. One key consequence of JAK-STAT activation is overactivity of STAT3, a STAT family transcription factor which results in high expression of the antiapoptotic protein Bcl-x_L [94], a protein correlated to chemoresistance in myeloma patients [96]. With this, inhibition of STAT3 with compounds such as curcumin, atiprimod, and the JAK2 kinase inhibitor AG490 are associated with inhibition of IL-6-induced myeloma survival *in vitro* [97–99]. Furthermore, inhibition of STAT3 has been shown to sensitize the U266 myeloma cell line to apoptosis induced through conventional chemotherapy agents [100]. Development of STAT3 inhibitors may therefore facilitate improved results with conventional chemotherapy agents in the future.

4.2.3. The Phosphatidylinositol-3 Kinase (PI3K) Pathway. A range of molecular signals, such as IL-6 and IGF-1, acting on tyrosine kinase receptors can activate the PI3K pathway leading to phosphorylation of the serine-threonine-specific kinase AKT. AKT then subsequently activates several downstream targets including mTOR, GSK-3B and FKHR which influence many processes including cell proliferation and apoptosis resistance. Deregulation of the PI3K pathway is thought to be important in myeloma as phosphorylated AKT, an indicative marker of pathway activity, is observed in approximately 50% of cases [101]. Additionally, DEPTOR, a positive regulator of the PI3K pathway is commonly upregulated in myeloma, especially in those with *MAF* translocations [102], further demonstrating pathway activity. Of interest, unlike the MAPK pathway, the PI3K pathway is rarely mutated in myeloma [5]. However, as the pathway is known to be active, therapeutic targeting of PI3K is of interest within myeloma research.

4.3. Cell Cycle Deregulation. Alongside the overexpression of cyclin D genes in myeloma, the loss of function to negative cell cycle regulatory genes also proves to be a key event which destabilises cell cycle regulation. For example, the downregulation of *CDKN2C* through del(1p), or the inactivation of *CDKN2A* via DNA methylation changes may both deregulate the G_1/S transition as these genes encode cyclin-dependent kinase inhibitors [65, 103]. Inactivation of the tumour suppressor gene *RB1*, a negative cell cycle regulator, also affects the G_1/S transition and may occur frequently due to monosomy 13 or infrequently due to homozygous deletion or mutational inactivation [57]. The disruption of *RB1* is known to be a key pathological event in many cancers and the development of anti-cancer drugs targeting cell cycle regulators, including *RB1*, is a rapidly growing field.

4.4. Abnormal DNA Repair. Chromosomal instability is a defining feature of myeloma and contributes to the perpetual accumulation of genetic aberrations during disease progression. Despite this, consistent mutations of DNA repair genes have not been demonstrated in the disease, with loss of *TP53* function through del(17p), found in 10% of cases, the most common finding. Another gene of emerging importance however is *PARP1*, a gene encoding the PARP1 enzyme which contributes to repairing ssDNA breaks. A recent GEP study has demonstrated that increased expression of *PARP1* is associated with shortened survival in myeloma patients [104], whereas another GEP study identified the gene as one of 15 which may be used as an expression signature to define high-risk disease [105]. Investigations in this area may prove pivotal for myeloma, as PARP inhibitors have shown promising activity in clinical trials [106]. This activity is especially prominent in cancers with defective homologous recombination (HR)-mediated DNA repair mechanisms, as cells with defects in this system are sensitized to PARP inhibitors [107]. Although not a recognised *de novo* finding for myeloma, it has been shown that bortezomib can induce a HR-mediated DNA repair defective state, a so called "BRCAness", through interference of BRCA1 and RAD51 recruitment to the sites of dsDNA breaks *in vitro* [104]. Thus, bortezomib and a PARP inhibitor may induce synthetic lethality and be utilised as a future combined treatment for myeloma.

4.5. Abnormal RNA Editing.

4.5. Abnormal RNA Editing. A recent study revealed that nearly half of 38 myeloma samples contained mutations in genes involved in RNA processing, protein translation and the unfolded protein response (UPR) [5]. Four different mutations of *DIS3*, a gene encoding an exonuclease serving as the catalytic component of the exosome complex involved in regulating the abundance of RNA species [108, 109], were observed in 11% of samples [5]. The *DIS3* gene has been mapped to 13q22.1, and in three out the four mutations identified loss of function was exhibited by monoallelic mutation coupled to deletion of the remaining allele [5]. This demonstrates the key contribution del(13) is likely to play to *DIS3* mutations and suggests another implication of this genetic aberration alongside *RB1* haploinsufficiency. Furthermore, two of the four mutations in *DIS3* have been functionally characterised in microorganisms where they result in loss of enzymatic activity with consequential accumulation of RNA targets [110, 111]. As it has been shown that the exosome plays a vital role in regulating the available pool of mRNAs for translation [112], these mutational findings indicate that loss of *DIS3* activity may contribute to myelomagenesis through deregulation of protein translation. Another gene, *FAM46C*, implicated in del(1p) and previously discussed, gives further support for the role of translational control in myeloma pathogenesis, as WGS/WES found this gene to be mutated in 13% of samples [5]. This frequency supports the implication of *FAM46C* in myeloma pathogenesis as recurrently mutated genes are likely to be of biological significance.

4.6. Protein Homeostasis: The Unfolded Protein Response. The UPR is essential for the normal functioning of plasma cells as it serves a critical function in the efficient production of immunoglobulin by regulating cellular responses to unfolded/misfolded protein in the endoplasmic reticulum. Of interest, sequencing has revealed mutations of the *LRRK2* gene at a frequency of 8% [5]. *LRRK2* encodes

a serine-threonine kinase responsible for phosphorylating the eukaryotic translation initiation factor 4E-binding protein 1 (EIF4EBP1), a protein which functions in regulating protein translation. *LRRK2* is predominantly known for its association with Parkinson's disease, where mutations in the gene are linked to a predisposition for the condition [113, 114]. As with other neurodegenerative conditions, Parkinson's disease is in part characterised by a dysfunctional UPR and abrogated protein, and as myeloma has a vastly increased rate of immunoglobulin production [115, 116], any changes in protein homeostasis are likely to be pathogenically important. Of related interest, sequencing data has also revealed mutations in the UPR gene *XBP1*, although at a low frequency of 3% [5]. When over-expressed in transgenic mice, a splice form of *XBP1* has been shown to induce a myeloma-like syndrome [117], whereas in mice deficient of *XBP1* B cells are able to proliferate and construct germinal centres but are unable to differentiate into immunoglobulin secreting plasma cells [118]. The exact role of *XBP1* in human myeloma pathogenesis is unclear, although a recent study has shown that finding a high ratio between un-spliced and spliced variants of *XBP1* in myeloma samples is linked to a poor outcome and serves as an independent prognostic factor [119].

4.7. Abnormal Plasma Cell Differentiation. One method to establish biologically significant gain-of-function changes in cancer genomes is to use WGS/WES to search for recurrent identical mutations in candidate oncogenes. Utilising this method, Chapman et al. found two myeloma patients from 38 harboured an identical mutation (K123R) in the DNA-binding domain of the interferon regulatory factor 4 (*IRF4*) [5]. As its name suggests, *IRF4* is involved in regulating the transcription of interferon's whilst it also plays an important role in B cell proliferation and differentiation. Interestingly, a recent RNA-inference-based genetic screen revealed that *IRF4* function is required for myeloma cell line survival as inhibition of the gene proved toxic to the malignant cells [120], an *in vitro* finding supporting the genes role in pathogenesis. One way in which *IRF4* acts is as a transcription factor for *BLIMP1*, also a transcription factor itself which plays a key role in plasma cell differentiation. The Chapman et al. study identified two mutations in the *BLIMP1* gene from their 38 samples, and as loss-of-function mutations in *BLIMP1* are known to occur in diffuse large B-cell lymphoma [121], this suggests *BLIMP1* mutations may be of pathogenic importance to myeloma. Of consideration, as myeloma is a malignancy of terminally differentiated plasma cells, the importance of dysfunction within differentiation pathways may be of less importance than in cancers of immature cells, further studies are however required to investigate this.

4.8. Myeloma Bone Disease. Bone disease occurs in 80–90% of patients with myeloma and can be either focal or diffuse resulting in pain, pathological factures, cord compression and hypercalcaemia. A recent GEP study aimed to identify the molecular basis of patients presenting with bone disease in order to elucidate whether a gene expression signature could identify those at high-risk of skeletal-related events after randomization into one of two bisphosphonate arms [122]. The study identified that 50 genes were significantly associated with presenting bone disease, mostly from pathways involved in growth factor signalling, apoptosis and transcription regulation. The two most significantly differently expressed genes were the Wnt pathway inhibitors *DKK1* and *FRZB*. The Wnt pathway is known to be important in regulating bone turnover and *DKK1* has been shown to both inhibit osteoblast differentiation and increase bone resorption through an increase in the RANKL/OPG ratio [123, 124]. An antibody against DKK1 is now being tested in clinical trials after showing promise by improving bone disease and inhibiting myeloma cell growth in a murine model [125]. The GEP study was also able to make more generalised observations of which some have been previously been reported [72, 126]. For example, bone disease is more prevalent in those with a hyperdiploidy signature and less associated with *t*(4; 14) and *MAF* translocations. Interestingly, this study found that *DKK1* and *FRZB* were more highly expressed in hyperdiploid tumours, providing a potential explanation for this finding. Secondly, patients with bone disease have shorter OS compared to those without [127], a finding which suggests bone disease significantly contributes to the impaired outcome of these patients, or, alternatively, that disease biology in myeloma with bone disease is distinctly different.

5. Epigenetic Changes in Myeloma

The study of epigenetics is an emerging field in myeloma and one which is demonstrating an increasing amount of influence on pathogenesis [128]. As outlined in Figure 5, the three main areas of epigenetic regulation include histone modification, RNA interference and DNA methylation.

5.1. DNA Methylation. DNA Methylation changes occur at CpG dinucleotides which are generally found at higher frequencies in promoter regions, repeat sequences and transposable elements. Changes in DNA methylation act to regulate gene expression and are known to be important in contributing to cell development and differentiation as well as the progression of many cancers. Myeloma genomes, as for many other cancers, often follow a recognised pattern of methylation represented by global DNA hypomethylation and gene-specific hypermethylation [129]. A recent study using a genome-wide methylation microarray built on this knowledge to demonstrate that a marked loss methylation occurred at the transition from MGUS to myeloma [129]. Furthermore, gene-specific hypo and hypermethylation was demonstrated at this transition with the genes affected involved in the cell cycle, transcriptional and cell development pathways [129]. During progression from myeloma to PCL, rather than finding global DNA hypomehtylation, gene-specific hypermethylation was found in genes involved in cell adhesion and cell signalling [129]. This finding suggests these methylation changes may contribute to destabilisation of the stromal-clone relationship and promotion of clonal transition into the circulation and a proliferating leukaemic phase.

The most significant DNA methylation changes, influencing cell survival, cell cycle progression and DNA repair, are seen in *t*(4; 14) tumours [33, 130], presumably as they over-express the *MMSET* gene which encodes a HMT transcription repressor.

5.2. Histone Modification. Other genes involved in methylation and chromatin modification are also deregulated in myeloma, including *KDM6A*, *MLL* genes and *HOXA9* [5]. Recent sequencing observed that *HOXA9* was ubiquitously expressed across 38 myeloma samples and hypothesised whether this gene represented a candidate oncogene [5]. The *HOXA9* gene is primarily regulated by HMTs and encodes a DNA-binding transcription factor which contributes to regulating gene expression, morphogenesis and differentiation. As the majority of cases over-expressing *HOXA9* in the study exhibited bi-allelic expression, consistent with deregulation of an upstream HMT event, genes involved in regulating *HOXA9* were evaluated for mutations with findings revealing mutations in several genes: *MLL, MLL2, MLL3*, and *MMSET* [5]. To establish the functional importance of *HOXA9* expression in myeloma, gene knockdown studies in a range of myeloma cell lines was performed and demonstrated that *HOXA9*-depleted cells incurred a competitive disadvantage against those with remaining *HOXA9* function [5]. These findings indicate that the expression of *HOXA9* has a role in myeloma pathogenesis and that these epigenetic changes may represent new therapeutic targets in myeloma.

5.3. MicroRNA Changes. MicroRNA (miRNA) genes encode a class of small RNAs (17–25 base pairs) which function to regulate the translation of other proteins by forming complementary base parings to specific mRNA transcripts. Studies have shown that miRNAs can act as both tumour suppressors and oncogenes in a range of cancers and that their transcriptional control is regulated by promoter methylation changes [131]. A substantial amount of work has been completed to investigate which miRNAs are differentially expressed in myeloma [132–134], and it has been shown that miRNA changes can deregulate genes and pathways relevant to myeloma pathogenesis including cell cycle progression, *TP53* and *MYC* [135–137]. Although there is some discrepancy between which miRNAs are differentially expressed, and when, in myeloma, the overall conclusion is that miRNA deregulation is likely to be an important contributor to the malignancy and that further investigation is warranted to improve understanding and to highlight potential treatment targets.

6. Conclusion

Myeloma is a highly heterogeneous disease and one which may progress from an indolent, asymptomatic phase, to an aggressive extramedullary phase as genetic "hits" are acquired over time. The primary genetic events contributing towards plasma cell immortalisation can be broadly divided into a hyperdiploid group, characterised by trisomies of odd

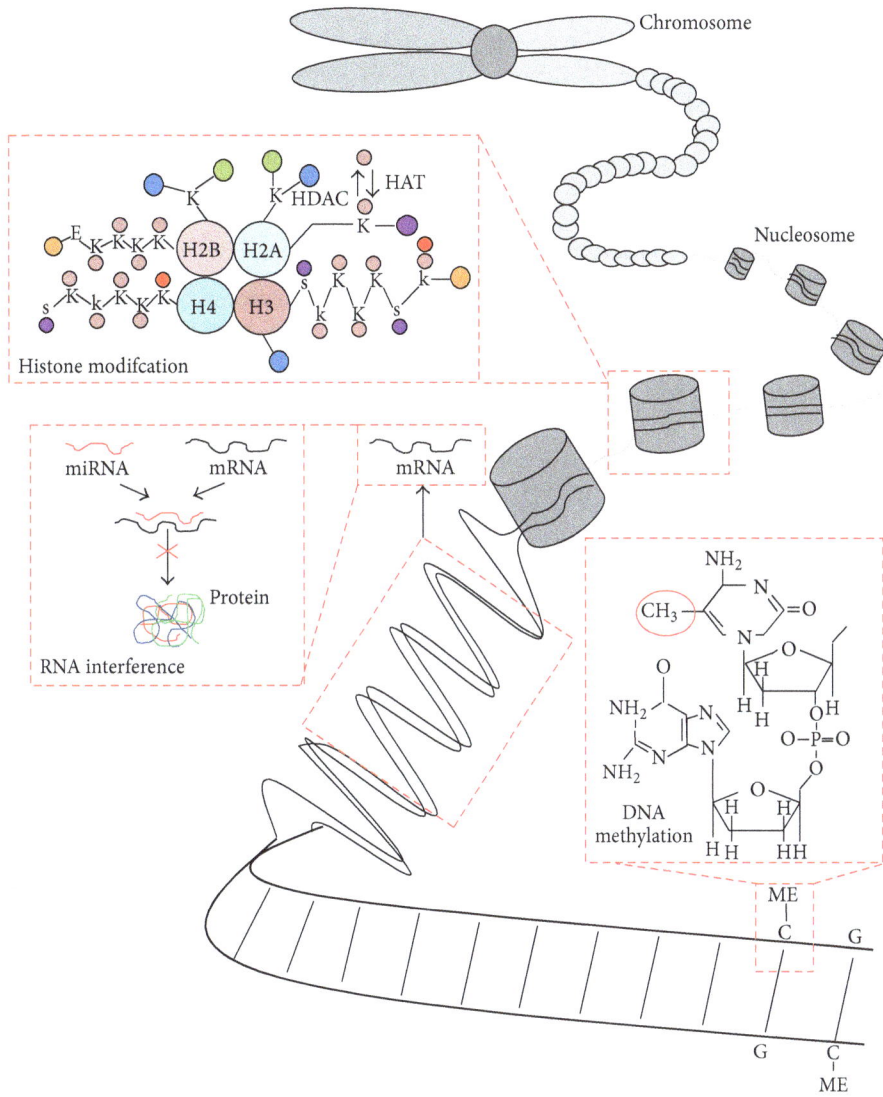

FIGURE 5: *Mechanisms of epigenetic regulation.* Three main forms of epigenetic modification include histone modification, RNA interference, and DNA methylation. Histone (chromatin) modification refers to the covalent posttranslational modifications to the N-terminal tails of the four core histone proteins; this modification is commonly acetylation/deacetylation changes at lysine residues mediated by histone acetyltransferases (HATs) and histone deacetylases (HDACs). RNA interference is predominantly mediated through microRNAs, which inhibit the translation of mRNA into protein. DNA methylation occurs at cytosine residues of CpG dinucleotides and acts to regulate gene expression. Pink circle = acetyl group, purple circle = phosphate group, red circle = methyl group, blue circle = carboxyl terminus, green circle = ubiquitin, orange circle = amino terminus, k = lysine, E = glutamic acid, S = serine. H2A, histone 2A; H2B, histone 2B; H3, histone 3; H4, histone 4.

numbered chromosomes, and a nonhyperdiploid group, characterised by IGH@ translocations to various partner chromosomes; it appears that overexpression of the cyclin D family of genes is an almost universal sequelae of primary events. Secondary genetic events, contributing to disease progression, are complex and involve secondary translocations, CNVs, acquired mutations, LOH, and epigenetic modification. From the use of molecular techniques to investigate myeloma, many of these primary and secondary events are now well characterised, and from this characterisation, it is apparent that disease behaviour can be correlated to the genetic makeup of a patient's disease. With this, it is therefore essential that genetic research remains focused in translating molecular characterisation into clinically useful advances.

Conflict of Interests

The authors declare that there is no conflict of interests regarding the publication of this paper.

References

[1] R. A. Kyle, B. G. Durie, S. V. Rajkumar et al., "Monoclonal gammopathy of undetermined significance (MGUS) and smoldering (asymptomatic) multiple myeloma: IMWG consensus

perspectives risk factors for progression and guidelines for monitoring and management," *Leukemia*, vol. 24, no. 6, pp. 1121–1127, 2010.

[2] R. A. Kyle, T. M. Therneau, S. V. Rajkumar et al., "Prevalence of monoclonal gammopathy of undetermined significance," *The New England Journal of Medicine*, vol. 354, no. 13, pp. 1362–1369, 2006.

[3] R. A. Kyle, T. M. Therneau, S. Vincent Rajkumar et al., "A long-term study of prognosis in monoclonal gammopathy of undetermined significance," *The New England Journal of Medicine*, vol. 346, no. 8, pp. 564–569, 2002.

[4] R. A. Kyle, E. D. Remstein, T. M. Therneau et al., "Clinical course and prognosis of smoldering (asymptomatic) multiple myeloma," *The New England Journal of Medicine*, vol. 356, no. 25, pp. 2582–2590, 2007.

[5] M. A. Chapman, M. S. Lawrence, J. J. Keats et al., "Initial genome sequencing and analysis of multiple myeloma," *Nature*, vol. 471, no. 7339, pp. 467–472, 2011.

[6] J. B. Egan, C. X. Shi, W. Tembe et al., "Whole-genome sequencing of multiple myeloma from diagnosis to plasma cell leukemia reveals genomic initiating events, evolution, and clonal tides," *Blood*, vol. 120, no. 5, pp. 1060–1066, 2012.

[7] K. Anderson, C. Lutz, F. W. van Delft et al., "Genetic variegation of clonal architecture and propagating cells in leukaemia," *Nature*, vol. 469, no. 7330, pp. 356–361, 2011.

[8] G. J. Morgan, B. A. Walker, and F. E. Davies, "The genetic architecture of multiple myeloma," *Nature Reviews Cancer*, vol. 12, no. 5, pp. 335–348, 2012.

[9] W. M. Kuehl and P. L. Bergsagel, "Early genetic events provide the basis for a clinical classification of multiple myeloma," *Hematology*, pp. 346–352, 2005.

[10] P. L. Bergsagel and W. M. Kuehl, "Molecular pathogenesis and a consequent classification of multiple myeloma," *Journal of Clinical Oncology*, vol. 23, no. 26, pp. 6333–6338, 2005.

[11] N.-V. Smadja, C. Fruchart, F. Isnard et al., "Chromosomal analysis in multiple myeloma: cytogenetic evidence of two different diseases," *Leukemia*, vol. 12, no. 6, pp. 960–969, 1998.

[12] J. Gould, R. Alexanian, A. Goodacre, S. Pathak, B. Hecht, and B. Barlogie, "Plasma cell karyotype in multiple myeloma," *Blood*, vol. 71, no. 2, pp. 453–456, 1988.

[13] J. R. Sawyer, J. A. Waldron, S. Jagannath, and B. Barlogie, "Cytogenetic findings in 200 patients with multiple myeloma," *Cancer Genetics and Cytogenetics*, vol. 82, no. 1, pp. 41–49, 1995.

[14] N. V. Smadja, C. Bastard, C. Brigaudeau, D. Leroux, and C. Fruchart, "Hypodiploidy is a major prognostic factor in multiple myeloma," *Blood*, vol. 98, no. 7, pp. 2229–2238, 2001.

[15] G. W. Dewald, R. A. Kyle, G. A. Hicks, and P. R. Greipp, "The clinical significance of cytogenetic studies in 100 patients with multiple myeloma, plasma cell leukemia, or amyloidosis," *Blood*, vol. 66, no. 2, pp. 380–390, 1985.

[16] P. L. Bergsagel, W. M. Kuehl, F. Zhan, J. Sawyer, B. Barlogie, and J. Shaughnessy Jr., "Cyclin D dysregulation: an early and unifying pathogenic event in multiple myeloma," *Blood*, vol. 106, no. 1, pp. 296–303, 2005.

[17] W. M. Kuehl and P. L. Bergsagel, "Molecular pathogenesis of multiple myeloma and its premalignant precursor," *Journal of Clinical Investigation*, vol. 122, no. 10, pp. 3456–3463, 2012.

[18] P. Neri, L. Ren, A. K. Azab et al., "Integrin β7-mediated regulation of multiple myeloma cell adhesion, migration, and invasion," *Blood*, vol. 117, no. 23, pp. 6202–6213, 2011.

[19] S. K. Brennan, Q. Wang, R. Tressler et al., "Telomerase inhibition targets clonogenic multiple myeloma cells through telomere length-dependent and independent mechanisms," *PLoS ONE*, vol. 5, no. 9, Article ID 12487, 2010.

[20] W. M. Kuehl and P. L. Bergsagel, "Multiple myeloma: evolving genetic events and host interactions," *Nature Reviews Cancer*, vol. 2, no. 3, pp. 175–187, 2002.

[21] T. Hideshima, C. Mitsiades, G. Tonon, P. G. Richardson, and K. C. Anderson, "Understanding multiple myeloma pathogenesis in the bone marrow to identify new therapeutic targets," *Nature Reviews Cancer*, vol. 7, no. 8, pp. 585–598, 2007.

[22] G. D. Roodman, "Targeting the bone microenvironment in multiple myeloma," *Journal of Bone and Mineral Metabolism*, vol. 28, no. 3, pp. 244–250, 2010.

[23] T. Rasmussen, J. Haaber, I. M. Dahl et al., "Identification of translocation products but not K-RAS mutations in memory B cells from patients with multiple myeloma," *Haematologica*, vol. 95, no. 10, pp. 1730–1737, 2010.

[24] O. Landgren, R. A. Kyle, R. M. Pfeiffer et al., "Monoclonal gammopathy of undetermined significance (MGUS) consistently precedes multiple myeloma: a prospective study," *Blood*, vol. 113, no. 22, pp. 5412–5417, 2009.

[25] A. Altieri, B. Chen, J. L. Bermejo, F. Castro, and K. Hemminki, "Familial risks and temporal incidence trends of multiple myeloma," *European Journal of Cancer*, vol. 42, no. 11, pp. 1661–1670, 2006.

[26] P. Broderick, D. Chubb, D. C. Johnson et al., "Common variation at 3p22.1 and 7p15.3 influences multiple myeloma risk," *Nature Genetics*, vol. 44, no. 1, pp. 58–61, 2012.

[27] F. Zhan, Y. Huang, S. Colla et al., "The molecular classification of multiple myeloma," *Blood*, vol. 108, no. 6, pp. 2020–2028, 2006.

[28] J. J. Keats, T. Reiman, C. A. Maxwell et al., "In multiple myeloma, t(4;14)(p16;q32) is an adverse prognostic factor irrespective of FGFR3 expression," *Blood*, vol. 101, no. 4, pp. 1520–1529, 2003.

[29] R. Fonseca, E. Blood, M. Rue et al., "Clinical and biologic implications of recurrent genomic aberrations in myeloma," *Blood*, vol. 101, no. 11, pp. 4569–4575, 2003.

[30] H. Chang, S. Sloan, D. Li et al., "The t(4;14) is associated with poor prognosis in myeloma patients undergoing autologous stem cell transplant," *British Journal of Haematology*, vol. 125, no. 1, pp. 64–68, 2004.

[31] M. Chesi, E. Nardini, R. S. C. Lim, K. D. Smith, W. Michael Kuehl, and P. L. Bergsagel, "The t(4;14) translocation in myeloma dysregulates both FGFR3 and a novel gene, MMSET, resulting in IgH/MMSET hybrid transcripts," *Blood*, vol. 92, no. 9, pp. 3025–3034, 1998.

[32] M. Santra, F. Zhan, E. Tian, B. Barlogie, and J. Shaughnessy Jr., "A subset of multiple myeloma harboring the t(4;14)(p16;q32) translocation lacks FGFR3 expression but maintains an IGH/MMSET fusion transcript," *Blood*, vol. 101, no. 6, pp. 2374–2376, 2003.

[33] E. Martinez-Garcia, R. Popovic, D.-J. Min et al., "The MMSET histone methyl transferase switches global histone methylation and alters gene expression in t(4;14) multiple myeloma cells," *Blood*, vol. 117, no. 1, pp. 211–220, 2011.

[34] H. Pei, L. Zhang, K. Luo et al., "MMSET regulates histone H4K20 methylation and 53BP1 accumulation at DNA damage sites," *Nature*, vol. 470, no. 7332, pp. 124–128, 2011.

[35] J. F. San Miguel, R. Schlag, N. K. Khuageva et al., "Bortezomib plus melphalan and prednisone for initial treatment of multiple myeloma," *The New England Journal of Medicine*, vol. 359, no. 9, pp. 906–917, 2008.

[36] H. Avet-Loiseau, X. Leleu, M. Roussel et al., "Bortezomib plus dexamethasone induction improves outcome of patients with t(4;14) myeloma but not outcome of patients with del(17p)," *Journal of Clinical Oncology*, vol. 28, no. 30, pp. 4630–4634, 2010.

[37] R. A. Kyle, J. A. Child, K. Anderson et al., "Criteria for the classification of monoclonal gammopathies, multiple myeloma and related disorders: a report of the International Myeloma Working Group," *British Journal of Haematology*, vol. 121, no. 5, pp. 749–757, 2003.

[38] J. Shaughnessy Jr., A. Gabrea, Y. Qi et al., "Cyclin D3 at 6p21 is dysregulated by recurrent chromosomal translocations to immunoglobulin loci in multiple myeloma," *Blood*, vol. 98, no. 1, pp. 217–223, 2001.

[39] M. Chesi, P. L. Bergsagel, L. A. Brents, C. M. Smith, D. S. Gerhard, and W. M. Kuehl, "Dysregulation of cyclin D1 by translocation into an IgH gamma switch region in two multiple myeloma cell lines," *Blood*, vol. 88, no. 2, pp. 674–681, 1996.

[40] L. B. Baughn, M. di Liberto, K. Wu et al., "A novel orally active small molecule potently induces G1 arrest in primary myeloma cells and prevents tumor growth by specific inhibition of cyclin-dependent kinase 4/6," *Cancer Research*, vol. 66, no. 15, pp. 7661–7667, 2006.

[41] X. Mao, B. Cao, T. E. Wood et al., "A small-molecule inhibitor of D-cyclin transactivation displays preclinical efficacy in myeloma and leukemia via phosphoinositide 3-kinase pathway," *Blood*, vol. 117, no. 6, pp. 1986–1997, 2011.

[42] H. Avet-Loiseau, M. Attal, P. Moreau et al., "Genetic abnormalities and survival in multiple myeloma: the experience of the Intergroupe Francophone du Myélome," *Blood*, vol. 109, no. 8, pp. 3489–3495, 2007.

[43] E. M. Hurt, A. Wiestner, A. Rosenwald et al., "Overexpression of c-maf is a frequent oncogenic event in multiple myeloma that promotes proliferation and pathological interactions with bone marrow stroma," *Cancer Cell*, vol. 5, no. 2, pp. 191–199, 2004.

[44] F. M. Ross, A. H. Ibrahim, A. Vilain-Holmes et al., "Age has a profound effect on the incidence and significance of chromosome abnormalities in myeloma," *Leukemia*, vol. 19, no. 9, pp. 1634–1642, 2005.

[45] H. Avet-Loiseau, F. Malard, L. Campion et al., "Translocation t(14;16) and multiple myeloma: is it really an independent prognostic factor?" *Blood*, vol. 117, no. 6, pp. 2009–2011, 2011.

[46] F. M. Ross, L. Chiecchio, G. Dagrada et al., "The t(14;20) is a poor prognostic factor in myeloma but is associated with long-term stable disease in monoclonal gammopathies of undetermined significance," *Haematologica*, vol. 95, no. 7, pp. 1221–1225, 2010.

[47] A. Dib, A. Gabrea, O. K. Glebov, P. L. Bergsagel, and W. M. Kuehl, "Characterization of MYC translocations in multiple myeloma cell lines," *Journal of the National Cancer Institute*, no. 39, pp. 25–31, 2008.

[48] H. Avet-Loiseau, F. Gerson, F. Magrangeas, S. Minvielle, J.-L. Harousseau, and R. Bataille, "Rearrangements of the c-myc oncogene are present in 15% of primary human multiple myeloma tumors," *Blood*, vol. 98, no. 10, pp. 3082–3086, 2001.

[49] P. R. Greipp, J. San Miguel, B. G. Durie et al., "International staging system for multiple myeloma," *Journal of Clinical Oncology*, vol. 23, no. 15, pp. 3412–3420, 2005.

[50] A. Gabrea, M. L. Martelli, Y. Qi et al., "Secondary genomic rearrangements involving immunoglobulin or MYC loci show similar prevalences in hyperdiploid and nonhyperdiploid myeloma

tumors," *Genes Chromosomes and Cancer*, vol. 47, no. 7, pp. 573–590, 2008.

[51] M. Chesi, D. F. Robbiani, M. Sebag et al., "AID-dependent activation of a MYC transgene induces multiple myeloma in a conditional mouse model of post-germinal center malignancies," *Cancer Cell*, vol. 13, no. 2, pp. 167–180, 2008.

[52] H. Avet-Loiseau, C. Li, F. Magrangeas et al., "Prognostic significance of copy-number alterations in multiple myeloma," *Journal of Clinical Oncology*, vol. 27, no. 27, pp. 4585–4590, 2009.

[53] N. Onodera, N. R. McCabe, and C. M. Rubin, "Formation of a hyperdiploid karyotype in childhood acute lymphoblastic leukemia," *Blood*, vol. 80, no. 1, pp. 203–208, 1992.

[54] W. J. Chng, S. Kumar, S. VanWier et al., "Molecular dissection of hyperdiploid multiple myeloma by gene expression profiling," *Cancer Research*, vol. 67, no. 7, pp. 2982–2989, 2007.

[55] L. Agnelli, S. Bicciato, M. Mattioli et al., "Molecular classification of multiple myeloma: a distinct transcriptional profile characterizes patients expressing CCND1 and negative for 14q32 translocations," *Journal of Clinical Oncology*, vol. 23, no. 29, pp. 7296–7306, 2005.

[56] K. D. Boyd, F. M. Ross, L. Chiecchio et al., "A novel prognostic model in myeloma based on co-segregating adverse FISH lesions and the ISS: analysis of patients treated in the MRC Myeloma IX trial," *Leukemia*, vol. 26, no. 2, pp. 349–355, 2012.

[57] B. A. Walker, P. E. Leone, L. Chiecchio et al., "A compendium of myeloma-associated chromosomal copy number abnormalities and their prognostic value," *Blood*, vol. 116, no. 15, pp. e56–e65, 2010.

[58] H. Chang, X. Qi, A. Jiang, W. Xu, T. Young, and D. Reece, "1p21 deletions are strongly associated with 1q21 gains and are an independent adverse prognostic factor for the outcome of high-dose chemotherapy in patients with multiple myeloma," *Bone Marrow Transplantation*, vol. 45, no. 1, pp. 117–121, 2010.

[59] R. Fonseca, P. L. Bergsagel, J. Drach et al., "International Myeloma Working Group molecular classification of multiple myeloma: spotlight review," *Leukemia*, vol. 23, no. 12, pp. 2210–2221, 2009.

[60] J. Shaughnessy, "Amplification and overexpression of CKS1B at chromosome band 1q21 is associated with reduced levels of p27Kip1 and an aggressive clinical course in multiple myeloma," *Hematology*, vol. 10, supplement 1, pp. 117–126, 2005.

[61] J. D. Shaughnessy Jr., F. Zhan, B. E. Burington et al., "A validated gene expression model of high-risk multiple myeloma is defined by deregulated expression of genes mapping to chromosome 1," *Blood*, vol. 109, no. 6, pp. 2276–2284, 2007.

[62] L. Shi, S. Wang, M. Zangari et al., "Over-expression of CKS1B activates both MEK/ERK and JAK/STAT3 signaling pathways and promotes myeloma cell drug-resistance," *Oncotarget*, vol. 1, no. 1, pp. 22–33, 2010.

[63] K. D. Boyd, F. M. Ross, B. A. Walker et al., "Mapping of chromosome 1p deletions in myeloma identifies FAM46C at 1p12 and CDKN2C at 1p32.3 as being genes in regions associated with adverse survival," *Clinical Cancer Research*, vol. 17, no. 24, pp. 7776–7784, 2011.

[64] H. Chang, A. Jiang, C. Qi, Y. Trieu, C. Chen, and D. Reece, "Impact of genomic aberrations including chromosome 1 abnormalities on the outcome of patients with relapsed or refractory multiple myeloma treated with lenalidomide and dexamethasone," *Leukemia and Lymphoma*, vol. 51, no. 11, pp. 2084–2091, 2010.

[65] P. E. Leone, B. A. Walker, M. W. Jenner et al., "Deletions of CDKN2C in multiple myeloma: biological and clinical

implications," *Clinical Cancer Research*, vol. 14, no. 19, pp. 6033–6041, 2008.

[66] R. Fonseca, M. M. Oken, D. Harrington et al., "Deletions of chromosome 13 in multiple myeloma identified by interphase FISH usually denote large deletions of the q arm or monosomy," *Leukemia*, vol. 15, no. 6, pp. 981–986, 2001.

[67] H. Avet-Loiseau, J.-Y. Li, N. Morineau et al., "Monosomy 13 is associated with the transition of monoclonal gammopathy of undetermined significance to multiple myeloma. Intergroupe Francophone du Myélome," *Blood*, vol. 94, no. 8, pp. 2583–2589, 1999.

[68] L. Chiecchio, R. K. M. Protheroe, A. H. Ibrahim et al., "Deletion of chromosome 13 detected by conventional cytogenetics is a critical prognostic factor in myeloma," *Leukemia*, vol. 20, no. 9, pp. 1610–1617, 2006.

[69] H. Avet-Loiseau, A. Daviet, S. Saunier, and R. Bataille, "Chromosome 13 abnormalities in multiple myeloma are mostly monosomy 13," *British Journal of Haematology*, vol. 111, no. 4, pp. 1116–1117, 2000.

[70] G. Tricot, B. Barlogie, S. Jagannath et al., "Poor prognosis in multiple myeloma is associated only with partial or complete deletions of chromosome 13 or abnormalities involving 11q and not with other karyotype abnormalities," *Blood*, vol. 86, no. 11, pp. 4250–4256, 1995.

[71] J. A. Pérez-Simón, R. García-Sanz, M. D. Tabernero et al., "Prognostic value of numerical chromosome aberrations in multiple myeloma: a FISH analysis of 15 different chromosomes," *Blood*, vol. 91, no. 9, pp. 3366–3371, 1998.

[72] W. J. Chng, R. Santana-Dávila, S. A. van Wier et al., "Prognostic factors for hyperdiploid-myeloma: effects of chromosome 13 deletions and IgH translocations," *Leukemia*, vol. 20, no. 5, pp. 807–813, 2006.

[73] G. Gahrton, S. Iacobelli, B. Björkstrand et al., "Autologous/reduced-intensity allogeneic stem cell transplantation vs autologous transplantation in multiple myeloma: long-term results of the EBMT-NMAM2000 study," *Blood*, vol. 121, no. 25, pp. 5055–5063, 2013.

[74] R. E. Tiedemann, N. Gonzalez-Paz, R. A. Kyle et al., "Genetic aberrations and survival in plasma cell leukemia," *Leukemia*, vol. 22, no. 5, pp. 1044–1052, 2008.

[75] L. Lodé, M. Eveillard, V. Trichet et al., "Mutations in TP53 are exclusively associated with del(17p) in multiple myeloma," *Haematologica*, vol. 95, no. 11, pp. 1973–1976, 2010.

[76] J. Drach, J. Ackermann, E. Fritz et al., "Presence of a p53 gene deletion in patients with multiple myeloma predicts for short survival after conventional-dose chemotherapy," *Blood*, vol. 92, no. 3, pp. 802–809, 1998.

[77] M. W. Jenner, P. E. Leone, B. A. Walker et al., "Gene mapping and expression analysis of 16q loss of heterozygosity identifies WWOX and CYLD as being important in determining clinical outcome in multiple myeloma," *Blood*, vol. 110, no. 9, pp. 3291–3300, 2007.

[78] C. M. Annunziata, R. E. Davis, Y. Demchenko et al., "Frequent engagement of the classical and alternative NF-κB pathways by diverse genetic abnormalities in multiple myeloma," *Cancer Cell*, vol. 12, no. 2, pp. 115–130, 2007.

[79] J. J. Keats, R. Fonseca, M. Chesi et al., "Promiscuous mutations activate the noncanonical NF-κB pathway in multiple myeloma," *Cancer Cell*, vol. 12, no. 2, pp. 131–144, 2007.

[80] T. Sutlu, E. Alici, M. Jansson et al., "The prognostic significance of 8p21 deletion in multiple myeloma," *British Journal of Haematology*, vol. 144, no. 2, pp. 266–268, 2009.

[81] K. Neben, A. Jauch, U. Bertsch et al., "Combining information regarding chromosomal aberrations t(4;14) and del(17p13) with the international staging system classification allows stratification of myeloma patients undergoing autologous stem cell transplantation," *Haematologica*, vol. 95, no. 7, pp. 1150–1157, 2010.

[82] A. Gmidène, A. Saad, and H. Avet-Loiseau, "8p21.3 deletion suggesting a probable role of TRAIL-R1 and TRAIL-R2 as candidate tumor suppressor genes in the pathogenesis of multiple myeloma," *Medical Oncology*, vol. 30, no. 2, p. 489, 2013.

[83] Y. Gazitt, "TRAIL is a potent inducer of apoptosis in myeloma cells derived from multiple myeloma patients and is not cytotoxic to hematopoietic stem cells," *Leukemia*, vol. 13, no. 11, pp. 1817–1824, 1999.

[84] K. Takeda, M. J. Smyth, E. Cretney et al., "Critical role for tumor necrosis factor-related apoptosis-inducing ligand in immune surveillance against tumor development," *Journal of Experimental Medicine*, vol. 195, no. 2, pp. 161–169, 2002.

[85] H. Liu, S. Tamashiro, S. Baritaki et al., "TRAF6 activation in multiple myeloma: a potential therapeutic target," *Clinical Lymphoma Myeloma and Leukemia*, vol. 12, no. 3, pp. 155–163, 2012.

[86] D. Chauhan, H. Uchiyama, Y. Akbarali et al., "Multiple myeloma cell adhesion-induced interleukin-6 expression in bone marrow stromal cells involves activation of NF-κB," *Blood*, vol. 87, no. 3, pp. 1104–1112, 1996.

[87] Y.-T. Tai, X.-F. Li, I. Breitkreutz et al., "Role of B-cell-activating factor in adhesion and growth of human multiple myeloma cells in the bone marrow microenvironment," *Cancer Research*, vol. 66, no. 13, pp. 6675–6682, 2006.

[88] W. J. Chng, N. Gonzalez-Paz, T. Price-Troska et al., "Clinical and biological significance of RAS mutations in multiple myeloma," *Leukemia*, vol. 22, no. 12, pp. 2280–2284, 2008.

[89] T. Rasmussen, M. Kuehl, M. Lodahl, H. E. Johnsen, and I. M. S. Dahl, "Possible roles for activating RAS mutations in the MGUS to MM transition and in the intramedullary to extramedullary transition in some plasma cell tumors," *Blood*, vol. 105, no. 1, pp. 317–323, 2005.

[90] E. Tiacci, V. Trifonov, G. Schiavoni et al., "BRAF mutations in hairy-cell leukemia," *The New England Journal of Medicine*, vol. 364, no. 24, pp. 2305–2315, 2011.

[91] S. Patrawala and I. Puzanov, "Vemurafenib, (RG67204, PLX4032): a potent, selective BRAF kinase inhibitor," *Future Oncology*, vol. 8, no. 5, pp. 509–523, 2012.

[92] A. C. Bharti, S. Shishodia, J. M. Reuben et al., "Nuclear factor-κB and STAT3 are constitutively active in CD138+ cells derived from multiple myeloma patients, and suppression of these transcription factors leads to apoptosis," *Blood*, vol. 103, no. 8, pp. 3175–3184, 2004.

[93] R. Catlett-Falcone, T. H. Landowski, M. M. Oshiro et al., "Constitutive activation of Stat3 signaling confers resistance to apoptosis in human U266 myeloma cells," *Immunity*, vol. 10, no. 1, pp. 105–115, 1999.

[94] M. Kawano, T. Hirano, T. Matsuda et al., "Autocrine generation and requirement of BSF-2/IL-6 for human multiple myelomas," *Nature*, vol. 332, no. 6159, pp. 83–85, 1988.

[95] B. Klein, X.-G. Zhang, Z.-Y. Lu, and R. Bataille, "Interleukin-6 in human multiple myeloma," *Blood*, vol. 85, no. 4, pp. 863–872, 1995.

[96] Y. Tu, S. Renner, F.-H. Xu et al., "BCL-X expression in multiple myeloma: possible indicator of chemoresistance," *Cancer Research*, vol. 58, no. 2, pp. 256–262, 1998.

[97] A. C. Bharti, N. Donato, and B. B. Aggarwal, "Curcumin (diferuloylmethane) inhibits constitutive and IL-6-inducible STAT3 phosphorylation in human multiple myeloma cells," *Journal of Immunology*, vol. 171, no. 7, pp. 3863–3871, 2003.

[98] M. Amit-Vazina, S. Shishodia, D. Harris et al., "Atiprimod blocks STAT3 phosphorylation and induces apoptosis in multiple myeloma cells," *British Journal of Cancer*, vol. 93, no. 1, pp. 70–80, 2005.

[99] J. de Vos, M. Jourdan, K. Tarte, C. Jasmin, and B. Klein, "JAK2 tyrosine kinase inhibitor tyrphostin AG490 downregulates the mitogen-activated protein kinase (MAPK) and signal transducer and activator of transcription (STAT) pathways and induces apoptosis in myeloma cells," *British Journal of Haematology*, vol. 109, no. 4, pp. 823–828, 2000.

[100] S. Alas and B. Bonavida, "Inhibition of constitutive STAT3 activity sensitizes resistant non-Hodgkin's lymphoma and multiple myeloma to chemotherapeutic drug-mediated apoptosis," *Clinical Cancer Research*, vol. 9, no. 1, pp. 316–326, 2003.

[101] L. Aronson, E. Davenport, S. Giuntoli et al., "Autophagy is a key myeloma survival pathway that can be manipulated therapeutically to enhance apoptosis," *ASH Annula Meeting Abstracts*, vol. 116, no. 21, p. 4083, 2010.

[102] K. D. Boyd, B. A. Walker, C. P. Wardell et al., "High expression levels of the mammalian target of rapamycin inhibitor DEPTOR are predictive of response to thalidomide in myeloma," *Leukemia and Lymphoma*, vol. 51, no. 11, pp. 2126–2129, 2010.

[103] A. Dib, B. Barlogie, J. D. Shaughnessy Jr., and W. M. Kuehl, "Methylation and expression of the p16INK4A tumor suppressor gene in multiple myeloma," *Blood*, vol. 109, no. 3, pp. 1337–1338, 2007.

[104] P. Neri, L. Ren, K. Gratton et al., "Bortezomib-induced "BRCAness" sensitizes multiple myeloma cells to PARP inhibitors," *Blood*, vol. 118, no. 24, pp. 6368–6379, 2011.

[105] O. Decaux, L. Lodé, F. Magrangeas et al., "Prediction of survival in multiple myeloma based on gene expression profiles reveals cell cycle and chromosomal instability signatures in high-risk patients and hyperdiploid signatures in low-risk patients: a study of the Intergroupe Francophone du Myélome," *Journal of Clinical Oncology*, vol. 26, no. 29, pp. 4798–4805, 2008.

[106] B. A. Gibson and W. L. Kraus, "New insights into the molecular and cellular functions of poly(ADP-ribose) and PARPs," *Nature Reviews Molecular Cell Biology*, vol. 13, no. 7, pp. 411–424, 2012.

[107] S. Kummar, A. Chen, R. E. Parchment et al., "Advances in using PARP inhibitors to treat cancer," *BMC Medicine*, vol. 10, article 25, 2012.

[108] A. Dziembowski, E. Lorentzen, E. Conti, and B. Séraphin, "A single subunit, Dis3, is essentially responsible for yeast exosome core activity," *Nature Structural and Molecular Biology*, vol. 14, no. 1, pp. 15–22, 2007.

[109] M. Schmid and T. H. Jensen, "The exosome: a multipurpose RNA-decay machine," *Trends in Biochemical Sciences*, vol. 33, no. 10, pp. 501–510, 2008.

[110] C. Schneider, J. T. Anderson, and D. Tollervey, "The exosome subunit Rrp44 Plays a direct role in RNA substrate recognition," *Molecular Cell*, vol. 27, no. 2, pp. 324–331, 2007.

[111] A. Barbas, R. G. Matos, M. Amblar, E. López-Viñas, P. Gomez-Puertas, and C. M. Arraiano, "Determination of key residues for catalysis and RNA cleavage specificity. One mutation turns RNase II Into a 'super-enzyme'," *Journal of Biological Chemistry*, vol. 284, no. 31, pp. 20486–20498, 2009.

[112] H. Ibrahim, J. Wilusz, and C. J. Wilusz, "RNA recognition by 3ʹ-to-5ʹ exonucleases: the substrate perspective," *Biochimica et Biophysica Acta*, vol. 1779, no. 4, pp. 256–265, 2008.

[113] A. Zimprich, S. Biskup, P. Leitner et al., "Mutations in LRRK2 cause autosomal-dominant parkinsonism with pleomorphic pathology," *Neuron*, vol. 44, no. 4, pp. 601–607, 2004.

[114] C. Paisán-Ruíz, S. Jain, E. W. Evans et al., "Cloning of the gene containing mutations that cause PARK8-linked Parkinson's disease," *Neuron*, vol. 44, no. 4, pp. 595–600, 2004.

[115] S. Masciarelli, A. M. Fra, N. Pengo et al., "CHOP-independent apoptosis and pathway-selective induction of the UPR in developing plasma cells," *Molecular Immunology*, vol. 47, no. 6, pp. 1356–1365, 2010.

[116] S. Cenci and R. Sitia, "Managing and exploiting stress in the antibody factory," *FEBS Letters*, vol. 581, no. 19, pp. 3652–3657, 2007.

[117] D. R. Carrasco, K. Sukhdeo, M. Protopopova et al., "The differentiation and stress response factor XBP-1 drives multiple myeloma pathogenesis," *Cancer Cell*, vol. 11, no. 4, pp. 349–360, 2007.

[118] A. M. Reimold, N. N. Iwakoshi, J. Manis et al., "Plasma cell differentiation requires the transcription factor XBP-1," *Nature*, vol. 412, no. 6844, pp. 300–307, 2001.

[119] T. Bagratuni, P. Wu, D. Gonzalez de Castro et al., "XBP1s levels are implicated in the biology and outcome of myeloma mediating different clinical outcomes to thalidomide-based treatments," *Blood*, vol. 116, no. 2, pp. 250–253, 2010.

[120] A. L. Shaffer, N. C. T. Emre, L. Lamy et al., "IRF4 addiction in multiple myeloma," *Nature*, vol. 454, no. 7201, pp. 226–231, 2008.

[121] J. Mandelbaum, G. Bhagat, H. Tang et al., "BLIMP1 Is a tumor suppressor gene frequently disrupted in activated B cell-like diffuse large B cell lymphoma," *Cancer Cell*, vol. 18, no. 6, pp. 568–579, 2010.

[122] P. Wu, B. A. Walker, D. Brewer et al., "A gene expression-based predictor for myeloma patients at high risk of developing bone disease on bisphosphonate treatment," *Clinical Cancer Research*, vol. 17, no. 19, pp. 6347–6355, 2011.

[123] E. Tian, F. Zhan, R. Walker et al., "The role of the Wnt-signaling antagonist DKK1 in the development of osteolytic lesions in multiple myeloma," *The New England Journal of Medicine*, vol. 349, no. 26, pp. 2483–2494, 2003.

[124] Y.-W. Qiang, Y. Chen, O. Stephens et al., "Myeloma-derived dickkopf-1 disrupts Wnt-regulated osteoprotegerin and RANKL production by osteoblasts: a potential mechanism underlying osteolytic bone lesions in multiple myeloma," *Blood*, vol. 112, no. 1, pp. 196–207, 2008.

[125] M. Fulciniti, P. Tassone, T. Hideshima et al., "Anti-DKK1 mAb (BHQ880) as a potential therapeutic agent for multiple myeloma," *Blood*, vol. 114, no. 2, pp. 371–379, 2009.

[126] D. F. Robbiani, M. Chesi, and P. L. Bergsagel, "Bone lesions in molecular subtypes of multiple myeloma," *The New England Journal of Medicine*, vol. 351, no. 2, pp. 197–198, 2004.

[127] G. J. Morgan, F. E. Davies, W. M. Gregory et al., "First-line treatment with zoledronic acid as compared with clodronic acid in multiple myeloma (MRC Myeloma IX): a randomised controlled trial," *The Lancet*, vol. 376, no. 9757, pp. 1989–1999, 2010.

[128] C. Sawan, T. Vaissière, R. Murr, and Z. Herceg, "Epigenetic drivers and genetic passengers on the road to cancer," *Mutation Research*, vol. 642, no. 1-2, pp. 1–13, 2008.

[129] B. A. Walker, C. P. Wardell, L. Chiecchio et al., "Aberrant global methylation patterns affect the molecular pathogenesis and prognosis of multiple myeloma," *Blood*, vol. 117, no. 2, pp. 553–562, 2011.

[130] J. L. R. Brito, B. Walker, M. Jenner et al., "MMSET deregulation affects cell cycle progression and adhesion regulons in t(4;14) myeloma plasma cells," *Haematologica*, vol. 94, no. 1, pp. 78–86, 2009.

[131] A. Rouhi, D. L. Mager, R. K. Humphries, and F. Kuchenbauer, "MiRNAs, epigenetics, and cancer," *Mammalian Genome*, vol. 19, no. 7-8, pp. 517–525, 2008.

[132] Y. Zhoua, L. Chena, B. Barlogiea et al., "High-risk myeloma is associated with global elevation of miRNAs and overexpression of EIF2C2/AGO2," *Proceedings of the National Academy of Sciences of the United States of America*, vol. 107, no. 17, pp. 7904–7909, 2010.

[133] M. Lionetti, M. Biasiolo, L. Agnelli et al., "Identification of microRNA expression patterns and definition of a microRNA/mRNA regulatory network in distinct molecular groups of multiple myeloma," *Blood*, vol. 114, no. 25, pp. e20–e26, 2009.

[134] N. C. Gutiérrez, M. E. Sarasquete, I. Misiewicz-Krzeminska et al., "Deregulation of microRNA expression in the different genetic subtypes of multiple myeloma and correlation with gene expression profiling," *Leukemia*, vol. 24, no. 3, pp. 629–637, 2010.

[135] F. Pichiorri, S.-S. Suh, A. Rocci et al., "Downregulation of p53-inducible microRNAs 192, 194, and 215 impairs the p53/MDM2 autoregulatory loop in multiple myeloma development," *Cancer Cell*, vol. 18, no. 4, pp. 367–381, 2010.

[136] F. Pichiorri, S.-S. Suh, M. Ladetto et al., "MicroRNAs regulate critical genes associated with multiple myeloma pathogenesis," *Proceedings of the National Academy of Sciences of the United States of America*, vol. 105, no. 35, pp. 12885–12890, 2008.

[137] T.-C. Chang, D. Yu, Y.-S. Lee et al., "Widespread microRNA repression by Myc contributes to tumorigenesis," *Nature Genetics*, vol. 40, no. 1, pp. 43–50, 2008.

25

Evaluation of Prothrombin Time and Activated Partial Thromboplastin Time in Hypertensive Patients Attending a Tertiary Hospital in Calabar, Nigeria

Nnamani Nnenna Adaeze,[1] Anthony Uchenna Emeribe,[2] Idris Abdullahi Nasiru,[3] Adamu Babayo,[4] and Emmanuel K. Uko[1]

[1] *Department of Medical Laboratory Science (Haematology and Blood Group Serology Unit), University of Calabar, PMB 1115, Calabar, Cross River State, Nigeria*
[2] *Department of Chemical Pathology, University of Abuja Teaching Hospital, PMB 228, Gwagwalada, Abuja, Nigeria*
[3] *Department of Medical Microbiology, University of Abuja Teaching Hospital, PMB 228, Gwagwalada, Abuja, Nigeria*
[4] *Department of Medical Laboratory Science, University of Maiduguri, PMB 1069, Maiduguri, Nigeria*

Correspondence should be addressed to Idris Abdullahi Nasiru; eedris888@yahoo.com

Academic Editor: Bashir A. Lwaleed

Introduction. Several biomedical findings have established the effects of hypertension on haemostasis and roles of blood coagulation products in the clinical course of hypertension. *Methods.* This cross-sectional study aimed at determining effects of hypertension on prothrombin time (PT) and activated partial thromboplastin time (APTT) in hypertensive patients in comparison with normotensive subjects attending a tertiary hospital in Calabar. Forty-two (42) hypertensive patients and thirty-nine (39) normotensive control subjects were investigated for PT and APTT using Quick one-stage methods. *Results.* Systolic blood pressure (SBP) and diastolic blood pressure (DBP) correlated positively with APTT ($r = 0.3072$, $r = 0.4988$; $P < 0.05$) in hypertensive patients. DBP, SBP, PT, and APTT were significantly higher in hypertensive patients when compared to normotensive subjects ($P < 0.05$). DBP correlated negatively with duration of illness ($r = -0.3097$; $P < 0.05$) in hypertensive patients and positively with age of normotensive subjects ($r = 0.3523$; $P < 0.05$). *Conclusion.* The results obtained indicated that measurements of PT and APTT may serve as indices for evaluating hemostatic abnormalities in hypertensive patients and guide for antihypertensive therapy. However, to have better understanding of hemostatic activities in hypertension, it is recommended to conduct D-dimer, platelet factors, and protein assays.

1. Introduction

Cardiovascular diseases account for about one-third of premature deaths in men and one-quarter in women and arterial hypertension is one of the most significant risk factors for cardiovascular diseases [1]. Despite current knowledge, extensive clinical and experimental research, the cause of hypertension remains unknown in about 95% of all cases [1]. Hypertension is a chronic medical condition in which the blood pressure is indisputably elevated ($\geq 140/90$ mmHg). It is one of the most common worldwide diseases afflicting humans. Globally cardiovascular disease accounts for approximately 17 million deaths a year, nearly one-third of the total. Of these, complications of hypertension account for 9.4 million deaths worldwide every year. Hypertension is responsible for at least 45% of deaths due to heart disease [2]. Due to several associated morbidity, mortality, and economic cost to society, hypertension is now a serious public health challenge to both developed and developing nations [3, 4].

According to recent epidemiologic data, the overall prevalence of 28% of the general population is suffering from hypertension in Sub-Saharan Africa, the prevalence rate in Nigeria is put at 22% with steady annual increase [5].

Hypertension is classified as either primary or secondary. It is primary when no medical cause can be found to explain the raised blood pressure. This type represents between 90 and 95% of hypertension cases [6]. Secondary hypertension represents approximately 10% of all hypertension cases. Identifiable underlying causes of secondary hypertension are kidney disease, renal hyperaldosteronism, and pheochromocytoma. Secondary hypertension has specific therapy; it is potentially curable and often distinguishable from primary one on clinical grounds [7].

Risk factors associated with hypertension include age, race, family history, obesity, sedentary lifestyle, alcohol abuse, and stress among others. Hypertension increases hardening of the arteries and predisposes individuals to heart disease, peripheral vascular disease, and strokes [7–10].

Hypertensive patients are at high risk for the development of cardiovascular diseases [11], whereas several studies have shown that treatment of hypertension diminishes the prevalence of cardiovascular diseases [12–14]. The existence of hypertension, especially in combination with other risk factors, is disadvantageous for the prognosis of cardiovascular diseases [15]. The integrity of the blood vessels is essential because damage of the intima, which may occur in hypertension, can finally cause atherosclerosis. This kind of patient is likely to develop increased platelet aggregation with heart and blood vessel problems as possible sequelae [16]. Moreover, blood vessel damage activates the coagulation system, which may also stimulate the progress of atherosclerosis.

Coagulation abnormalities in pregnant women have been reported to be more serious in women with hypertension (preeclampsia) than in those without hypertension [17]. In patients with borderline hypertension, even before the appearance of clinical manifestations of vascular damages [18], coagulation activation seems to be already present [18].

Besides platelet aggregability and coagulation activation, fibrinolysis, that is, plasma tissue-type plasminogen activator activity, appears to be a major factor related to the risk of cardiovascular disease [19–22].

Prothrombin time (PT) and activated partial thromboplastin time (APTT) have been shown to be associated with elevated systolic and diastolic blood pressures in hypertensive and normotensive patients [23]. In a study which involved the inclusion of one hundred and one patients with hypertension of mild to moderate grades, attending Al-Najaf Teaching Hospital, Iraq, significant differences were found in PT and APTT between hypertensive and normotensive patients [24]. The prothrombin time (PT) and its derived measures of prothrombin ratio (PR) and international normalized ratio (INR) are measures of the extrinsic pathway of coagulation. The APTT in contrast to the PT measures the activity of the intrinsic pathways of coagulation. Endothelial damage, platelet hyperactivity, and other changes of blood coagulation may play a role in the vascular complications of essential hypertension [25–27].

The main aim of this study is to assess possible association between prothrombin time and activated partial thromboplastin time with effects of blood pressures in hypertensive and normotensive subjects and their significant utility for screening hemostatic dysfunction in hypertensive patients.

2. Materials and Methods

2.1. Study Area. The study was conducted at the University of Calabar Teaching Hospital, Calabar, Cross River State. Calabar is the capital city of Cross River State which is divided into Calabar Municipal and Calabar South Local Governments and is located at the coastal southeastern area ($4°57'$N $8°19'$E) of Nigeria. It has an area of $604\,km^2$ and a population of 371,022 at the 2006 census.

2.2. Study Population. A total of eighty-onesubjects were enrolled into the study. Forty-two (42) hypertensive patients aged between 30 and 80 years and thirty-nine (39) normotensive control subjects were investigated for PT and APTT using Quick one-stage methods. The selection of patients was done with the support of the physician and nursing staff of the Medical Outpatient Department (MOPD) of University of Calabar Teaching Hospital (UCTH), Calabar. The procedures employed consisted of a questionnaire interview, taking of patient's history, and blood pressure measurement.

2.3. Inclusion Criteria for Hypertensive Patients. The inclusion criteria are as follows:

(i) the presence of the history of primary hypertension;

(ii) elevated blood pressure (≥140/90 mmHg);

(iii) no history of administration of anticoagulant therapy;

(iv) no history of chronic viral infection and/or liver diseases (HBV, HCV, HIV, and alcohol consumption);

(v) having not been on long-term drug regimen;

(vi) must be within normal range body mass index;

(vii) being with no trace of underlying causes.

2.4. Exclusion Criteria for Hypertensive Patients. The exclusion criteria are as follows:

(i) the absence of family history of primary hypertension;

(ii) normal blood pressure (<140/90 mmHg);

(iii) those on anticoagulant therapy;

(iv) those with chronic viral infections and/or liver diseases such as HBV, HCV, HIV, and alcoholism;

(v) obese individuals.

2.5. Inclusion Criteria for Normotensive Control Subjects. The inclusion criteria are as follows:

(i) the absence of family history of hypertension;

(ii) normal blood pressure (<140/90 mmHg);

(iii) no history of administration of anticoagulant therapy;

(iv) no history of chronic viral infection and/or liver diseases (HBV, HCV, HIV, and alcohol consumption);

(v) having not been on long-term drug regimen;

(vi) must be within normal body mass index;

(vii) with no trace of underlying causes.

2.6. Exclusion Criteria for Normotensive Control Subjects. The exclusion criteria are as follows:

(i) the presence of family history of hypertension;

(ii) elevated blood pressure (≥140/90 mmHg);

(iii) the absence of family history of primary hypertension;

(iv) normal blood pressure (<140/90 mmHg);

(v) those on anticoagulant therapy;

(vi) those with chronic viral infections and/or liver diseases such as HBV, HCV, HIV, and alcoholism;

(vii) obese individuals.

2.7. Ethical Clearance and Informed Consent. The ethical clearance was obtained from the Ethical Committee of UCTH, Calabar, Cross River State, Nigeria. Informed consent was obtained from all participating subjects. This was done via an informed consent form duly completed by all the subjects.

2.8. Questionnaire. Semistructured administered questionnaires were used to obtain data such as age, marital status, clinical signs and symptoms, and provisional diagnosis.

2.9. Sample Collection. Four and a half-millilitres (4.5 mL) of blood sample was drawn from hypertensive and normotensive subjects and discharged into a 0.5 mL of 3.13% trisodium citrate sample bottle. The anticoagulated samples were centrifuged at 4000 rpm for 10 minutes and platelet poor plasma stored in a deep freezer at −20°C until assayed. Standard method of Quick one-stage analysis by [28] was used for PT and APTT.

2.10. Statistical Method. The generated data was systematically analysed as appropriate for means, standard deviation, Student's t-test, Pearson's correlation analysis, and analysis of variance on Microsoft Excel and SPSS software version 18 (California Inc.). Results were presented as the mean ± standard deviation. A two-sided $P < 0.05$ was considered statistically significant for t-test (used to determine the differences between the groups) and Pearson's correlation analysis was used to determine the intervariable associations of the various groups.

3. Results

Table 1 shows the mean and standard deviation for the systolic pressure, diastolic pressure, prothrombin time test, and activated partial thromboplastin time test of hypertensives and normotensives including the duration of hypertensive subjects enrolled in the study. The mean and standard deviation for systolic blood pressure, diastolic blood pressure, prothrombin time test, activated partial thromboplastin time test, and duration of hypertensives were 157.02 ± 18.78 mmHg, 95.12 ± 13.00 mmHg, 14.45 ± 1.97 seconds, 35.43±5.05 seconds, and 4.06±5.93 years, respectively, while

TABLE 1: Mean systolic pressure, diastolic pressure, prothrombin time test (PTT), and partial thromboplastin time test kaolin (PTTK) of hypertensive patients (test) and normotensive subjects (control) of the University of Calabar Teaching Hospital.

Parameters	Hypertensive patients ($n_1 = 42$)	Normotensive subjects ($n_2 = 30$)	P value
Systolic blood pressure (mmHg)	157.02 ± 18.77	117.66 ± 11.65	$P < 0.05$
Diastolic blood pressure (mmHg)	95.11 ± 12.99	79.16 ± 10.99	$P < 0.05$
PTT (seconds)	14.45 ± 1.96	13.60 ± 1.19	$P < 0.05$
PTTK (seconds)	35.42 ± 5.04	32.56 ± 3.23	$P < 0.05$

Student's t-test analysis.
$P < 0.05$ is significant.
$P < 0.05$ is not significant.
n_1 = number of hypertensive patients.
n_2 = number of normotensive subjects.

TABLE 2: Comparison of the prothrombin time test (PTT) and partial thromboplastin time test kaolin (PTTK) based on duration of illness of hypertensive patients attending the University of Calabar Teaching Hospital.

Parameters	Groups			P value
	≤3 years ($n_1 = 28$)	4–7 years ($n_2 = 8$)	≥8 years ($n_3 = 6$)	
PTT (seconds)	14.28 ± 1.80	15.00 ± 2.67	14.50 ± 1.87	$P > 0.05$
PTTK (seconds)	34.89 ± 4.57	37.37 ± 6.07	35.33 ± 6.05	$P > 0.05$

Analysis of variance.
$P < 0.05$ is significant.
$P < 0.05$ is not significant.
n_1 = number of hypertensive patients with duration of illness ≤3 years.
n_2 = number of hypertensive patients with duration of illness 4–7 years.
n_3 = number of hypertensive patients with duration of illness ≥8 years.

the mean and standard deviation for the systolic pressure, diastolic pressure, prothrombin time test, and activated partial thromboplastin time test of normotensives studied were 117.67 ± 11.65 mmHg, 79.17 ± 10.99 mmHg, 13.60 ± 1.19 seconds, and 32.57 ± 3.23 seconds, respectively.

Diastolic blood pressures, systolic blood pressures, Prothrombin Time Test and Activated Partial Thromboplastin Time Test were significantly higher in hypertensive patients when compared to normotensives ($P < 0.05$).

Based on the duration of hypertension, the hypertensive patients were grouped into three different groups (≤3 years, 4–7 years, and ≥8 years); their prothrombin time was 14.28 ± 1.80, 15.00±2.67, and 14.50±1.87 seconds, respectively, while their activated partial thromboplastin time was 34.89 ± 4.57, 37.37 ± 6.07, and 35.33 ± 6.05 seconds, respectively, as shown in Table 2.

Systolic blood pressure correlated positively with PTTK ($r = 0.3072$; $P < 0.05$) (Figure 4) and with diastolic blood pressure ($r = 0.4988$; $P < 0.05$) (Figure 2) in hypertensive patients, respectively. Diastolic blood pressure correlated negatively with duration of illness ($r = -0.3097$;

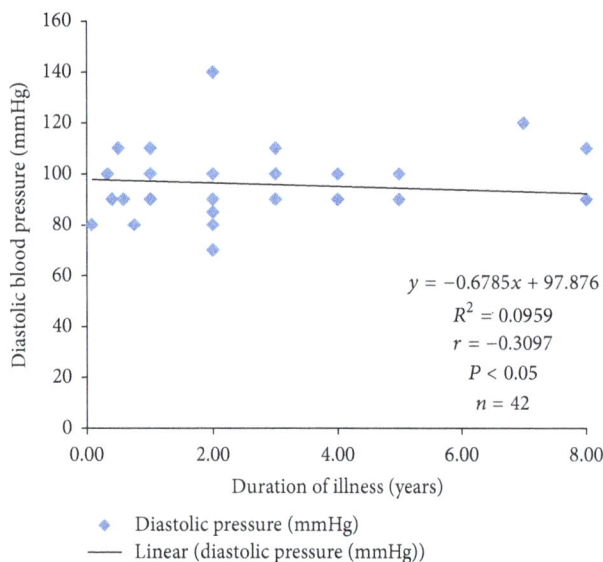

FIGURE 1: Correlation plot of diastolic blood pressure against duration of illness in hypertensive patients.

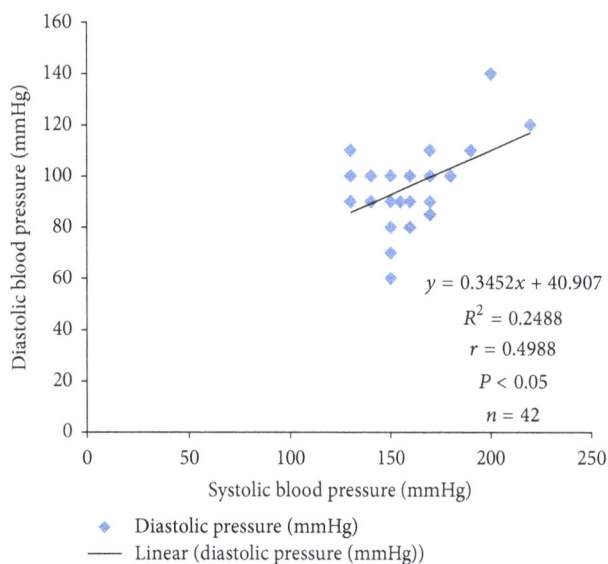

FIGURE 2: Correlation plot of systolic blood pressure against diastolic blood pressure in hypertensive patients.

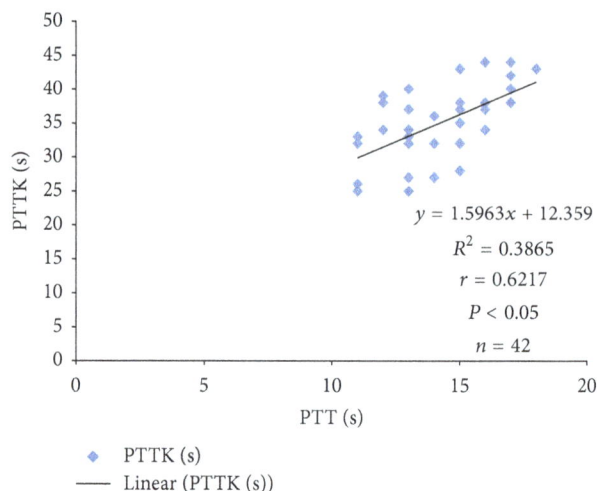

FIGURE 3: Correlation plot of PTTK against PTT in hypertensive patients.

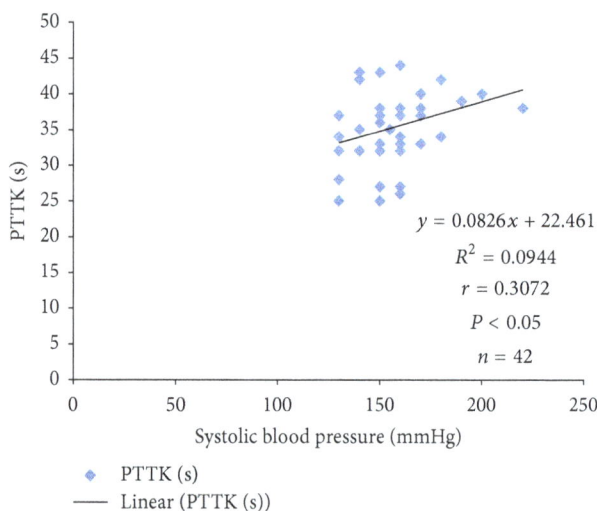

FIGURE 4: Correlation plot of PTTK against systolic blood pressure in hypertensive patients.

$P < 0.05$) in hypertensive patients (Figure 1) and positively with age ($r = 0.3523$; $P < 0.05$) in normotensive subjects (Figure 5). A positive correlation was observed between PTT and PTTK both in hypertensive patients ($r = 0.6217$; $P < 0.05$) (Figure 3) and in normotensive subjects ($r = 0.5886$; $P < 0.05$) (Figure 6). More so positive correlation of systolic and diastolic blood pressure of normotensive subjects was observed across gender distribution (Figure 8) but negative correlation between systolic blood pressure and male hypertensive subjects (Figure 7). There was a statistical relationship between PT and APTT and age of hypertensive patients ($P < 0.05$) (Table 3). However there was no statistical relationship between PTT and APTT across ages of normotensive patients (Table 4).

4. Discussion

Haemostatic system is directly involved in the atherosclerotic process. Hypertension is an atherosclerotic risk factor causing endothelial dysfunction; therefore, endothelial damage, platelets hyperactivation, and drugs are involved in the coagulation and fibrinolytic system [29, 30]. Prothrombin time and activated partial thromboplastin time are important clinical parameters for assessing extrinsic and intrinsic factors/pathways of the coagulation system [30].

The findings of this study show significant increases in the prothrombin time and activated partial thromboplastin time of hypertensive patients when compared to those of the normotensives (control). This increase could be due to endothelial damage as a result of atherosclerosis caused by hypertension on these patients ($P < 0.05$) [31].

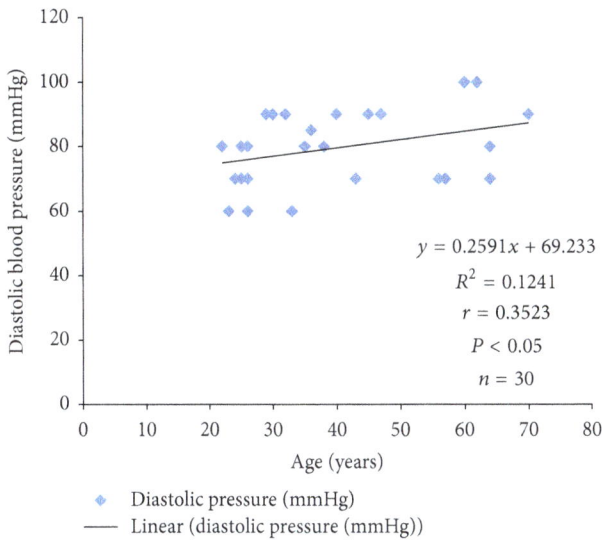

FIGURE 5: Correlation plot of diastolic blood pressure against age in normotensive subjects.

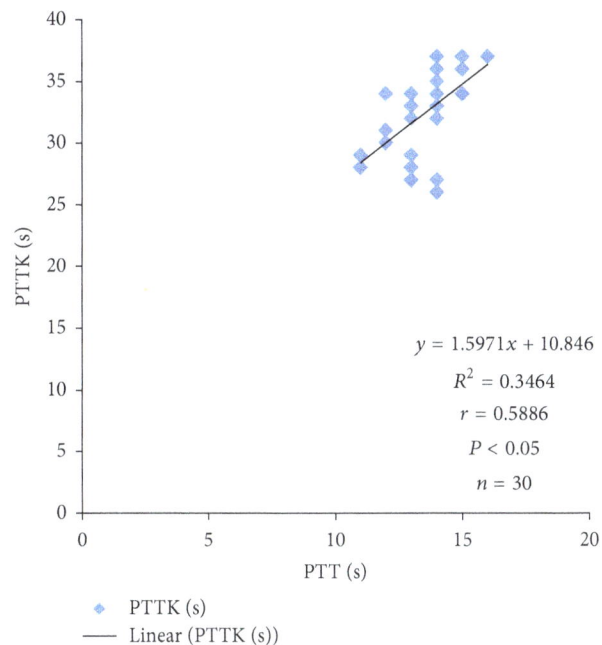

FIGURE 6: Correlation plot of PTTK against PTT in normotensive subjects.

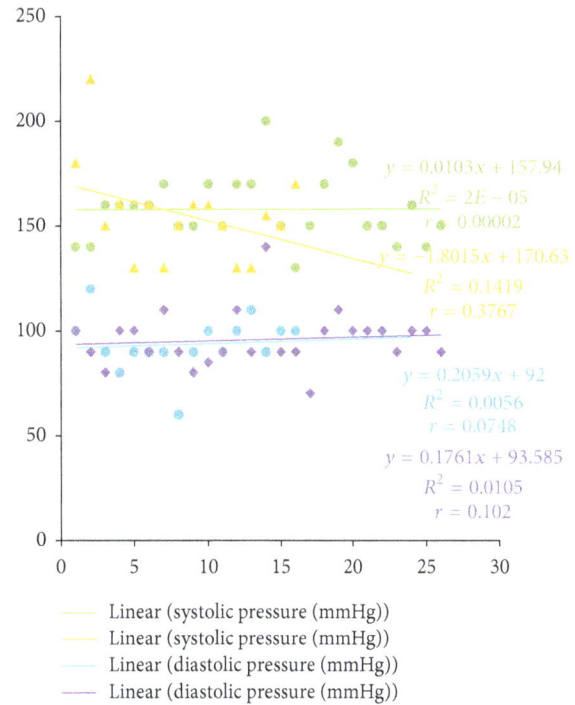

FIGURE 7: Correlation of systolic and diastolic blood pressure of hypertensive subjects across gender distribution. Purple lines and points: females. Blue line and points: males. Green line and points: females. Yellow line and points: males. Number of male hypertensive subjects (n) = 16. Number of female hypertensive subjects (n) = 26.

TABLE 3: Comparison of the prothrombin time test (PTT) and partial thromboplastin time test kaolin (PTTK) across ages of hypertensive patients attending the University of Calabar Teaching Hospital.

Parameters	Age range			P value
	≤35 years ($n_1 = 5$)	36–50 years ($n_2 = 14$)	≥51 years ($n_3 = 23$)	
PTT (seconds)	13.80 ± 1.92	15.00 ± 1.96	14.26 ± 1.98	$P < 0.05$
PTTK (seconds)	32.60 ± 4.39	38.29 ± 3.60	34.3 ± 5.29	$P < 0.05$

Analysis of variance.
$P < 0.05$ is significant.
$P < 0.05$ is not significant.
n_1 = number of hypertensive patients with age range ≤35 years.
n_2 = number of hypertensive patients with age range 36–50 years.
n_3 = number of hypertensive patients with age range ≥51 years.

The prothrombin time and activated partial thromboplastin time of hypertensive patients increase with increase in duration of hypertension which may be due to prolonged endothelial wall effect as this will lead to sustained release of vasoactive substances that interfere coagulation cascades, and these indices eventually decrease as the antihypertensive therapy continues, even lower than before they started treatment; this finding is in consonance with Lee's work and that of Mirsaiedi et al. [32, 33].

There was a positive correlation between systolic pressure and activated partial thromboplastin time in hypertensive patients which could be due to the risk factors associated with hypertension, for example, atherosclerosis, endothelial dysfunction and antihypertensive drugs [34, 35].

There was a negative correlation between diastolic pressure and duration of illness and a probable explanation to this could be that reduced exposure of the vascular walls to pressure in those with lower duration will give a higher pressure than those who have higher exposure to this tension because their blood vessels might be weaker and cannot exert

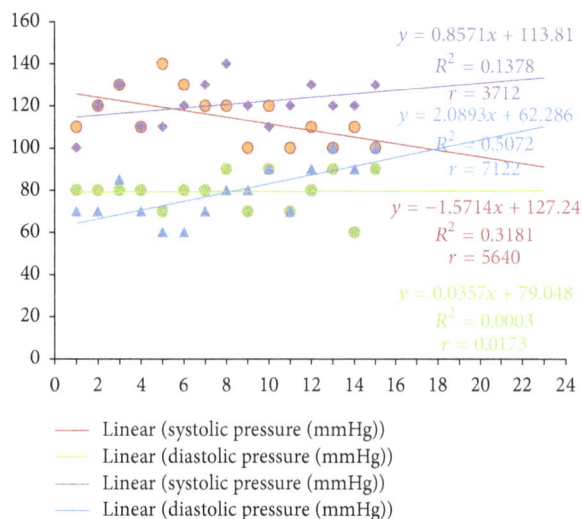

FIGURE 8: Correlation of systolic and diastolic blood pressure of normotensive subjects across gender distribution. Purple lines and points: females. Blue line and points: females. Green line and points: males. Red line and points: males. Number of male normotensive subjects (n) = 15. Number of female normotensive subjects (n) = 15.

TABLE 4: Comparison of the prothrombin time test (PTT) and partial thromboplastin time test kaolin (PTTK) across ages of normotensive patients attending the University of Calabar Teaching Hospital.

Parameters	Age range			P value
	≤35 years (n_1 = 16)	32–50 years (n_2 = 7)	≥51 years (n_3 = 7)	
PTT (seconds)	13.75 ± 1.24	13.00 ± 1.154	13.86 ± 1.069	$P > 0.05$
PTTK (seconds)	29.19 ± 8.06	27.14 ± 10.75	32.71 ± 4.46	$P > 0.05$

Analysis of variance.
$P < 0.05$ is significant.
$P < 0.05$ is not significant.
n_1 = number of normotensive patients with age range ≤35 years.
n_2 = number of normotensive patients with age range 36–50 years.
n_3 = number of normotensive patients with age range ≥51 years.

resistance or pressure against blood flow when compared to those with lower duration [35–38].

Positive correlation of systolic and diastolic blood pressure of normotensive subjects was observed across gender distribution, but negative correlation between systolic blood pressure in male hypertensive subjects; these findings are in conformity with previous studies [38–41]. There was a statistical relationship between PT and APTT and age distribution of hypertensive patients ($P < 0.05$); this supports the findings of Akputuzor et al. and Mirsaiedi et al. [33, 42]. Prolonged PT and APTT were common with elderly hypertensive subjects; one could speculate that this phenomenon is due to diminished prostacyclin synthesis and/or release by the endothelial cells during old age.

Due to the fact that there was significant increase in prothrombin time and activated partial thromboplastin time of hypertensive patients when compared with normotensive (control) subjects, assessment of these parameters may serve as prognostic indices for evaluating hypertensive patients in whom there was clinical evidence of hemostatic abnormality and guide for antihypertensive therapy. However, to have complete understanding of hemostatic activities in hypertension, it is recommended to conduct D-dimer, platelet factors, and protein assays.

Conflict of Interests

The authors declare that there is no conflict of interests regarding the publication of this paper.

Acknowledgments

The authors would like to acknowledge the staff of Medical Laboratory Department, University of Calabar Teaching Hospital, Nigeria, for their technical support and Pharmacist Ibrahim Abdulkadir for typesetting the final paper.

References

[1] I. Bernatova, "Endothelial dysfunction in experimental models of arterial hypertension: cause or consequence?" *BioMed Research International*, vol. 2014, Article ID 598271, 14 pages, 2014.

[2] A. V. Chobanian, G. L. Bakris, H. R. Black et al., "Seventh report of the joint national committee on prevention, detection, evaluation, and treatment of high blood pressure," *Hypertension*, vol. 42, no. 6, pp. 1206–1252, 2003.

[3] P. M. Kearney, M. Whelton, K. Reynolds, P. Muntner, P. K. Whelton, and J. He, "Global burden of hypertension: analysis of worldwide data," *The Lancet*, vol. 365, no. 9455, pp. 217–223, 2005.

[4] I. Hajjar and T. A. Kotchen, "Trends in prevalence, awareness, treatment, and control of hypertension in the United States, 1988–2000," *Journal of the American Medical Association*, vol. 290, no. 2, pp. 199–206, 2003.

[5] World Health Organisation, *Global Health Observatory Data Repository*, World Health Organisation, Geneva, Switzerland, 2013, http://apps.who.int/gho/data/view.main.

[6] O. A. Carretero and S. Oparil, "Essential hypertension. Part I: definition and etiology," *Circulation*, vol. 101, no. 3, pp. 329–335, 2000.

[7] M. Mayo, *Foundation for Medical Education and Research on Secondary Hypertension*, McGraw-Hill, London, UK, 2008.

[8] E. Agabiti-Rosei, "From macro- to microcirculation: benefits in hypertension and diabetes," *Journal of Hypertension*, vol. 26, no. 3, pp. 15–19, 2008.

[9] D. R. J. Singer and A. Kite, "Management of hypertension in peripheral arterial disease: does the choice of drugs matter?" *European Journal of Vascular and Endovascular Surgery*, vol. 35, no. 6, pp. 701–708, 2008.

[10] W. B. White, "Defining the problem of treating the patient with hypertension and arthritis pain," *The American Journal of Medicine*, vol. 122, no. 5, supplement, pp. S3–S9, 2009.

[11] G. M. Patrassi, F. Fallo, A. Santarossa, M. T. Sartori, A. Casonato, and A. Girolami, "Clotting changes in borderline hypertension," *Journal of Human Hypertension*, vol. 1, no. 2, pp. 101–103, 1987.

[12] M. A. DeWood, J. Spores, R. Notske et al., "Prevalence of total coronary occlusion during the early hours of transmural myocardial infarction," *The New England Journal of Medicine*, vol. 303, no. 16, pp. 897–902, 1980.

[13] J. Gram and J. Jespersen, "A selective depression of tissue plasminogen activator (t-PA) activity in euglobulins characterises a risk group among survivors of acute myocardial infarction," *Thrombosis and Haemostasis*, vol. 57, no. 2, pp. 137–139, 1987.

[14] J. Franzen, B. Nilsson, B. W. Johansson, and I. M. Nilsson, "Fibrinolytic activity in men with acute myocardial infarction before 60 years of age," *Acta Medica Scandinavica*, vol. 214, no. 5, pp. 339–344, 1983.

[15] A. Hamsten, M. Blomback, B. Wiman et al., "Haemostatic function in myocardial infarction," *British Heart Journal*, vol. 55, no. 1, pp. 58–66, 1986.

[16] T. K. Nilsson and O. Johnson, "The extrinsic fibrinolytic system in survivors of myocardial infarction," *Thrombosis Research*, vol. 48, no. 6, pp. 621–630, 1987.

[17] M. C. Stone and J. M. Thorp, "Plasma fibrinogen—a major coronary risk factor," *The Journal of the Royal College of General Practitioners*, vol. 35, no. 281, pp. 565–569, 1985.

[18] L. Wilhelmsen, K. Svärsudd, L. Korsan-Bengtsenj, B. Larsson, L. Welin, and G. Tibblin, "Fibrinogen as a risk factor for stroke and myocardial infarction," *Northern England Journal of Medicine*, vol. 377, pp. 501–505, 1984.

[19] K. S. Sakariassen, P. A. Bolhuis, and J. J. Sixma, "Human blood platelet adhesion to artery subendothelium is mediated by factor VIII-Von Willebrand factor bo und to the subendothelium," *Nature*, vol. 279, no. 5714, pp. 636–638, 1979.

[20] T. Jensen, "Increased plasma concentration of von Willebrand factor in insulin dependent diabetics with incipient nephropathy," *British Medical Journal*, vol. 298, no. 6665, pp. 27–28, 1989.

[21] J. A. Panza, A. A. Quyyumi, J. E. Brush Jr., and S. E. Epstein, "Abnormal endothelium-dependent vascular relaxation in patients with essential hypertension," *The New England Journal of Medicine*, vol. 323, no. 1, pp. 22–27, 1990.

[22] J. R. Vane, E. E. Anggard, and R. M. Botting, "Regulatory functions of the vascular endothelium," *The New England Journal of Medicine*, vol. 323, no. 1, pp. 27–36, 1990.

[23] N. Uren and D. Rutherford, High blood pressure (hypertension), Net Doctor, 2004, http://www.netdoctor.co.uk/diseases/facts/hypertension.htm.

[24] G. Giacchetti, F. Turchi, M. Boscaro, and V. Ronconi, "Management of primary aldosteronism: its complications and their outcomes after treatment," *Current Vascular Pharmacology*, vol. 7, no. 2, pp. 244–249, 2009.

[25] J. Schrader, "Stroke and hypertension," *Der Internist*, vol. 50, no. 4, pp. 423–432, 2009.

[26] J. A. Blumenthal, M. A. Babyak, A. Hinderliter et al., "Effects of the DASH diet alone and in combination with exercise and weight loss on blood pressure and cardiovascular biomarkers in men and women with high blood pressure: the ENCORE study," *Archives of Internal Medicine*, vol. 170, no. 2, pp. 126–135, 2010.

[27] O. M. Alhamami, J. Y. AL-Mayah, N. R. AL-Mousawi, and H. I. AL-Mousawi, "Pleiotropic effects of antihypertensive drugs," *The Islamic University Journal (Series of National Studies and Engineering)*, vol. 15, no. 1, pp. 1–12, 2007.

[28] M. Laffan and R. Manning, "Investigation of haemostasis," in *Practical Haematology*, S. M. Lewis, B. J. Bain, and I. Bates, Eds., pp. 380–463, Elsevier, Philadelphia, Pa, USA, 10th edition, 2006.

[29] R. Junker, J. Heinrich, H. Schulte, M. Erren, and G. Assmann, "Hemostasis in normotensive and hypertensive men: results of the PROCAM study," *Journal of Hypertension*, vol. 16, no. 7, pp. 917–923, 1998.

[30] J. E. Deanfield, J. P. Halcox, and T. J. Rabelink, "Endothelial function and dysfunction: testing and clinical relevance," *Circulation*, vol. 115, no. 10, pp. 1285–1295, 2007.

[31] A. H. Kamal, A. Tefferi, and R. K. Pruthi, "How to interpret and pursue an abnormal prothrombin time, activated partial thromboplastin time, and bleeding time in adults," *Mayo Clinic Proceedings*, vol. 82, no. 7, pp. 864–873, 2007.

[32] A. J. Lee, "The role of rheological and haemostatic factors in hypertension," *Journal of Human Hypertension*, vol. 11, no. 12, pp. 767–776, 1997.

[33] M. Mirsaiedi, Z. Fallah, P. Farzanegi, and M. B. Khameslu, "Comparing the fibrinogen, prothrombin time, Partial thromboplastin time and Platelets number and d-dimerin aerobic, control and resistance groups in Sari elderly sedentary men," *Annals of Biological Research*, vol. 3, no. 5, pp. 2087–2090, 2087.

[34] P. M. Vanhoutte, M. Feletou, and S. Taddei, "Endothelium-dependent contractions in hypertension," *British Journal of Pharmacology*, vol. 144, no. 4, pp. 449–458, 2005.

[35] G. S. Berenson, S. R. Srinivasan, S. Hunter MacD et al., "Risk factors in early life as predictors of adult heart disease: the Bogalusa Heart Study," *The American Journal of the Medical Sciences*, vol. 298, no. 3, pp. 141–151, 1989.

[36] A. W. Zieske, G. T. Malcom, and J. P. Strong, "Natural history and risk factors of atherosclerosis in children and youth: the PDAY study," *Pediatric Pathology and Molecular Medicine*, vol. 21, no. 2, pp. 213–237, 2002.

[37] S. Mendis, P. Nordet, J. E. Fernandez-Britto, and N. Sternby, "Atherosclerosis in children and young adults: an overview of the World Health Organization and International Society and Federation of Cardiology study on Pathobiological Determinants of Atherosclerosis in Youth study (1985–1995)," *Prevention and Control*, vol. 1, no. 1, pp. 3–15, 2005.

[38] S. S. Lim, T. Vos, A. D. Flaxman et al., "A comparative risk assessment of burden of disease and injury attributable to 67 risk factors and risk factor clusters in 21 regions, 1990–2010: a systematic analysis for the Global Burden of Disease Study 2010," *The Lancet*, vol. 380, pp. 2224–2260, 2010.

[39] E. Jervase, D. Barnabas, A. Emeka, and N. Osondu, "Sex differences and relationship between blood pressure and age among the Ibos of Nigeria," *The Internet Journal of Biological Anthropology*, no. 2, pp. 37–43, 2012.

[40] Y. S. Kusuma, B. V. Babu, and J. M. Naidu, "Blood pressure levels among cross-cultural populations of Visakhapatnam district, Andhra Pradesh, India," *Annals of Human Biology*, vol. 29, no. 5, pp. 502–512, 2002.

[41] T. S. Bowman, H. D. Sesso, and J. M. Gaziano, "Effect of age on blood pressure parameters and risk of cardiovascular death in men," *American Journal of Hypertension*, vol. 19, no. 1, pp. 47–52, 2006.

[42] J. O. Akputuzor, E. C. Akwiwu, and I. A. Udoh, "Prothrombin time and relative plasma viscosity of hypertensive patients attending university of Calabar teaching hospital, Calabar, Nigeria," *International Journal of Natural and Applied Sciences*, vol. 7, no. 2, 2011.

26

Treatment of Febrile Neutropenia and Prophylaxis in Hematologic Malignancies: A Critical Review and Update

Paola Villafuerte-Gutierrez,[1] Lucia Villalon,[2] Juan E. Losa,[3] and Cesar Henriquez-Camacho[3]

[1] Hospital Universitario Torrejón de Ardoz, Servicio de Hematología, Calle Mateo Inurria, 28850 Madrid, Spain
[2] Hospital Universitario Fundación Alcorcón, Servicio de Hematología, Calle Budapest 1, 28922 Madrid, Spain
[3] Unidad de Medicina Interna, Sección de Enfermedades Infecciosas, Hospital Universitario Fundación Alcorcón, Calle Budapest 1, 28922 Madrid, Spain

Correspondence should be addressed to Cesar Henriquez-Camacho; cajhenriquez@fhalcorcon.es

Academic Editor: Myriam Labopin

Febrile neutropenia is one of the most serious complications in patients with haematological malignancies and chemotherapy. A prompt identification of infection and empirical antibiotic therapy can prolong survival. This paper reviews the guidelines about febrile neutropenia in the setting of hematologic malignancies, providing an overview of the definition of fever and neutropenia, and categories of risk assessment, management of infections, and prophylaxis.

1. Introduction

Febrile neutropenia (FN) is one of the most serious adverse events in patients with haematological malignancies and chemotherapy. Infections in neutropenic patients can rapidly progress, leading to life-threatening complications. A prompt initiation of empirical antibiotic therapy is favourable for patients with FN in order to avoid progression to sepsis and regardless of the detection of bacteraemia [1].

FN is considered a medical emergency, as infections can rapidly progress without a broad spectrum antibiotic treatment within 1 hour of fever [2]. The spectrum of bacterial pathogens isolated from FN patients has shifted from Gram-negative (1970s) species to Gram-positive organisms (since mid-1980), related to the use of antibacterial prophylaxis with fluoroquinolone and the use of indwelling catheter. Actually, the most common species isolated are Gram-positive pathogens: *Coagulase-negative staphylococci, Staphylococcus aureus* (including methicillin-resistant strains), *Enterococcus* spp. (including vancomycin-resistant strains), *Viridans group streptococci, Streptococcus pneumoniae,* and *Streptococcus pyogenes,* and drug-resistant Gram-negative pathogens:

Escherichia coli, Klebsiella spp., *Enterobacter* spp., *Pseudomonas aeruginosa, Acinetobacter* spp., *Citrobacter* spp., and *Stenotrophomonas maltophilia* [3, 4].

An overview of the risk assessment of patients with neutropenic fever and neutropenic fever syndromes and the use of empiric antibacterial and antifungal therapy for neutropenic adults will be discussed.

2. Definitions

Fever in neutropenic patients is classically defined as a single oral temperature of >38.3°C (101°F) [1]. Although, it is known that a neutropenic patient can be infected without fever or stay subfebrile, the definition of neutropenia is an absolute neutrophil count (ANC) < 1500 cells/microL, and severe neutropenia is usually defined as an ANC < 500 cells/microL or that is expected to decrease below 500 cells/microL during the next 48 hours, and profound neutropenia is an ANC < 100 cells/microL [1]. The risk of clinically important infection rises as the neutrophil count falls below 500 cells/microL and is higher in those with a prolonged duration of neutropenia (>7 days).

TABLE 1: MASCC score [8].

Clinical parameters	Score*
Burden of illness: no or mild symptoms[†]	5
No hypotension	5
No chronic obstructive pulmonary disease[‡]	4
Solid tumour or no previous fungal infection[§]	4
No dehydration	3
Outpatient status	3
Burden of illness: moderate symptoms	3
Patient's age < 60 years	2

MASCC: Multinational Association for Supportive Care in Cancer.
Scores > 21 indicate a low risk for medical complications.
*The maximum theoretical score is 26.
[†]Burden of FN refers to the general clinical status of the patient as influenced by the febrile neutropenic episode. It should be evaluated on the following scale: no or mild symptoms (score of 5), moderate symptoms (score of 3), and severe symptoms or moribund (score of 0). Scores of 3 and 5 are not cumulative.
[‡]Chronic obstructive pulmonary disease means active chronic bronchitis, emphysema, decrease in forced expiratory volumes, or need for oxygen therapy and/or steroids and/or bronchodilators requiring treatment at the presentation of the febrile neutropenic episode.
[§]Previous fungal infection means demonstrated fungal infection or empirically treated suspected fungal infection.

3. Risk of Complications

Patients who develop neutropenia can be categorized as at low risk or high risk of complications and thus poor outcome. The risk assessment has practical implications to dictate the management (including the need for inpatient admission, choice of antibiotics, and prolonged hospitalization).

Some guidelines (ESMO [5], ASCO [6], and NCCN [7]) recommend the use of the Multinational Association for Supportive Care in Cancer (MASCC) index to identify patients at low risk of complications to be treated as outpatients (see Table 1) [8]. In the MASCC study, factors associated with good prognosis in cancer patients were burden of the illness (mild or moderate clinical symptoms at presentation): absence of hypotension; absence of chronic obstructive pulmonary disease; presence of solid tumour or, in patients with hematologic malignancies, absence of previous fungal infection; outpatient status, absence of dehydration; and age lower than 60 years. A patient with a MASCC score > 21 points is considered "low risk" with positive and negative predictive values of 91% and 36%, respectively. Those patients can be treated using oral antibiotics. The IDSA guideline favours the expert clinical criteria and considers low-risk patients as those who are expected to be neutropenic (ANC < 500 cells/microL) for ≤7 days and those who have no active comorbidities or evidence of significant hepatic or renal dysfunction. Similarly, high-risk patients are those who are expected to be neutropenic (ANC < 500 cells/microL) for >7 days. Patients with neutropenic fever who have on-going comorbidities or evidence of significant hepatic or renal dysfunction are also considered to be high risk, regardless of the duration of neutropenia. The NCCN guidelines consider other risk factors but they also support the use of the MASCC

index [7] (see Table 2). ASCO guideline presents a list of conditions which makes the outpatients high risk without considering the MASCC score [6].

4. Antibiotic Prophylaxis

Bacterial infections are a major cause of morbidity and mortality in patients who are neutropenic following chemotherapy for malignancy [9]. Trials have shown the efficacy of antibiotic prophylaxis in reducing the incidence of bacterial infections [10]. The IDSA [1], ESMO [5], ASCO [6], and NCCN [7] recommend antibacterial prophylaxis with a fluoroquinolone for high-risk patients (who are going to be neutropenic for >7 days), although the Australian Consensus Guidelines consider that the evidence was not strong enough to recommend antibiotic prophylaxis, except for stem cell transplantation patients and palliative patients with BM failure [11].

Meta-analyses have indicated that antibiotic prophylaxis with fluoroquinolone may reduce the overall mortality in neutropenic patients of an intermediate- to high-risk group as well as the incidence of fever and bacteraemia [12, 13]. A Cochrane review (109 trials, 13579 participants) showed that prophylaxis significantly reduced the risk of death from all causes (RR: 0.66, 95% CI 0.55 to 0.79), the risk of infection-related death (RR 0.61, 95% CI 0.48 to 0.77), the occurrence of fever (RR 0.80, 95% CI 0.74 to 0.87), and clinically documented infection (RR 0.65, 95% CI 0.56 to 0.76). There were no significant differences between fluoroquinolone prophylaxis and TMP-SMX prophylaxis with regard to death from all causes or infection; however, fluoroquinolone prophylaxis was associated with fewer side effects leading to discontinuation. Antibiotic prophylaxis in afebrile neutropenic patients significantly reduced all-cause mortality [14].

Some controversy remains regarding precisely which patient groups are the most appropriate candidates for fluoroquinolone prophylaxis. Some randomized trial did not include allogeneic HSCT recipients. Accordingly, many experts do not recommend fluoroquinolone prophylaxis for neutropenic autologous HSCT recipients [1].

Another quinolone, moxifloxacin, has been used as antibacterial prophylaxis for autologous HSCT, showing in a small double blind and placebo controlled randomized clinical trial that is superior to prevent bacteraemia and shortened febrile episodes. No significant increase of adverse events in the moxifloxacin arm was observed (adverse events reported were diarrhoea, C. difficile associated diarrhoea, exanthema, and QT prolongation) [15].

Although fluoroquinolone agents are widely used for prevention and management of infections in neutropenic patients, there is a main concern about the emergence of fluoroquinolone-resistant bacteria [16]. Fluoroquinolone resistance is linked to community fluoroquinolone consumption and the prophylaxis efficacy is reduced when the prevalence of fluoroquinolone Gram-negative bacillary resistance exceeds 20% [17]. The emergence of methicillin-resistant Staphylococcus aureus (MRSA) is associated with the use

TABLE 2: Initial risk assessment for febrile neutropenic patients (adapted from NCCN guideline) [7].

Low risk (score > 21 on the MASCC risk score) OR:	High risk (score < 21 on the MASCC risk score) OR:
Outpatient status at time of development of fever	Inpatient status at time of development of fever
No associated acute comorbid illness	Significant medical comorbidity or clinically unstable
Anticipated short duration of severe neutropenia (less than 7 days)	Anticipated prolonged severe neutropenia (ANC < 100 cells and >7 days)
Good performance status (ECOG 01)	Hepatic insufficiency
No hepatic insufficiency	Renal insufficiency
No renal insufficiency	Pneumonia or other complex infections at clinical presentation
	Alemtuzumab
	Mucositis grade 3-4

of multiple antibiotics, particularly with fluoroquinolones. The same occurs with the colonization by *C. difficile* and vancomycin-resistant enterococci (VRE) [17, 18].

In contrast, some cohort studies show that quinolone prophylaxis did not affect the emergence of quinolone-resistant Gram-negative isolates from blood cultures in FN patients. Probably, the resistance is not induced by quinolone alone [19, 20].

Finally, the antibiotic prophylaxis is effective and the emergence of resistant bacteria should be continuously monitored for the detection of local antibiotic resistance bacteria and discriminate the appropriate antibiotic that can be used based on different settings.

5. Antifungal Prophylaxis

Invasive fungal infections produced by yeasts and molds are the main infectious cause of mortality in patients with haematological malignancies. In the era preantifungal prophylaxis, *Candida* spp. accounted for the majority of fungal infections that occurred during neutropenia, followed by *Aspergillus* spp. Actually, *Aspergillus* has surpassed *Candida* as a cause of invasive fungal infections due to the use of antifungal prophylaxis against *Candida* spp. [21].

5.1. Candida Infection. Meta-analyses and randomized trials have determined that fluconazole is efficacious in preventing *Candida* infections in high-risk patients [22, 23]. Among lower-risk patient populations, invasive candidiasis is rare and generally does not merit routine fluconazole prophylaxis.

5.2. Aspergillus Infection. The efficacy of antifungal agents with activity against *Aspergillus* spp. and other molds (voriconazole, posaconazole, amphotericin B) has been evaluated, suggesting that prophylaxis prevents invasive fungal infections. Cornely et al. showed that prophylaxis with Posaconazole was superior to prophylaxis with fluconazole or itraconazole in the prevention of invasive fungal infection and resulted in lower mortality in patients with acute myelogenous leukemia or myelodysplastic syndromes who are undergoing remission-induction chemotherapy [24]. Aspergillus prophylaxis with posaconazole shows benefit in patients with graft-versus-host disease (GVHD) who were receiving

immunosuppressive therapy [25]. All of the agents with activity against molds also have activity against *Candida* spp.

Fluconazole was the first azole used for antifungal prophylaxis, having high systemic activity, excellent tolerability, low toxicity, and cheap generic formulations and prevents infection with all species of Candida except for *C. krusei* or *C. glabrata* [26]. It is important to note that Fluconazole has no activity against *Aspergillus* or other molds.

Other agents such as itraconazole, voriconazole, posaconazole, and caspofungin are all acceptable alternatives [1]. The other echinocandins (anidulafungin and micafungin) have not been studied specifically for empiric antifungal therapy; however, NCCN panel members consider them to likely be effective, based on the data for caspofungin [7].

The echinocandins have a broader spectrum of activity than fluconazole and an excellent safety record. Micafungin was compared to fluconazole in a prospective, randomized, double blind comparative trial study showing that it is being superior during the neutropenic phase after haemopoietic stem cell transplant [27]. The drawback of this antifungal class is its availability only as an intravenous formulation and its high cost.

Voriconazole is available since 2003 and was initially approved for treatment of *Aspergillus* spp. infections but not against the agents of mucormycosis. Voriconazole has been best evaluated for the treatment of invasive aspergillosis and it is the preferred agent for treatment. Some trials have demonstrated its efficacy also as antifungal prophylaxis. Randomized, double blind trails compared fluconazole against voriconazole for the prevention of IFI, showing no significant difference in incidence of IFI or survival [28]. Another randomized, open-label, multicentre study comparing voriconazole and itraconazole showed no difference in terms of incidence or IFI or survival [29]. Voriconazole has both oral and IV formulations but has been noted to cause transient visual disturbances (which are not permanent or serious). A major drawback is its potential interactions with certain chemotherapy agents.

Itraconazole is active against *Aspergillus* spp. and it is available as an oral formulation. Two studies compared to fluconazole showed the prophylactic activity for fungal infections [30, 31]. A meta-analysis (including 13 randomized trials, 3597 neutropenic patients) evaluated the efficacy of itraconazole versus other forms of prophylaxis for the prevention of IFI, showing a significant reduction in the incidence of IFI, of invasive yeast infections and mortality [32]. A major drawback is its potential interactions with certain chemotherapy agents (best documented with cyclophosphamide and vinca alkaloids).

Posaconazole is available as an oral suspension since 2007. Recently, the FDA has approved the intravenous presentation of posaconazole. It is active against *Candida* spp., *Aspergillus* spp., *Zygomycetes,* and *Fusarium*. A randomized, multicentre single-blind study evaluated the efficacy and safety of posaconazole compared to fluconazole or itraconazole as prophylaxis for each cycle of chemotherapy in patients with AML or myelodysplastic syndrome and prolonged neutropenia. Posaconazole was superior over standard triazoles in preventing IFIs and significantly better in preventing invasive aspergillosis. Survival was significantly longer among recipients of posaconazole than among recipients of fluconazole or itraconazole [24]. Another randomized double-blind trial found no difference between posaconazole and fluconazole to prevent IFIs but posaconazole was superior to fluconazole preventing invasive aspergillosis. Mortality was similar between both groups but the number of deaths from IFI was lower in posaconazole group [25].

Its major drawbacks of oral suspension of posaconazole include variability of blood levels after oral admission. It should be taken with a full meal or with liquid nutritional supplements or an acidic carbonated beverage. If the patient is not eating, absorption is greatly impeded. In that case, the delayed-release tablets result in higher plasma drug concentrations than the oral suspension regardless of food intake. Patients who are unable to take medications orally or who are expected not to absorb oral medications should be given IV posaconazole.

The other disadvantage is its potential interactions with certain chemotherapy agents, such as cyclophosphamide, and the vinca alkaloids, such as vincristine. The NCCN Guidelines panel advises that prophylaxis with posaconazole, itraconazole and voriconazole should be avoided in patients receiving vinca alkaloid-based regimens (such as vincristine in acute lymphoblastic leukemia) because of the potential of these azoles to inhibit the cytochrome P3A4 isoenzyme reducing clearance of vinca alkaloids [7].

Finally, it is important to note that antifungal prophylaxis could decrease the sensitivity of biomarkers such as galactomannan [33]. Theoretically, the use of prophylaxis could impact the choice of the strategy during the neutropenia but few data are available [34].

6. When to Start Antibiotics?

ESMO, IDSA, and ASCO guidelines recommend antibiotic prophylaxis with a fluoroquinolone for patients who are going to be neutropenic for >7 days [1, 5, 6].

In all febrile neutropenic patients, empiric broad-spectrum antibacterial therapy should be initiated immediately after blood cultures have been obtained and before any other investigations have been completed [35]. Antimicrobial therapy should be administered within 60 minutes of presentation [36]. Mortality in neutropenic patients with

TABLE 3: Intravenous antibiotics for empirical therapy of fever in neutropenic patients.

Monotherapy	Two-drug regimen
Piperacillin-tazobactam	Piperacillin-tazobactam + amikacin
Imipenem-cilastatin	Imipenem-cilastatin + amikacin
Meropenem	Meropenem + amikacin
Ceftazidime	Ceftazidime + amikacin
Cefepime	Ceftriaxone + amikacin

Gram-negative bacteraemia can approach 40%, if an empirical treatment is not promptly undertaken [37].

The specific empirical regimen remains controversial. Actual guidelines recommend, for high-risk patients, starting monotherapy with a beta-lactam with activity against *Pseudomonas aeruginosa* (piperacillin-tazobactam, meropenem, imipenem-cilastatin, ceftazidime, and cefepime) [38]. Regarding the choice of beta-lactam, no single agent is clearly superior, although, in a meta-analysis (44 trials included), mortality was significantly lower with piperacillin-tazobactam compared to other antibiotics (RR 0.56, 95% CI 0.34 to 0.92, 8 trials, 1314 participants), without heterogeneity. Carbapenems resulted in a higher rate of antibiotic-associated and *Clostridium difficile*-associated diarrhoea, and the all-cause mortality was higher with cefepime compared to other beta-lactams [38]. Concerns regarding increased overall mortality with cefepime have been largely dismissed by the IDSA and ASCO after a reanalysis of the cefepime data by the FDA [39].

A two-drug regimen can be chosen in patients suspected of infection caused by resistant Gram-negative. Thus, a second gram-negative antibiotic should be added. Although a recent meta-analysis (seventy-one trials published between 1983 and 2012) showed that beta-lactam monotherapy is advantageous compared with beta-lactam-aminoglycoside combination therapy with regard to survival (RR 0.80, 95% CI 0.64 to 0.99), adverse events (numbers needed to harm 4; 95% CI 4 to 5), and fungal superinfections (RR 0.70, 95%CI 0.49 to 1.00) [40] (see Tables 3 and 4).

All the guidelines recommend not including vancomycin routinely in the initial regimen and not adding it empirically for persistent fever, although the IDSA guideline strongly recommends adding vancomycin in cases of hemodynamic instability, pneumonia, clinically evident catheter-related infection, skin and soft tissue infections, severe mucositis when fluoroquinolone prophylaxis has been used and ceftazidime is used empirically, and known colonization with methicillin-resistant *Staphylococcus aureus* [1].

For low risk patients eligible for outpatient management, the regimen of choice is the combination of fluoroquinolone and amoxicillin-clavulanic acid (or clindamycin for penicillin-allergic patients) as long as no fluoroquinolone prophylaxis was used, the patient tolerates oral medication, and the rate of resistance to fluoroquinolone is less than 20% [6]. Ciprofloxacin should not be employed as a solo agent because of its poor coverage of Gram-positive organisms [1]. When a fluoroquinolone cannot be used, a broad-spectrum beta-lactam active against *Pseudomonas* and suitable for

TABLE 4: Dosages of administrations of intravenous antibiotics for empirical treatment of febrile neutropenia.

Antibiotics	Doses
Amikacin	15–20 mg/kg every 24 h
Gentamicin	5–7 mg/kg every 24 h
Tobramycin	5–7 mg/kg every 24 h
Piperacillin-tazobactam	3.375 g/500 mg every 8 h or every 6 h
Ceftazidime	2 g every 8 h
Cefepime	2 g every 8 h
Imipenem-cilastatin	1 g every 8 h or every 6 h
Meropenem	1-2 g every 8 h
Vancomycin	15–20 mg/kg every 12 h
Linezolid	600 mg every 12 h
Daptomycin	6 mg/kg every 24 h
Teicoplanin	0.4–1.2 g qid (2 doses within the first 24 hours)
Ciprofloxacin	400 mg every 8 h or every 12 h
Levofloxacin	500–750 mg every 24 h

outpatient use should be used. Recently, a randomized, double-blind, multicenter clinical trial (intention to treat analysis: 169 patients in the moxifloxacin group versus 164 patients in the combination therapy) using a single daily oral dose of Moxifloxacin 400 mg in low-risk febrile neutropenic patients (MASCC score > 20) compared with ciprofloxacin (750 mg every 12 hours) plus amoxicillin/clavulanic acid (1000 mg every 12 hours) showed similar efficacy and safety (80% versus 82%, resp.). The most common adverse event was diarrhea in the combination therapy arm (42 versus 21 patients), but more neurologic events (eg, dizziness, vertigo, sleep disorder) were seen in the moxifloxacin arm [41].

If an infectious source of fever is identified, antibiotics should be continued for at least the standard duration indicated for the specific infection (e.g., 14 days for *Escherichia coli* bacteraemia); antibiotics should also continue at least until the absolute neutrophil count (ANC) is ≥500 cells/microL or longer if clinically indicated [1]. In case of no source of infection is identified and cultures are negative, the timing of discontinuation of antibiotics is usually dependent on resolution of fever and clear evidence of bone marrow recovery. If the patient has been a febrile for at least two days and the ANC is >500 cells/microL and is showing a consistent increasing trend, antibiotics may be stopped [1]. If the patient is still neutropenic and antibiotic therapy is stopped, the patient should be kept hospitalized under close observation for at least 24–48 hours. If fever recurs, antibiotics should be restarted urgently after obtaining blood cultures and performing other relevant evaluation based on clinical judgment [42].

7. Persistent Fever

Persistent fever is an episode of fever during neutropenia that does not resolve after 5 days of broad-spectrum antibacterial agents. The median time to defervescence following the initiation of empiric antibiotics in patients with hematologic malignancies is five days, in contrast with only two days for patients with solid tumours [1]. Modification of the initial antibacterial therapy is not needed for persistent fever alone if the patient is in good clinical condition. In that case, the best clinical option should be watchful waiting. However, patients who remain febrile after the initiation of empiric antibiotics should be revaluated for possible infectious sources.

Management algorithms have been developed for the reassessment of neutropenic patients with persistent fever after two to four days and after four or more days [1]. Consideration should be given to invasive fungal infection identified as a common cause of persistent fever in neutropenic patients [43]. To avoid the onset of invasive fungal infection in neutropenic patients, three approaches have been developed, which are often combined: antifungal prophylaxis, empirical antifungal therapy, and preemptive antifungal approaches. Before efficient antifungal prophylaxis was available and before indirect biological markers and effective imaging were assessed, the only acceptable approach was empirical antifungal therapy in patients with persistent or recurrent unexplained fever refractory to broad-spectrum antibiotics [34].

Based on trials adding amphotericin B after 4 to 7 days of persistent fever, [44, 45] the guidelines recommend adding an empiric antifungal agent after four to seven days in high-risk neutropenic patients who are expected to have a total duration of neutropenia >7 days who have persistent or recurrent fever and in whom reassessment does not yield a cause [1]. Additionally, sepsis status (severe sepsis or septic shock), focused infection (lung, central nervous system, sinus, abdominal, or skin), and clinical judgment can be used to decide empiric antifungal therapy and avoid unnecessary treatment [46].

The incidence of fungal infection (especially those caused by *Candida* or *Aspergillus* spp.) rises after patients have experienced more than seven days of persistent neutropenic fever [47]. In patients who are clinically unstable or have a suspected fungal infection, antifungal therapy should be considered even earlier than what is recommended for empiric therapy.

The choice of agent for empiric antifungal therapy depends upon which fungi are most likely to be causing infection, as well as the toxicity profiles and cost [1]. The IDSA guideline for empiric antifungal therapy recommends lipid formulation of amphotericin B, caspofungin, voriconazole, or itraconazole as suitable options for empiric antifungal therapy in neutropenic patients [1, 48–50] (see Table 5).

For persistently febrile patients with pulmonary nodules or nodular pulmonary infiltrates, invasive mold infection should be strongly suspected, and prompt assessment frequently requires bronchoscopy with bronchoalveolar lavage with cultures, stains, and *Aspergillus* galactomannan antigen testing to distinguish bacterial from mold pathogens, while simultaneously initiating antibacterial and antimold therapy until the specific aetiology is established. Voriconazole or a lipid formulation of amphotericin B is the drug of choices for invasive mold infection. Caspofungin is not preferred because of high failure rates in preventing and treating invasive aspergillosis. If mucormycosis is suspected, an

TABLE 5: Dosages of administrations of antifungal agents for empirical treatment of febrile neutropenia.

Antifungal	Doses
Fluconazole	400 mg/24 h IV/PO
Itraconazole	400 mg/24 h PO
Voriconazole	6 mg/kg every 12 h × 2 doses, then 4 mg/kg every 12 h; 200 mg/12 h PO
Posaconazole	Prophylaxis: 200 mg PO every 8 h
Caspofungin	70 mg IV initial doses, then 50 mg/24 h IV
Micafungin	100 mg/24 h IV for candidemia and 50 mg/24 h IV as prophylaxis; 150 mg/24 h IV for *Aspergillus* spp. infection
Anidulafungin	200 mg IV initial doses, then 100 mg/24 h IV

amphotericin B formulation should be given since voriconazole has no activity against *Mucor* species [51] There is insufficient evidence to conclusively determine the superiority of any agent; the choice of the initial antifungal agent may vary based on epidemiology and local susceptibility patterns. IDSA guideline recommends a diagnostic imaging workup (chest and/or sinus computed tomography) to rule out fungal infections in patients with neutropenia expected to last >7 days and persistent fever [1].

In case of febrile neutropenic patients who have been receiving antimold prophylaxis, a different class of antifungal agent with activity against molds should be used for empiric therapy. Finally, caspofungin and other echinocandins are not active against *Cryptococcus* spp., *Trichosporon* spp., and filamentous molds other than *Aspergillus* spp., such as *Fusarium* spp. In addition, some yeast can demonstrate relative resistance to these drugs (*C. parapsilosis*, *C. rugosa*, *C. guilliermondii*, and noncandidal yeasts). Moreover, the clinical efficacy of the echinocandins for endemic fungi (*Histoplasma*, *Blastomyces*, *Coccidioides* spp.) has not been demonstrated.

8. Preemptive Antifungal Therapy

In recent years, some authors have suggested that limiting antifungal therapy to selected patients may reduce the perceived unnecessary use of overempirical antifungal treatment, reduce toxicity, and reduce costs without increasing IFI-related mortality [52, 53].

There is no consensual definition of a preemptive therapy, but the common goal is to use the current screening tests (serum galactomannan, beta-D-glucan assay, and high-resolution chest CT) to postpone starting antifungal therapy until IFI is more likely. This approach is best suited for patients receiving prophylaxis with an antiyeast agent, such as fluconazole, where the concern is mainly mold pathogens and broadening the coverage to include antimold agents is appropriate.

In 2005, Maertens et al. evaluated the feasibility of a "preemptive" approach based on the incorporation of sensitive, noninvasive diagnostic tests (galactomannan and CT-scanning) for high-risk neutropenic patients who had

received fluconazole prophylaxis while avoiding empirical therapy. This approach reduced the rate of antifungal use for FN from 35% to 7.7%, lowering the exposure to expensive and potentially toxic drugs and led to the early initiation of antifungal therapy in about 7% of episodes that had not been clinically suspected of being related to an invasive fungal disease [54].

In 2009, Cordonnier et al. published a randomized open label trial comparing an empirical antifungal strategy with a preemptive one in high-risk neutropenic patients using a galactomannan and a chest CT. This trial showed that preemptive treatment increased the incidence of invasive fungal disease, without increasing mortality, and decreased the costs of antifungal drugs but empirical treatment showed better survival rates for patients receiving induction chemotherapy [55].

Girmenia et al. showed that an intensive clinically driven diagnostic strategy based on galactomannan tests and CT scans in selected patients with neutropenic fever reduced the use of antifungal treatment by 43% compared to that used with a standard empirical approach. At the 3-month follow-up, 63% of the patients with invasive fungal disease had survived, and no cases of undetected invasive fungal disease were found [56].

Controversy about the reduction of antifungal consumption by the preemptive strategy is not resolved. The larger observational study, including 190 patients treated with empirical antifungal therapy (neutropenic patients with fever without known source of infection and unresponsive to antibacterial agents) and 207 with preemptive antifungal therapy (patients with laboratory tests or radiographic signs indicative of invasive fungal disease, without culture or histology proof) published by Pagano et al., showed that the rate of invasive fungal disease was higher in the preemptive antifungal therapy (23.7% versus 7.4%, $P < 0.001$) as well as the overall mortality rates (15.9% versus 6.3%, $P = 0.002$) [57]. Of note, the definition for an early preemptive therapy, in the included population, was not used (screening tests to postpone starting antifungal therapy until IFI is more likely).

Recently, Morrissey et al. in an open label randomized controlled trial (240 patients), compared an empirical strategy (culture and histology), with a preemptive approach using twice-weekly blood testing with galactomannan and PCR to detect *Aspergillus* spp. A CT scan was performed in the case of positive biomarker(s) or of persistent fever. The use of empirical antifungal drugs was significantly lower in the preemptive compared with the empirical group (15% versus 32%; $P = 0.002$). Overall survival was not different between groups. IFD were significantly more frequent in the preemptive group than in the standard group (24.5% versus 4.1%; $P < 0.0001$) [58].

Despite the risk of overtreatment in patients who do not have an invasive fungal disease, the empirical approach seems able to guarantee a better outcome in hematologic patients, remains easy, reproducible, safe, and cheap in terms of diagnostic methods, probably making it the best choice when adequate microbiological and radiological support is lacking and neutropenia lasts more than 10–15 days. For neutropenia of shorter duration (<10 days), the benefit of both strategies is similar and both are even debatable considering the low risk of IFD in that setting [55].

9. Catheter Removal

Central venous catheter- (CVC-) related infections are common in patients with neutropenic fever. Differential time to positivity 120 min of qualitative blood cultures performed on specimens simultaneously drawn from the CVC and a vein suggests a central line associated bacteraemia. In addition to 14 days of systemic antibiotics, CVC removal is recommended in which any of the following organisms is implicated: *S. aureus*, *P. aeruginosa*, *Candida* spp., other fungi, and rapidly growing nontuberculous mycobacteria. This recommendation is based upon observational studies showing improved clearance of infection among patients with *S. aureus*, *P. aeruginosa*, or *Candida* spp. bloodstream infections in which the CVC was removed [59, 60]. In a study of cancer patients with bacteraemia caused by rapidly growing mycobacteria, CVC removal was associated with a significantly reduced rate of relapse of bacteraemia [61].

Catheter removal is also recommended for tunnel infection, port pocket infection, septic thrombosis, endocarditis, sepsis with hemodynamic instability, and bloodstream infection that persists despite ≥72 hours of therapy with appropriate antibiotics, even when pathogens other than those described above are isolated [1]. Prolonged treatment (4–6 weeks) is recommended for complicated infection, defined as the presence of deep tissue infection, endocarditis, septic thrombosis, or persistent bacteraemia or fungemia occurring 72 h after catheter removal in a patient who has received appropriate antimicrobials.

For CVC-associated bacteraemia caused by coagulase-negative staphylococci, the CVC may be retained if the patient is stable, using systemic therapy with or without antibiotic lock therapy [1, 5].

10. Conclusion

(i) FN is a medical emergency with high mortality without an appropriate treatment. It is imperative to assess the risk for serious complications in neutropenic patients to decide the use of prophylaxis and an antimicrobial therapy and the need for inpatient admission.

(ii) Low-risk patients with FN are those in whom the duration of neutropenia (ANC < 500 cells/microL) is expected to be ≤7 days and those with no comorbidities. Those patients can be treated as outpatients.

(iii) High-risk patients with FN are those who are expected to be neutropenic (ANC < 500 cells/microL) for >7 days and those with comorbidities. Those patients should be admitted to hospitalization.

(iv) Blood stream infection is a serious complication in neutropenic patients. Gram-positive bacteria are the most common causes of infection, but drug-resistant Gram-negative bacteria are generally associated with the most serious infections.

(v) Prophylaxis is not necessary in all patients and should only be used in high-risk patients to avoid the emergence of resistant pathogens.

(vi) Empiric broad-spectrum antibacterial therapy should be initiated immediately after blood cultures have been obtained in high-risk patients with FN. Empiric antibacterial therapy should be started within 60 minutes of presentation in all patients presenting with neutropenic fever. Preemptive antifungal therapy strategy seems to be similar to empirical approach in low-risk patients with FN.

(vii) Fungal pathogens are more common in high-risk patients. *Candida* spp. and *Aspergillus* spp. account for the most invasive fungal infections during neutropenia.

(viii) Selecting antimicrobial agents for prophylaxis and/or empirical therapy should be based on the local susceptibility and resistance patterns of microorganisms.

Conflict of Interests

The authors declare that they have no conflict of interests regarding the publication of this paper.

Acknowledgment

The authors would like to express their gratitude to Myriam Labopin for the review of this paper and to all editorial staff. They would like to thank Eulalia Grifol for providing invaluable research support in compiling the bibliography.

References

[1] A. G. Freifeld, E. J. Bow, K. A. Sepkowitz et al., "Clinical practice guideline for the use of antimicrobial agents in neutropenic patients with cancer: 2010 update by the infectious diseases society of america," *Clinical Infectious Diseases*, vol. 52, no. 4, pp. e56–e93, 2011.

[2] M. K. Keng and M. A. Sekeres, "Febrile neutropenia in hematologic malignancies," *Current Hematologic Malignancy Reports*, vol. 8, no. 4, pp. 370–378, 2013.

[3] T. Goulenok and B. Fantin, "Antimicrobial treatment of febrile neutropenia: pharmacokinetic-pharmacodynamic considerations," *Clinical Pharmacokinetics*, vol. 52, no. 10, pp. 869–883, 2013.

[4] L. Pagano, M. Caira, G. Rossi et al., "A prospective survey of febrile events in hematological malignancies," *Annals of Hematology*, vol. 91, no. 5, pp. 767–774, 2012.

[5] J. de Naurois, I. Novitzky-Basso, M. J. Gill, F. M. Marti, M. H. Cullen, and F. Roila, "Management of febrile neutropenia: ESMO Clinical Practice Guidelines," *Annals of Oncology*, vol. 21, no. 5, pp. v252–v256, 2010.

[6] C. R. Flowers, J. Seidenfeld, E. J. Bow et al., "Antimicrobial prophylaxis and outpatient management of fever and neutropenia in adults treated for malignancy: American society of clinical oncology clinical practice guideline," *Journal of Clinical Oncology*, vol. 31, no. 6, pp. 794–810, 2013.

[7] L. R. Baden, W. Bensinger, M. Angarone et al., "Prevention and treatment of cancer-related infections," *Journal of the National Comprehensive Cancer Network*, vol. 10, no. 11, pp. 1412–1445, 2012.

[8] J. Klastersky, M. Paesmans, E. B. Rubenstein et al., "The multinational association for supportive care in cancer risk index: a multinational scoring system for identifying low-risk febrile neutropenic cancer patients," *Journal of Clinical Oncology*, vol. 18, no. 16, pp. 3038–3051, 2000.

[9] E. J. Bow, "Management of the febrile neutropenic cancer patient: lessons from 40 years of study," *Clinical Microbiology and Infection, Supplement*, vol. 11, no. 5, pp. 24–29, 2005.

[10] G. Bucaneve, A. Micozzi, F. Menichetti et al., "Levofloxacin to prevent bacterial infection in patients with cancer and neutropenia," *The New England Journal of Medicine*, vol. 353, no. 10, pp. 977–987, 2005.

[11] M. A. Slavin, S. Lingaratnam, L. Mileshkin et al., "Use of antibacterial prophylaxis for patients with neutropenia," *Internal Medicine Journal*, vol. 41, no. 1, pp. 102–109, 2011.

[12] L. Leibovici, M. Paul, M. Cullen et al., "Antibiotic prophylaxis in neutropenic patients: new evidence, practical decisions," *Cancer*, vol. 107, no. 8, pp. 1743–1751, 2006.

[13] A. Gafter-Gvili, A. Fraser, M. Paul, and L. Leibovici, "Meta-analysis: antibiotic prophylaxis reduces mortality in neutropenic patients," *Annals of Internal Medicine*, vol. 142, no. 12 I, pp. 979–995, 2005.

[14] A. Gafter-Gvili, A. Fraser, M. Paul, M. van de Wetering, L. Kremer, and L. Leibovici, "Antibiotic prophylaxis for bacterial infections in afebrile neutropenic patients following chemotherapy," *The Cochrane Database of Systematic Reviews*, vol. 1, Article ID CD004386, 2005.

[15] J. J. Vehreschild, G. Moritz, M. J. G. T. Vehreschild et al., "Efficacy and safety of moxifloxacin as antibacterial prophylaxis for patients receiving autologous haematopoietic stem cell transplantation: a randomised trial," *International Journal of Antimicrobial Agents*, vol. 39, no. 2, pp. 130–134, 2012.

[16] F. G. De Rosa, I. Motta, E. Audisio et al., "Epidemiology of bloodstream infections in patients with acute myeloid leukemia undergoing levofloxacin prophylaxis," *BMC Infectious Diseases*, vol. 13, no. 1, article 563, 2013.

[17] E. J. Bow, "Fluoroquinolones, antimicrobial resistance and neutropenic cancer patients," *Current Opinion in Infectious Diseases*, vol. 24, no. 6, pp. 545–553, 2011.

[18] C. Kjellander, M. Björkholm, H. Cherif, M. Kalin, and C. G. Giske, "Hematological: low all-cause mortality and low occurrence of antimicrobial resistance in hematological patients with bacteremia receiving no antibacterial prophylaxis: a single-center study," *European Journal of Haematology*, vol. 88, no. 5, pp. 422–430, 2012.

[19] Y. Chong, H. Yakushiji, Y. Ito, and T. Kamimura, "Clinical impact of fluoroquinolone prophylaxis in neutropenic patients with hematological malignancies," *International Journal of Infectious Diseases*, vol. 15, no. 4, pp. e277–e281, 2011.

[20] E. M. Trecarichi and M. Tumbarello, "Antimicrobial-resistant Gram-negative bacteria in febrile neutropenic patients with cancer: current epidemiology and clinical impact," *Current Opinion in Infectious Diseases*, vol. 27, no. 2, pp. 200–210, 2014.

[21] L. Pagano, M. Caira, A. Candoni et al., "The epidemiology of fungal infections in patients with hematologic malignancies: the SEIFEM-2004 study," *Haematologica*, vol. 91, no. 8, pp. 1068–1075, 2006.

[22] E. Robenshtok, A. Gafter-Gvili, E. Goldberg et al., "Antifungal prophylaxis in cancer patients after chemotherapy or hematopoietic stem-cell transplantation: systematic review and meta-analysis," *Journal of Clinical Oncology*, vol. 25, no. 34, pp. 5471–5489, 2007.

[23] E. J. Bow, M. Laverdière, N. Lussier, C. Rotstein, M. S. Cheang, and S. Ioannou, "Antifungal prophylaxis for severely neutropenic chemotherapy recipients: a meta-analysis of randomized-controlled clinical trials," *Cancer*, vol. 94, no. 12, pp. 3230–3246, 2002.

[24] O. A. Cornely, J. Maertens, D. J. Winston et al., "Posaconazole vs. fluconazole or itraconazole prophylaxis in patients with neutropenia," *The New England Journal of Medicine*, vol. 356, no. 4, pp. 348–359, 2007.

[25] A. J. Ullmann, J. H. Lipton, D. H. Vesole et al., "Posaconazole or fluconazole for prophylaxis in severe graft-versus-host disease," *The New England Journal of Medicine*, vol. 356, no. 4, pp. 335–347, 2007.

[26] R. Hachem, H. Hanna, D. Kontoyiannis, Y. Jiang, and I. Raad, "The changing epidemiology of invasive candidiasis: candida glabrata and candida krusei as the leading causes of candidemia in hematologic malignancy," *Cancer*, vol. 112, no. 11, pp. 2493–2499, 2008.

[27] J.-A. H. van Burik, V. Ratanatharathorn, D. E. Stepan et al., "Micafungin versus fluconazole for prophylaxis against invasive fungal infections during neutropenia in patients undergoing hematopoietic stem cell transplantation," *Clinical Infectious Diseases*, vol. 39, no. 10, pp. 1407–1416, 2004.

[28] J. R. Wingard, S. L. Carter, T. J. Walsh et al., "Randomized, double-blind trial of fluconazole versus voriconazole for prevention of invasive fungal infection after allogeneic hematopoietic cell transplantation," *Blood*, vol. 116, no. 24, pp. 5111–5118, 2010.

[29] D. I. Marks, A. Pagliuca, C. C. Kibbler et al., "Voriconazole versus itraconazole for antifungal prophylaxis following allogeneic haematopoietic stem-cell transplantation," *British Journal of Haematology*, vol. 155, no. 3, pp. 318–327, 2011.

[30] K. A. Marr, F. Crippa, W. Leisenring et al., "Itraconazole versus fluconazole for prevention of fungal infections in patients receiving allogeneic stem cell transplants," *Blood*, vol. 103, no. 4, pp. 1527–1533, 2004.

[31] D. J. Winston, R. T. Maziarz, P. H. Chandrasekar et al., "Intravenous and oral itraconazole versus intravenous and oral fluconazole for long-term antifungal prophylaxis in allogeneic hematopoietic stem-cell transplant recipients. A multicenter, randomized trial," *Annals of Internal Medicine*, vol. 138, no. 9, pp. 705–713, 2003.

[32] A. Glasmacher, A. Prentice, M. Gorschlüter et al., "Itraconazole prevents invasive fungal infections in neutropenic patients treated for hematologic malignancies: evidence from a meta-analysis of 3,597 patients," *Journal of Clinical Oncology*, vol. 21, no. 24, pp. 4615–4626, 2003.

[33] K. A. Marr, M. Laverdiere, A. Gugel, and W. Leisenring, "Antifungal therapy decreases sensitivity of the *Aspergillus* galactomannan enzyme immunoassay," *Clinical Infectious Diseases*, vol. 40, no. 12, pp. 1762–1769, 2005.

[34] C. Cordonnier, C. Robin, A. Alanio, and S. Bretagne, "Antifungal pre-emptive strategy for high-risk neutropenic patients: why the story is still ongoing," *Clinical Microbiology and Infection*, vol. 20, supplement 6, pp. 27–35, 2014.

[35] H. Link, A. Böhme, O. A. Cornely et al., "Antimicrobial therapy of unexplained fever in neutropenic patients–guidelines of the Infectious Diseases Working Party (AGIHO) of the German Society of Hematology and Oncology (DGHO), Study Group Interventional Therapy of Unexplained Fever, Arbeitsgemeinschaft Supportivmassnahmen in der Onkologie (ASO) of the Deutsche Krebsgesellschaft (DKG-German Cancer Society),"

Annals of Hematology, vol. 82, supplement 2, pp. S105–S117, 2003.

[36] K. V. I. Rolston, "Challenges in the treatment of infections caused by gram-positive and gram-negative bacteria in patients with cancer and neutropenia," *Clinical Infectious Diseases*, vol. 40, no. 4, pp. S246–S252, 2005.

[37] J. Klastersky, "Concept of empiric therapy with antibiotic combinations. Indications and limits," *The American Journal of Medicine*, vol. 80, no. 5, pp. 2–12, 1986.

[38] M. Paul, D. Yahav, A. Bivas, A. Fraser, and L. Leibovici, "Antipseudomonal beta-lactams for the initial, empirical, treatment of febrile neutropenia: comparison of beta-lactams," *Cochrane Database of Systematic Reviews*, vol. 11, 2010.

[39] J. Gea-Banacloche, "Evidence-based approach to treatment of febrile neutropenia in hematologic malignancies," *Hematology/the Education Program of the American Society of Hematology*, vol. 2013, no. 1, pp. 414–422, 2013.

[40] M. Paul, Y. Dickstein, A. Schlesinger, S. Grozinsky-Glasberg, K. Soares-Weiser, and L. Leibovici, "Beta-lactam versus beta-lactam-aminoglycoside combination therapy in cancer patients with neutropenia," *The Cochrane Database of Systematic Reviews*, vol. 6, Article ID CD003038, 2013.

[41] W. V. Kern, O. Marchetti, L. Drgona et al., "Oral antibiotics for fever in low-risk neutropenic patients with cancer: a double-blind, randomized, multicenter trial comparing single daily moxifloxacin with twice daily ciprofloxacin plus amoxicillin/clavulanic acid combination therapy—EORTC infectious diseases group trial XV," *Journal of Clinical Oncology*, vol. 31, no. 9, pp. 1149–1156, 2013.

[42] D. Averbuch, C. Cordonnier, D. M. Livermore et al., "Targeted therapy against multi-resistant bacteria in leukemic and hematopoietic stem cell transplant recipients: guidelines of the 4th European conference on Infections in Leukemia (ECIL-4, 2011)," *Haematologica*, vol. 98, no. 12, pp. 1836–1847, 2013.

[43] R. S. Stein, J. Kayser, and J. M. Flexner, "Clinical value of empirical amphotericin B in patients with acute myelogenous leukemia," *Cancer*, vol. 50, no. 11, pp. 2247–2251, 1982.

[44] P. A. Pizzo, K. J. Robichaud, F. Gill, and F. G. Witebsky, "Empiric antibiotic and antifungal therapy for cancer patients with prolonged fever and granulocytopenia," *The American Journal of Medicine*, vol. 72, no. 1, pp. 101–111, 1982.

[45] F. Meunier, "Empirical antifungal therapy in febrile granulocytopenic patients. EORTC International Antimicrobial Therapy Cooperative Group," *The American Journal of Medicine*, vol. 86, no. 6, pp. 668–672, 1989.

[46] M. Aguilar-Guisado, I. Espigado, E. Cordero et al., "Empirical antifungal therapy in selected patients with persistent febrile neutropenia," *Bone Marrow Transplantation*, vol. 45, no. 1, pp. 159–164, 2010.

[47] J. R. Wingard and H. L. Leather, "Empiric antifungal therapy for the neutropenic patient," *Oncology*, vol. 15, no. 3, pp. 351–363, 2001.

[48] T. J. Walsh, R. W. Finberg, C. Arndt et al., "Liposomal amphotericin b for empirical therapy in patients with persistent fever and neutropenia," *The New England Journal of Medicine*, vol. 340, no. 10, pp. 764–771, 1999.

[49] T. J. Walsh, H. Teppler, G. R. Donowitz et al., "Caspofungin versus liposomal amphotericin B for empirical antifungal therapy in patients with persistent fever and neutropenia," *The New England Journal of Medicine*, vol. 351, no. 14, pp. 1391–1402, 2004.

[50] T. J. Walsh, P. Pappas, D. J. Winston et al., "Voriconazole compared with liposomal amphotericin B for empirical antifungal therapy in patients with neutropenia and persistent fever," *The New England Journal of Medicine*, vol. 346, no. 4, pp. 225–234, 2002.

[51] A. Madureira, A. Bergeron, C. Lacroix et al., "Breakthrough invasive aspergillosis in allogeneic haematopoietic stem cell transplant recipients treated with caspofungin," *International Journal of Antimicrobial Agents*, vol. 30, no. 6, pp. 551–554, 2007.

[52] B. H. Segal, N. G. Almyroudis, M. Battiwalla et al., "Prevention and early treatment of invasive fungal infection in patients with cancer and neutropenia and in stem cell transplant recipients in the era of newer broad-spectrum antifungal agents and diagnostic adjuncts," *Clinical Infectious Diseases*, vol. 44, no. 3, pp. 402–409, 2007.

[53] H. Cherif, M. Kalin, and M. Björkholm, "Antifungal therapy in patients with hematological malignancies: how to avoid overtreatment?" *European Journal of Haematology*, vol. 77, no. 4, pp. 288–292, 2006.

[54] J. Maertens, K. Theunissen, G. Verhoef et al., "Galactomannan and computed tomography-based preemptive antifungal therapy in neutropenic patients at high risk for invasive fungal infection: a prospective feasibility study," *Clinical Infectious Diseases*, vol. 41, no. 9, pp. 1242–1250, 2005.

[55] C. Cordonnier, C. Pautas, S. Maury et al., "Empirical versus preemptive antifungal therapy for high-risk, febrile, neutropenic patients: a randomized, controlled trial," *Clinical Infectious Diseases*, vol. 48, no. 8, pp. 1042–1051, 2009.

[56] C. Girmenia, A. Micozzi, G. Gentile et al., "Clinically driven diagnostic antifungal approach in neutropenic patients: a prospective feasibility study," *Journal of Clinical Oncology*, vol. 28, no. 4, pp. 667–674, 2010.

[57] L. Pagano, M. Caira, A. Nosari et al., "The use and efficacy of empirical versus pre-emptive therapy in the management of fungal infections: the HEMA e-Chart project," *Haematologica*, vol. 96, no. 9, pp. 1366–1370, 2011.

[58] C. O. Morrissey, S. C.-A. Chen, T. C. Sorrell et al., "Galactomannan and PCR versus culture and histology for directing use of antifungal treatment for invasive aspergillosis in high-risk haematology patients: a randomised controlled trial," *The Lancet Infectious Diseases*, vol. 13, no. 6, pp. 519–528, 2013.

[59] H. Hanna, C. Afif, B. Alakech et al., "Central venous catheter-related bacteremia due to gram-negative bacilli: significance of catheter removal in preventing relapse," *Infection Control and Hospital Epidemiology*, vol. 25, no. 8, pp. 646–649, 2004.

[60] I. Raad, H. Hanna, M. Boktour et al., "Management of central venous catheters in patients with cancer and candidemia," *Clinical Infectious Diseases*, vol. 38, no. 8, pp. 1119–1127, 2004.

[61] G. El Helou, R. Hachem, G. M. Viola et al., "Management of rapidly growing mycobacterial bacteremia in cancer patients," *Clinical Infectious Diseases*, vol. 56, no. 6, pp. 843–846, 2013.

27

In Vitro Whole Blood Clot Lysis for Fibrinolytic Activity Study Using D-Dimer and Confocal Microscopy

Abuzar Elnager,[1] Wan Zaidah Abdullah,[1] Rosline Hassan,[1] Zamzuri Idris,[2] Nadiah Wan Arfah,[3] S. A. Sulaiman,[4] and Zulkifli Mustafa[2]

[1] *Department of Haematology, School of Medical Sciences, Universiti Sains Malaysia, Health Campus,*
  16150 Kubang Kerian, Kelantan, Malaysia
[2] *Department of Neurosciences, School of Medical Sciences, Universiti Sains Malaysia, Health Campus,*
  16150 Kubang Kerian, Kelantan, Malaysia
[3] *Unit of Biostatistics and Research Methodology, School of Medical Sciences, Universiti Sains Malaysia, Health Campus,*
  16150 Kubang Kerian, Kelantan, Malaysia
[4] *Department of Pharmacology, School of Medical Sciences, Universiti Sains Malaysia, Health Campus,*
  16150 Kubang Kerian, Kelantan, Malaysia

Correspondence should be addressed to Wan Zaidah Abdullah; wzaidah@kb.usm.my

Academic Editor: Frits R. Rosendaal

This study aimed to evaluate *in vitro* whole blood (WB) clot lysis method for the assessment of fibrinolytic activity. Standardized unresected (uncut) retracted WB clot was incubated in pool platelet poor plasma (PPP) for varying incubation times and in streptokinase (SK) at different concentrations. The fibrinolytic activity was assessed by D-dimer (DD), confocal microscopy, and clot weight. DD was measured photometrically by immunoturbidimetric method. There was a significant difference in mean DD levels according to SK concentrations ($P = 0.007$). The mean DD $\pm$ SD according to the SK concentrations of 5, 30, 50, and 100 IU/mL was: 0.69 ± 0.12, 0.78 ± 0.14, 1.04 ± 0.14 and $2.40 \pm 1.09\,\mu g/mL$. There were no significant changes of clot weight at different SK concentrations. Gradual loss and increased branching of fibrin in both PPP and SK were observed. Quantitation of DD and morphology of fibrin loss as observed by the imaging features are in keeping with fibrinolytic activity. Combination of DD levels and confocal microscopic features was successfully applied to evaluate the *in vitro* WB clot lysis method described here.

1. Introduction

Fibrinolysis is a mechanism of fibrin breakdown in blood clot occurring *in vivo* or *in vitro* through a physiological process or by therapeutic induction. Naturally, fibrinolysis is a result of plasmin serine protease pathway activation. Fibrinolytic agent induces enzymatic activation of plasminogen to plasmin which cleaves the fibrin molecules [1–4].

The quantity of DD reflects intravascular levels of fibrin turnover, without significant interference from fibrinogen or soluble fibrin degradation products, indicating that both thrombin generation and plasmin generation have occurred [5].

Prasad et al. in 2006 developed an *in vitro* clot lytic model using streptokinase (SK) based on the percentage of clot lysis and found that increased percentage of lysis occurred according to the concentrations of SK [6]. Other *in vitro* studies investigated the association of blood plasma flow characteristics using recombinant tissue-plasminogen activator (rt-PA) or SK on the degradation of retracted (aged) and nonretracted (fresh) WB clot under a special perfusion system. They concluded that the size of clot fragments and the frequency of their removal increase with direct flow of plasma or flow velocity [4, 7, 8].

A few other *in vitro* studies of WB clot lysis reported the use of ^{125}I-fibrin labeled rt-PA, recombinant two chain urokinase-type plasminogen activator (rtcu-PA), and SK. They found that the rate of release of ^{125}I-fibrin was an indicator of clot lysis [9–11]. Other researchers used the rate of hemoglobin release as determined by cyanomethemoglobin technique as indicator of clot dissolution which was expressed as percentage of lysis [12]. On the other hand, a few studies reported on plasma clot containing washed red blood cells (RBCs) with different concentrations to determine the effects of RBCs on fibrin clot structure as assisted by confocal microscopy. They noted that different concentrations had an effect on fibrin arrangement in a clot structure [13, 14].

There are very few reports that have highlighted the *in vitro* procedure for WB clot lysis by using DD and structural evaluation for fibrinolytic activity assessment. It is thought that WB clot structure (compared to fibrin clot) has an advantage to reflect the closest similarity between *in vitro* and *in vivo* process of lytic activity with the exception of the vascular milieu. WB clot mimics the *in vivo* clot which contains all the components of blood such as RBCs, platelets, and white blood cells.

The aim of the present study was to validate and standardize an *in vitro* WB clot method for fibrinolysis related studies. The validation method used SK as an inducer of fibrinolysis and PPP as controls for time factor. The fibrinolytic activity was assessed quantitatively by measurement of DD concentrations (a specific fibrinolytic marker) and clot weight and qualitatively by WB clot morphology using confocal microscopy. These tools were used to validate the procedure for *in vitro* WB clot lysis method for fibrinolytic activity which could be performed in a clinical laboratory. With the advances of laboratory automation (measuring DD, etc.), more works for research purposes could be applied as a preliminary study. So far no report had combined the structural and molecular measurement of fibrinolysis from a WB clot for the *in vitro* fibrinolytic activity study.

2. Methodology

2.1. In Vitro WB Clot Procedure for Fibrinolytic Activity Studies

2.1.1. Preparation of Normal Pool Plasma.
Following local Institutional Ethical Board approval of the protocol, an informed consent was obtained and then human PPP was prepared and processed strictly using O blood group as a source of plasma by collecting about 9 mL of WB from each donor into two trisodium citrate tubes (4.5 mL each). Blood free from HIV and hepatitis B antigen (Ag) was drawn from volunteers using evacuated system with multisample needle green sterile 21GX1(1/2). Immediately after collection, samples were spun using a centrifuge (Eppendorf, 5810 R, Germany) at 1500 g for 15 minutes at room temperature and then the supernatant was spun down at 1200 g for 15 min. The procedure was carried out according to the Clinical Laboratory Standardization Institute (CLSI) guideline for coagulation tests. Next, the PPP of all donors was pooled and the coagulation profile including fibrinolytic markers was measured to obtain standardized pool PPP especially tested with prothrombin time, activated partial prothrombin time, fibrinogen, and DD using STA compact, and ACL Elite-Procoagulation Analyzers (Diagnostic STAGO, France, and Instrumentation Laboratory, Italy, resp.). The standardized pool PPP was aliquot into small volume (1 mL) in cryogenic vial and stored at −80°C for further study.

2.1.2. WB Clot Preparation.
Venous blood (4.5 mL) was drawn from one healthy volunteer from blood group O donor so as to maintain the consistency of the results. The blood was then transferred into three preweighed sterile siliconized glass tubes 12 × 75 mm without anticoagulant. It was first allowed to clot at room temperature for approximately 10 min. The tube was covered by parafilm to prevent contamination and haemolysis from water when it was incubated in water bath. It was then incubated at 37°C in controlled temperature water bath (Grant SUB6 England) for 3 hrs to ensure complete clot retraction. After the WB clot completely retracted from the edges of the glass tube, the serum was removed using Pasteur pipette. The tubes were dried by using filter paper and each tube with clot was again weighed to determine the clot weight (clot weight = weight of clot containing tube − weight of tube alone) using electronic analytical balance (AND FR-200 MK II, Japan) and the tube containing WB clot was appropriately labeled.

In the early part of this study we have validated the unresected (uncut) and resected (cut) WB clots to ensure a uniform clot weight. The unresected clot showed more consistent results of DD trends when suspended in pool PPP for a period of time than the resected clot.

The quantitation of DD was done using STA Compact Coagulation Analyzer (STAGO) and was determined photometrically by the immunoturbidimetric method using Liatest kit (STAGO).

2.1.3. Procedure for WB Clot Lysis Incubated in Pool PPP.
This procedure was used as a control test when duration of incubation was assessed for fibrinolytic activity. To each of the tubes containing retracted WB clot, 1 mL of prepared pool PPP was added after thawing at 37°C. The tubes were covered by parafilm and incubated at 37°C for 3, 6, and 9 hrs. Four groups of tests were analyzed as follows: Group 1 as baseline (0 hour incubation), Group 2 incubated for 3 hrs, Group 3 for 6 hrs of incubation, and Group 4 for 9 hrs of incubation. Following incubation, the plasma was obtained after gentle shaking of the clot and was then removed by Pasteur pipette in microcentrifuge tube (bullet tube) and each glass tube containing clot was again weighed after pool PPP incubation the difference in weight before and after clot lysis was then subsequently recorded. The previously removed plasma containing RBCs and other particles due to WB clot lysis was spun at 1200 g for 5 min (Eppendorf 5424, USA) and then the supernatant was tested for the DD levels. These procedures were repeated 10 times to assess the DD and clot weight changes.

2.1.4. Procedure for WB Clot Lysis Incubated in SK.
Commercial lyophilized SK vial (15, 00,000 IU, CLS Behring GmbH, 35041 Marburg, Germany) was purchased as a powder. The powder was dissolved with 5 mL normal saline, as per the manufacturer's instruction. This solution was used as a stock from which suitable dilutions were made to study the fibrinolytic activity using *in vitro* WB clot performed in our laboratory. The stock solution was aliquot into small volumes in cryogenic vials and stored at −80°C until use. The solution was thawed at room temperature (~22°C) whenever needed

and the unused portion was discarded. For the validation of the WB clot lysis procedure, four dilutions of thrombolytic drug (5, 30, 50, and 100 IU/mL) using SK were prepared using pool PPP as diluents with defined volume of 1 mL. WB clots were exposed to the SK in the above-mentioned dilutions. Following 1 hr incubation, the DD level and WB clot weight were measured as described above. The function of SK is to convert plasminogen to plasmin which in turn degrades the fibrin clot [15]. The normal range of plasminogen level in plasma is 0.75–1.60 μ/mL [16]. In the present study, we used PPP from apparently normal subjects who were expected to have normal plasminogen level. In pathological fibrinolysis such as disseminated intravascular coagulation (DIC), plasminogen level is usually low [16]. In this study, different concentrations of SK (mentioned above) were used and expected to have different fibrinolytic effects on the WB clot. A local intracoronary infusion of 20,000 IU by bolus maintained at 2000 units/minute was used in the treatment of myocardial infarction. The highest concentration, that is, 100 IU/mL, used in this study is 14.3 times more than the therapeutic dose for test tube equivalent (taking into consideration the fact that the WB clot is placed in a static milieu). Another reason for choosing these concentrations is because, at concentration more than 100 IU/mL, SK has a potent effect on the clot lysis difficult for assessment of DD linearity. The same procedure was performed for each concentration of SK and repeated 10 times to assess the DD and clot weight changes.

2.2. Confocal Microscopy Protocol and Staining Procedure. Confocal microscopic studies on WB clot have been reported and previously described in a few studies [2, 13, 14]. The reagents used in this study are fibrinogen fluorescence dye (Alexa Fluor 488 human fibrinogen conjugates (F-13191) purchased from Molecular Probes and prepared as per manufacturer's instructions. Stock solution was prepared by dissolving 5 mg of fibrinogen in 3.3 mL of 0.1 M sodium bicarbonate (NaHCO$_3$) (PH 8.3) at room temperature. The working solution was prepared by adding 100 μL fibrinogen (stock) dye to 6 mL distilled water. The complete solubilization was done with occasional gentle mixing for one hour. Stock solution was stored at 4°C for further use. The working solution (0.3 M) of merocyanine 540 fluorescent (MC-540) 25 mg/(MW = 569.67) (erythrocyte dye) was prepared by dissolving 3.4 mg in 20 mL distilled water. Commercially available phosphate buffered saline (PBS) was used as the main washing buffer in this study. The other buffer 0.1 M sodium bicarbonate (NaHCO$_3$) was used as diluents for fibrinogen fluorescence dye.

Venous blood was collected strictly from O blood group volunteers and 180 μL of WB was put in each well of 8-chambers polystyrene vessel tissue culture treated glass slide (BD falcon cultures, USA) according to the ratio used for WB clot lysis in the method described above. The WB clot was incubated at 37°C for 3 hrs to ensure complete clot retraction (as above). The serum was completely and gently removed from the chambers after 3 hrs. After that 120 μL of the pool

PPP (Group 1), stock solution of SK (Group 2) and SK + plasma, that is Group 3, at different concentrations (5, 30, 50, and 100 IU/mL) were added to the retracted WB clots which were formed in each well of the chambers. The labeling was done according to the period of incubation in pool PPP: 0, 3, 6, and 9 hrs at 37°C. On the other hand the labeling was done according to the SK concentration and incubated for one hour. The plasma was removed after each incubation period of time. The WB clot was washed by PBS three times for 3–5 min for each wash. The fibrin fibres were labeled with 600 μL working concentration of the primary antibody (Alexa Fluor 488 human fibrinogen conjugate F-13191, Molecular Probes 5 mg, Invitrogen Life Technologies) which was freshly prepared using sodium bicarbonate buffer (PH 8.3) and it was incubated and added to the clot at room temperature for 15 min in dark area to avoid direct light. The stain was removed and the clot was washed 3 times using PBS, after which it was incubated with buffer for 5 min. Following that the buffer was then removed. Subsequently, 600 μL of the merocyanine-labeled RBC-emission wavelength 520 nm (Molecular Probe USA) was added to the WB clot as RBC staining and incubated at room temperature for 45 min in dark room. After that the dye was washed using PBS 3 times for 3–5 min for each washing. The antifade fluorescence mounting medium was added before being examined by confocal microscopy. Images for fibrin and RBCs for each group were obtained on a Pascal 5 Axiovert inverted laser confocal microscope with a 63X lens using an argon and HeNe laser (Carl Zeiss, Germany). For confocal image of retracted WB clot, Alexa 488 labeled fibrin fibers in green, while the merocyanine 540 fluorescent dye (MC-540) labeled the RBC membranes in red colour.

2.3. Statistical Analysis. Statistical analyses were performed using PASW Statistics 19 (SPSS, Chicago, IL). Data were expressed as mean difference of DD within group for WB clot lysis, when incubated with plasma at different time and SK at different concentrations. The relationship between them was investigated by using repeated measures ANOVA within group analysis followed by pairwise comparison and one way ANOVA test followed by posthoc comparison, respectively. The WB clot weight between before and after plasma and SK incubation was compared using Wilcoxon Signed Rank test. A P value ≤ 0.05 was considered to be statistically significant.

3. Results

There was a significant mean difference of DD within the group of unresected WB clot lysis in pool PPP (without SK) when compared between 0 and 3 hrs, 0 and 6 hrs, 0 and 9 hrs, 3 and 6 hrs, 3 and 9 hrs, and lastly 6 and 9 hrs (P values <0.007). These findings reflect a proportional increase in DD according to the incubation time. The mean DD (SD) according to time recorded at 3, 6, and 9 hrs is 1.30 (0.26), 1.77 (0.48), and 2.31 (0.37) μg/mL, respectively (Figure 1).

There was a significant difference of median clot weight of unresected clot between before and after PPP incubation at 3, 6 and 9 hrs. The median (interquartile range) (IQR) weight

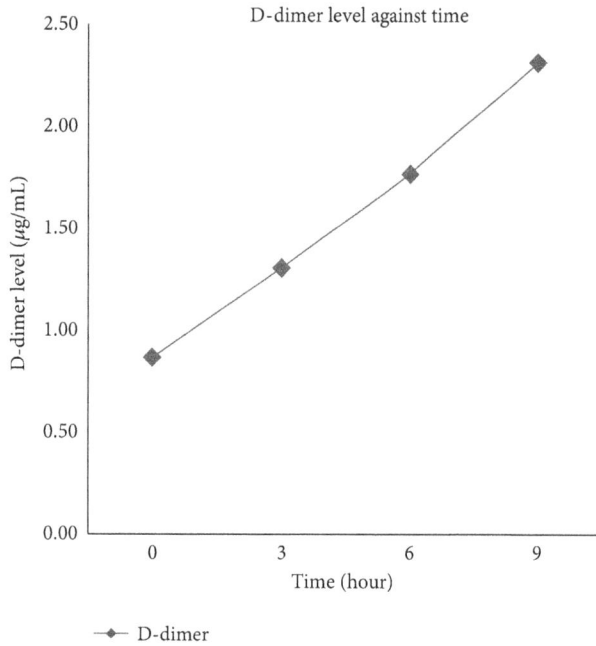

FIGURE 1: Line graph of D-dimer level against time of whole blood clot lysis in plasma.

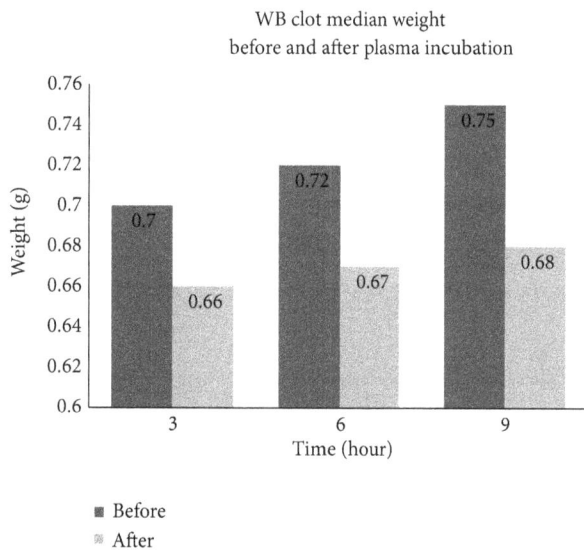

FIGURE 2: The difference in clot median weight between before and after pool PPP incubation.

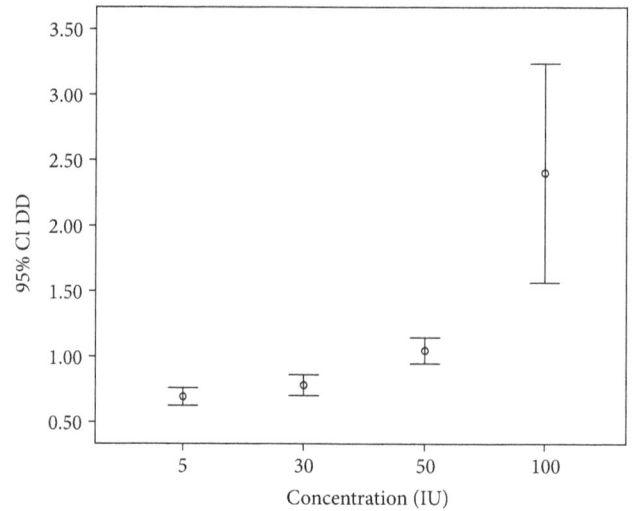

FIGURE 3: D-dimer level (μg/mL) against various concentrations (IU/mL) of streptokinase using Box-and-Whisker plot.

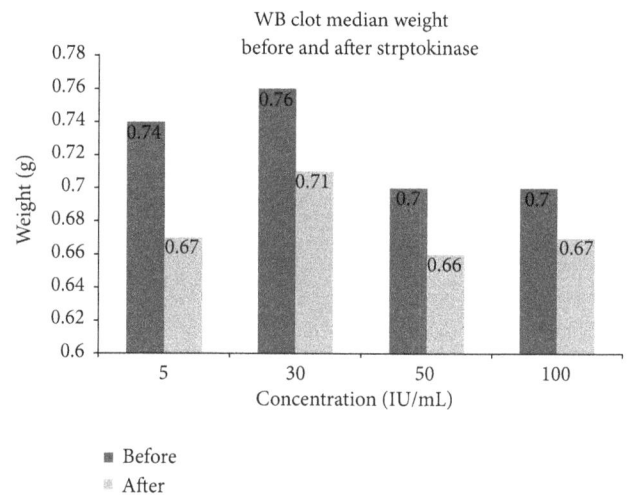

FIGURE 4: The difference in clot median weight between before and after SK induced fibrinolysis.

before versus after incubation at 3 hrs was 0.7 (0.06) versus 0.66 (0.04); at 6 hrs 0.72 (0.06) versus 0.67 (0.07); at 9 hrs 0.75 (0.07) versus 0.68 (0.06) gram, respectively (P values <0.001). These findings reflect WB clot lysis activity before and after incubation in PPP in their respective groups (Figure 2). However there were no significant changes of clot weight after incubation between different times (0.66–0.68 g) as depicted in Figure 2.

The results for WB clot incubated in SK at different concentrations are demonstrated in Figure 3. The baseline

level of DD from pool PPP for SK dilution was <0.50 μg/mL. This reflects a proportional increase in DD level according to the SK concentrations. There was significant mean difference of DD between all concentrations except for concentration of 5 versus 30 IU/mL. The mean DD (SD) according to the SK concentrations for 5, 30, 50, and 100 IU/mL was 0.69 (0.12), 0.78 (0.14), 1.04 (0.14), and 2.40 (1.09) μg/mL, respectively.

There was also a significant difference in median clot weight between before and after SK for each concentration: 5, 30, 50, and 100 IU/mL (P values <0.01). The median (IQR) weight before versus after SK incubation for each concentration at 5 IU/mL was 0.74 (0.08) versus 0.67 (0.06), at 30 IU/mL 0.76 (0.10) versus 0.71 (0.8), at 50 IU/mL 0.70 (0.10) versus 0.66 (0.12), and at 100 IU/mL 0.70 (0.09) versus 0.67 (0.10) gram, respectively (Figure 4).

While there was significant difference between before and after incubation at individual SK concentration, the median

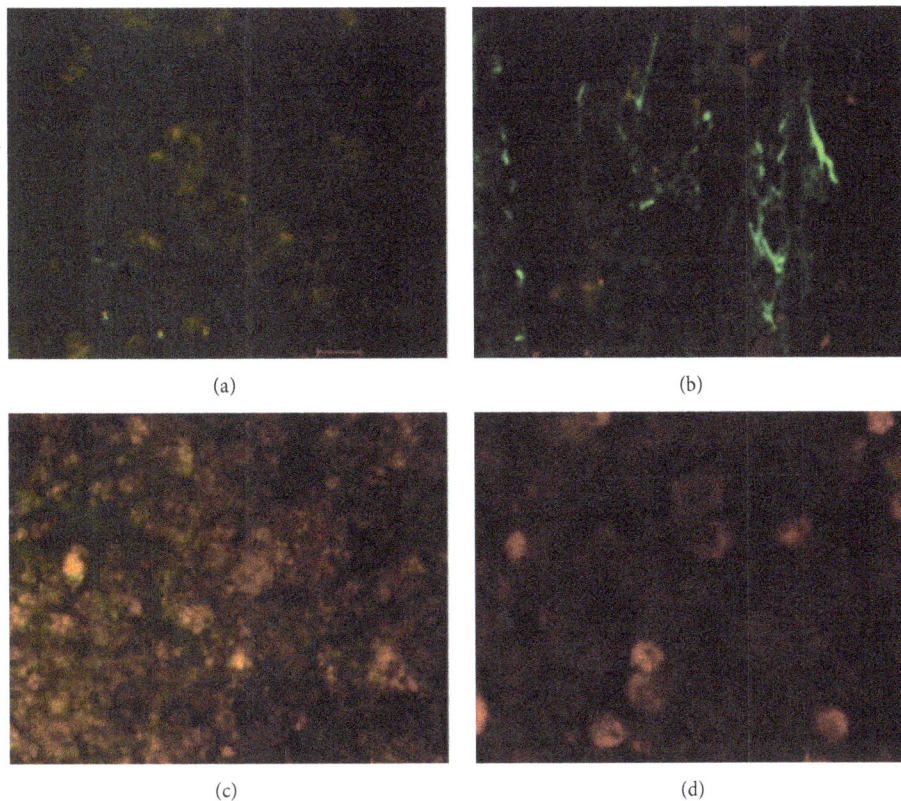

FIGURE 5: Confocal images for retracted WB clot incubated in pool PPP. (a) showed confocal image of normal retracted WB clot. (b), (c), and (d) showed retracted WB clot after 3, 6, and 9 hrs incubation in pool PPP, respectively. (a) shows confocal images of normal retracted WB clot showing fibrin mass surrounded and covered by RBCs (control untreated). (b) demonstrates a clear separation of fibrin from the RBCs after 3 hrs of WB clot incubation in PPP. (c) shows fibrin separation from the RBCs and a gradual loss of fibrin fibres after 6 hrs of incubation. (d) shows at 9 hrs of incubation in PPP minimal fibrin fibres with some remaining RBCs.

clot weight showed little or no difference between 5, 50 and 100 IU/mL post SK incubation. This indicates that the clot weight changes were not significant between the SK concentrations designed for this study.

3.1. Confocal Microscopy. Parallel experiments were performed *in vitro* in the presence of retracted WB clot incubated in pool PPP and SK. There was a gradual loss of fibrin fibres in WB clot according to the incubation time for pool PPP and concentrations of SK as shown in Figures 5 and 6, respectively.

4. Discussion

In this study combination of D-dimer, WB clot morphology, and WB clot weight were used for the validation of *in vitro* WB clot lysis method. The present method was modified from previously published articles and validated independently using the above-mentioned parameters [6, 17, 18]. The plasma was used as a medium to immerse the WB clot for the purpose of monitoring the coagulation parameters or products such as DD. The retracted WB clot when suspended in a plasma milieu became more sensitive to lysis with fibrinolytic agents than in buffer reagent. The plasma proteins such as plasminogen and fibrin that were entrapped in the clots might have

contributed to their sensitivity to lysis; in addition, the plasma milieu contains soluble proteins such as plasminogen, tissue plasminogen activators, and α_2 antiplasmin all of which also play crucial role in clot lysis [9]. The O blood group donors were used to ensure compatibility because the WB clot was created from O blood group individuals (however, plasma from A, B, and AB blood groups could also be used as sources of plasma because they do not usually produce haemolysis as a result of minor ABO incompatibility).

The present study used retracted WB clot as fresh WB clot was found not suitable for fibrinolytic studies [9]. The quantity of unbound plasminogen inside the clot (plasminogen/fibrin ratio) is higher in nonretracted clots than in retracted ones. This high ratio (which is as a result of high number of plasminogen molecules in close proximity to fibrin that can bind to partially degraded fibrin) makes the non retracted clots more prone to lysis with any type of activator. The ratio is even lesser in retracted clots as the pool of plasminogen is mainly located at the external surface of the clot [10]. Retracted WB clot increases the concentration of fibrin network and bound fibrinolytic inductors. Also fibrin induces the conversion of plasminogen to plasmin by plasminogen activators. In addition, the fibrin formed due to the clot retraction may stimulate the lysis activity [11]. Thrombolytic agents such as rt-PA cleave the fibrinogen and fibrin of

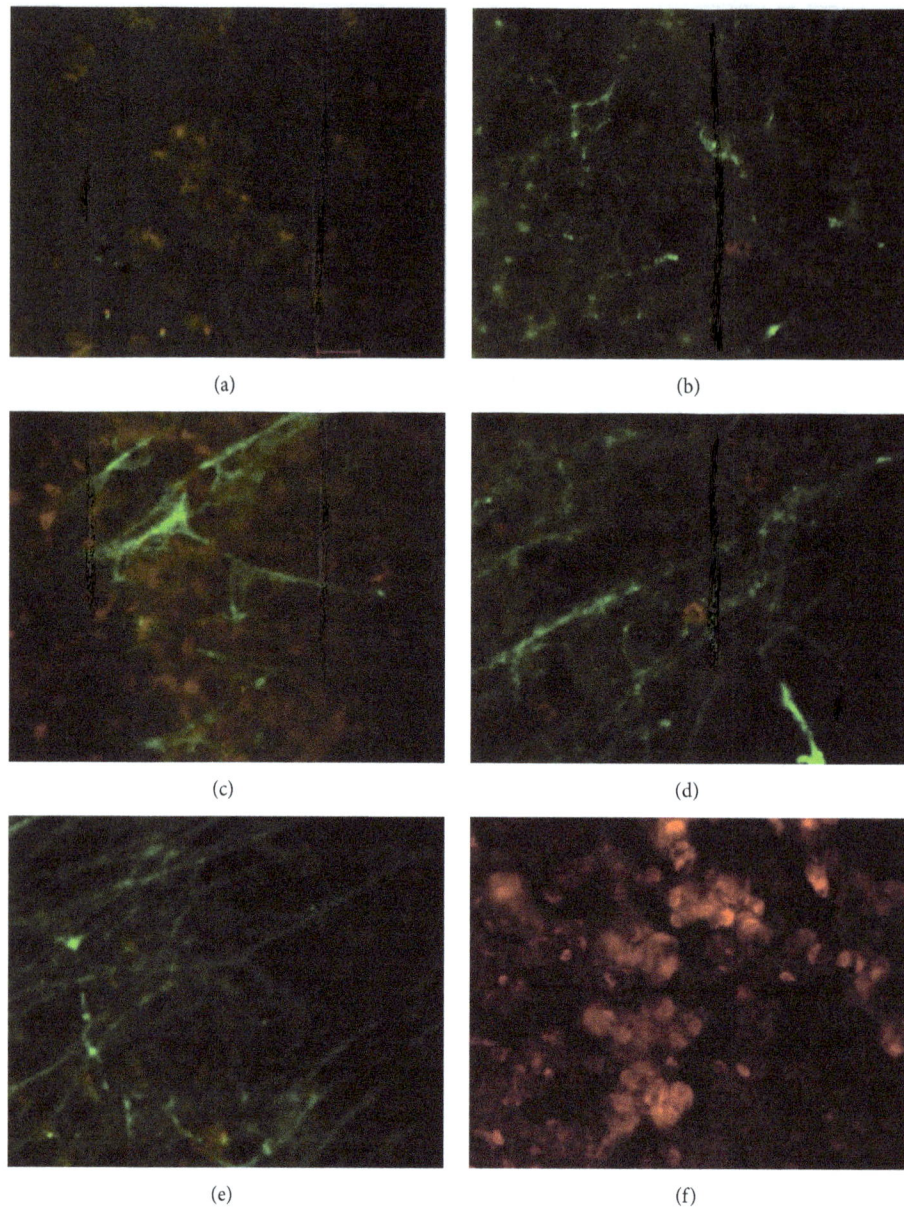

FIGURE 6: Confocal images for retracted WB clot treated with SK. (a) showed image of normal retracted WB clot. (b), (c), (d), (e) and (f) showed retracted WB clot treated with 5 IU/mL, 30 IU/mL, 50 IU/mL, 100 IU/mL, and 1500,000 IU (stock) of SK concentrations after 1-hour incubation, respectively. (a) demonstrates fibrin integrated with RBCs in retracted WB clot (control untreated). (b) shows 5 IU/mL concentration of SK where the fibrin started to separate from the RBCs. (c) depicts 30 IU/mL concentration of SK showing the fibrin that separated from the RBCs and a gradual thinning of fibrin fibres. (d) shows 50 IU/mL concentration of SK demonstrating fibrin separation from the RBCs and the fibrin fibres became much thinner and increased branching than 30 IU/mL. (e) shows 100 IU/mL concentration of SK where the fibrin almost separated from the RBCs and fibrin fibres became much thinner and increased branching than the 50 IU/mL SK. (f) shows 1500,000 IU (stock) of SK showing complete disappearance of fibrin from the RBCs.

the thrombus into fragments D and E, and these products are represented by the concentration of DD as a specific fibrin degradation product. Determination of DD concentration is a valid measure for quantifying the efficacy of fibrinolytic therapy [19].

In this method validation, retracted WB clot lysis in PPP was used as control test in which the lysis was allowed to occur spontaneously with time. The rate and concentrations of DD were lower than the treated clot using SK. This finding

is supported by previous studies, which used spontaneous clot lysis activity in buffer or plasma as control [11, 12]. Our study showed that DD levels increased with time of incubation in plasma and with increasing concentrations of SK which were also statistically significant ($P < 0.05$). A comparable finding with the plasma clot has been reported previously [19]. This study found that DD provides more discriminative results for assessment of *in vitro* whole blood clot lysis activity than clot weight. Increasing trend of DD but not the clot weight was observed when the clot was allowed to undergo natural lysis with time. This finding suggests that DD is a suitable and sensitive marker for assessment of *in vitro* WB clot lysis activity. The increasing trend of DD agrees with the previous report that used haemoglobin and radioactive method to evaluate the clot lysis activity [11, 12].

As mentioned earlier in the methods, there were differences between resected and unresected WB clot. There was a problem in standardizing the clot weight. Although the same blood volume was used from healthy donors with normal haemoglobin level, it was observed that, the clot weight after retraction varied from one tube to another. It was difficult to get an acceptable uniform weight unless the clots were resected so as to fix their weight. On the bases of this, the value of clot weight was fixed in the preliminary study by resecting the clots to standardize their weight. It was suggested that by using resected WB clot, fibrinolytic activity might be affected probably as a result of exposing the inner layer of the clot to PPP. This in turn leads to inconsistencies in the results of the resected clot compared with the unresected one. Previous studies have reported clot weight in the form of ranges for *in vitro* studies [17, 18].

In the present study we included WB clot weight as previous studies had used it as indicator of clot lysis activity. The median weights the whole blood clot after PPP incubation and with SK were significantly lower than before PPP and SK incubation. This result correlates with the previous studies [6, 18]. However we observed that, at different concentrations of SK (5, 50, and 100 IU/mL), there was not much difference in weight changes. This could probably imply that the SK doses used here were inappropriate or the lytic activity has reached its plateau despite of the different concentrations used. This effect is probably due to a limiting factor from natural inducers of fibrinolysis such as plasminogen which control the clot to continue the lytic process. However, the concentrations of DD increased significantly with SK in these concentrations (5, 50, and 100 IU/mL). This finding also explained the sensitivity of the two different methods in detecting fibrinolytic activity particularly at molecular level.

The branching of fibrin fibres was found to be larger in size, thinner, and separated from RBC with the higher levels of DD. The size of the fibrin branching increased and then disappeared with the increasing concentration of SK. In PPP, fibrin was separated from RBC and disappeared with time. A study has shown increased porosity of fibrin when treated with thrombin and factor Xa inhibitors using 3D confocal microscopy [20]. This study applied qualitative assessment of the blood clot morphology and hence the finding was not reported in quantitative measurement (such as grading system). In future, evaluation of the WB clot morphology subjected to fibrinolysis could be improved by applying appropriate quantitative measurements for more objective results.

The effect of SK on fibrin imaging was evaluated by optimization of the untreated fibrin as shown by the representative image in Figures 5(a) and 6(a). It was found that fibrin of WB clot incubated in PPP at 3 and 6 hrs showed highly branching feature and loss of fibres at 9 hrs. The WB clot on confocal images also demonstrated that the fibrin fibres were thicker in PPP than in the SK treated clot. WB clot underwent gradual loss of fibrin fibres when incubated in PPP according to the incubation time and there was minimal or no fibrin fibres at 9 hrs.

In contrast, there was a gradual loss of fibrin fibres in WB clot treated in SK at different concentrations: 5, 30, 50, 100 IU/mL, and 1,500,000 IU (stock solution). There was also increasing branching and loss of scaffolding features (red cells integrated in the fibrin mass) at 100 IU/mL and eventually the fibres disappeared with higher concentration of SK such as at 250, 1000 IU/mL and stock solution.

Previous study indicated that the fibres ends are rarely seen in an undamaged normal fibrin clot. This is because the protofibrils lateral aggregation produces clots with thick fibres and few branch points. However, the inhibition of lateral aggregation due to fibrinolytic process tends to produce clots with thin fibres and numerous branching points which is in agreement with our findings where increased branching is seen at 30 IU/mL compared to 5 IU/mL [1].

In this study the fibrin fibres were thinner in SK incubation than with the control test (incubated in PPP) at 5 IU/mL and 30 IU/mL versus 3 hrs of incubation in PPP. This shows the effect of penetration of SK into the WB clot. WB clot incubated in PPP undergoes natural fibrinolysis induced by plasma proteins. In these two methods, the structure of the fibrin networks underwent significant changes in architecture during the lytic process. The fibrin fibres became thinner and, underwent gradual loss based on the increasing concentrations of SK and time of incubation in PPP [13, 14, 20]. While optimizing SK concentrations for the method, we found that 100 IU/mL was more suitable for *in vitro* method. The highest concentration (100 IU/mL) used in this study is 14.3 times more than the therapeutic dose for test tube equivalent. There are limitations in this study; for example, the concentration of streptokinase used was probably low and difficult to optimize with the size of the blood clot. In addition the time for incubation with plasma containing streptokinase was short (1 hour). Although increased levels of D-dimer could be a marker of initiation of biochemical reactions involved in fibrinolysis after incubating clots with plasma containing streptokinase, under conditions used in this experiment one would not expect significant reduction of blood clot weight regardless of concentration of streptokinase used. In future studies, it would be interesting to compare D-dimer levels after same period of time (e.g., 1 hour or longer) in clots exposed only to plasma on one hand and in clots exposed to plasma and streptokinase on the other hand.

5. Conclusion

The modified *in vitro* WB clot lysis method has been evaluated using combination of DD and confocal microscopy. Unresected retracted WB clot was found suitable for this method validation. DD is more appropriate than clot weight in discriminating the fibrinolytic activity. This WB clot method is useful for investigation of factors affecting the WB clot lysis or for exploring the potential fibrinolytic agents in a clinical laboratory as a preliminary research work.

Conflict of Interests

There is no conflict of financial interests related to this study.

Acknowledgments

This work was supported by Research University (RU) Grant 1001/PPSP/812111 from Universiti Sains Malaysia. The first author is supported by the Graduate Assistant Scheme, School of Medical Sciences, Universiti Sains Malaysia. The authors would like to thank the staff of the Haematology Laboratory and Blood Bank of Hospital Universiti Sains Malaysia for their support and cooperation especially to Miss Ang Cheng Yong and Mr. Khairul Putra. They would like to thank the late Madam Wan Soriany Wan Md. Zain, for her technical assistance and ideas for this study.

References

[1] J. W. Weisel, "Structure of fibrin: impact on clot stability," *Journal of Thrombosis and Haemostasis*, vol. 5, no. 1, pp. 116–124, 2007.

[2] R. C. Carroll, J. M. Gerrard, and J. M. Gilliam, "Clot retraction facilitates clot lysis," *Blood*, vol. 57, no. 1, pp. 44–48, 1981.

[3] L. T. Couto, J. L. Donato, and G. de Nucci, "Analysis of five streptokinase formulations using the euglobulin lysis test and the plasminogen activation assay," *Brazilian Journal of Medical and Biological Research*, vol. 37, no. 12, pp. 1889–1894, 2004.

[4] G. Tratar, A. Blinc, M. Štrukelj, U. Mikac, and I. Serša, "Turbulent axially directed flow of plasma containing rt-PA promotes thrombolysis of non-occlusive whole blood clots *in vitro*," *Thrombosis and Haemostasis*, vol. 91, no. 3, pp. 487–496, 2004.

[5] E. Bruinstroop, M. A. van de Ree, and M. V. Huisman, "The use of D-dimer in specific clinical conditions: a narrative review," *European Journal of Internal Medicine*, vol. 20, no. 5, pp. 441–446, 2009.

[6] S. Prasad, R. S. Kashyap, J. Y. Deopujari, H. J. Purohit, G. M. Taori, and H. F. Daginawala, "Development of an *in vitro* model to study clot lysis activity of thrombolytic drugs," *Thrombosis Journal*, vol. 4, article 14, 2006.

[7] F. Bajd, J. Vidmar, A. Blinc, and I. Serša, "Microscopic clot fragment evidence of biochemo-mechanical degradation effects in thrombolysis," *Thrombosis Research*, vol. 126, no. 2, pp. 137–143, 2010.

[8] W. W. Jeong, A. S. Jang, and K. Rhee, "Whole blood clot dissolution: *in vitro* study on the effects of permeation pressure," *Proceedings of the Institution of Mechanical Engineers H*, vol. 221, no. 4, pp. 357–364, 2007.

[9] M. Sabovic, H. R. Lijnen, D. Keber, and D. Collen, "Effect of retraction on the lysis of human clots with fibrin specific and non-fibrin specific plasminogen activators," *Thrombosis and Haemostasis*, vol. 62, no. 4, pp. 1083–1087, 1989.

[10] M. Sabovic and D. Keber, "*In-vitro* synergism between t-PA and scu-PA depends on clot retraction," *Fibrinolysis*, vol. 9, no. 2, pp. 101–105, 1995.

[11] M. López, A. Ojeda, and C. L. Arocha-Piñango, "*In vitro* clot lysis: a comparative study of two methods," *Thrombosis Research*, vol. 97, no. 2, pp. 85–87, 2000.

[12] E. Coll-Sangrona and C. L. Arocha-Piñango, "Fibrinolytic action on fresh human clots of whole body extracts and two semipurified fractions from Lonomia achelous caterpillar," *Brazilian Journal of Medical and Biological Research*, vol. 31, no. 6, pp. 779–784, 1998.

[13] K. C. Gersh, C. Nagaswami, and J. W. Weisel, "Fibrin network structure and clot mechanical properties are altered by incorporation of erythrocytes," *Thrombosis and Haemostasis*, vol. 102, no. 6, pp. 1169–1175, 2009.

[14] N. Wohner, P. Sótonyi, R. MacHovich et al., "Lytic resistance of fibrin containing red blood cells," *Arteriosclerosis, Thrombosis, and Vascular Biology*, vol. 31, no. 10, pp. 2306–2313, 2011.

[15] A. Banerjee, Y. Chisti, and U. C. Banerjee, "Streptokinase—a clinically useful thrombolytic agent," *Biotechnology Advances*, vol. 22, no. 4, pp. 287–307, 2004.

[16] S. S. M. Lewis, B. J. Bain, and I. Bates, *Dacie and Lewis Practical Haematology*, Churchill Livingstone, New York, NY, USA, 2006.

[17] G. J. Shaw, N. Bavani, A. Dhamija, and C. J. Lindsell, "Effect of mild hypothermia on the thrombolytic efficacy of 120 kHz ultrasound enhanced thrombolysis in an *in-vitro* human clot model," *Thrombosis Research*, vol. 117, no. 5, pp. 603–608, 2006.

[18] G. J. Shaw, A. Dhamija, N. Bavani, K. R. Wagner, and C. K. Holland, "Arrhenius temperature dependence of *in vitro* tissue plasminogen activator thrombolysis," *Physics in Medicine and Biology*, vol. 52, no. 11, pp. 2953–2967, 2007.

[19] H. Schwarzenberg, S. Müller-Hülsbeck, J. Brossman, C. C. Glüer, H. D. Bruhn, and M. Heller, "Hyperthermic fibrinolysis with rt-PA: *in vitro* results," *CardioVascular and Interventional Radiology*, vol. 21, no. 2, pp. 142–145, 1998.

[20] M. Blombäck, S. He, N. Bark, H. N. Wallen, and M. Elg, "Effects on fibrin network porosity of anticoagulants with different modes of action and reversal by activated coagulation factor concentrate," *The British Journal of Haematology*, vol. 152, no. 6, pp. 758–765, 2011.

28

The Bone Marrow Microenvironment as Niche Retreats for Hematopoietic and Leukemic Stem Cells

Felix Nwajei[1,2] and Marina Konopleva[3]

[1] Department of Immunology, The University of Texas MD Anderson Cancer Center, 1515 Holcombe Boulevard, Unit 0902, Houston, TX 77030, USA
[2] Graduate School of Biomedical Sciences, The University of Texas Health Science Center at Houston, 6767 Bertner Avenue, 3rd Floor, Houston, TX 77030, USA
[3] Department of Leukemia, The University of Texas MD Anderson Cancer Center, 1515 Holcombe Boulevard, Unit 428, Houston, TX 77030, USA

Correspondence should be addressed to Marina Konopleva; mkonople@mdanderson.org

Academic Editor: Karl-Anton Kreuzer

Leukemia poses a serious challenge to current therapeutic strategies. This has been attributed to leukemia stem cells (LSCs), which occupy endosteal and sinusoidal niches in the bone marrow similar to those of hematopoietic stem cells (HSCs). The signals from these niches provide a viable setting for the maintenance, survival, and fate specifications of these stem cells. Advancements in genetic engineering and microscopy have enabled us to critically deconstruct and analyze the anatomic and functional characteristics of these niches to reveal a wealth of new knowledge in HSC biology, which is quite ahead of LSC biology. In this paper, we examine the present understanding of the regulatory mechanisms governing HSC niches, with the goals of providing a framework for understanding the mechanisms of LSC regulation and suggesting future strategies for their elimination.

1. Introduction

A dysfunctional stem cell microenvironment, or niche, contributes significantly to disease pathology, particularly in cancer [1]. Characterization of the cells that form this niche and the mechanisms by which they regulate stem cell function is imperative for understanding the pathophysiology of diseases that arise in this setting. Stem cells have the unique ability to self-renew, differentiate into multiple lineages, and withstand stress signals to survive and function [2, 3]. In the bone marrow, hematopoietic stem cells (HSCs) are essential for the production of both lymphoid and myeloid cells, which are necessary for the body's immune integrity, oxygen delivery, blood clotting, waste removal, and a multitude of physiologic processes necessary for survival.

For some time, the intracellular regulatory environment of HSCs has been studied in the isolation of its confines in the bone marrow, with little emphasis on the effects this environment might have on these cells' survival and fate specifications [4]. Testing of the prevailing theory, proposed by Schofield, regarding the underlying indispensable role of the bone marrow structure in engineering hematopoiesis [5] became possible only with the advent and introduction of new *in vivo* technological tools such as intravital multiphoton microscopy (IVM), which is powerful in optical sectioning of deep tissues and providing real-time visualization of cellular interactions [5, 6]. This has led to a radical revolution in the way stem cells are studied in the bone marrow. IVM studies have shown that hematopoiesis depends not only on the cellular biology of HSCs, but also on the microenvironment where they reside, buttressing the "stem cell niche" hypothesis [5].

HSCs reside in two distinct niches in the bone marrow, the endosteal and vascular [7–13]. These niches are complex, encompassing a broad range of bone marrow cells that includes bone lining cells (osteoblasts and osteoclasts), mesenchymal stem cells (MSCs), sinusoidal endothelium and perivascular stromal cells, immune cells, and several others that play different roles in HSC regulation [14]. In the context of the "seed and soil" hypothesis, studies in solid organs of nonhuman mammals have shown that MSCs fuel the growth of cancerous cells and contribute to the therapy resistance and metastatic potential of tumors by shielding cancer stem cells [15–18]. However, because of its anatomy, the bone marrow is a more complex system that includes both an endosteal bone surface stem cell microenvironment and a vascular niche.

The biology of HSCs shares many similarities with that of leukemia stem cells (LSCs). Despite these similarities, LSCs are able to outcompete HSCs, hijacking the bone marrow microenvironment and subverting it to a relatively more hypoxic state suitable for their survival and proliferation [19–22] (illustrated in Figure 1). Previous review articles from our group and others have critically analyzed the role of the bone marrow microenvironment in acute myeloid leukemia (AML) [23–25]. In this paper, we dissect the biology of HSC niches and the impact of the immune system, oxygenation/hypoxia, and MSCs on the maintenance of HSCs. In this context, we discuss LSC niches, using chronic myeloid leukemia (CML) as a model and providing insight into potential therapeutic strategies.

2. Niche Retreats for HSCs in the Bone Marrow

The bone marrow endosteum and sinusoids are the two predominant niches for HSCs. Prevailing early studies had suggested the bone marrow endosteum as the major HSC niche. This was demonstrated by utilizing hematopoietic progenitor cells stained with nonspecific markers that did not specifically label HSCs. However, *in vivo* studies of HSCs became possible when it was discovered that a unique array of surface adhesion markers, the signaling lymphocyte activation molecule (SLAM) family receptors, comprising $CD150^+CD244^-CD48^-$, could be used to select and purify HSCs with great specificity [10]. With this capability, most HSCs were shown to reside adjacent to sinusoidal endothelium in the spleen and bone marrow, while a few were observed to show preference for the bone marrow endosteum, as shown in Figure 1. Therefore, two specialized niches in the bone marrow support HSCs. Elucidating the functions of these two niches is crucial to the understanding of the behavior of HSCs and to exploiting this knowledge for clinical applications.

2.1. Endosteal HSC Niche. The endosteum is the inner surface of the bone marrow cavity, made up of both cortical and trabecular bone types, where hematopoiesis occurs actively. This surface is lined by bone cells such as osteoblasts and osteoclasts. Osteoblasts are progenitor bone-forming cells that work in tandem with osteoclasts in the process of osteogenesis [26]. They are transient cells that actively provide mineralization during bone development and replace lost bone tissues in adults. IVM revealed the homing of fluorescently labeled HSCs to the bone marrow endosteum, suggesting a preference for this anatomical site for their survival and maintenance [14]. Previous studies have shown direct associations between osteoblasts and HSCs. For instance, in a fascinating study conducted by Chan and

colleagues, the knockdown of osterix, an osteoblast-specific transcription factor, essential for endochondral ossification, led to impairment of bone formation and the absence of the HSC niche at an ectopic kidney site [27]. Again, HSC number was decreased by conditionally depleting osteoblasts in transgenic mice [28]. However, an expansion in the osteoblast number requires other factors to mediate a proportionate increase in the HSC pool [29]. Some of these factors can be expressed by osteoblasts *in vitro*, including several cytokines, chemokines, and adhesion molecules, such as CXCL12, angiopoietin-1, stem cell factor (SCF), and thrombopoietin, to maintain HSCs. In the process of validating some of these *in vivo*, in conditional knockout mice, Ding and colleagues demonstrated that conditional deletion of SCF from osteoblasts does not affect HSC number, whereas its deletion from endothelial and leptin receptor- (lepr-) expressing perivascular stromal cells significantly reduces HSC number [9]. This suggests that the regulation of HSCs in their niche is very cell specific, or rather niche specific. The HSCs that associate with osteoblasts are quiescent in nature, giving them the ability to survive and contribute to hematopoiesis over a long period of time [30–33].

Osteoclasts are bone-resorbing cells that coordinate with osteoblasts in bone formation [26]. They are less well characterized than osteoblasts in the context of HSC niche formation and maintenance. Nevertheless, new findings are beginning to emerge on the role of osteoclasts in the process of hematopoiesis. Osteoblast expansion had been observed to cause a proportionate increase in HSC number [8, 13]. Lymperi and colleagues demonstrated, however, that HSC number did not increase on administration of strontium, an element with the dual effects of osteoblast expansion and osteoclast depletion [34]. They hypothesized that this observation could be explained by the reduction in osteoclast number and activity. In line with this, they showed that bisphosphonates inhibit osteoclasts in mice and that this inhibition severely depresses HSCs and delays hematopoietic recovery [35]. More recently, osteoclast impairment reduced osteoblast differentiation and HSC localization in the oc/oc mouse model, in which endochondral ossification is impaired because of osteoclast deficiency [28]. These findings reveal a greater complexity of hematopoiesis regulation than was previously known; more studies are needed to clarify how osteoclastic involvement in this process connects to the better understood osteoblast involvement.

2.2. Immune Privilege. Regardless of the bone marrow's role in the production of immune cells, which maintain the immune integrity of the body, there is limited data on the activity of immune cells in the HSC microenvironment in the bone marrow. An IVM study suggested that regulatory T cells (Tregs) contribute to the formation of a localized zone and relative sanctuary for hematopoietic stem/progenitor cells (HSPCs), which provides a safe environment for HSPC maintenance and survival from immune attacks [14]. In that study, HSPCs from allogeneic donor mice survived as long as 30 days in nonirradiated immunocompetent mice, similar to the survival of syngeneic HSPCs. IVM revealed

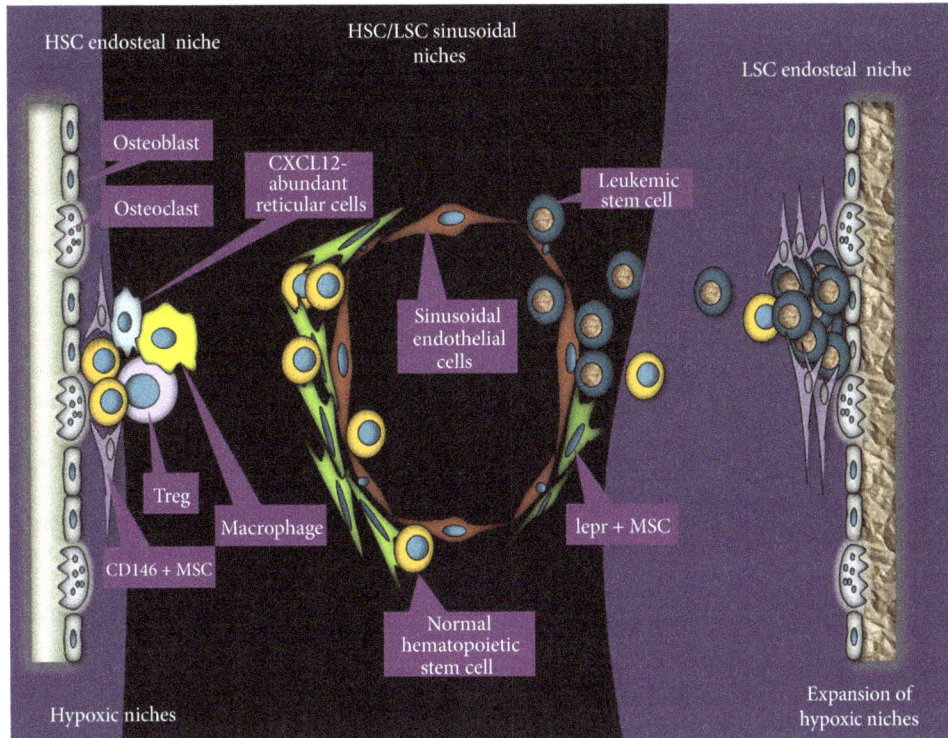

FIGURE 1: Organization of normal hematopoietic stem cell (HSC) and leukemic stem cell (LSC) niches in the bone marrow. Both HSCs and LSCs establish niches around the bone marrow endosteum and sinusoids. In normal hematopoiesis, the endosteal niche is formed and regulated by osteoblasts, osteoclasts, mesenchymal stromal cells (MSCs), T-regulatory cells (Tregs), and macrophages, while in leukemia, LSCs associate with osteoblasts and mesenchymal stromal cells. HSCs form sinusoidal niches with sinusoidal endothelial cells and leptin receptor- (lepr+-) expressing-perivascular stromal cells. LSCs form sinusoidal niches with sinusoidal endothelial cells. Oxygen gradient decreases from the sinusoids to the endosteum. The normal HSC endosteal niches are hypoxic, while there is an expansion of hypoxic niches in LSC endosteal niches due to LSC proliferation.

that Tregs lodge around the HSPC microenvironment in the bone marrow endosteum and protect them by creating an immune privilege sanctuary akin to those in the testis, eye, and brain as depicted in Figure 1. These HSPCs were lost following depletion of Tregs [14]. In a different study, depletion of macrophages disengaged HSCs from their endosteal niche into the circulation by reducing osteoblast number and cytokines that mediate the adhesion of HSCs to this niche [36, 37]. Our increasing understanding of the role of immune activity in the HSC niche shows great promise for development of novel strategies that will be more effective than the current approaches in harvesting HSCs and in preventing graft-versus-host disease in patients undergoing HSC transplant for a hematologic malignancy.

2.3. Sinusoidal HSC Niche. Bone marrow sinusoids are thin-walled vessels that serve as the medium for communication between the marrow cavity and blood circulation. They are lined by a single layer of endothelium and directly continue from arterioles to venules. A broad range of cells, including adventitial reticular cells, perivascular stromal cells, MSCs, and neurons, associate with sinusoids to form a niche that can sustain and regulate HSCs. Identification of HSCs in this niche (by the SLAM family receptors $CD150^+CD244^-CD48^-$

[10]) provided a link between the maintenance of HSCs in sinusoidal niches of the liver/spleen and the bone marrow and suggested that the HSC niche is perivascular. The cells that support this niche have been suggested to express a range of cytokines, such as SCF, CXCL12, and alkaline phosphatase, which have been shown to support the maintenance of HSCs *in vitro*.

Uncertainty about which specific sinusoidal or endosteal niche cell is functionally important in producing any of these molecules and sufficient to maintain HSCs led Ding et al. to conduct the study already mentioned in which cre-lox conditional knockout mice were used to delete SCF *in vivo* from osteoblasts, sinusoidal endothelium, perivascular stromal cells, and nestin-positive MSCs [9]. Their results showed that sinusoidal endothelium and lepr-expressing perivascular stromal cells, but not osteoblasts or nestin-cre- or nestin-creER-expressing cells, are directly responsible for the expression of SCF and functionally regulate HSCs in the sinusoidal niche; their deletion resulted in decreased hematopoiesis in the liver, spleen, and bone marrow. Indeed, SCF deletion by genetic knockout in embryos led to lethality due to hematopoietic deficiencies. This pivotal study paved the way for studying the functional specificity of cells that make up HSC niches.

3. HSCs and Hypoxia

HSCs that reside in the vascular niche are short term, actively cycling and replenishing circulating cells by differentiating into hematopoietic cell types [38]. This metabolic state is thought to be due to the sinusoidal HSC niche being oxygen rich relative to the hypoxic endosteal niche (depicted in Figure 1), in which HSCs are mainly quiescent [39–41]. Hypoxia is necessary for the long-term maintenance of HSCs and is regulated by hypoxia-inducible factor (HIF)-1α [42]. The metabolic activity of these long-term HSCs is dependent on glycolysis, which is driven by Meis1 via transcriptional activation of HIF-1α [43]. The same HIF-1α stabilizes endosteal HSCs and maintains them in a state of quiescence, enabling them to withstand stressful conditions. This maintenance and survival of HSCs occurs via HIF regulation of vascular endothelial growth factor alpha (VEGF-α), Cripto/GRP78 signaling, and upregulation of CXCR4 [44, 45].

Osteoblastic cells, whose major role in the endosteal HSC niche has already been described, have been shown to regulate hematopoiesis by expanding the HSC pool and erythroid cells via a heretofore unknown ability to produce erythropoietin, which was previously thought to be produced only in the kidney [46]. This role is mediated by upstream HIF signaling in osteoprogenitors. Thus, HIF-1α is critical for the survival of HSCs.

4. Mesenchymal Stromal Cells

Mesenchymal stromal cells (MSCs) have the ability to differentiate in culture into multilineage precursors of bone, fat, and cartilage [47]. They provide a sustainable framework or scaffold in which the endosteal and sinusoidal HSC niches take root, as shown in Figure 1. Nestin expression identified a subset of MSCs that has been shown to be important in HSC niche formation [48]. These nestin-positive MSCs associate with HSCs and sympathetic nerve fibers. They express genes that maintain HSCs, and their depletion caused a proportionate drop in the HSC pool, suggesting an essential role in HSC niche formation. The interaction between MSCs and HSCs is mediated by N-cadherin [49]. MSCs have been shown to express agrin, a proteoglycan that plays a role at the neuromuscular junction, to enable hematopoietic cell proliferation [50]. Furthermore, MSCs have been shown to express CXCL12/SDF-1 ligand, which is crucial for HSC homing via CXCR4 [51]. This finding has been buttressed by the finding that HSCs are mobilized into the circulation by administration of CXCR4 antagonists [52]. MSCs are also able to form osteoblasts for the endosteum.

Despite the ability of MSCs to differentiate into multilineage cells *in vitro*, recent evidence suggests that the fate of MSCs may be restricted in bone marrow *in vivo*, with an ability to replenish only the osteogenic lineage, such as the osteoblasts that form part of the endosteal niche [53]. Therefore, the survival and maintenance of HSCs is tightly controlled by MSCs that associate with the HSC niche.

5. Chronic Myeloid Leukemia and LSCs

Chronic myeloid leukemia (CML) arises consequently to the reciprocal translocation of chromosomes 9 and 22, t(9:22), leading to expression of the fusion gene *BCR-ABL*. This gene encodes an oncoprotein that expresses a constitutively active tyrosine kinase and generates clonal leukemic cells [54, 55]. CML progresses through three major phases, from chronic phase to accelerated phase to blast crisis [56]. The chronic phase is the most treatment-responsive phase, while the blast crisis is an acute transformation of the disease process in which mature CML cells revert to immature forms that are insensitive to therapy, and can lead rapidly to host death. Identification of the *BCR-ABL* gene has led to specific targeting with tyrosine kinase inhibitor imatinib (Gleevec), which has achieved great success in depleting *BCR-ABL*-positive leukemia cells [57].

Actively cycling leukemia cells are especially vulnerable to imatinib therapy [58]. In contrast, quiescent leukemia cells are resistant to imatinib therapy [59, 60]. They persist in the bone marrow, constituting CML "minimal residual disease" and accounting for relapse or transition to the accelerated or blast crisis phase [61]. Newer tyrosine kinase inhibitors such as nilotinib or dasatinib are effective in eliminating *BCR-ABL* leukemia cells that have acquired additional mutations and keeping them in check. Like imatinib, however, these newer agents are unable to eradicate the quiescent CML cells [62]. Therefore, patients may have to be on chemotherapy for the rest of their life to prevent relapse [63]. Such long-term treatment poses major challenges, including uncomfortable side effects, costs, and noncompliance [64]. Thus, newer strategies that target not only the intrinsic regulatory mechanisms of residual leukemia cells, but also supporting factors that enhance their survival will be necessary for improved therapeutic efficacy and complete eradication of residual CML cells.

Understanding how CML minimal residual disease evades chemotherapy is best discussed in the context of CML stem cells. The CML cells that resist therapy have been shown to exhibit stem cell characteristics and are referred to as leukemia stem cells. LSCs are akin to HSCs in several ways. They can self-renew via wnt/β-catenin and hedgehog signaling, differentiate into different myeloid lineages that account for CML bone marrow pathology, and resist stressful conditions that threaten their survival [65–68].

A major hindrance in studying LSC biology is the lack of a clear method of detecting them in an unaltered bone marrow milieu. However, advancement in the knowledge of LSC biology has been made possible by harvesting leukemia cells from humans or mice, identifying the fraction of LSCs that meet the requirements for stem cell properties and using that fraction for *in vitro* and transplantation *in vivo* studies, whose purposes are to better understand the behavior of these cells and to apply them in developing new treatment strategies.

6. LSC Bone Marrow Niches

Like normal HSCs, LSCs are thought to harbor specialized microenvironments in the bone marrow cavity, including the endosteal and sinusoidal niches [69, 70] (illustrated in Figure 1). The endosteal niche has received more emphasis in LSC studies because the treatment-resistant cells are thought to lodge here and utilize metabolic programs that sustain their survival. Indeed, human or mouse LSCs have been transplanted *in vivo* and been shown to home to the epiphyseal osteoblastic surface of the endosteum before later dispersion to perivascular niches in vessels near the endosteum and diaphysis [71].

LSCs localize and associate with cells around the endosteum to form discrete niches. Other cell types, including MSCs, that contribute to this niche play a major role in LSC biology. In a pivotal study, Raaijmakers et al. showed that a specific deletion of Dicer1 in mouse osteoprogenitors prevents expression of the *SBDS* gene, a genetic mishap responsible for Scwachman-Bodian-Diamond syndrome, and gives rise to myelodysplasia and AML [72]. This suggests that genetic changes in bone marrow stromal cells that contribute to the endosteal niche are not trivial, because they are able to differentiate into osteolineage progenitors (osteoblast precursors) and initiate a malignant process in the normal HSC endosteal niche.

Importantly, this LSC endosteal microenvironment has been suggested to mirror the HSC hypoxic endosteal niche. In this context, BCR-ABL has been shown to induce, upregulate, and stabilize HIF-1α in CML stem cells [73, 74]. This enables the cells to survive in a quiescent state by undergoing metabolic changes, such as abandoning mitochondrial oxidative phosphorylation and switching to glycolysis [75]. We demonstrated that, unlike the HSCs, LSCs expand hypoxic bone marrow areas (depicted in Figure 1) and become resistant to chemotherapy. However, a hypoxia-activated dinitrobenzamide mustard, PR-104, reduced leukemic cell numbers and significantly extended host survival [76]. Thus, targeting hypoxia niches presents a novel opportunity for killing LSCs.

Using *in vivo* dynamic imaging, Sipkins et al. revealed that LSCs home and form perivascular niches in cranial bone marrow vasculature [70]. HSCs have been shown to use chemokine-mediated mechanisms such as CXCR4/SDF-1 to interact with the vasculature [51]. In fact, the interaction of LSCs with the vasculature was shown by Sipkins et al. to be strongly dependent on their expression of CXCR4 and binding to SDF-1 expressed by vessel endothelium. E-selectin was found to contribute to LSC vessel homing, but to a lesser extent than CXCR4. Interestingly, this site of LSC localization overlapped with the HSPC site. We demonstrated that, besides decimating CML cells, imatinib also upregulates CXCR4 in CML cells, helping them to migrate to shelter sites in bone marrow stroma, where they revert to a G_0-G_1 cell cycle state and survive therapy [77].

This upregulation of CXCR4 by imatinib was mechanistically dissected by showing a redistribution of CXCR4 in the lipid raft fraction of CML cells, where it colocalized with phosphorylated Lyn, suggesting that therapeutic targeting of the CML cell lipid raft is a viable option in preventing chemoresistance [78]. In another study, plerixafor, a CXCR4 antagonist, disengaged CML cells from bone marrow stroma and extracellular matrix and made them vulnerable

to nilotinib therapy [79]. Yamamoto-Sugitani and colleagues showed that bone marrow stroma is capable of upregulating galectin-3, which caused activation of Akt and Erk, allowed accumulation of Mcl-1, and provided resistance to BCR-ABL tyrosine kinase inhibitors by subverting apoptotic induction [80]. Therefore, strategies that target these adhesion molecules may provide an opening for effective therapeutic tyrosine kinase inhibition.

Colmone et al. showed that LSCs adopted hematopoietic progenitor cell niches as "foster homes" and altered the residential dynamics of hematopoietic progenitor cells in a normal bone marrow microenvironment, as shown in Figure 1 [81]. The LSCs expressed stem cell factor, which enabled creation of new microenvironments, termed "malignant niches." The new niches appeared to provide alternative homes for hematopoietic progenitor cells, distorting their migration patterns and dislodging them into the circulation on introduction of granulocyte colony-stimulating factor. Whether these new hematopoietic progenitor cell niches provide cues that may drive these progenitors toward malignancy is yet to be explored. In a recent study, Zhang et al. demonstrated that CML cells produce granulocyte colony-stimulating factor, which reduced expression of CXCL12 in CML bone marrow [82]. This made long-term HSCs present in CML bone marrow exhibit more mobility and reduced growth. However, imatinib reversed this effect and restored long-term HSC growth. Thus, LSCs appear to crosstalk with bone marrow stroma to secure their survival while preventing and outcompeting normal HSCs from benefiting from bone marrow resources.

In support of this crosstalk mechanism, a recent study showed that bone marrow stroma expresses high levels of placental growth factor in CML [83]. Previous studies have shown that BCR-ABL upregulates VEGF and induces angiogenesis to promote its survival [73]. However, Schmidt et al. demonstrated that stroma-derived placental growth factor, which also induces angiogenesis and enhances CML proliferation and metabolism, is independent of BCR-ABL regulation. Inhibition of placental growth factor was effective in prolonging survival of imatinib-sensitive and -resistant CML mice [83], thus identifying another target that is crucial in the survival and growth of CML.

7. Conclusions

We have highlighted the successes and obstacles in combating LSCs, drawing from parallels in HSC studies. Several new targets have been identified within the supporting bone marrow microenvironment; the challenge lies in finding therapies that can specifically address these targets in a combinatorial manner with other therapies targeting intrinsic pathways. More needs to be accomplished to develop novel therapeutic strategies that can completely eradicate residual LSCs. Recent discoveries indicate that elucidation of the molecular mechanisms of leukemia-microenvironment interactions will provide a framework for the identification of novel-targeted therapies aimed at destroying LSC without adversely affecting normal stem cell properties. Finally, it may be worthwhile to determine the role of the immune system in LSC biology, especially as immunotherapy of solid tumors is gaining prominence.

References

[1] Z. Ju, H. Jiang, M. Jaworski et al., "Telomere dysfunction induces environmental alterations limiting hematopoietic stem cell function and engraftment," *Nature Medicine*, vol. 13, no. 6, pp. 742–747, 2007.

[2] H. Lin, "The stem-cell niche theory: lessons from flies," *Nature Reviews Genetics*, vol. 3, no. 12, pp. 931–940, 2002.

[3] M. R. Wallenfang and E. Matunis, "Orienting stem cells," *Science*, vol. 301, no. 5639, pp. 1490–1491, 2003.

[4] A. Spradling, D. Drummond-Barbosa, and T. Kai, "Stem cells find their niche," *Nature*, vol. 414, no. 6859, pp. 98–104, 2001.

[5] R. Schofield, "The stem cell system," *Biomedicine & Pharmacotherapy*, vol. 37, no. 8, pp. 375–380, 1983.

[6] C. Lo Celso, H. E. Fleming, J. W. Wu et al., "Live-animal tracking of individual haematopoietic stem/progenitor cells in their niche," *Nature*, vol. 457, no. 7225, pp. 92–96, 2009.

[7] G. B. Adams, K. T. Chabner, I. R. Alley et al., "Stem cell engraftment at the endosteal niche is specified by the calcium-sensing receptor," *Nature*, vol. 439, no. 7076, pp. 599–603, 2006.

[8] L. M. Calvi, G. B. Adams, K. W. Weibrecht et al., "Osteoblastic cells regulate the haematopoietic stem cell niche," *Nature*, vol. 425, no. 6960, pp. 841–846, 2003.

[9] L. Ding, T. L. Saunders, G. Enikolopov, and S. J. Morrison, "Endothelial and perivascular cells maintain haematopoietic stem cells," *Nature*, vol. 481, no. 7382, pp. 457–462, 2012.

[10] M. J. Kiel, Ö. H. Yilmaz, T. Iwashita, O. H. Yilmaz, C. Terhorst, and S. J. Morrison, "SLAM family receptors distinguish hematopoietic stem and progenitor cells and reveal endothelial niches for stem cells," *Cell*, vol. 121, no. 7, pp. 1109–1121, 2005.

[11] S. K. Nilsson, H. M. Johnston, and J. A. Coverdale, "Spatial localization of transplanted hemopoietic stem cells: inferences for the localization of stem cell niches," *Blood*, vol. 97, no. 8, pp. 2293–2299, 2001.

[12] D. Visnjic, Z. Kalajzic, D. W. Rowe, V. Katavic, J. Lorenzo, and H. L. Aguila, "Hematopoiesis is severely altered in mice with an induced osteoblast deficiency," *Blood*, vol. 103, no. 9, pp. 3258–3264, 2004.

[13] J. Zhang, C. Niu, L. Ye et al., "Identification of the haematopoietic stem cell niche and control of the niche size," *Nature*, vol. 425, no. 6960, pp. 836–841, 2003.

[14] J. Fujisaki, J. Wu, A. L. Carlson et al., "In vivo imaging of T reg cells providing immune privilege to the haematopoietic stem-cell niche," *Nature*, vol. 474, no. 7350, pp. 216–219, 2011.

[15] A. E. Karnoub, A. B. Dash, A. P. Vo et al., "Mesenchymal stem cells within tumour stroma promote breast cancer metastasis," *Nature*, vol. 449, no. 7162, pp. 557–563, 2007.

[16] D. Hanahan and L. M. Coussens, "Accessories to the crime: functions of cells recruited to the tumor microenvironment," *Cancer Cell*, vol. 21, no. 3, pp. 309–322, 2012.

[17] S. B. Coffelt, F. C. Marini, K. Watson et al., "The pro-inflammatory peptide LL-37 promotes ovarian tumor progression through recruitment of multipotent mesenchymal stromal cells," *Proceedings of the National Academy of Sciences of the United States of America*, vol. 106, no. 10, pp. 3806–3811, 2009.

[18] E. Cukierman and D. Bassi, "The mesenchymal tumor microenvironment: a drug resistant niche," *Cell Adhesion & Migration*, vol. 6, no. 3, pp. 285–296, 2012.

[19] E. Passegué, E. F. Wagner, and I. L. Weissman, "JunB deficiency leads to a myeloproliferative disorder arising from hematopoietic stem cells," *Cell*, vol. 119, no. 3, pp. 431–443, 2004.

[20] J. Lessard and G. Sauvageau, "Bmi-1 determines the proliferative capacity of normal and leukaemic stem cells," *Nature*, vol. 423, no. 6937, pp. 255–260, 2003.

[21] I. K. Park, D. Qian, M. Kiel et al., "Bmi-1 is required for maintenance of adult self-renewing haematopoietic stem cells," *Nature*, vol. 423, no. 6937, pp. 302–305, 2003.

[22] Y. Kato, A. Iwama, Y. Tadokoro et al., "Selective activation of STAT5 unveils its role in stem cell self-renewal in normal and leukemic hematopoiesis," *Journal of Experimental Medicine*, vol. 202, no. 1, pp. 169–179, 2005.

[23] Y. Shiozawa, A. M. Havens, K. J. Pienta, and R. S. Taichman, "The bone marrow niche: habitat to hematopoietic and mesenchymal stem cells, and unwitting host to molecular parasites," *Leukemia*, vol. 22, no. 5, pp. 941–950, 2008.

[24] S. W. Lane, D. T. Scadden, and D. G. Gilliland, "The leukemic stem cell niche: current concepts and therapeutic opportunities," *Blood*, vol. 114, no. 6, pp. 1150–1157, 2009.

[25] M. Y. Konopleva and C. T. Jordan, "Leukemia stem cells and microenvironment: biology and therapeutic targeting," *Journal of Clinical Oncology*, vol. 29, no. 5, pp. 591–599, 2011.

[26] H. C. Schröder, X. H. Wang, M. Wiens et al., "Silicate modulates the cross-talk between osteoblasts (SaOS-2) and osteoclasts (RAW 264.7 cells): inhibition of osteoclast growth and differentiation," *Journal of Cellular Biochemistry*, vol. 113, no. 10, pp. 3197–3206, 2012.

[27] C. K. F. Chan, C. C. Chen, C. A. Luppen et al., "Endochondral ossification is required for haematopoietic stem-cell niche formation," *Nature*, vol. 457, no. 7228, pp. 490–494, 2009.

[28] A. Mansour, G. Abou-Ezzi, E. Sitnicka, S. E. Jacobsen, A. Wakkach, and C. Blin-Wakkach, "Osteoclasts promote the formation of hematopoietic stem cell niches in the bone marrow," *Journal of Experimental Medicine*, vol. 209, no. 3, pp. 537–549, 2012.

[29] L. M. Calvi, O. Bromberg, Y. Rhee et al., "Osteoblastic expansion induced by parathyroid hormone receptor signaling in murine osteocytes is not sufficient to increase hematopoietic stem cells," *Blood*, vol. 119, no. 11, pp. 2489–2499, 2012.

[30] K. Kataoka, T. Sato, A. Yoshimi et al., "Evi1 is essential for hematopoietic stem cell self-renewal, and its expression marks hematopoietic cells with long-term multilineage repopulating activity," *Journal of Experimental Medicine*, vol. 208, no. 12, pp. 2403–2416, 2011.

[31] A. Mullally, L. Poveromo, R. K. Schneider, F. Al-Shahrour, S. W. Lane, and B. L. Ebert, "Distinct roles for long-term hematopoietic stem cells and erythroid precursor cells in a murine model of Jak2V617F-mediated polycythemia vera," *Blood*, vol. 120, no. 1, pp. 166–172, 2012.

[32] F. Notta, S. Doulatov, E. Laurenti, A. Poeppl, I. Jurisica, and J. E. Dick, "Isolation of single human hematopoietic stem cells capable of long-term multilineage engraftment," *Science*, vol. 333, no. 6039, pp. 218–221, 2011.

[33] S. J. Morrison and A. C. Spradling, "Stem cells and niches: mechanisms that promote stem cell maintenance throughout life," *Cell*, vol. 132, no. 4, pp. 598–611, 2008.

[34] S. Lymperi, N. Horwood, S. Marley, M. Y. Gordon, A. P. Cope, and F. Dazzi, "Strontium can increase some osteoblasts without increasing hematopoietic stem cells," *Blood*, vol. 111, no. 3, pp. 1173–1181, 2008.

[35] S. Lymperi, A. Ersek, F. Ferraro, F. Dazzi, and N. J. Horwood, "Inhibition of osteoclast function reduces hematopoietic stem cell numbers in vivo," *Blood*, vol. 117, no. 5, pp. 1540–1549, 2011.

[36] I. G. Winkler, N. A. Sims, A. R. Pettit et al., "Bone marrow macrophages maintain hematopoietic stem cell (HSC) niches and their depletion mobilizes HSCs," *Blood*, vol. 116, no. 23, pp. 4815–4828, 2010.

[37] A. Chow, D. Lucas, A. Hidalgo et al., "Bone marrow CD169$^+$ macrophages promote the retention of hematopoietic stem and progenitor cells in the mesenchymal stem cell niche," *The Journal of Experimental Medicine*, vol. 208, no. 2, pp. 261–271, 2011.

[38] I. G. Winkler, V. Barbier, R. Wadley, A. C. W. Zannettino, S. Williams, and J. P. Lévesque, "Positioning of bone marrow hematopoietic and stromal cells relative to blood flow in vivo: serially reconstituting hematopoietic stem cells reside in distinct nonperfused niches," *Blood*, vol. 116, no. 3, pp. 375–385, 2010.

[39] D. C. Chow, L. A. Wenning, W. M. Miller, and E. T. Papoutsakis, "Modeling pO$_2$ distributions in the bone marrow hematopoietic compartment. II. Modified Kroghian models," *Biophysical Journal*, vol. 81, no. 2, pp. 685–696, 2001.

[40] D. C. Chow, L. A. Wenning, W. M. Miller, and E. T. Papoutsakis, "Modeling pO$_2$ distributions in the bone marrow hematopoietic compartment. I. Krogh's model," *Biophysical Journal*, vol. 81, no. 2, pp. 675–684, 2001.

[41] K. Parmar, P. Mauch, J. A. Vergilio, R. Sackstein, and J. D. Down, "Distribution of hematopoietic stem cells in the bone marrow according to regional hypoxia," *Proceedings of the National Academy of Sciences of the United States of America*, vol. 104, no. 13, pp. 5431–5436, 2007.

[42] G. L. Semenza, "Oxygen-dependent regulation of mitochondrial respiration by hypoxia-inducible factor 1," *Biochemical Journal*, vol. 405, no. 1, pp. 1–9, 2007.

[43] T. Simsek, F. Kocabas, J. Zheng et al., "The distinct metabolic profile of hematopoietic stem cells reflects their location in a hypoxic niche," *Cell Stem Cell*, vol. 7, no. 3, pp. 380–390, 2010.

[44] K. Miharada, G. Karlsson, M. Rehn, E. Rörby, K. Siva, and S. Karlsson, "Cripto regulates hematopoietic stem cells as a hypoxic-niche-related factor through cell surface receptor GRP78," *Cell Stem Cell*, vol. 9, no. 4, pp. 330–344, 2011.

[45] M. Rehn, A. Olsson, K. Reckzeh, E. Diffner, P. Carmeliet, and G. Landberg, "Hypoxic induction of vascular endothelial growth factor regulates murine hematopoietic stem cell function in the low-oxygenic niche," *Blood*, vol. 118, no. 6, pp. 1534–1543, 2011.

[46] E. B. Rankin, C. Wu, R. Khatri et al., "The HIF signaling pathway in osteoblasts directly modulates erythropoiesis through the production of EPO," *Cell*, vol. 149, no. 1, pp. 63–74, 2012.

[47] M. Crisan, S. Yap, L. Casteilla et al., "A perivascular origin for mesenchymal stem cells in multiple Human Organs," *Cell Stem Cell*, vol. 3, no. 3, pp. 301–313, 2008.

[48] S. Méndez-Ferrer, T. V. Michurina, F. Ferraro et al., "Mesenchymal and haematopoietic stem cells form a unique bone marrow niche," *Nature*, vol. 466, no. 7308, pp. 829–834, 2010.

[49] F. Wein, L. Pietsch, R. Saffrich et al., "N-Cadherin is expressed on human hematopoietic progenitor cells and mediates interaction with human mesenchymal stromal cells," *Stem Cell Research*, vol. 4, no. 2, pp. 129–139, 2010.

[50] C. Mazzon, A. Anselmo, J. Cibella et al., "The critical role of agrin in the hematopoietic stem cell niche," *Blood*, vol. 118, no. 10, pp. 2733–2742, 2011.

[51] T. Sugiyama, H. Kohara, M. Noda, and T. Nagasawa, "Maintenance of the hematopoietic stem cell pool by CXCL12-CXCR4 chemokine signaling in bone Marrow Stromal Cell Niches," *Immunity*, vol. 25, no. 6, pp. 977–988, 2006.

[52] H. E. Broxmeyer, C. M. Orschell, D. W. Clapp et al., "Rapid mobilization of murine and human hematopoietic stem and progenitor cells with AMD3100, a CXCR4 antagonist," *Journal of Experimental Medicine*, vol. 201, no. 8, pp. 1307–1318, 2005.

[53] D. Park, J. A. Spencer, B. I. Koh et al., "Endogenous bone marrow MSCs are dynamic, fate-restricted participants in bone maintenance and regeneration," *Cell Stem Cell*, vol. 10, no. 3, pp. 259–272, 2012.

[54] J. D. Rowley, "A new consistent chromosomal abnormality in chronic myelogenous leukaemia identified by quinacrine fluorescence and Giemsa staining," *Nature*, vol. 243, no. 5405, pp. 290–293, 1973.

[55] C. L. Sawyers, "Chronic myeloid leukemia," *New England Journal of Medicine*, vol. 340, no. 17, pp. 1330–1340, 1999.

[56] D. Perrotti, C. Jamieson, J. Goldman, and T. Skorski, "Chronic myeloid leukemia: mechanisms of blastic transformation," *Journal of Clinical Investigation*, vol. 120, no. 7, pp. 2254–2264, 2010.

[57] A. Hochhaus, S. G. O'Brien, F. Guilhot et al., "Six-year follow-up of patients receiving imatinib for the first-line treatment of chronic myeloid leukemia," *Leukemia*, vol. 23, no. 6, pp. 1054–1061, 2009.

[58] M. S. Holtz, M. L. Slovak, F. Zhang, C. L. Sawyers, S. J. Forman, and R. Bhatia, "Imatinib mesylate (STI571) inhibits growth of primitive malignant progenitors in chronic myelogenous leukemia through reversal of abnormally increased proliferation," *Blood*, vol. 99, no. 10, pp. 3792–3800, 2002.

[59] A. S. Corbin, A. Agarwal, M. Loriaux, J. Cortes, M. W. Deininger, and B. J. Druker, "Human chronic myeloid leukemia stem cells are insensitive to imatinib despite inhibition of BCR-ABL activity," *Journal of Clinical Investigation*, vol. 121, no. 1, pp. 396–409, 2011.

[60] L. J. Elrick, H. G. Jorgensen, J. C. Mountford, and T. L. Holyoake, "Punish the parent not the progeny," *Blood*, vol. 105, no. 5, pp. 1862–1866, 2005.

[61] S. Chu, T. McDonald, A. Lin et al., "Persistence of leukemia stem cells in chronic myelogenous leukemia patients in prolonged remission with imatinib treatment," *Blood*, vol. 118, no. 20, pp. 5565–5572, 2011.

[62] T. Skorski, "Chronic myeloid leukemia cells refractory/resistant to tyrosine kinase inhibitors are genetically unstable and may cause relapse and malignant progression to the terminal disease state," *Leukemia and Lymphoma*, vol. 52, supplement 1, pp. 23–29, 2011.

[63] F. X. Mahon, D. Réa, J. Guilhot et al., "Discontinuation of imatinib in patients with chronic myeloid leukaemia who have maintained complete molecular remission for at least 2 years: the prospective, multicentre Stop Imatinib (STIM) trial," *The Lancet Oncology*, vol. 11, no. 11, pp. 1029–1035, 2010.

[64] J. Cortes, A. Hochhaus, T. Hughes, and H. Kantarjian, "Front-line and salvage therapies with tyrosine kinase inhibitors and

other treatments in chronic myeloid leukemia," *Journal of Clinical Oncology*, vol. 29, no. 5, pp. 524–531, 2011.

[65] Y. Wang, A. V. Krivtsov, A. U. Sinha et al., "The wnt/β-catenin pathway is required for the development of leukemia stem cells in AML," *Science*, vol. 327, no. 5973, pp. 1650–1653, 2010.

[66] C. Zhao, A. Chen, C. H. Jamieson et al., "Hedgehog signalling is essential for maintenance of cancer stem cells in myeloid leukaemia," *Nature*, vol. 458, no. 7239, pp. 776–779, 2009.

[67] T. Suda and F. Arai, "Wnt signaling in the niche," *Cell*, vol. 132, no. 5, pp. 729–730, 2008.

[68] L. Mandal, J. A. Martinez-Agosto, C. J. Evans, V. Hartenstein, and U. Banerjee, "A Hedgehog- and Antennapedia-dependent niche maintains Drosophila haematopoietic precursors," *Nature*, vol. 446, no. 7133, pp. 320–324, 2007.

[69] F. Ishikawa, S. Yoshida, Y. Saito et al., "Chemotherapy-resistant human AML stem cells home to and engraft within the bone-marrow endosteal region," *Nature Biotechnology*, vol. 25, no. 11, pp. 1315–1321, 2007.

[70] D. A. Sipkins, X. Wei, J. W. Wu et al., "In vivo imaging of specialized bone marrow endothelial microdomains for tumour engraftment," *Nature*, vol. 435, no. 7044, pp. 969–973, 2005.

[71] M. Ninomiya, A. Abe, A. Katsumi et al., "Homing, proliferation and survival sites of human leukemia cells in vivo in immunodeficient mice," *Leukemia*, vol. 21, no. 1, pp. 136–142, 2007.

[72] M. H. G. P. Raaijmakers, S. Mukherjee, S. Guo et al., "Bone progenitor dysfunction induces myelodysplasia and secondary leukaemia," *Nature*, vol. 464, no. 7290, pp. 852–857, 2010.

[73] M. Mayerhofer, P. Valent, W. R. Sperr, J. D. Griffin, and C. Sillaber, "BCR/ABL induces expression of vascular endothelial growth factor and its transcriptional activator, hypoxia inducible factor-1α, through a pathway involving phosphoinositide 3-kinase and the mammalian target of rapamycin," *Blood*, vol. 100, no. 10, pp. 3767–3775, 2002.

[74] H. Zhang, H. Li, H. S. Xi, and S. Li, "HIF1α is required for survival maintenance of chronic myeloid leukemia stem cells," *Blood*, vol. 119, no. 11, pp. 2595–2607, 2012.

[75] F. Zhao, A. Mancuso, T. V. Bui et al., "Imatinib resistance associated with BCR-ABL upregulation is dependent on HIF-1α-induced metabolic reprograming," *Oncogene*, vol. 29, no. 20, pp. 2962–2972, 2010.

[76] J. Benito, Y. Shi, B. Szymanska et al., "Pronounced hypoxia in models of murine and human leukemia: high efficacy of hypoxia-activated prodrug PR-104," *PLoS One*, vol. 6, no. 8, Article ID e23108, 2011.

[77] L. Jin, Y. Tabe, S. Konoplev et al., "CXCR4 up-regulation by imatinib induces chronic myelogenous leukemia (CML) cell migration to bone marrow stroma and promotes survival of quiescent CML cells," *Molecular Cancer Therapeutics*, vol. 7, no. 1, pp. 48–58, 2008.

[78] Y. Tabe, L. Jin, K. Iwabuchi et al., "Role of stromal microenvironment in nonpharmacological resistance of CML to imatinib through Lyn/CXCR4 interactions in lipid rafts," *Leukemia*, vol. 26, no. 5, pp. 883–892, 2012.

[79] E. Weisberg, A. K. Azab, P. W. Manley et al., "Inhibition of CXCR4 in CML cells disrupts their interaction with the bone marrow microenvironment and sensitizes them to nilotinib," *Leukemia*, vol. 26, no. 5, pp. 985–990, 2012.

[80] M. Yamamoto-Sugitani, J. Kuroda, E. Ashihara et al., "Galectin-3 (Gal-3) induced by leukemia microenvironment promotes drug resistance and bone marrow lodgment in chronic myelogenous leukemia," *Proceedings of the National Academy of Sciences of the United States of America*, vol. 108, no. 42, pp. 17468–17473, 2011.

[81] A. Colmone, M. Amorim, A. L. Pontier, S. Wang, E. Jablonski, and D. A. Sipkins, "Leukemic cells create bone marrow niches that disrupt the behavior of normal hematopoietic progenitor cells," *Science*, vol. 322, no. 5909, pp. 1861–1865, 2008.

[82] B. Zhang, Y. W. Ho, Q. Huang et al., "Altered microenvironmental regulation of leukemic and normal stem cells in chronic myelogenous leukemia," *Cancer Cell*, vol. 21, no. 4, pp. 577–592, 2012.

[83] T. Schmidt, B. K. Masouleh, S. Loges et al., "Loss or inhibition of stromal-derived PlGF prolongs survival of mice with imatinib-resistant Bcr-Abl1$^+$ leukemia," *Cancer Cell*, vol. 19, no. 6, pp. 740–753, 2011.

29

Dendritic Cell Development:
A Choose-Your-Own-Adventure Story

Amanda J. Moore[1,2] **and Michele K. Anderson**[1,2]

[1] *Division of Biological Sciences, Sunnybrook Research Institute, 2075 Bayview Avenue, Toronto, ON, Canada M4N 3M5*
[2] *Department of Immunology, University of Toronto, Toronto, ON, Canada M5S 1A8*

Correspondence should be addressed to Michele K. Anderson; manderso@sri.utoronto.ca

Academic Editor: Sheila Dias

Dendritic cells (DCs) are essential components of the immune system and contribute to immune responses by activating or tolerizing T cells. DCs comprise a heterogeneous mixture of subsets that are located throughout the body and possess distinct and specialized functions. Although numerous defined precursors from the bone marrow and spleen have been identified, emerging data in the field suggests many alternative routes of DC differentiation from precursors with multilineage potential. Here, we discuss how the combinatorial expression of transcription factors can promote one DC lineage over another as well as the integration of cytokine signaling in this process.

1. Introduction

Dendritic cells (DCs) are professional antigen-presenting cells that bridge the gap between the innate and adaptive immune systems by acting as sentinels throughout the body to capture, process, and present antigen to T cells. Their ability to distinguish between self and nonself molecules allows them to deliver tolerizing or activating signals to T cells accordingly. Scientific exploration of DCs has become increasingly complex with the recognition that DCs exist as a heterogenous mixture of populations. Named for their cellular size and morphology [1], DCs all share the ability to activate naïve T cells but exhibit unique functions within each subset. These DC populations have primarily been defined by their combinatorial cell surface marker expression, but they also differ in their developmental origins, transcriptional regulation, patterns of migration or residence, and anatomical and microenvironmental localization. DCs can be broadly classified as two major subsets: the inflammatory or infection-derived DCs, which develop from monocytes in response to stimulation, and the steady-state DCs, which are present at all times. The DCs present under steady state conditions include CD8$^+$ and CD8$^-$ conventional DCs

(cDCs), plasmacytoid DCs (pDCs), and migratory CD103$^+$ CD11b$^-$ DCs, CD103$^-$ CD11b$^+$ DCs, and Langerhans cells (LCs) (Table 1). The CD8$^-$ cDCs can be further classified as CD4$^+$ or CD4$^-$ DCs, which both express high levels of CD11b [2]. However, the majority of gene perturbation analyses that have examined CD8$^+$ cDCs, CD8$^-$ cDC, and pDCs as well as global gene analysis have shown mostly congruent gene expression between the CD4$^+$ and CD4$^-$ subsets [3]; thus, we will classify CD4$^+$ and CD4$^-$ DCs as CD8$^-$ DCs for simplicity.

The cDCs and pDCs are found throughout the primary and secondary lymphoid organs. In the spleen and lymph nodes (LNs), the CD8$^-$ cDCs constitute the majority of the resident DCs, whereas the CD8$^+$ cDCs are the predominant DC subset within the thymus. Initially termed interferon-producing cells (IPCs) in humans, pDCs are known for their hallmark function of detecting virus by TLR7 or TLR9 and producing vast amounts of type I interferons [4, 5]. CD8$^+$ cDCs are specialized for efficient cross-presentation of antigen to CD8$^+$ T cells, resulting in heightened viral and antitumor responses [6, 7]. Since cross-presentation has been associated with more efficient negative selection, it is likely that the higher proportion of CD8$^+$ cDCs within the thymus can be attributed to this unique function [8, 9]. Although

TABLE 1: Surface molecule expression of steady state dendritic cell subsets. Phenotype of lymphoid-resident CD8+ cDC, CD8− cDC, pDC, nonlymphoid tissue-resident CD11b+, CD103+, CD103+ CD11b+ DCs, and Langerhans cells. CD103+ CD11b+ DCs only exist in the lamina propria of the intestine. Transcription factors important for each DC lineage and known human DC equivalent subsets are listed. *Thymic CD8+ cDCs express Langerin. #CD103+ DCs in the peyer's patches also express CD8α. Abbreviations, CD numeration, and alternate names: DEC-205 (CD205), B220 (CD45R), PDCA-1 (plasmacytoid DC Ag-1; CD317; Bst2), Siglec H (Sialic acid-binding immunoglobulin-like lectin H), Langerin (CD207), CD141 (BDCA-3), CD1c (BDCA-1), and CD303 (BDCA-2).

	CD11c	MHC class II	CD8α	CD11b	CD4	DEC-205	B220	PDCA-1	Siglec-H	CD103	Langerin	Master regulators	Minor regulators	Human DC subset equivalent
CD8+ cDC	+	+	+	−	−	+	−	−	−	−	−*	PU.1, Id2, Batf3, E4BP4, IRF-8, Flt3	Gfi1, IRF-1, IRF-2	CD11c^lo, CD141+, CD11b−, XCR1+
CD8− cDC	+	+	−	+	+/−	−	−	−	−	−	−	PU.1, RelB, Flt3	Gfi1, Id2, IRF-1, IRF-4, IRF-7	CD11c^hi, CD11b+, CD1c+
pDC	int	int	−	−	−	+	+	+	+	−	−	E2-2, PU.1, Ikaros, IRF-8, Flt3	Spi-B, Gfi1, IRF-2	CD123+, CD303+, CD304+
CD103+	+	+	−#	−	−	+	−	−	−	+	+	Id2, Batf3, IRF-8		
CD11b+	+	+	−	+	−	+/−	−	−	−	−	−			
CD103+	+	+	−	+	−	+	−	−	−	+	−			
CD11b+	+	+	−	+	−	+	−	−	−	−	−			
Langerhans cells	int	+	−	+	−	+	−	−	−	−	+	Id2, M-CSFR	IRF-8	

CD1c = BDCA-1.
CD303 = BDCA-2.
CD141 = BDCA-3.
CD103+ are CD8+ in the peyer's patches.
CD11b+ only in lamina propria.

thymic DCs (tDCs) can participate in negative selection [10], a definitive requirement for tDCs in this process is still debated [11]. CD8$^-$ cDCs are distinguished by their superior phagocytic abilities which lead to enhanced presentation of antigen to MHC class II-restricted CD4$^+$ T cells [12, 13].

In nonlymphoid organs, the roles of CD103$^+$ CD11b$^-$ DCs and CD103$^-$ CD11b$^+$ DCs mirror the specialized functions of CD8$^+$ and CD8$^-$ cDCs, respectively. A unique CD103$^+$ CD11b$^+$ subset also exists, but only in the lamina propria of the intestine [14]. There are also CD103$^+$ (dermal DCs) and CD11b$^+$ subsets, which monitor peripheral locations and migrate to draining LNs upon activation. The epithelium-resident LCs are another type of DC that responds to activation by migrating to skin-draining LNs where they present antigen to T cells [15, 16].

Human DC subsets within the peripheral blood, where pDCs were first discovered, have been extensively studied, but due to practical limitations lymphoid and nonlymphoid tissue-resident DCs are less well understood. However, the vast amounts of data on murine DC subsets have enabled the identification of equivalent human DC populations by correlative functional characterization, gene profiling, and by the identification of genetic mutations resulting in human DC deficiency (reviewed in [17]) [18–22]. A summary of the designations of murine DC subsets as defined by cell surface molecules and the transcriptional regulators involved in the development of each subset is shown in Table 1. The equivalent human populations of cDCs and pDCs are also summarized.

Although DC classification has historically been defined by cell surface markers, it is important to note that molecules, such as B220, CD8α, and DEC-205, can be upregulated or downregulated following activation or stimulus. DC researchers remain in a quandary, as it is difficult to ascertain whether the identification of DC subsets by surface marker expression relates to discrete lineages or specific physiological states due to the plasticity of DC populations. For example, cells displaying a pDC phenotype can upregulate CD8α, downregulate B220, and manifest a classical DC morphology upon stimulation with CpG [23, 24]. Similarly, although Langerin is historically a marker for skin-resident or migratory DCs, it was recently shown that the majority of CD8$^+$ tDCs also express Langerin [25]. In order to truly understand the capabilities of these DC subsets, we will need to move beyond cell surface markers and define the transcriptional regulators that govern their genetic programming. Here, we will focus on the origins and development of CD8$^+$ cDCs, CD8$^-$ cDCs, and pDCs, with an emphasis on the transcription factors that control lineage choice and differentiation of these DC subsets.

2. Dendritic Cell Progenitors

2.1. Laying the Groundwork. Although considerable advances have been made in identifying upstream DC precursors in the past decade, much is still unknown. An understanding of the cellular origins of peripheral lymphoid tissue-resident DCs largely began with the advent of the identification of common lymphoid progenitors (CLPs; Lin$^-$ IL-7R$^+$ Thy-1$^-$ Sca-1^{int} c-Kit^{int}) and common myeloid progenitors (CMPs; Lin$^-$ IL-7Rα^- Sca-1$^-$ c-Kit$^+$ FcRγRII/III^{lo} CD34$^+$) at the turn of the century [36, 37]. Following intravenous injections into lethally irradiated recipients, CLPs, CMPs, and granulocyte/macrophage precursors (GMPs; Sca-1$^-$ c-Kit$^+$ IL-7Ra$^-$ FcRγRII/III$^+$ CD34$^+$) all gave rise to splenic DCs [38–40]. Interestingly, CLPs produced greater absolute numbers of DCs and a higher proportion of CD8$^+$ DCs in the spleen than CMPs [40]. Moreover, Flt3, a cytokine receptor required for peripheral lymphoid tissue DC development [41], was expressed at higher levels on CLPs relative to CMPs [42]. Fate-mapping mice, in which cells expressing IL-7R were irreversibly labeled with YFP, revealed that only one tenth of thymic and splenic CD8$^+$ and CD8$^-$ cDCs had arisen from IL-7R$^+$ precursors, suggesting that most of these cells did not arise from CLPs [43]. In contrast, the majority of thymic and splenic pDCs were YFP$^+$. However, these pDCs also expressed *IL7r* mRNA, thereby confounding the determination of whether they had arisen from CLPs. Nevertheless, the reconstitution of irradiated recipients with each of these precursors did not collectively regenerate the same numbers of DCs observed following injection of whole bone marrow, foreshadowing the presence of unidentified DC precursor(s) [40].

2.2. The Common DC Precursor with Conventional and Plasmacytoid DC Potential. The identification of a more defined DC precursor was inspired by observations that Flt3 ligand (Flt3L), GM-CSF, and M-CSF could support DC development *in vitro*. Subsequent pursuits of DC lineage precursors identified a bipotent macrophage/DC precursor (MDP; Lin$^-$ c-Kit^{hi} CD115$^+$ CX$_3$CR1$^+$ Flt3$^+$) [44] that gives rise to a common DC precursor (CDP; Lin$^-$ c-Kit^{lo} CD115$^+$ CX$_3$CR1$^+$ Flt3$^+$) [45–47] in which macrophage lineage potential is lost. The CDP can then diverge into pre-cDCs (Lin$^-$ CD11c$^+$ MHC class II$^-$ SIRPα^{int} Flt3$^+$) or a yet unidentified precursor leading to pDCs [47]. All cDC populations in lymphoid organs and tissue-resident CD103$^+$ DCs can arise from pre-cDCs [47, 48]. However, this pathway is not mutually exclusive from the CLP or CMP pathways nor does it eliminate other alternative pathways of DC differentiation. Instead, it appears that there are different developmental routes that converge to give rise to the same functional subsets of DCs.

2.3. Development of Thymic Dendritic Cells. There has been much controversy over the origins of the three major subsets of tDCs (CD8$^+$ cDCs, CD8$^-$ cDCs, and pDCs) and whether they develop within the thymus [25, 35, 43, 49–51]. There are three major developmental routes by which these tDCs could arise. First, they could develop extrathymically and migrate in as mature DCs. Secondly, they could arrive in the thymus as committed DC precursors and differentiate within the thymus. Thirdly, they could arise within the thymus from an uncommitted precursor that shares T cell and DC potential. Development into tDCs has been proposed to occur outside of the thymus for some subsets, namely, CD8$^-$ cDCs, and pDCs [52, 53]. In fact, bone marrow-derived MDP, CDP, and pre-DC populations can give rise to tDCs following intravenous injections [25]. In addition, a model of CCR9-dependent pDC migration to the thymus suggests that peripheral self-antigen can be transported from the periphery to the thymus by pDCs and cDCs, in the absence of activation [54]. However, other studies have suggested that intrathymic DC development occurs, as well [25, 35]. The environment of the thymus, which is the primary site of T cell development, provides a vastly different set of microenvironmental cues for DC development than those available to other peripheral tissue-resident DC precursors (reviewed in [55]) [56]. Fortunately, the ongoing search for thymic seeding progenitors has resulted in the progressive elucidation of putative tDCs precursors as well. The populations that are thought to seed the thymus include multipotent progenitors (MPPs), lymphoid-primed multipotent progenitors (LMPPs), CLPs, and circulating T cell progenitors (CTPs) [57]. Early studies showed that the majority of thymic and splenic pDCs had undergone IgH gene D-J rearrangements, and that they expressed CD3 and preTα, which provided evidence for DC development from CLPs or a similar precursor [58]. A minority population of CD8$^+$ tDCs also exhibited these characteristics, which would coincide with the low percentage of CD8$^+$ tDCs labeled in the IL-7R fate-mapping experiments [59]. Overall, it appears that cDCs do not arise from a CLP or CLP-similar precursor, whereas pDCs likely do.

2.4. Intrathymic Precursors of tDCs. The ability of some T cell precursors to develop into DCs when removed from the thymus has suggested that these cells could be physiological precursors of tDCs. T cell precursors within the thymus are characterized as double negative (DN; CD8$^-$ CD4$^-$) and develop from DN1 (CD44$^+$ CD25$^-$) into DN2a cells (c-Kit^{hi} DN44$^+$ CD25$^+$), which is the point of T cell specification. DN2a cells retain the ability to differentiate *in vitro* into natural killer (NK) cells and DCs [60, 61]. Next, DN2a cells give rise to T-lineage committed DN2b cells (c-Kit$^+$ CD44$^+$ CD25$^+$) and eventually differentiate to DN3 cells (c-Kit$^-$ CD44$^-$ CD25$^+$), which must receive survival signals through the pre-T cell receptor to progress further through T cell development. The DN1 cells can be further subdivided into early T cell progenitors (ETPs; DN1a/b; c-Kit^{hi} CD24$^{-/lo}$), DN1c (cKit^{int} CD24^{hi}), DN1d (cKit$^-$ CD24$^+$), and DN1e (cKit$^-$ CD24$^-$) subsets based on their surface expression of c-Kit and CD24 [62]. ETPs are the canonical T cell precursors and contain some NK cell potential, whereas DN1c and DN1d cells exhibit B cell potential. Little is known about the lineage potential of DN1e cells.

Many studies have provided evidence that T cell precursors have DC [63] and myeloid [64, 65] lineage potential. During specification, T-lineage genes are upregulated, and genes influencing development towards other lineages are downregulated. Interestingly, the minimal myeloid potential present in DN1 subsets is lost in DN2 cells, whereas DC potential is still present in DN2 cells which have not yet upregulated the T cell specific gene, *lck* [63]. Moreover, numerous *in vivo* studies have shown that intrathymic

precursors, prior to T cell commitment at the β-selection checkpoint, can develop into tDCs [35, 49, 66].

Additional *in vivo* studies have supported the ability of distinct T cell precursors to give rise to DCs. Early studies characterized a "low-CD4 precursor" (CD4^{lo} CD8$^-$ CD3$^-$ CD24^{hi}), which contained what are now referred to as DN1c and DN1d cells, that could give rise to CD8$^+$ tDCs following intravenous injections into irradiated mice [49]. One progenitor within the thymus expressing CD24, c-Kit, CD11c, and Langerin can arise from MDPs, CDPs, and pre-DCs from the bone marrow and spleen and has been shown to give rise to Langerin$^+$ CD8$^+$ tDCs [25]. Studies by our laboratory have shown that ETP, DN1d, and DN1e subsets can all give rise to tDCs *in vivo*, which localize to the medulla in nonirradiated mice [35]. Unquestionably, there are many developmental routes by which DCs can arise, depending on a variety of factors such as their localization and surrounding stimuli, which in turn influences the transcriptional regulators that orchestrate cellular fate.

3. Context-Dependent Transcriptional Regulators of Lymphoid Tissue-Resident DCs

Despite the differences in the location of DC development, specific subsets share transcriptional regulatory programs, which indicates an intrinsic requirement for certain transcription factors for the DC lineage [67]. Interestingly, to date there is no known single transcription factor that is universally required for the development of all DCs, analogous to the requirement of Pax-5 for the development of all B cells [68], highlighting the versatility and plasticity of DC development and homeostasis.

3.1. The Multitasking Transcriptional Regulators:
    Ets Transcription Factors

3.1.1. PU.1. The two Ets transcription factor family members PU.1 and Spi-B have been intensely studied in myeloid and lymphoid cells owing to their expression in many progenitors and their roles in multiple lineages. PU.1 is expressed during the earliest stages of hematopoiesis onwards in CMP, CLP, CDP, preDC, DN1 cells, cDCs, and pDCs [37, 69, 70]. Early studies of the functions of PU.1 in DCs were conflicting due to the generation of two independent lines of PU.1 knockout mice, one of which was embryonic lethal, whereas the other one allowed survival until about two weeks after birth [71, 72]. Neither PU.1-deficient mouse strain, however, enabled analysis of the adult splenic and thymic DC compartments which are established 3–5 weeks after birth [73]. PU.1 (*Spi-1*)-deficient E14.5 and E16.5 embryos exhibited a lack of CD11c$^+$ CD8$^-$ tDCs, while CD11c$^+$ CD8$^+$ tDCs remained intact in one study [71]. However, another study demonstrated a reduction in DEC-205$^+$ tDCs (equivalent to CD8$^+$ tDCs; see Table 1) in 10- to 12-day old mice [72]. Subsequently, a polyI:C inducible PU.1-knockout clarified the requirement for PU.1 in splenic and thymic cDC and pDC populations and in the generation of these subsets from CDPs [74]. However, the involvement of

PU.1 in other DC subsets and the generation of upstream precursors remain unclear. Interestingly, the context-dependent roles of PU.1 are emphasized by its ability to upregulate Flt3 in DCs [74], while exhibiting an equally important role in upregulating IL-7R in B cells [75]. Moreover, the dose of PU.1 is critical for lineage determination, as highlighted by a higher level of PU.1 favouring macrophage development over B cell and granulocyte development [76, 77]. PU.1 also plays a role in the macrophage/DC lineage decision, in part by binding to and inhibiting Mafb, which is a bZip transcription factor that promotes macrophage and monocyte development [78].

The roles of PU.1 in early thymocyte development are complex. PU.1 inhibits T cell development from DN2 cells [79] but is required for the generation of T cell precursors [80]. Interestingly, there is an accumulation of CD24^{hi} cKit^{int} Sca1$^-$ DN1 precursors, corresponding phenotypically to the DN1c population, in PU.1$^{-/-}$ animals [80], suggesting that it is needed for the developmental progression of DN1c cells to CD8$^+$ tDCs. PU.1 induces the expression of many DC-promoting factors, such as M-CSFR, GM-CSFR, and CD11b [26, 27, 81, 82]. Thus, the decrease of PU.1 during early T cell development correlates with the loss of DC potential and likely results in the downregulation of a DC-specific gene program. The complexity of the functions of PU.1 in the intrathymic T/DC lineage choice is highlighted by a recent study, which amalgamated global transcript analysis with chromatin structure data over the early stages of T cell development. These results revealed, surprisingly, that during the stages of PU.1 expression from DN1 to DN2b cells, there were just as many targets of PU.1 in T cells as there were in B cells and macrophages. Importantly, however, these targets were unique and corresponded to genes active in early T cell development [83]. Therefore, PU.1 plays very important but divergent roles in DC and T cell development, by coordinating the expression of target genes required for each lineage. The ability of PU.1 to direct T-lineage gene expression is likely due to collaboration with Notch signals [84]. Other factors that may collaborate with PU.1 in the T/DC choice are under investigation.

3.1.2. Spi-B.

Spi-B is another Ets family transcription factor that is closely related to PU.1. Initially, Spi-B was identified as a lymphoid-specific factor involved in B cell receptor signaling [85]. Surprisingly, however, a knock-in of Spi-B into the PU.1 locus showed that it was able to rescue myeloid but not B cell development [86], and it was subsequently found to be expressed specifically in pDCs [87]. Further studies using RNA interference techniques showed that Spi-B is required for pDC development from human precursors [88], and it has recently been shown to be influential in bone marrow-derived pDC development [89]. Curiously, Spi-B does not appear to play a role in the generation of splenic pDCs, suggesting that its main roles are developmentally upstream of the immature DC precursors found in the spleen. Interestingly, Spi-B activates the production of type I IFN in concert with interferon regulatory factor-7 (IRF-7), a factor important for pDC function [89]. Unlike PU.1, which is normally expressed in DN1 and DN2 cells and decreases as T cells develop, Spi-B increases in expression during the DN1-3 stages, suggesting a role in T cell commitment [70]. Furthermore, Spi-B$^{-/-}$ animals exhibit slightly lower cellularity and delayed T cell development in the thymus. However, overexpression of Spi-B at the DN3 stage interrupts β-selection resulting in greater DC development within fetal thymic organ culture (FTOC) [90] and inhibits T cell, B cell, and NK cell development from human precursors in vitro [87]. The impact of Spi-B overexpression on lymphocyte development may be due to the levels driven by PU.1-locus regulatory elements or retroviral elements in these studies, enabling Spi-B, which binds to the same promoter site as PU.1, to act in a PU.1-like manner. The presence of DC subsets therefore in PU.1$^{-/-}$ and Spi-B$^{-/-}$ mice is further evidence of a compensatory role for these two factors. Accordingly, there is a complete lack of tDCs in PU.1$^{-/-}$ Spi-B$^{-/-}$ E18 fetal thymic lobes in contrast to a reduction of DC subsets in PU.1$^{-/-}$ lobes [90]. Adult Spi-B$^{-/-}$ tDCs, however, appear normal (unpublished data), suggesting that PU.1 is capable of compensating for a loss of Spi-B specifically in tDCs, whereas the reverse relationship is not present.

3.2. Controlling the DC versus Macrophage Lineage Choice

3.2.1. Ikaros.

Ikaros is a zinc finger transcription factor that acts as a dimer with itself and with the other family members, Aiolos and Helios. Ikaros is critical for early stages of hematopoiesis [91], which has complicated analysis of developmental defects in different lineages in Ikaros-deficient mice. Ikaros dominant negative mutant mice, which lack activity of all Ikaros family members, exhibit a loss of cDCs and an increase in monocytes and macrophages [92], suggesting a requirement for Ikaros in cDC development. Interestingly, however, Ikaros null mice only lack CD8$^-$ cDCs and pDCs, while retaining their CD8$^+$ DC population, indicating that Ikaros is either needed in each lineage independently or that Ikaros null CD8$^+$ DCs arise independently of the CDP. In another mouse model in which only low levels of Ikaros were expressed in hematopoietic cells only, pDCs were absent, indicating that pDCs require high levels of Ikaros whereas cDCs do not [93]. This defect was cell autonomous and was linked to inappropriate upregulation of a large array of genes and a failure to respond to Flt3L. Interestingly, Flt3 expression was missing in Ikaros null LMPP cells [94]. Therefore, part of the role of Ikaros in pDCs is to silence alternative lineage genes and to upregulate Flt3 on DC precursor populations. Interestingly, Ikaros can bind to promoter elements in the PU.1 gene locus to activate or repress PU.1 transcription in myeloid cells, depending on the regulatory site [95]. Overall, these data support a role for Ikaros in pDC development as well as the divergence of the cDC and monocyte-derived DC lineages prior to the CDP stage of DC development.

3.2.2. Gfi1.

Gfi1 is another transcriptional regulator with important roles in DC development. One of the main roles of Ikaros in the B/macrophage lineage choice is to upregulate Gfi1, promoting B cell development and repressing myeloid development [32]. It is therefore possible that

Gfi1 is downstream of Ikaros in DCs as well. However, Gfi1$^{-/-}$ mice exhibit a more striking DC deficiency than Ikaros$^{-/-}$ mice, with a reduction in all splenic, thymic, and peripheral LN DC populations, correlated with an increase in LCs [96]. Gfi1$^{-/-}$ mice also exhibit defects in early T cell development, reduced thymic cellularity, and increased Id2 mRNA levels [33]. Gfi1 represses Id2 in B and myeloid cells. This might also occur in developing T cells, since it is expressed throughout T cell development [97, 98]. In the context of multipotent progenitors, Gfi1 promotes the B cell lineage over the macrophage lineage by repressing PU.1 [32]. Moreover, *in vitro* experiments showed an increase in macrophage potential from Gfi1$^{-/-}$ precursors. Collectively, these results indicate that Gfi1, like Ikaros, likely play a role in the DC/macrophage lineage choice.

3.3. cDC-Specific Regulators

3.3.1. Zbtb46. Recently, two independent studies identified a novel transcription factor, Zbtb46 (also known as Btbd4 or zDC), exclusively expressed in pre-cDC, CD8$^+$ cDC, and CD8$^-$ cDC cells, but not in pDCs [99, 100]. Although Zbtb46 expression was restricted to these lineages, it was not required for their development, but rather to modulate their activation status [100–102]. Zbtb46 acts primarily as a transcriptional repressor in cDCs, with targets including many MHC class II genes. Once cDCs are stimulated with TLR agonists, Zbtb46 protein is downregulated, allowing MHC class II molecules to be expressed at higher levels, thereby conferring an activated status to these cDCs [102]. Zbtb46 might also play a role in promoting the development of CD8$^+$ cDCs over CD8$^-$ cDCs in the spleen [102]. However, the deletion of Zbtb46$^+$ cells using diptheria toxin did not affect tumour or parasitic immunity, thus illuminating the compensatory roles of the remaining DC compartment in these functional capacities [100]. Certainly, the ability to label Zbtb46-expressing cells with GFP has provided a valuable tool for clarifying DC classification and enabling the identification of cells committed to the cDC lineage fate.

3.3.2. Bcl6. Bcl6, another zinc finger transcription factor, is also known to be a transcriptional repressor [103, 104] of many target genes, including p53 [105]. This transcriptional regulator is involved in modulating Th2 immune responses [106, 107] and inhibiting plasma cell differentiation [108] and has recently been implicated in DC development [109]. Bcl6$^{-/-}$ mice exhibit a reduction in the splenic CD4$^+$CD8$^-$ and CD8$^+$ subsets. Additionally, as shown by adoptive transfer studies, Bcl6$^{-/-}$ BM-derived precursors possessed a decreased capacity to develop into cDCs. This was attributed to increased p53 expression, leading to increased apoptosis [109]. Bcl6$^{-/-}$ DCs also secreted greater amounts of IL-6 and IL-12, which led to a greater activation of CD4$^+$ T cells, likely skewing to a Th2 inflammatory response [109]. Thus, Bcl6 plays a role in the differentiation and survival of cDCs.

3.4. Controlling the cDC versus pDC Lineage Choice

3.4.1. Id2. Id factors, which contain helix-loop-helix domains, can dimerize with and inhibit E proteins including HEB (HEBAlt, HEBCan), E2A (E12, E47), and E2-2 (E2-2Can, E2-2Alt). The major cDC-specific Id regulator is Id2. Id2 is not expressed in LSK, LMPPs, or CLPs, or in the CDP or pre-cDC DC progenitors, but is present in all cDCs, regardless of anatomical location [110]. However, Id2 is only required for epidermal LCs, splenic CD8$^+$, and nonlymphoid tissue resident CD103$^+$ DCs [48, 111]. Interestingly, the DN1e subset within the thymus also expresses high levels of Id2 indicating that these cells might have an increased propensity to develop into cDCs, in particular CD8$^+$ tDCs [35]. Thus, Id2 appears to have a role in the later stages of DC development. However, unlike Zbtb46, Id2 expression is not restricted to the DC lineage, since it is also important for the development of other lineages, such as NK and myeloid cells.

3.4.2. E Proteins. In contrast to cDCs, pDCs require the E protein E2-2 for their development and homeostasis [34]. Interestingly, E2-2 can activate pDC-specific regulators, such as Spi-B, IRF-7, and IRF-8, as well as Bcl11a. Furthermore, the deletion of E2-2 from pDCs converts them to cDCs, as determined by surface marker phenotype, function, gene expression, and morphology [34, 112]. Since E2-2-dependent upregulation of these genes would be inhibited by Id2, the Id2/E2-2 dichotomy is likely at the top of the hierarchy that splits the pDC/cDC gene programs. Another E protein that is expressed specifically in thymic pDCs is HEBCan [35]. HEB-Can is also expressed throughout thymocyte development, while the shorter form of HEB, HEBAlt, is expressed only during early T-lineage developmental stages. HEBAlt has defined roles in promoting T cell development [113, 114], and decreasing DC development from bone marrow precursors *in vitro* [35]. However, constitutive expression of HEBAlt in T cell precursors does not alter tDC development in the adult thymus, perhaps due to additional microenvironmental factors present in the thymus that are not available *in vitro* (A. J. Moore and M. K. Anderson, unpublished data). Therefore, further study is needed to assess the roles of HEBCan and HEBAlt in the T cell/tDC lineage choice.

3.5. CD8$^+$ DC-Specific Regulators

3.5.1. Batf3. Global gene expression analyses of DC populations have led to the discovery of many DC subset-specific genes, including the transcription factor Batf3 [7]. Studies of Batf3-deficient mice showed that Batf3 is required for CD8$^+$ cDC development during steady state. The lack of splenic and LN CD8$^+$ cDCs in Batf3$^{-/-}$ mice demonstrated that these cells are required for cross-presentation of antigen to CD8$^+$ T cells. Furthermore, these mice had defective antiviral and antitumor immunity [7]. Interestingly, Batf3 was also required for the generation of CD103$^+$ CD11b$^-$ DCs within the skin and mesenteric LN, dermis, lung, and intestine, which emphasizes the similarities in transcriptional regulation between CD8$^+$ cDC and CD103$^+$ nonlymphoid tissue DCs [115]. *In vitro* studies showed that the cultured equivalents to CD8$^+$ DCs were not hampered by a lack of Batf3 until later timepoints, suggesting more of a homeostatic role than a developmental role of Batf3 in CD8$^+$ DC development and also foreshadowing recent work highlighting the redundancy of Batf factors [110]. Interestingly, when challenged by intracellular pathogens or administration of IL-12, CD8$^+$ DCs were restored by 3 weeks in Batf3$^{-/-}$ mice by an alternative pathway whereby Batf and Batf2 compensate for the lack of Batf3 [31]. This study also showed that Batf could interact directly with IRF-4 and IRF-8. Thus, it appears that Batf3 is important in the terminal stages of CD8$^+$ cDC development and plays a role in maintaining this subset.

3.5.2. E4BP4. Recently, E4BP4 (NFIL3), a basic leucine zipper transcription factor, which was first recognized for its importance in NK cell development [116, 117], has been implicated in CD8$^+$ DC development. Despite higher E4BP4 mRNA expression levels in pDCs than CD8$^+$ cDCs, E4BP4$^{-/-}$ mice specifically lacked splenic and thymic CD8$^+$ cDCs [30]. The defect in development appears to take place at the pre-cDC to CD8$^+$ cDC developmental transition since precursors, such as LSK, CLP, CMP, GMP, CDP, and pre-cDC populations, are not affected by the absence of E4BP4 [30]. *In vitro* studies showed that E4BP4$^{-/-}$ bone marrow cells could be partially rescued by retroviral transduction with a Batf3-containing vector into CD24$^+$ Sirpα$^-$ DCs (CD8$^+$ cDC equivalent), thus indicating that Batf3 is involved directly or indirectly with the CD8$^+$ DC-promoting effects of E4BP4 expression.

3.6. CD8$^-$ DC-Specific Regulator: RelB. Despite the identification of many regulators for the CD8$^+$ cDC and pDC lineages, the regulation of the CD8$^-$ cDC subset by unique transcription factors remains elusive. Initially, tDCs were reported absent in RelB$^{-/-}$ mice, but this was attributed to a lack of medullary thymic epithelial cells which tDCs normally localize to [118, 119]. RelB, a subunit of the NFkB complex, is a downstream signaling mediator of immune cell activation via pattern recognition receptors, such as Toll-like receptors [120]. RelB is specifically expressed in splenic CD8$^-$ cDCs and is required for their development [119]. Although functional roles pertaining to DC activation have been attributed to RelB in DCs [121, 122], the influence RelB has on lineage decisions is largely unknown.

3.7. Interferon Regulatory Factors. As their names suggest, IRFs are transcription factors known for their ability to induce the expression of interferons in response to stimulus, such as the activation of toll-like receptors (reviewed in [123]). IRF-1, IRF-2, IRF-4, IRF-7, and IRF-8 have been implicated in DC development across many subsets.

3.7.1. IRF-8. In addition to Batf3, Id2, and E4BP4, CD8$^+$ cDCs also require IRF-8 (ICSBP; interferon consensus-binding protein) for their development [124, 125]. IRF-8 also plays a major role in CD103$^+$ DCs and a minor role

in pDC, LC, and dermal DC development with a more pronounced defect in pDCs [48, 124]. IRF8$^{-/-}$ mice were unable to produce type I IFNs following viral challenge and exhibited delayed migration of LCs to the draining LNs in steady state and inflammatory conditions [124, 126, 127]. Interestingly, a single point mutation within the IRF association domain (IAD) of IRF-8, which confers the ability to interact with other IRFs, replicates the loss of CD8$^+$ cDCs, but not pDCs, in IRF-8$^{-/-}$ mice. Although the wildtype IRF-8 could interact with IRF-2 or PU.1 and Spi-B to bind to interferon-stimulated response element (ISRE) or Ets/IRF promoter sites, respectively, the mutated IRF8^{R294C} could not [128]. Therefore, IRF-8 is involved in the development of CD8$^+$ cDCs, CD103$^+$ DCs, and pDCs but likely act through different mechanisms in each subset.

3.7.2. Other IRFs. Another factor implicated in DC development is IRF-4. IRF-4-deficient mice lacked the majority of splenic CD11b$^+$ CD4$^+$ CD8$^-$ cDCs and had a slight reduction in pDCs [129, 130]. In addition to developmental defects, the lack of IRF-4 impaired the migration of LCs and CD103$^+$ dermal DCs to the cutaneous LN following skin inflammation [131]. IRF-1$^{-/-}$ mice also differ from wildtype mice in that they exhibit a slight reduction in CD8$^+$ and CD8$^-$ cDCs and an increase in pDCs [132]. Further complexity is added by the severe decrease of CD8$^-$ cDCs and a partial lack of CD8$^+$ cDCs and pDCs in IRF-2$^{-/-}$ mice [133]. Interestingly, IRF-4 mRNA expression levels were greater in E4BP4$^{-/-}$ pre-cDCs compared to the wildtype counterparts, suggesting that E4BP4 might act by restricting the IRF4-mediated development of other DC lineages [30]. Thus, in addition to IRF-8, IRF-1 and IRF-2 play minor roles in CD8$^+$ DC development, whereas IRF-2, IRF-4, and, to a lesser extent, IRF-1 are important for CD8$^-$ DC development. The increase in pDCs in IRF1$^{-/-}$ mice suggests that IRF-1 might repress or inhibit IRF-8. IRF-2 and IRF-4 also play minor roles in pDC development. Interestingly, ChIP analysis has shown that human E2-2, which is required for pDC development, is capable of binding to promoter regions upstream *Irf*-7 and *Irf*-8 gene loci [34].

4. Cytokines Involved in DC Development

4.1. GM-CSF, M-CSF, and Flt3. Cytokines, secreted by surrounding tissues and immune cells, provide many developmental cues that influence the transcriptional regulation and functions of the receiving cells. Initial *in vitro* studies of cytokines in DC development revealed distinct and important roles for the receptor tyrosine kinases, GM-CSF, M-CSF and Flt3L, in the generation of DCs [134–138]. Flt3L and M-CSF, in particular, have been shown to influence many discrete DC subsets. Flt3L-supplemented cultures can induce the differentiation of CD8$^+$cDCs, CD8$^-$ cDCs, and pDCs from a variety of precursors [23, 135–137, 139]. M-CSF-supplemented cultures can also generate CD8$^+$ cDCs, CD8$^-$ cDCs, and pDCs, albeit with lower efficiency than Flt3L cultures [138]. Moreover, Flt3$^+$ precursors including

LMPPs, MDPs, CDPs, pre-cDCs and a proportion of CLPs, CMPs, and ETPs, in addition to progenitors transduced to express Flt3, possess greater DC potential than their Flt3$^-$ counterparts [42, 139–142]. Correspondingly, Flt3-deficient mice exhibit decreased cDCs and pDCs [41]. However, the degree of reduction in cDC and pDC subsets in Flt3$^{-/-}$ mice does not reflect the severe decrease of these populations in Flt3L$^{-/-}$ mice [23, 143], suggesting the presence of another, as of yet unidentified, receptor for Flt3L.

Interestingly, this speculation reflects recent findings in the M-CSF/M-CSF1R pathway. Mice carrying a mutated M-CSF gene (op/op mice) exhibited a reduction in splenic CD11c^{dim} B220$^+$ pDCs, but LCs and microglia remained intact [144–146]. Microglia, the resident macrophages within the central nervous system (reviewed in [147]), and some LCs arise from progenitors in the embryonic yolk sac and thus exhibit similar developmental requirements [146, 148]. By contrast, LCs and microglia were completely absent from M-CSF1R$^{-/-}$ mice [146, 149]. The disparity in DC developmental defects in M-CSF$^{-/-}$ and M-CSF1R$^{-/-}$ mice was clarified by the discovery of an alternate ligand for M-CSF1R, IL-34 [150]. IL-34 is secreted by keratinocytes and neurons to foster the development of steady state LCs and microglia, respectively [151]. Accordingly, IL-34$^{-/-}$ mice lack LCs and exhibit reduced microglia, thereby replicating the results in M-CSF1R$^{-/-}$ mice [151]. Comparable populations of monocytes and DCs were observed between IL-34$^{-/-}$ and WT mice [152]. By contrast, there are no significant LC deficiencies in Flt3$^{-/-}$ or Flt3L$^{-/-}$ mice [48, 153]. In addition to M-CSF1R expression on MDPs and CDPs, it is also expressed by yolk sac macrophages, adult macrophages, LCs, and splenic cDC and pDC subsets [145, 154]. Although Flt3 and M-CSFR are both expressed on MDPs and CDPs, they clearly influence different DC lineage fates.

Although GM-CSF is commonly added to many in vitro cultures to stimulate DC development from bone marrow progenitors, GM-CSF$^{-/-}$ and GM-CSFR$^{-/-}$ mice do not show any significant deficiencies in DC populations in lymphoid tissues [155]. Splenic CD8$^+$ cDCs were slightly increased in GM-CSF$^{-/-}$ mice, indicating that GM-CSF inhibits the generation of this subset [156]. There are many conflicting reports on the involvement of GM-CSF in nonlymphoid tissue DC subsets. One study shows that CD103$^+$ CD11b$^-$ dermal DCs are reduced in GM-CSF$^{-/-}$ mice and GM-CSFR$^{-/-}$ mice [157], which is confirmed by another report, whereby CD103$^+$ CD11b$^+$ lamina propria DCs and CD103$^+$ DCs from skin and lung draining LN were also decreased in both GM-CSF$^{-/-}$ and GM-CSFR$^{-/-}$ mice [158]. A third report observed that DC populations remained similar to WT in GM-CSFR$^{-/-}$ mice, but CD103 surface expression was slightly downregulated on GM-CSFR$^{-/-}$ DCs [159]. Although GM-CSF does not seem to be unequivocally required for many, if any, DC subsets, GM-CSFR transgenic mice exhibit an increase in cellularity in the thymus and spleen, which is echoed by an increase in cDCs as well [155, 156]. Conversely, the presence of GM-CSF inhibits the development of CD8$^+$ cDC equivalent cells and pDCs in vitro [136, 156]. Moreover,

GM-CSF does not enhance DC development from early T cell precursors as Flt3L does [160]. GM-CSF does, however, seem to play a role in the function of DCs. The addition of GM-CSF to in vitro cultures resulted in the upregulation of CD103 and an increase in cross-presentation abilities of DCs [161], which was confirmed ex vivo and in vivo using GM-CSF-transgenic and GM-CSFR$^{-/-}$ mice [162].

Therefore, GM-CSF signaling directs different developmental outcomes than Flt3L signaling. Although many other cytokines, such as SCF, TGF-β, IL-3, IL-4, or IL-7, have been studied and can modify the outcomes of in vitro cultures, they do not appear to play an overarching, essential role for DC development.

4.2. STATs. The signal transducer and activator of transcription (STAT) family of transcription factors has been implicated downstream of the cytokine receptors, Flt3 and GM-CSFR, thus bridging the gap between extracellular signals and transcriptional regulation. Signaling through the Flt3 receptor induces the phosphorylation of STAT3, which is required for DC development as evidenced by the lack of splenic DCs and reduced CLP and CMP precursors in STAT3$^{-/-}$ mice [28]. This defect was not restored by treating mice with Flt3L, indicating that the requirement for STAT3 is downstream of Flt3 signaling [28]. STAT1, STAT3, and STAT5 are all phosphorylated in response to administration of GM-CSF to bone marrow cultures [28]. GM-CSF blocks pDC development in vitro through STAT5, which inhibits IRF-8 transcription [29]. Clearly, the Flt3L and GM-CSF pathways are connected, since Flt3 can induce the transcription of GM-CSFR, as well as M-CSFR and PU.1 [142]. Thus, this experimental evidence suggests that Flt3 is required during earlier stages of DC development, whereas the function of GM-CSF might be to favour the cDC lineage over pDCs. The point in DC differentiation at which M-CSF influences developmental outcomes is likely during the MDP to CDP conversion when M-CSF1R is expressed, but this has not yet been directly examined. Determining the cellular sources of Flt3L, GM-CSF, and M-CSF will provide important insights into the homeostatic versus infection-induced mechanisms of DC development.

5. cDC and pDC Gene Regulatory Networks

Once organized into lineage-specific gene regulatory maps, the similarities and differences between cDCs and pDCs become more apparent (Figure 1). The networks are separated based on the stage of development in which each factor is proposed to function. PU.1 is a master regulator of both cDCs and pDCs, and, based on experimental evidence, it likely functions early in DC development at or immediately prior to the CDP stage. The main function of PU.1 is to turn on regulatory genes that are responsible for proper DC development, such as Id2, Flt3L, and GM-CSFR. Since signaling through GM-CSFR can activate STAT5, which inhibits IRF-8 transcription, GM-CSF might be an environmental cue to favour CD8$^-$ cDC development. Indeed, GM-CSF promotes the development of CD8$^-$ CD11b$^+$ DCs in vitro

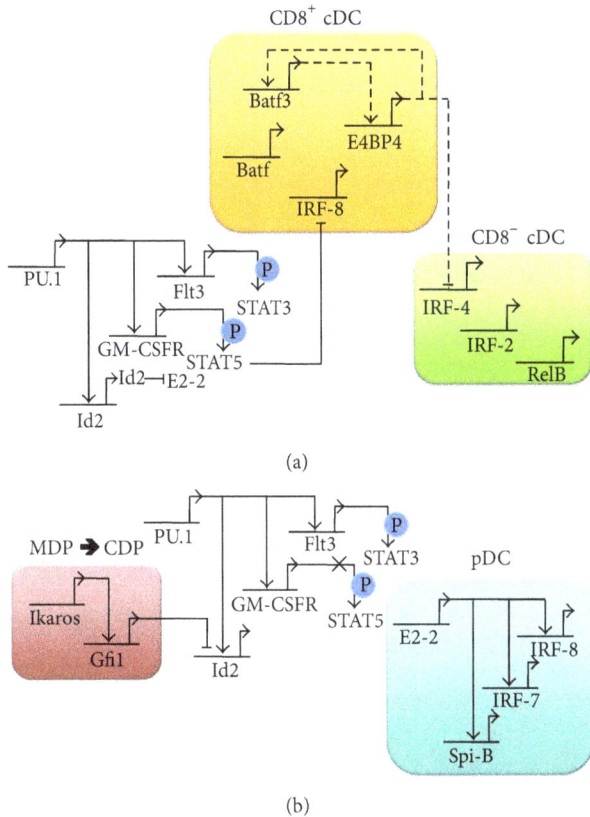

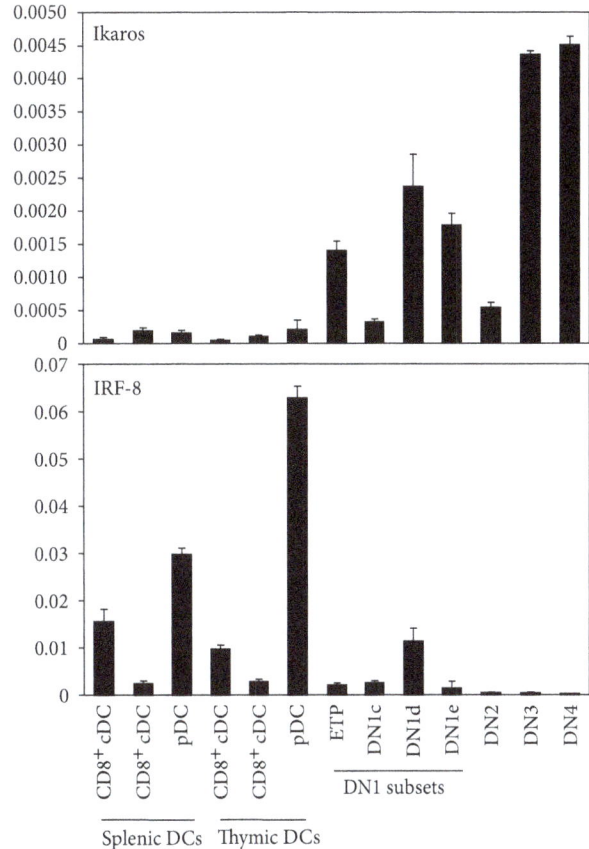

FIGURE 1: Gene regulatory networks for cDC and pDC development. Shared gene regulation patterns in (a) and (b). PU.1 upregulates many factors important for DC development, including Id2, GM-CSFR, and Flt3L [26, 27]. The Flt3 pathway phosphorylates STAT3, which can upregulate/downregulate target genes [28]. (a) Gene regulation in cDCs. Id2 expression inhibits E2-2 via protein interaction. GM-CSFR phosphorylates STAT5, which can inhibit IRF-8 expression [29]. Batf3 upregulates E4BP4 [30]. Batf expression in CD8+ cDCs compensates for a lack of Batf3 [31]. E4BP4 negatively modulates IRF-4 expression [30]. (b) Gene regulation in pDCs. Ikaros upregulates Gfi1 [32], which can inhibit Id2 expression [33], allowing for E2-2 function. E2-2 binds to the promoter of Spi-B, IRF-7, and IRF-8 to upregulate gene expression [34]. A yet unidentified mechanism prevents the downstream events of GM-CSFR in pDCs, since STAT5 has been shown to downregulate IRF-8, which is required for pDC development. Proven interactions are indicated in solid bars. Hypothesized interactions are shown in dashed lines.

FIGURE 2: IRF-8 and Ikaros gene expression in early T cell precursors. Cell subsets were sorted, and qRT-PCR was performed as previously described [35]. Gene expression levels, as determined by qRT-PCR, were normalized to β-actin. Values shown are mean $\pm$ standard deviation ($n = 3$).

[29]. The partial restoration of a wildtype phenotype by transducing E4BP4$^{-/-}$ cells with Batf3 suggests that either E4BP4 and Batf3 have similar transcriptional targets or Batf3 is upregulated by E4BP4. Conversely, the elevated levels of IRF-4 mRNA in E4BP4$^{-/-}$ cells indicate that E4BP4 inhibits IRF-4, directly or indirectly (Figure 1(a)).

Clearly, Id2 functions to inhibit pDC development by binding to and inhibiting E2-2, which is required for pDCs. Although the earlier Ikaros mutant studies were contradictory, a model in which Ikaros is expressed only at low levels elucidates its role in the pDC lineage. In this model, Ikaros upregulates Gfi1, and Gfi1 inhibits Id2 transcription (Figure 1(b)). The repression of Id2 would result in functioning E2-2 protein, which can reprogram precursors for the pDC lineage fate by upregulating Spi-B, IRF-7, and IRF-8. There must be mechanisms in place to restrict GM-CSF signals from inhibiting IRF-8 through STAT5 to allow for CD8$^+$ cDC development, as well as pDCs. Future studies examining the environmental cues and resulting transcriptional regulation will allow us to further understand the mechanisms that govern homeostatic DC development and infection- or inflammatory-induced DC differentiation.

Many of the major DC regulators, such as PU.1, Spi-B, Gfi1, Id2, and IRF-4, are expressed by developing T cell precursors [70, 163]. However, with the exception of PU.1, the gene targets and roles of each factor have not been explored in T cell progenitors versus DC progenitors. Here, we examined the gene expression profiles of Ikaros, IRF-8, and Batf3 in ETP, DN1c, DN1d, DN1e, DN2, DN3, and DN4 cells to determine whether DC gene network components were present in these precursors (Figure 2). Batf3 was not expressed at high levels, if at all, in these T cell precursors (unpublished data). However, Ikaros was expressed and increased as precursors became committed to the T cell lineage (Figure 2). Earlier work showed that fetal T cells, but not adult T cells, were absent from Ikaros null mutant mice [164]. The presence of Ikaros could upregulate Gfi1, which is known to be expressed in T cell precursors, to inhibit Id2 and promote pDC development. Interestingly, mature splenic and thymic DC subsets do not express high levels of Ikaros or Gfi1 (Figure 2; unpublished data), agreeing with the speculation that Ikaros and Gfi1 play roles early in DC development but not in mature DCs. DN1d cells, which we have previously determined, express high levels of Spi-B [35], contained the highest levels of IRF-8 when compared to the remaining T cell precursors (Figure 2). These results indicate that DN1d cells might have a greater pDC lineage potential. Overall, the expression of multiple DC-essential transcription factors within T cell precursors suggests these cells are partially equipped to develop into DCs.

6. Discussion

Although the properties varying between distinct DC subsets are vast, there is emerging evidence linking DC populations by common gene expression profiles [67]. These comparisons show that lymphoid tissue-resident $CD8^+$ cDC and nonlymphoid tissue-resident $CD103^+$ DCs are more closely related to each other than they are to $CD8^-$ cDCs and pDCs. Similarly, migratory DCs differ from all other DC subsets and uniquely upregulate genes expressing immunomodulatory molecules, which could regulate immune response to self-antigen [67]. It is probable that the transcriptional regulators expressed earlier in DC development, such as PU.1, Ikaros, and Gfi1, primarily function to modulate precursor responsiveness to cytokine signals, growth factors, and inflammatory signals. These events allow for the production of steady state DC subsets and prompt alternative pathways of DC development during infection [31, 165]. By contrast, while the transcription factors expressed during the terminal stages of DC differentiation might be required for DC subset development, they are often also essential for specialized functions. In particular, $RelB^{-/-}$ and $IRF-8^{-/-}$ DCs express lower levels of MHC class II and costimulatory molecules, such as CD40, CD80, and CD86, following microbial or CD40L stimulation [122, 125]. The tolerogenic cytokines TGF-β and IL-10 were secreted at higher concentrations from $IRF-1^{-/-}$ DCs [132]. Furthermore, the transcriptional marker of cDCs, Zbtb46, has been shown to play important functions by promoting tolerogenic phenotypes of steady state cDCs until stimulated by antigen [102]. Certainly, the duality of these transcription factors for developmental and functional inputs makes targeted experiments more challenging to design. Despite the availability of many high throughput methods, such as RNA-seq or ChIP-seq, flaws in data interpretation can still arise from purifying DCs according to their surface cellular phenotypes. If a method for typing single cells by transcriptome signatures was available, it would be interesting to see how DC subsets that emerged from this analysis would compare with established DC subsets grouped by combinatorial cell surface receptor expression.

List of Abbreviations

DC: Dendritic cell
tDC: Thymic DC
cDC: Conventional DC
pDC: Plasmacytoid DC
LC: Langerhans cell
LNs: Lymph nodes
IPCs: Interferon-producing cells
CLP: Common lymphoid progenitor
CMP: Common myeloid progenitor
GMP: Granulocyte/macrophage precursor
MDP: Macrophage/DC precursor
CDP: Common DC precursor
MPP: Multipotent progenitor
LMPP: Lymphoid-primed multipotent progenitor
CTP: Circulating T cell progenitor
DN: Double negative
NK: Natural killer
ETP: Early T cell progenitor
FTOC: Fetal thymic organ culture
IFNs: Interferon regulatory factors
ICSBP: Interferon consensus-binding protein
IAD: IRF association domain
ISRE: Interferon-stimulated response element
Flt3L: Flt3 ligand
STAT: Signal transducer and activator of transcription.

Acknowledgments

The authors thank G. Knowles and C. McIntosh for sorting expertise and the Sunnybrook Comparative Research Facility for excellent animal care. This work was supported by research grants from the Canadian Institute for Health Research (MOP82861) and Sunnybrook Research Institute to M. K. Anderson, as well as funds from the Ontario Graduate Scholarship (OGSST and OGS) and the University of Toronto to A. J. Moore.

References

[1] R. M. Steinman and Z. A. Cohn, "Identification of a novel cell type in peripheral lymphoid organs of mice. I. Morphology, quantitation, tissue distribution," *The Journal of Immunology*, vol. 137, no. 5, pp. 1142–1162, 1973.

[2] D. Vremec, J. Pooley, H. Hochrein, L. Wu, and K. Shortman, "CD4 and CD8 expression by dendritic cell subtypes in mouse thymus and spleen," *The Journal of Immunology*, vol. 164, no. 6, pp. 2978–2986, 2000.

[3] A. D. Edwards, D. Chaussabel, S. Tomlinson, O. Schulz, A. Sher, and C. Reis e Sousa, "Relationships among murine CD11chigh dendritic cell subsets as revealed by baseline gene expression patterns," *The Journal of Immunology*, vol. 171, no. 1, pp. 47–60, 2003.

[4] F. Eckert and U. Schmid, "Identification of plasmacytoid T cells in lymphoid hyperplasia of the skin," *Archives of Dermatology*, vol. 125, no. 11, pp. 1518–1524, 1989.

[5] F. P. Siegal, N. Kadowaki, M. Shodell et al., "The nature of the principal type 1 interferon-producing cells in human blood," *Science*, vol. 284, no. 5421, pp. 1835–1837, 1999.

[6] J. M. M. den Haan, S. M. Lehar, and M. J. Bevan, "CD8⁺ but not CD8⁻ dendritic cells cross-prime cytotoxic T cells in vivo," *Journal of Experimental Medicine*, vol. 192, no. 12, pp. 1685–1696, 2000.

[7] K. Hildner, B. T. Edelson, W. E. Purtha et al., "Batf3 deficiency reveals a critical role for CD8α⁺ dendritic cells in cytotoxic T cell immunity," *Science*, vol. 322, no. 5904, pp. 1097–1100, 2008.

[8] C. Koble and B. Kyewski, "The thymic medulla: a unique microenvironment for intercellular self-antigen transfer," *Journal of Experimental Medicine*, vol. 206, no. 7, pp. 1505–1513, 2009.

[9] A. M. Gallegos and M. J. Bevan, "Central tolerance: good but imperfect," *Immunological Reviews*, vol. 209, pp. 290–296, 2006.

[10] T. Brocker, M. Riedinger, and K. Karjalainen, "Targeted expression of major histocompatibility complex (MHC) class II molecules demonstrates that dendritic cells can induce negative but not positive selection of thymocytes in vivo," *Journal of Experimental Medicine*, vol. 185, no. 3, pp. 541–550, 1997.

[11] T. Birnberg, L. Bar-On, A. Sapoznikov et al., "Lack of conventional dendritic cells is compatible with normal development and T cell homeostasis, but causes myeloid proliferative syndrome," *Immunity*, vol. 29, no. 6, pp. 986–997, 2008.

[12] B. Pulendran, J. Lingappa, M. K. Kennedy et al., "Developmental pathways of dendritic cells in vivo: distinct function, phenotype, and localization of dendritic cell subsets in FLT3 ligand-treated mice," *The Journal of Immunology*, vol. 159, no. 5, pp. 2222–2231, 1997.

[13] D. Dudziak, A. O. Kamphorst, G. F. Heidkamp et al., "Differential antigen processing by dendritic cell subsets in vivo," *Science*, vol. 315, no. 5808, pp. 107–111, 2007.

[14] M. Bogunovic, F. Ginhoux, J. Helft et al., "Origin of the lamina propria dendritic cell network," *Immunity*, vol. 31, no. 3, pp. 513–525, 2009.

[15] M. Merad, F. Ginhoux, and M. Collin, "Origin, homeostasis and function of Langerhans cells and other langerin-expressing dendritic cells," *Nature Reviews Immunology*, vol. 8, no. 12, pp. 935–947, 2008.

[16] N. Romani, B. E. Clausen, and P. Stoitzner, "Langerhans cells and more: langerin-expressing dendritic cell subsets in the skin," *Immunological Reviews*, vol. 234, no. 1, pp. 120–141, 2010.

[17] M. Collin, V. Bigley, M. Haniffa, and S. Hambleton, "Human dendritic cell deficiency: the missing ID?" *Nature Reviews Immunology*, vol. 11, no. 9, pp. 575–583, 2011.

[18] A. Dzionek, A. Fuchs, P. Schmidt et al., "BDCA-2, BDCA-3, and BDCA-4: three markers for distinct subsets of dendritic cells in human peripheral blood," *The Journal of Immunology*, vol. 165, no. 11, pp. 6037–6046, 2000.

[19] A. Bachem, S. Güttler, E. Hartung et al., "Superior antigen cross-presentation and XCR1 expression define human CD11c⁺CD141⁺ cells as homologues of mouse CD8⁺ dendritic cells," *Journal of Experimental Medicine*, vol. 207, no. 6, pp. 1273–1281, 2010.

[20] K. Crozat, R. Guiton, V. Contreras et al., "The XC chemokine receptor 1 is a conserved selective marker of mammalian cells homologous to mouse CD8α⁺ dendritic cells," *Journal of Experimental Medicine*, vol. 207, no. 6, pp. 1283–1292, 2010.

[21] S. L. Jongbloed, A. J. Kassianos, K. J. McDonald et al., "Human CD141⁺ (BDCA-3)⁺ dendritic cells (DCs) represent a unique myeloid DC subset that cross-presents necrotic cell antigens," *Journal of Experimental Medicine*, vol. 207, no. 6, pp. 1247–1260, 2010.

[22] L. F. Poulin, M. Salio, E. Griessinger et al., "Characterization of human DNGR-1⁺ BDCA3⁺ leukocytes as putative equivalents of mouse CD8α⁺ dendritic cells," *Journal of Experimental Medicine*, vol. 207, no. 6, pp. 1261–1271, 2010.

[23] P. Brawand, D. R. Fitzpatrick, B. W. Greenfield, K. Brasel, C. R. Maliszewski, and T. De Smedt, "Murine plasmacytoid pre-dendritic cells generated from Flt3 ligand-supplemented bone marrow cultures are immature APCs," *The Journal of Immunology*, vol. 169, no. 12, pp. 6711–6719, 2002.

[24] M. O'Keeffe, H. Hochrein, D. Vremec et al., "Mouse plasmacytoid cells: Long-lived cells, heterogeneous in surface phenotype and function, that differentiate into CD8⁺ dendritic cells only after microbial stimulus," *Journal of Experimental Medicine*, vol. 196, no. 10, pp. 1307–1319, 2002.

[25] H. Luche, L. Ardouin, P. Teo et al., "The earliest intrathymic precursors of CD8α⁺ thymic dendritic cells correspond to myeloid-type double-negative 1c cells," *European The Journal of Immunology*, vol. 41, no. 8, pp. 2165–2175, 2011.

[26] R. P. DeKoter, J. C. Walsh, and H. Singh, "PU.1 regulates both cytokine-dependent proliferation and differentiation of granulocyte/macrophage progenitors," *EMBO Journal*, vol. 17, no. 15, pp. 4456–4468, 1998.

[27] H. L. Pahl, R. J. Scheibe, D. E. Zhang et al., "The proto-oncogene PU. 1 regulates expression of the myeloid-specific CD11b promoter," *The Journal of Biological Chemistry*, vol. 268, no. 7, pp. 5014–5020, 1993.

[28] Y. Laouar, T. Welte, X. Y. Fu, and R. A. Flavell, "STAT3 is required for Flt3L-dependent dendritic cell differentiation," *Immunity*, vol. 19, no. 6, pp. 903–912, 2003.

[29] E. Esashi, Y. H. Wang, O. Perng, X. F. Qin, Y. J. Liu, and S. S. Watowich, "The signal transducer STAT5 inhibits plasmacytoid dendritic cell development by suppressing transcription factor IRF8," *Immunity*, vol. 28, no. 4, pp. 509–520, 2008.

[30] M. Kashiwada, N. L. L. Pham, L. L. Pewe, J. T. Harty, and P. B. Rothman, "NFIL3/E4BP4 is a key transcription factor for CD8α⁺ dendritic cell development," *Blood*, vol. 117, no. 23, pp. 6193–6197, 2011.

[31] R. Tussiwand, W. L. Lee, T. L. Murphy et al., "Compensatory dendritic cell development mediated by BATF-IRF interactions," *Nature*, vol. 490, no. 421, pp. 502–507, 2012.

[32] C. J. Spooner, J. X. Cheng, E. Pujadas, P. Laslo, and H. Singh, "A recurrent network involving the transcription factors PU.1 and Gfi1 orchestrates innate and adaptive immune cell fates," *Immunity*, vol. 31, no. 4, pp. 576–586, 2009.

[33] R. Yücel, H. Karsunky, L. Klein-Hitpass, and T. Möröy, "The transcriptional repressor Gfi1 affects development of early, uncommitted c-Kit⁺ T cell progenitors and CD4/CD8 lineage decision in the thymus," *Journal of Experimental Medicine*, vol. 197, no. 7, pp. 831–844, 2003.

[34] B. Cisse, M. L. Caton, M. Lehner et al., "Transcription factor E2-2 is an essential and specific regulator of plasmacytoid dendritic cell development," *Cell*, vol. 135, no. 1, pp. 37–48, 2008.

[35] A. J. Moore, J. Sarmiento, M. Mohtashami et al., "Transcriptional priming of intrathymic precursors for dendritic cell development," *Development*, vol. 139, no. 2, pp. 373–384, 2011.

[36] M. Kondo, I. L. Weissman, and K. Akashi, "Identification of clonogenic common lymphoid progenitors in mouse bone marrow," *Cell*, vol. 91, no. 5, pp. 661–672, 1997.

[37] K. Akashi, D. Traver, T. Miyamoto, and I. L. Weissman, "A clonogenic common myeloid progenitor that gives rise to all myeloid lineages," *Nature*, vol. 404, no. 6774, pp. 193–197, 2000.

[38] D. Traver, K. Akashi, M. Manz et al., "Development of CD8α-positive dendritic cells from a common myeloid progenitor," *Science*, vol. 290, no. 5499, pp. 2152–2154, 2000.

[39] M. G. Manz, D. Traver, T. Miyamoto, I. L. Weissman, and K. Akashi, "Dendritic cell potentials of early lymphoid and myeloid progenitors," *Blood*, vol. 97, no. 11, pp. 3333–3341, 2001.

[40] L. Wu, A. D'Amico, H. Hochrein, M. O'Keeffe, K. Shortman, and K. Lucas, "Development of thymic and splenic dendritic cell populations from different hemopoietic precursors," *Blood*, vol. 98, no. 12, pp. 3376–3382, 2001.

[41] C. Waskow, K. Liu, G. Darrasse-Jèze et al., "The receptor tyrosine kinase Flt3 is required for dendritic cell development in peripheral lymphoid tissues," *Nature Immunology*, vol. 9, no. 6, pp. 676–683, 2008.

[42] A. D'Amico and L. Wu, "The early progenitors of mouse dendritic cells and plasmacytoid predendritic cells are within the bone marrow hemopoietic precursors expressing Flt3," *Journal of Experimental Medicine*, vol. 198, no. 2, pp. 293–303, 2003.

[43] S. M. Schlenner, V. Madan, K. Busch et al., "Fate mapping reveals separate origins of T cells and myeloid lineages in the thymus," *Immunity*, vol. 32, no. 3, pp. 426–436, 2010.

[44] D. K. Fogg, C. Sibon, C. Miled et al., "A clonogenic bone harrow progenitor specific for macrophages and dendritic cells," *Science*, vol. 311, no. 5757, pp. 83–87, 2006.

[45] S. H. Naik, P. Sathe, H. Y. Park et al., "Development of plasmacytoid and conventional dendritic cell subtypes from single precursor cells derived in vitro and in vivo," *Nature Immunology*, vol. 8, no. 11, pp. 1217–1226, 2007.

[46] N. Onai, A. Obata-Onai, M. A. Schmid, T. Ohteki, D. Jarrossay, and M. G. Manz, "Identification of clonogenic common Flt3+M-CSFR+ plasmacytoid and conventional dendritic cell progenitors in mouse bone marrow," *Nature Immunology*, vol. 8, no. 11, pp. 1207–1216, 2007.

[47] K. Liu, G. D. Victora, T. A. Schwickert et al., "In vivo analysis of dendritic cell development and homeostasis," *Science*, vol. 324, no. 5925, pp. 392–397, 2009.

[48] F. Ginhoux, K. Liu, J. Helft et al., "The origin and development of nonlymphoid tissue CD103+ DCs," *Journal of Experimental Medicine*, vol. 206, no. 13, pp. 3115–3130, 2009.

[49] C. Ardavin, L. Wu, C. L. Li, and K. Shortman, "Thymic dendritic cells and T cells develop simultaneously in the thymus from a common precursor population," *Nature*, vol. 362, no. 6422, pp. 761–763, 1993.

[50] F. Radtke, I. Ferrero, A. Wilson, R. Lees, M. Aguet, and H. R. MacDonald, "Notch1 deficiency dissociates the intrathymic development of dendritic cells and T cells," *Journal of Experimental Medicine*, vol. 191, no. 7, pp. 1085–1094, 2000.

[51] T. B. Feyerabend, G. Terszowski, A. Tietz et al., "Deletion of Notch1 converts pro-T cells to dendritic cells and promotes thymic B cells by cell-extrinsic and cell-intrinsic mechanisms," *Immunity*, vol. 30, no. 1, pp. 67–79, 2009.

[52] E. Donskoy and I. Goldschneider, "Two developmentally distinct populations of dendritic cells inhabit the adult mouse thymus: demonstration by differential importation of hematogenous precursors under steady state conditions," *The Journal of Immunology*, vol. 170, no. 7, pp. 3514–3521, 2003.

[53] J. Li, J. Park, D. Foss, and I. Goldschneider, "Thymus-homing peripheral dendritic cells constitute two of the three major subsets of dendritic cells in the steady-state thymus," *Journal of Experimental Medicine*, vol. 206, no. 3, pp. 607–622, 2009.

[54] H. Hadeiba, K. Lahl, A. Edalati et al., "Plasmacytoid dendritic cells transport peripheral antigens to the thymus to promote central tolerance," *Immunity*, vol. 36, no. 3, pp. 438–450, 2012.

[55] H. T. Petrie and J. C. Zúñiga-Pflücker, "Zoned out: functional mapping of stromal signaling microenvironments in the thymus," *Annual Review of Immunology*, vol. 25, no. 1, pp. 649–679, 2007.

[56] A. V. Griffith, M. Fallahi, H. Nakase, M. Gosink, B. Young, and H. T. Petrie, "Spatial mapping of thymic stromal microenvironments reveals unique features influencing T lymphoid differentiation," *Immunity*, vol. 31, no. 6, pp. 999–1009, 2009.

[57] A. Bhandoola, H. von Boehmer, H. T. Petrie, and J. C. Zúñiga-Pflücker, "Commitment and developmental potential of extrathymic and intrathymic T cell precursors: plenty to choose from," *Immunity*, vol. 26, no. 6, pp. 678–689, 2007.

[58] L. Corcoran, I. Ferrero, D. Vremec et al., "The lymphoid past of mouse plasmacytoid cells and thymic dendritic cells," *The Journal of Immunology*, vol. 170, no. 10, pp. 4926–4932, 2003.

[59] S. M. Schlenner and H. R. Rodewald, "Early T cell development and the pitfalls of potential," *Trends in Immunology*, vol. 31, no. 8, pp. 303–310, 2010.

[60] M. A. Yui, N. Feng, and E. V. Rothenberg, "Fine-scale staging of T cell lineage commitment in adult mouse thymus," *The Journal of Immunology*, vol. 185, no. 1, pp. 284–293, 2010.

[61] L. Li, M. Leid, and E. V. Rothenberg, "An early T cell lineage commitment checkpoint dependent on the transcription factor Bcl11b," *Science*, vol. 329, no. 5987, pp. 89–93, 2010.

[62] H. E. Porritt, L. L. Rumfelt, S. Tabrizifard, T. M. Schmitt, J. C. Zúñiga-Pflücker, and H. T. Petrie, "Heterogeneity among DN1 prothymocytes reveals multiple progenitors with different capacities to generate T cell and non-T cell lineages," *Immunity*, vol. 20, no. 6, pp. 735–745, 2004.

[63] K. Masuda, K. Kakugawa, T. Nakayama, N. Minato, Y. Katsura, and H. Kawamoto, "T cell lineage determination precedes the initiation of TCRβ gene rearrangement," *The Journal of Immunology*, vol. 179, no. 6, pp. 3699–3706, 2007.

[64] J. J. Bell and A. Bhandoola, "The earliest thymic progenitors for T cells possess myeloid lineage potential," *Nature*, vol. 452, no. 7188, pp. 764–767, 2008.

[65] H. Wada, K. Masuda, R. Satoh et al., "Adult T-cell progenitors retain myeloid potential," *Nature*, vol. 452, no. 7188, pp. 768–772, 2008.

[66] L. Wu, C. L. Li, and K. Shortman, "Thymic dendritic cell precursors: relationship to the T lymphocyte lineage and phenotype of the dendritic cell progeny," *Journal of Experimental Medicine*, vol. 184, no. 3, pp. 903–911, 1996.

[67] J. C. Miller, B. D. Brown, T. Shay et al., "Deciphering the transcriptional network of the dendritic cell lineage," *Nature Immunology*, vol. 13, no. 9, pp. 888–899, 2012.

[68] J. Medvedovic, A. Ebert, and H. Tagoh, *Busslinger M. Pax5: A Master Regulator of B Cell Development and Leukemogenesis*, Elsevier, New York, NY, USA, 1st edition, 2011.

[69] S. Carotta, L. Wu, and S. L. Nutt, "Surprising new roles for PU.1 in the adaptive immune response," *Immunological Reviews*, vol. 238, no. 1, pp. 63–75, 2010.

[70] M. K. Anderson, G. Hernandez-Hoyos, R. A. Diamond, and E. V. Rothenberg, "Precise developmental regulation of Ets family transcription factors during specification and commitment to the T cell lineage," *Development*, vol. 126, no. 14, pp. 3131–3148, 1999.

[71] A. Guerriero, P. B. Langmuir, L. M. Spain, and E. W. Scott, "PU.1 is required for myeloid-derived but not lymphoid-derived dendritic cells," *Blood*, vol. 95, no. 3, pp. 879–885, 2000.

[72] K. L. Anderson, H. Perkin, C. D. Surh, S. Venturini, R. A. Maki, and B. E. Torbett, "Transcription factor PU.1 is necessary for development of thymic and myeloid progenitor-derived dendritic cells," *The Journal of Immunology*, vol. 164, no. 4, pp. 1855–1861, 2000.

[73] A. Dakic, Q. X. Shao, A. D'Amico et al., "Development of the dendritic cell system during mouse ontogeny," *The Journal of Immunology*, vol. 172, no. 2, pp. 1018–1027, 2004.

[74] S. Carotta, A. Dakic, A. D'Amico et al., "The transcription factor PU.1 controls dendritic cell development and Flt3 cytokine receptor expression in a dose-dependent manner," *Immunity*, vol. 32, no. 5, pp. 628–641, 2010.

[75] R. P. DeKoter, H. J. Lee, and H. Singh, "PU.1 regulates expression of the interleukin-7 receptor in lymphoid progenitors," *Immunity*, vol. 16, no. 2, pp. 297–309, 2002.

[76] R. P. DeKoter and H. Singh, "Regulation of B lymphocyte and macrophage development by graded expression of PU.1," *Science*, vol. 288, no. 5470, pp. 1439–1441, 2000.

[77] P. Laslo, C. J. Spooner, A. Warmflash et al., "Multilineage transcriptional priming and determination of alternate hematopoietic cell fates," *Cell*, vol. 126, no. 4, pp. 755–766, 2006.

[78] Y. Bakri, S. Sarrazin, U. P. Mayer et al., "Balance of MafB and PU.1 specifies alternative macrophage or dendritic cell fate," *Blood*, vol. 105, no. 7, pp. 2707–2716, 2005.

[79] M. K. Anderson, A. H. Weiss, G. Hernandez-Hoyos, C. J. Dionne, and E. V. Rothenberg, "Constitutive expression of PU.1 in fetal hematopoietic progenitors blocks T cell development at the pro-T cell stage," *Immunity*, vol. 16, no. 2, pp. 285–296, 2002.

[80] L. M. Spain, A. Guerriero, S. Kunjibettu, and E. W. Scott, "T cell development in PU.1-deficient mice," *The Journal of Immunology*, vol. 163, no. 5, pp. 2681–2687, 1999.

[81] D. E. Zhang, C. J. Hetherington, H. M. Chen, and D. G. Tenen, "The macrophage transcription factor PU.1 directs tissue-specific expression of the macrophage colony-stimulating factor receptor," *Molecular and Cellular Biology*, vol. 14, no. 1, pp. 373–381, 1994.

[82] S. Hohaus, M. S. Petrovick, M. T. Voso, Z. Sun, D. Zhang, and D. G. Tenen, "PU.1 (Spi-1) and C/EBPα regulate expression of the granulocyte-macrophage colony-stimulating factor receptor α gene," *Molecular and Cellular Biology*, vol. 15, no. 10, pp. 5830–5845, 1995.

[83] J. A. Zhang, A. Mortazavi, B. A. Williams, B. J. Wold, and E. V. Rothenberg, "Dynamic transformations of genome-wide epigenetic marking and transcriptional control establish T cell identity," *Cell*, vol. 149, no. 2, pp. 467–482, 2012.

[84] C. B. Franco, D. D. Scripture-Adams, I. Proekt et al., "Notch/δ signaling constrains reengineering of pro-T cells by PU. 1," *Proceedings of the National Academy of Sciences of the United States of America*, vol. 103, no. 32, pp. 11993–11998, 2006.

[85] G. H. Su, H. M. Chen, N. Muthusamy et al., "Defective B cell receptor-mediated responses in mice lacking the Ets protein, Spi-B," *The EMBO Journal*, vol. 16, no. 23, pp. 7118–7129, 1997.

[86] R. Dahl, D. L. Ramirez-Bergeron, S. Rao, and M. C. Simon, "Spi-B can functionally replace PU.1 in myeloid but not lymphoid development," *EMBO Journal*, vol. 21, no. 9, pp. 2220–2230, 2002.

[87] R. Schotte, M. C. Rissoan, N. Bendriss-Vermare et al., "The transcription factor Spi-B is expressed in plasmacytoid DC precursors and inhibits T-, B-, and NK-cell development," *Blood*, vol. 101, no. 3, pp. 1015–1023, 2003.

[88] R. Schotte, M. Nagasawa, K. Weijer, H. Spits, and B. Blom, "The ETS transcription factor Spi-B is required for human plasmacytoid dendritic cell development," *Journal of Experimental Medicine*, vol. 200, no. 11, pp. 1503–1509, 2004.

[89] I. Sasaki, K. Hoshino, T. Sugiyama et al., "Spi-B is critical for plasmacytoid dendritic cell function and development," *Blood*, vol. 120, no. 24, pp. 4733–4743, 2012.

[90] J. M. Lefebvre, M. C. Haks, M. O. Carleton et al., "Enforced expression of Spi-B reverses T lineage commitment and blocks beta-selection," *The Journal of Immunology*, vol. 174, no. 10, pp. 6184–6194, 2005.

[91] L. B. John and A. C. Ward, "The Ikaros gene family: transcriptional regulators of hematopoiesis and immunity," *Molecular Immunology*, vol. 48, no. 9-10, pp. 1272–1278, 2011.

[92] L. Wu, A. Nichogiannopoulou, K. Shortman, and K. Georgopoulos, "Cell-autonomous defects in dendritic cell populations of Ikaros mutant mice point to a developmental relationship with the lymphoid lineage," *Immunity*, vol. 7, no. 4, pp. 483–492, 1997.

[93] D. Allman, M. Dalod, C. Asselin-Paturel et al., "Ikaros is required for plasmacytoid dendritic cell differentiation," *Blood*, vol. 108, no. 13, pp. 4025–4034, 2006.

[94] A. Nichogiannopoulou, M. Trevisan, S. Neben, C. Friedrich, and K. Georgopoulos, "Defects in hemopoietic stem cell activity in Ikaros mutant mice," *Journal of Experimental Medicine*, vol. 190, no. 9, pp. 1201–1214, 1999.

[95] M. A. Zarnegar and E. V. Rothenberg, "Ikaros represses and activates PU.1 cell-type-specifically through the multifunctional Sfpi1 URE and a myeloid specific enhancer," *Oncogene*, vol. 31, no. 43, pp. 4647–4654, 2012.

[96] C. Rathinam, R. Geffers, R. Yücel et al., "The transcriptional repressor Gfi1 controls STAT3-dependent dendritic cell development and function," *Immunity*, vol. 22, no. 6, pp. 717–728, 2005.

[97] H. Li, M. Ji, K. D. Klarmann, and J. R. Keller, "Repression of Id2 expression by Gfi-1 is required for B-cell and myeloid development," *Blood*, vol. 116, no. 7, pp. 1060–1069, 2010.

[98] R. Yücel, C. Kosan, F. Heyd, and T. Möröy, "Gfi1:green fluorescent protein knock-in mutant reveals differential expression and autoregulation of the growth factor independence 1 (Gfi1) gene during lymphocyte development," *The Journal of Biological Chemistry*, vol. 279, no. 39, pp. 40906–40917, 2004.

[99] A. T. Satpathy, K. M. Murphy, and K. C. Wumesh, "Transcription factor networks in dendritic cell development," *Seminars in Immunology*, vol. 23, no. 5, pp. 388–397, 2011.

[100] M. M. Meredith, K. Liu, G. Darrasse-Jeze et al., "Expression of the zinc finger transcription factor zDC (Zbtb46, Btbd4) defines the classical dendritic cell lineage," *Journal of Experimental Medicine*, vol. 209, no. 6, pp. 1153–1165, 2012.

[101] A. T. Satpathy, K. C. Wumesh, J. C. Albring et al., "Zbtb46 expression distinguishes classical dendritic cells and their committed progenitors from other immune lineages," *Journal of Experimental Medicine*, vol. 209, no. 6, pp. 1135–1152, 2012.

[102] M. M. Meredith, K. Liu, A. O. Kamphorst et al., "Zinc finger transcription factor zDC is a negative regulator required to prevent activation of classical dendritic cells in the steady state," *Journal of Experimental Medicine*, vol. 209, no. 9, pp. 1583–1593, 2012.

[103] C. Deweindt, O. Albagli, F. Bernardin et al., "The LAZ3/BCL6 oncogene encodes a sequence-specific transcriptional inhibitor: a novel function for the BTB/POZ domain as an autonomous repressing domain," *Cell Growth and Differentiation*, vol. 6, no. 12, pp. 1495–1503, 1995.

[104] O. Albagli, P. Dhordain, F. Bernardin, S. Quief, J. P. Kerckaert, and D. Leprince, "Multiple domains participate in distance-independent LAZ3/BCL6-mediated transcriptional repression," *Biochemical and Biophysical Research Communications*, vol. 220, no. 3, pp. 911–915, 1996.

[105] R. T. Phan and R. Dalla-Favera, "The BCL6 proto-oncogene suppresses p53 expression in germinal-centre B cells," *Nature*, vol. 432, no. 7017, pp. 635–639, 2004.

[106] A. L. Dent, A. L. Shaffer, X. Yu, D. Allman, and L. M. Staudt, "Control of inflammation, cytokine expression, and germinal center formation by BCL-6," *Science*, vol. 276, no. 5312, pp. 589–592, 1997.

[107] B. H. Ye, G. Cattoretti, Q. Shen et al., "The BCL-6 proto-oncogene controls germinal-centre formation and Th2-type inflammation," *Nature Genetics*, vol. 16, no. 2, pp. 161–170, 1997.

[108] M. Shapiro-Shelef and K. C. Calame, "Regulation of plasma-cell development," *Nature Reviews Immunology*, vol. 5, no. 3, pp. 230–242, 2005.

[109] H. Ohtsuka, A. Sakamoto, J. Pan et al., "Bcl6 is required for the development of mouse CD4$^+$ and CD8α^+ dendritic cells," *The Journal of Immunology*, vol. 186, no. 1, pp. 255–263, 2011.

[110] J. T. Jackson, Y. Hu, R. Liu et al., "Id2 expression delineates differential checkpoints in the genetic program of CD8α^+ and CD103$^+$ dendritic cell lineages," *EMBO Journal*, vol. 30, no. 13, pp. 2690–2704, 2011.

[111] C. Hacker, R. D. Kirsch, X. S. Ju et al., "Transcriptional profiling identifies Id2 function in dendritic cell development," *Nature Immunology*, vol. 4, no. 4, pp. 380–386, 2003.

[112] H. S. Ghosh, B. Cisse, A. Bunin, K. L. Lewis, and B. Reizis, "Continuous expression of the transcription factor E2-2 maintains the cell fate of mature plasmacytoid dendritic cells," *Immunity*, vol. 33, no. 6, pp. 905–916, 2010.

[113] D. Wang, C. L. Claus, G. Vaccarelli et al., "The basic helix-loop-helix transcription factor HEBAlt is expressed in pro-T cells and enhances the generation of t cell precursors," *The Journal of Immunology*, vol. 177, no. 1, pp. 109–119, 2006.

[114] M. Braunstein and M. K. Anderson, "HEB in the spotlight: transcriptional regulation of T-cell specification, commitment, and developmental plasticity," *Clinical and Developmental Immunology*, vol. 2012, Article ID 678705, 15 pages, 2012.

[115] B. T. Edelson, K. C. Wumesh, R. Juang et al., "Peripheral CD103$^+$ dendritic cells form a unified subset developmentally related to CD8α^+ conventional dendritic cells," *Journal of Experimental Medicine*, vol. 207, no. 4, pp. 823–836, 2010.

[116] D. M. Gascoyne, E. Long, H. Veiga-Fernandes et al., "The basic leucine zipper transcription factor E4BP4 is essential for natural killer cell development," *Nature Immunology*, vol. 10, no. 10, pp. 1118–1124, 2009.

[117] S. Kamizono, G. S. Duncan, M. G. Seidel et al., "Nfil3/E4bp4 is required for the development and maturation of NK cells in vivo," *Journal of Experimental Medicine*, vol. 206, no. 13, pp. 2977–2986, 2009.

[118] L. Burkly, C. Hession, L. Ogata et al., "Expression of relB is required for the development of thymic medulla and dendritic cells," *Nature*, vol. 373, no. 6514, pp. 531–536, 1995.

[119] L. Wu, A. D'Amico, K. D. Winkel, M. Suter, D. Lo, and K. Shortman, "RelB is essential for the development of myeloid-related CD8α^- dendritic cells but not of lymphoid-related CD8α^+ dendritic cells," *Immunity*, vol. 9, no. 6, pp. 839–847, 1998.

[120] S. C. Sun, "The noncanonical NF-κB pathway," *Immunological Reviews*, vol. 246, no. 1, pp. 125–140, 2012.

[121] A. Le Bon, M. Montoya, M. J. Edwards et al., "A role for the transcription factor RelB in IFN-α production and in IFN-α-stimulated cross-priming," *European The Journal of Immunology*, vol. 36, no. 8, pp. 2085–2093, 2006.

[122] M. Li, X. Zhang, X. Zheng et al., "Immune modulation and tolerance induction by RelB-silenced dendritic cells through RNA interference," *The Journal of Immunology*, vol. 178, no. 9, pp. 5480–5487, 2007.

[123] A. Battistini, "Interferon regulatory factors in hematopoietic cell differentiation and immune regulation," *Journal of Interferon and Cytokine Research*, vol. 29, no. 12, pp. 765–780, 2009.

[124] G. Schiavoni, F. Mattei, P. Sestili et al., "ICSBP is essential for the development of mouse type I interferon-producing cells and for the generation and activation of CD8α^+ dendritic cells," *Journal of Experimental Medicine*, vol. 196, no. 11, pp. 1415–1425, 2002.

[125] J. Aliberti, O. Schulz, D. J. Pennington et al., "Essential role for ICSBP in the in vivo development of murine CD8α^+ dendritic cells," *Blood*, vol. 101, no. 1, pp. 305–310, 2003.

[126] G. Schiavoni, F. Mattei, P. Borghi et al., "ICSBP is critically involved in the normal development and trafficking of Langerhans cells and dermal dendritic cells," *Blood*, vol. 103, no. 6, pp. 2221–2228, 2004.

[127] H. Tsujimura, T. Tamura, and K. Ozato, "Cutting edge: IFN consensus sequence binding protein/IFN regulatory factor 8 drives the development of type I IFN-producing plasmacytoid dendritic cells," *The Journal of Immunology*, vol. 170, no. 3, pp. 1131–1135, 2003.

[128] P. Tailor, T. Tamura, H. C. Morse, and K. Ozato, "The BXH2 mutation in IRF8 differentially impairs dendritic cell subset development in the mouse," *Blood*, vol. 111, no. 4, pp. 1942–1945, 2008.

[129] S. Suzuki, K. Honma, T. Matsuyama et al., "Critical roles of interferon regulatory factor 4 in CD11b^{high}CD8α^- dendritic cell development," *Proceedings of the National Academy of Sciences of the United States of America*, vol. 101, no. 24, pp. 8981–8986, 2004.

[130] T. Tamura, P. Tailor, K. Yamaoka et al., "IFN regulatory factor-4 and -8 govern dendritic cell subset development and their functional diversity," *The Journal of Immunology*, vol. 174, no. 5, pp. 2573–2581, 2005.

[131] S. Bajana, K. Roach, S. Turner, J. Paul, and S. Kovats, "IRF4 promotes cutaneous dendritic cell migration to lymph nodes during homeostasis and inflammation," *The Journal of Immunology*, vol. 189, no. 7, pp. 3368–3377, 2012.

[132] L. Gabriele, A. Fragale, P. Borghi et al., "IRF-1 deficiency skews the differentiation of dendritic cells toward plasmacytoid and tolerogenic features," *Journal of Leukocyte Biology*, vol. 80, no. 6, pp. 1500–1511, 2006.

[133] K. Honda, T. Mizutani, and T. Taniguchi, "Negative regulation of IFN-α/β signaling by IFN regulatory factor 2 for homeostatic development of dendritic cells," *Proceedings of the National Academy of Sciences of the United States of America*, vol. 101, no. 8, pp. 2416–2421, 2004.

[134] K. Inaba, M. Inaba, N. Romani et al., "Generation of large numbers of dendritic cells from mouse bone marrow cultures supplemented with granulocyte/macrophage colony-stimulating factor," *Journal of Experimental Medicine*, vol. 176, no. 6, pp. 1693–1702, 1992.

[135] K. Brasel, T. De Smedt, J. L. Smith, and C. R. Maliszewski, "Generation of murine dendritic cells from flt3-ligand-supplemented bone marrow cultures," *Blood*, vol. 96, no. 9, pp. 3029–3039, 2000.

[136] M. Gilliet, A. Boonstra, C. Paturel et al., "The development of murine plasmacytoid dendritic cell precursors is differentially regulated by FLT3-ligand and granulocyte/macrophage colony-stimulating factor," *Journal of Experimental Medicine*, vol. 195, no. 7, pp. 953–958, 2002.

[137] S. H. Naik, L. M. Corcoran, and L. Wu, "Development of murine plasmacytoid dendritic cell subsets," *Immunology and Cell Biology*, vol. 83, no. 5, pp. 563–570, 2005.

[138] B. Fancke, M. Suter, H. Hochrein, and M. O'Keeffe, "M-CSF: a novel plasmacytoid and conventional dendritic cell poietin," *Blood*, vol. 111, no. 1, pp. 150–159, 2008.

[139] H. Karsunky, M. Merad, A. Cozzio, I. L. Weissman, and M. G. Manz, "Flt3 ligand regulates dendritic cell development from Flt3$^+$ lymphoid and myeloid-committed progenitors to Flt3$^+$ dendritic cells in vivo," *Journal of Experimental Medicine*, vol. 198, no. 2, pp. 305–313, 2003.

[140] J. L. Christensen and I. L. Weissman, "Flk-2 is a marker in hematopoietic stem cell differentiation: a simple method to isolate long-term stem cells," *Proceedings of the National Academy of Sciences of the United States of America*, vol. 98, no. 25, pp. 14541–14546, 2001.

[141] E. Sitnicka, D. Bryder, K. Theilgaard-Mönch, N. Buza-Vidas, J. Adolfsson, and S. E. W. Jacobsen, "Key role of flt3 ligand in regulation of the common lymphoid progenitor but not in maintenance of the hematopoietic stem cell pool," *Immunity*, vol. 17, no. 4, pp. 463–472, 2002.

[142] N. Onai, A. Obata-Onai, R. Tussiwand, A. Lanzavecchia, and M. G. Manz, "Activation of the Flt3 signal transduction cascade rescues and enhances type I interferon-producing and dendritic cell development," *Journal of Experimental Medicine*, vol. 203, no. 1, pp. 227–238, 2006.

[143] H. J. McKenna, K. L. Stocking, R. E. Miller et al., "Mice lacking flt3 ligand have deficient hematopoiesis affecting hematopoietic progenitor cells, dendritic cells, and natural killer cells," *Blood*, vol. 95, no. 11, pp. 3489–3497, 2000.

[144] M. D. Witmer-Pack, D. A. Hughes, G. Schuler et al., "Identification of macrophages and dendritic cells in the osteopetrotic (op/op) mouse," *Journal of Cell Science*, vol. 104, no. 4, pp. 1021–1029, 1993.

[145] K. P. A. MacDonald, V. Rowe, H. M. Bofinger et al., "The colony-stimulating factor 1 receptor is expressed on dendritic cells during differentiation and regulates their expansion," *The Journal of Immunology*, vol. 175, no. 3, pp. 1399–1405, 2005.

[146] F. Ginhoux, M. Greter, M. Leboeuf et al., "Fate mapping analysis reveals that adult microglia derive from primitive macrophages," *Science*, vol. 330, no. 6005, pp. 841–845, 2010.

[147] R. M. Ransohoff and A. E. Cardona, "The myeloid cells of the central nervous system parenchyma," *Nature*, vol. 468, no. 7321, pp. 253–262, 2010.

[148] G. Hoeffel, Y. Wang, M. Greter et al., "Adult Langerhans cells derive predominantly from embryonic fetal liver monocytes with a minor contribution of yolk sac-derived macrophages," *Journal of Experimental Medicine*, vol. 209, no. 6, pp. 1167–1181, 2012.

[149] F. Ginhoux, F. Tacke, V. Angeli et al., "Langerhans cells arise from monocytes in vivo," *Nature Immunology*, vol. 7, no. 3, pp. 265–273, 2006.

[150] H. Lin, E. Lee, K. Hestir et al., "Discovery of a cytokine and its receptor by functional screening of the extracellular proteome," *Science*, vol. 320, no. 5877, pp. 807–811, 2008.

[151] Y. Wang, K. J. Szretter, W. Vermi et al., "IL-34 is a tissue-restricted ligand of CSF1R required for the development of Langerhans cells and microglia," *Nature Immunology*, vol. 13, no. 8, pp. 753–760, 2012.

[152] M. Greter, I. Lelios, P. Pelczar et al., "Stroma-derived interleukin-34 controls the development and maintenance of Langerhans cells and the maintenance of microglia," *Immunity*, vol. 37, no. 6, pp. 1050–1060, 2012.

[153] D. Kingston, M. A. Schmid, N. Onai, A. Obata-Onai, D. Baumjohann, and M. G. Manz, "The concerted action of GM-CSF and Flt3-ligand on in vivo dendritic cell homeostasis," *Blood*, vol. 114, no. 4, pp. 835–843, 2009.

[154] R. T. Sasmono, D. Oceandy, J. W. Pollard et al., "A macrophage colony-stimulating factor receptor-green fluorescent protein transgene is expressed throughout the mononuclear phagocyte system of the mouse," *Blood*, vol. 101, no. 3, pp. 1155–1163, 2003.

[155] D. Vremec, G. J. Lieschke, A. R. Dunn, L. Robb, D. Metcalf, and K. Shortman, "The influence of granulocyte/macrophage colony-stimulating factor on dendritic cell levels in mouse lymphoid organs," *European The Journal of Immunology*, vol. 27, no. 1, pp. 40–44, 1997.

[156] Y. Zhan, J. Vega-Ramos, E. M. Carrington et al., "The inflammatory cytokine, GM-CSF, alters the developmental outcome of murine dendritic cells," *European Journal of Immunology*, vol. 42, no. 11, pp. 2889–2900, 2012.

[157] I. L. King, M. A. Kroenke, and B. M. Segal, "GM-CSF-dependent, CD103$^+$ dermal dendritic cells play a critical role in Th effector cell differentiation after subcutaneous immunization," *Journal of Experimental Medicine*, vol. 207, no. 5, pp. 953–961, 2010.

[158] M. Greter, J. Helft, A. Chow et al., "GM-CSF controls nonlymphoid tissue dendritic cell homeostasis but is dispensable for the differentiation of inflammatory dendritic cells," *Immunity*, vol. 36, no. 6, pp. 1031–1046, 2012.

[159] B. T. Edelson, T. R. Bradstreet, K. C. Wumesh et al., "Batf3-dependent CD11blow/-peripheral dendritic cells are GM-CSF-independent and are not required for Th cell priming after subcutaneous immunization," *PLoS ONE*, vol. 6, no. 10, Article ID e25660, 2011.

[160] D. Saunders, K. Lucas, J. Ismaili et al., "Dendritic cell development in culture from thymic precursor cells in the absence of granulocyte/macrophage colony-stimulating factor," *Journal of Experimental Medicine*, vol. 184, no. 6, pp. 2185–2196, 1996.

[161] P. Sathe, J. Pooley, D. Vremec et al., "The acquisition of antigen cross-presentation function by newly formed dendritic cells," *The Journal of Immunology*, vol. 186, no. 9, pp. 5184–5192, 2011.

[162] Y. Zhan, E. M. Carrington, A. van Nieuwenhuijze et al., "GM-CSF increases cross-presentation and CD103 expression by mouse CD8$^+$ spleen dendritic cells," *European Journal of Immunology*, vol. 41, no. 9, pp. 2585–2595, 2011.

[163] E. V. Rothenberg, J. E. Moore, and M. A. Yui, "Launching the T-cell-lineage developmental programme," *Nature Reviews Immunology*, vol. 8, no. 1, pp. 9–21, 2008.

[164] J. H. Wang, A. Nichogiannopoulou, L. Wu et al., "Selective defects in the development of the fetal and adult lymphoid system in mice with an Ikaros null mutation," *Immunity*, vol. 5, no. 6, pp. 537–549, 1996.

[165] P. M. Domínguez and C. Ardavín, "Differentiation and function of mouse monocyte-derived dendritic cells in steady state and inflammation," *Immunological Reviews*, vol. 234, no. 1, pp. 90–104, 2010.

30

Thalassemia and Hemoglobin E in Southern Thai Blood Donors

Manit Nuinoon,[1] Kwanta Kruachan,[2] Warachaya Sengking,[1] Dararat Horpet,[3] and Ubol Sungyuan[2]

[1] *School of Allied Health Sciences and Public Health, Walailak University, Nakhon Si Thammarat 80161, Thailand*
[2] *Regional Blood Centre XI, National Blood Centre Thai Red Cross Society, Nakhon Si Thammarat 80110, Thailand*
[3] *Center for Scientific and Technological Equipment, Walailak University, Nakhon Si Thammarat 80161, Thailand*

Correspondence should be addressed to Manit Nuinoon; manit.nu@wu.ac.th

Academic Editor: John Roback

Thalassemia and hemoglobin E (Hb E) are common in Thailand. Individuals with thalassemia trait usually have a normal hemoglobin concentration or mild anemia. Therefore, thalassemic individuals who have minimum acceptable Hb level may be accepted as blood donors. This study was aimed at determining the frequency of α-thalassemia 1 trait, β-thalassemia trait, and Hb E-related syndromes in Southern Thai blood donors. One hundred and sixteen voluntary blood donors, Southern Thailand origin, were recruited for thalassemia and Hb E screening by red blood cell indices/dichlorophenolindophenol precipitation test. β-Thalassemia and Hb E were then identified by high performance liquid chromatography and 4 common α-thalassemia deletions were characterized by a single tube-multiplex gap-polymerase chain reaction. Overall frequency of hemoglobinopathies was 12.9%, classified as follows: homozygous α-thalassemia 2 (1.7%), heterozygous α-thalassemia 1 (1.7%), heterozygous β-thalassemia without α-thalassemia (0.9%), heterozygous Hb E without α-thalassemia (5.2%), double heterozygotes for Hb E/α-thalassemia 1 (1.7%), homozygous Hb E without α-thalassemia (0.9%), and homozygous Hb E with heterozygous α-thalassemia 2 (0.9%). The usefulness of thalassemia screening is not only for receiving highly effective red blood cells in the recipients but also for encouraging the control and prevention program of thalassemia in blood donors.

1. Introduction

α-Thalassemia, β-thalassemia, and Hb E ($\beta^{\text{codon 26, Glu} \rightarrow \text{Lys}}$), the most common genetic blood disorders, are considered not only public health problems but also socioeconomic problem in Thailand [1, 2]. The frequencies of α-thalassemia, β-thalassemia, and Hb E carriers in Thailand were ranged from 20 to 30%, 3 to 9% and 10 to 60%, respectively, and vary from region to region [3, 4]. These abnormal globin genes in different combinations lead to more than 60 thalassemia syndromes including three severe thalassemic diseases found in Thailand such as Hb Bart's hydrops fetalis (homozygous α-thalassemia 1, --/--), homozygous β-thalassemia (β^+/β^+, β^+/β^0, or β^0/β^0), and β-thalassemia/Hb E (β^+/β^E or β^0/β^E). Thai married couples are at risk of giving birth to babies with severe hemoglobinopathies about 5.6% [2]. To reduce the number of affected patients with severe thalassemia syndrome, the prevention and control program for thalassemia

in Thailand is necessary by screening the carriers of abnormal genes in general population [5]. Concerning the precision of thalassemia diagnosis, the red blood cells from Hb E donors (Hb E trait or homozygous Hb E) can cause the misdiagnosis of thalassemia in the normal recipients (false positive) or the red blood cells from normal donors can cause the misdiagnosis of thalassemia in the thalassemic recipients (false negative) [6]. The prevalence of thalassemia and abnormal hemoglobin in general population has been reported in several studies. In Thailand the hemoglobin concentration of thalassemia carriers is variable ranging from anemia to normal range because there are different numbers of globin gene defects and interactions of α-and β-thalassemia in a region with high frequency [7, 8]. According to AABB's (American Association of Blood Banks) Technical Manual, minimal hemoglobin concentration for accepting a blood donor is not less than 125 g/L for allogeneic donor and 110 g/L for autologous donor [9]. Therefore, the thalassemia traits with normal hemoglobin concentration could donate their blood. Nowadays, the study of thalassemia and abnormal hemoglobin in blood donors has been reported in several populations with different frequencies [10–15]. This report is the first published data in Thailand that provides the useful data for hemoglobinopathies among blood donors for reducing a number of severe thalassemia patients.

2. Materials and Methods

A cross-sectional study was conducted at Regional Blood Centre XI, National Blood Centre Thai Red Cross Society, Nakhon Si Thammarat from July to September 2013. The samples were collected from different hospitals located in Southern Thailand. The study protocol was reviewed and approved by the institutional review board of Walailak University, Thailand (IRB number 2013-011). Informed consent was confirmed by the IRB. After informed consent was obtained, peripheral blood samples anticoagulated with EDTA were collected from 116 Southern Thai voluntary blood donors who had passed the donor self-exclusion according to AABB criteria. Briefly, donors must be between the ages of 17 and 70 years and must weigh more than 45 kilograms and be in good health with no risks of infectious diseases. According to blood donor criteria of Thai Red Cross Society, minimal Hb concentration for accepting a blood donor is not less than 120 g/L and 130 g/L for female and male, respectively. Hb concentration was estimated by copper sulfate ($CuSO_4$) specific gravity method. Copper sulfate with specific gravity of 1.052 (representing Hb concentration of 120 g/L) was used for Hb screening in female donors and specific gravity of 1.053 (representing Hb concentration of 130 g/L) was used for Hb screening in female donors. The individuals who have a drop of blood floats or takes too long to sink are deferred and were excluded from this study.

Complete blood count (CBC) was determined by using an automated blood cell analyzer, MEK-8222 K (NIHON KOHDEN, Tokyo, Japan). Mean corpuscular volume (MCV) and dichlorophenolindophenol precipitation test by using the KKU-DCIP Clear Reagent Kit (PCL Holding, Bangkok, Thailand) were used as thalassemia and Hb E screening methods, respectively. The positive results of MCV (<80 fL) and/or DCIP were subsequently performed Hb typing by high performance liquid chromatography (HPLC). Hemoglobin type and quantitation of Hb A_2/E, Hb A, and Hb F were conducted by an automated hemoglobin cation exchange HPLC (Variant β-thalassemia short program, Bio-rad Laboratories, Hercules, CA).

Genomic DNA was extracted from peripheral blood leukocytes by using the Genomic DNA Extraction Kit (Geneaid, Taipei, Taiwan) according to the manufacturer's instructions. Concentration and quality of a sample of genomic DNA are measured with ND-1000 (NanoDrop Technologies, Wilmington, DE). To characterize the α-globin gene deletions, the 3.7 kb ($-\alpha^{3.7}$) and 4.2 kb ($-\alpha^{4.2}$) deletion types for α-thalassemia 2, Southeast Asian ($--^{SEA}$), and THAI ($--^{THAI}$) deletions' types for α-thalassemia 1 were performed by multiplex GAP-PCR [16] in the all samples with low MCV ($\leq$80 fL). Therefore, α-thalassemia 2 trait

was not separated from normal individuals by DNA testing in this study. PCR products were amplified by GeneAmp PCR system 9700 (Perkin Elmer, CT, USA). 8 μL of PCR products was electrophoresized in 1.5% agarose gel, stained with ethidium bromide, and visualized and photographed by a gel documentation system (G-Box, SynGene, Frederick, MD, USA).

2.1. Statistical Analysis. The data were presented as mean $\pm$ standard deviation (SD). Statistical comparison of hematological data was conducted with the nonparametric Kruskal-Wallis test using SPSS version 17.0 (SPSS, Chicago, IL, USA). P values < 0.05 were considered statistically significant.

3. Results

A total of 116 voluntary blood donors were recruited in this study, 65 males (56%) and 51 females (44%). All voluntary blood donors lived in Southern Thailand. The mean age ($\pm$ SD) was 33 $\pm$ 11.3 years (range: 17–58 years) old. The most common status of the subjects was single (55%). Blood groups "O" and "B" were found to be the codominant and all donors were positive Rh (D) blood group. The average values of all red cell parameters were ranged in the normal values. The high variation of red cell volume (MCV) was observed (SD = 6.94) because of hemoglobinopathies as shown in Table 1. Table 2 represents the prevalence of hemoglobinopathies in 116 Southern Thai blood donors. According to our study design, α-thalassemia 1, β-thalassemia, and Hb E were focused on and identified because they can cause the severe thalassemia in the next generation such as Hb Bart's hydrops fetalis, homozygous β-thalassemia, and β-thalassemia/Hb E disease. The normal individuals and α-thalassemia 2 traits were not differentiated by DNA analysis because of its high cost and its low importance. Out of 116 donors, 101 (87.1%) donors were diagnosed as normal or heterozygous α-thalassemia 2 and 15 (12.9%) donors were interpreted as thalassemia and/or abnormal hemoglobin. Among these hemoglobinopathies, Hb E-related disorders (both Hb E heterozygote and homozygote with and without α-thalassemia) are the most common form of hemoglobinopathies accounting for 8.6% (10/116), followed by heterozygous α-thalassemia 1 (both heterozygous α-thalassemia 1 [1.7%] and double heterozygote for Hb E and heterozygous α-thalassemia 1 [1.7%]) accounting for 3.4% (4/116) and heterozygous β-thalassemia accounting for 0.9% (1/116).

We divided the 116 Southern Thai blood donors into seven groups according to the type of thalassemia and Hb E (red cell indices, Hb type, and DNA analysis were used to interpret the phenotype). Hematological findings are listed and compared as shown in Table 3. Multiplex gap PCR for determining α-globin gene deletions as depicted in Figure 1. Normal and α-thalassemia 2 traits are the major component of the studied donors. We found statistically significant differences for all hematological parameters among the four groups (groups I, II, IV, and V); when they were analyzed using the nonparametric Kruskal-Wallis test, MCV, MCH, and % Hb A_2/E were most obvious (P < 0.001). In this

TABLE 1: Descriptive data and hematological findings of voluntary blood donors ($n = 116$).

Donor characteristics	Number of donors (%)
Gender	
Male	65 (56)
Female	51 (44)
Status	
Single	64 (55)
Married	47 (41)
Others	5 (4)
ABO blood group system	
A	29 (25)
B	41 (35)
O	38 (33)
AB	8 (7)
Rh (D) blood group system	
Positive	116 (100)
Negative	0 (0)
Age (years)*	33 ± 11.3 (17–58)
Hematological data**	
RBC (10^{12}/L)	5.0 ± 0.60
Hemoglobin (g/L)	140 ± 13.3
HCT (L/L)	0.41 ± 0.04
MCV (fL)	82.8 ± 6.94
MCH (pg)	28.2 ± 2.71
MCHC (g/dL)	34.0 ± 0.69
RDW (%)	12.5 ± 1.16

*Age is presented as mean ± standard deviation (range).
**Hematological data are expressed as mean ± standard deviation.

TABLE 2: Prevalence of thalassemia and Hb E among Southern Thai blood donors.

Diagnosis	Number of donors (%)
Normal and heterozygous α-thalassemia 2	101 (87.1)
Homozygous α-thalassemia 2	2 (1.7)
Heterozygous α-thalassemia 1	2 (1.7)
Heterozygous β-thalassemia without α-thalassemia	1 (0.9)
Heterozygous Hb E without α-thalassemia	6 (5.2)
Double heterozygotes for Hb E/α-thalassemia 1	2 (1.7)
Homozygous Hb E without α-thalassemia	1 (0.9)
Homozygous Hb E with heterozygous α-thalassemia 2	1 (0.9)
Total	116 (100)

study, homozygous Hb E without α-thalassemia interaction had the lowest MCV and MCH compared with other groups. Increased Hb A_2/E levels were observed in β-thalassemia trait, Hb E trait, and Hb E homozygote. Coinheritance of α-thalassemia in Hb E heterozygote was found to be decreased hematological parameters compared with Hb E heterozygote with no α-thalassemia interaction. In contrast, interaction

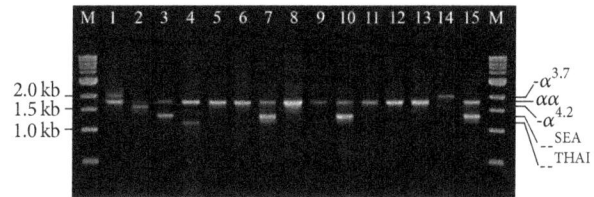

FIGURE 1: Representative 1.5% agarose gel electrophoresis of the amplified PCR products for characterizing α-globin gene deletion types by multiplex gap PCR. The 2 kb, 1.8 kb, 1.6 kb, 1.4 kb and 1.2 kb represent 3.7 kb deletion fragment ($-\alpha^{3.7}$), normal fragment ($\alpha\alpha$), 4.2 kb deletion fragment ($-\alpha^{4.2}$), SEA type deletion fragment ($--^{SEA}$), and THAI type deletion fragment ($--^{THAI}$), respectively. The M represents the 1 kb DNA ladder. Lanes 1–4 (positive controls) are genotypes as follows: $-\alpha^{3.7}/\alpha\alpha$, $-\alpha^{4.2}/\alpha\alpha$, $--^{SEA}/\alpha\alpha$, and $--^{THAI}/\alpha\alpha$, respectively. Lanes 5, 6, 8, 9, and 11–13 are normal α-globin genotype ($\alpha\alpha/\alpha\alpha$). Lanes 7, 10, and 15 are heterozygous α-thalassemia 1 ($--^{SEA}/\alpha\alpha$). Lane 14 is homozygous α-thalassemia 2 ($-\alpha^{3.7}/-\alpha^{3.7}$).

of α-thalassemia in Hb E homozygote was found to have improved hematological parameters (increased Hb, MCV, and MCH) compared with Hb E homozygote with no α-thalassemia. Microcytic (MCV < 80 fL) and/or hypochromic (MCH < 27 pg) red blood cells were 25.9% (30/116) and 26.7% (31/116), respectively. Among 30 blood donors with microcytic red blood cells, fifteen blood donors (50%) were found to have hemoglobinopathies and the left blood donors may be having an iron deficiency and/or α-thalassemia 2 trait.

HbA$_2$/E levels are used to diagnose the β-thalassemia trait (%HbA$_2$ = 4.0–8.0) and Hb E-related disorders (HbA$_2$/E > 10.0%). However, α-thalassemia and interaction of α-thalassemia in β-thalassemia and Hb E-related disorders, red blood cell indices, and Hb typing could not be used for interpretation. In this study, multiplex gap PCR was used to characterize the four common α-globin gene deletions (both α-thalassemia 1 allele [$--^{SEA}$ and $--^{THAI}$] and α-thalassemia 2 allele [$-\alpha^{3.7}$ and $-\alpha^{4.2}$]) as shown in Figure 1. Table 4 demonstrates the number of risk alleles among thalassemia or Hb E-related blood donors. From all blood donors, there are 17 alleles (from 13 blood donors) that can cause the severe thalassemia in the offspring (risk allele frequency = 3.7%). Among 17 risk alleles, Hb E allele (β^E) is the most common form of all risk alleles ($--/$, $\beta^{0/+}$ and β^E), 12/17 (70.6%), followed by α-thalassemia 1 allele ($--/$), 4/17 (23.5%), and β-thalassemia allele ($\beta^{0/+}$), 1/17 (5.9%).

4. Discussion

Blood donor selection is crucial to ensure the safety of both donors and recipients. According to the standards of the American Association of Blood Banks (AABB), hemoglobin concentration more than 125 g/L was accepted for blood donation [9]. The prevalence of thalassemia and abnormal hemoglobin varies from region to region, the frequency of α-thalassemia in Bangkok and northern Thailand was ranging from 20 to 30%, and β-thalassemia varies between 3 and 9%. Among abnormal hemoglobin, Hb E is the most

TABLE 3: Hematological findings of normal and different types of thalassemia and Hb E.

Group (n)	Hb (g/L)	MCV (fL)	MCH (pg)	Hb A$_2$/E (%)
I. Normal and heterozygous α-thalassemia 2 ($n = 101$)	141 ± 13.4	84.9 ± 4.31	30.0 ± 1.68	—
II. Homozygous α-thalassemia 2 and heterozygous α-thalassemia 1 ($n = 4$)	129 ± 10.5	65.1 ± 2.44	21.4 ± 0.90	2.9 ± 0.25
III. Heterozygous β-thalassemia without α-thalassemia ($n = 1$)	139	62.2	20.0	5.0
IV. Heterozygous Hb E without α-thalassemia ($n = 6$)	134 ± 9.6	75.1 ± 3.39	25.2 ± 1.16	26.2 ± 0.58
V. Double heterozygotes for Hb E/α-thalassemia 1 ($n = 2$)	123 ± 6.4	67.5 ± 1.84	21.8 ± 0.57	19.3 ± 0.64
VI. Homozygous Hb E without α-thalassemia ($n = 1$)	127	61.6	19.7	74.5
VII. Homozygous Hb E with heterozygous α-thalassemia 2 ($n = 1$)	139	67.6	22.0	75.4
P value*	0.05	<0.001	<0.001	<0.001

Hematological data are expressed either as mean ± standard deviation (SD) or raw data where appropriate ($n = 1$, groups III, VI, and VII).
Hb: hemoglobin; g/L: gram per liter; MCV: mean corpuscular volume; fL: femtoliter; MCH: mean corpuscular hemoglobin; pg: picogram.
*P value was calculated by using the nonparametric Kruskal-Wallis test (groups I, II, IV, and V were compared).

TABLE 4: Number of risk alleles and risk allele frequency in Southern Thai blood donors.

Diagnosis	α-Globin and β-globin genotypes	Number of alleles*	Number of risk alleles (risk allele)
Normal, heterozygous α-thalassemia 2, and homozygous α-thalassemia 2 ($n = 103$)	$\alpha\alpha/\alpha\alpha$, $-\alpha/\alpha\alpha$, $-\alpha/-\alpha$, and β^A/β^A	412	0
Heterozygous α-thalassemia 1 ($n = 2$)	$--^{SEA}/\alpha\alpha$, β^A/β^A	8	2 ($--^{SEA}$)
Heterozygous β-thalassemia without α-thalassemia ($n = 1$)	$\alpha\alpha/\alpha\alpha$, $\beta^{0/+}/\beta^A$	4	1 ($\beta^{0/+}$)
Heterozygous Hb E without α-thalassemia ($n = 6$)	$\alpha\alpha/\alpha\alpha$, β^E/β^A	24	6 (β^E)
Double heterozygotes for Hb E/α-thalassemia 1 ($n = 2$)	$--^{SEA}/\alpha\alpha$, β^E/β^A	8	4 ($2*\beta^E$ and $2*--^{SEA}$)
Homozygous Hb E with and without heterozygous α-thalassemia 2 ($n = 2$)	$-\alpha/\alpha\alpha$, $\alpha\alpha/\alpha\alpha$, and β^E/β^E	8	4 (β^E)
Total ($n = 116$)		464	17
Risk allele frequency = 17/464 * 100 = 3.7%			

$--^{SEA}$: α-thalassemia 1 allele with Southeast Asian type deletion; $\beta^{0/+}$: β^0 or β^+-thalassemia allele with uncharacterized β-globin gene mutation; β^A: normal β-globin gene; β^E: Hb E allele.
*The number of alleles was calculated from two alleles of α-globin genotype ($\alpha\alpha/\alpha\alpha$) and two alleles from β-globin genotype (β/β) [4 alleles were considered per one donor].

common, especially in the northeastern part of Thailand and the junction of Thailand with Laos and Cambodia where its prevalence can reach 50–60% [3, 4, 17]. The prevalence of β-thalassemia trait, Hb E trait, homozygous Hb E, and α-thalassemia 1 trait in Southern Thai couples was 2.22%, 12.08%, 1.11%, and 3.06%, respectively, and among Thai population; Southern Thai population was found to have the lowest prevalence of thalassemia and Hb E [18]. In this study similar pattern with lower frequency of thalassemia and Hb E was observed in blood donors because Hb concentration in thalassemia carriers (α-thalassemia 1 trait, β-thalassemia trait, and Hb E-related syndromes) varies ranging from normal value to very slight anemia [7, 19, 20]. Therefore, thalassemic individuals could or could not donate the blood and some thalassemic individuals who have anemia were excluded from this study. The frequencies of thalassemia in blood donors have been reported in several populations [10–12, 21]. For example, among 80 Malaysian blood donors, the frequency of thalassemia was 16.25% which is slightly higher than this study [12]. Tiwari and Chandola [22] reported that the prevalence of microcytosis in Indian blood donors was

5.4% (50/925). Alabdulaali et al. [23] published that sickle cell trait was found 2% (23/1,150) in King Khalid University Hospital (KKUH) in Riyadh. In addition, Bryant et al. [24] found that 2.8% (33/1,162) of the apheresis donors had low mean corpuscular volume values (MCV < 80 fL). In the present study, microcytosis was found to be 25.9% in blood donors. These blood donors could be having hemoglobinopathies and/or iron deficiency [25, 26]. For other red blood cell disorders, glucose-6-phosphate dehydrogenase deficiency was found to be 1.1% (33/3,004) in Italian blood donors [27], 0.3% (1/301) in a metropolitan transfusion service [28], and 0.78% (9/1,150) in King Khalid University Hospital (KKUH) in Riyadh. The importance of glucose-6-phosphate dehydrogenase deficiency is red blood cell destruction in response to several oxidative stresses [29]. Increased osmotic fragility of erythrocytes in 1,464 healthy German blood donors was 1.1% (16/1,464) [30]. Iron deficiency was also observed in blood donors [31, 32]. Donor selection is very important to protect both the donor and the recipient. In this study, two important issues are concerned and highlighted. Firstly, concerning the quality of red blood cells, it is common practice in many hospitals or transfusion service centers to accept blood for transfusion from donors with thalassemia minor . However, two donors with homozygous Hb E from this study have normal Hb levels (12.7 and 13.9 g/dL) with very low MCV (61.6 and 67.6 fL) and MCH (19.7 and 22.0 pg) consistent with the blood smear showing microcytic and hypochromic red blood cells. High quality of packed red cell (PRC) for regularly transfused patients such as severe β-thalassemia patients should be considered. The red blood cells from blood donors can cause the misdiagnosis of thalassemia in the recipients (false positive or false negative), for example, individuals who have received blood transfusions from Hb E-related donors (Hb E trait or Hb E homozygote) or Hb E-related individuals who have received transfusions from normal blood donors [6]. Therefore, not only quantitative screening but also qualitative evaluation is necessary for selecting blood for severe thalassemia patients. Secondly, blood donors may be carriers of the hemoglobinopathies without being aware of it because they can donate the blood. In Thailand prevention and control program of severe thalassemia has been established [32]. Screening of hemoglobinopathies in blood donors is one of strategies for prevention and control of severe thalassemia. Hemoglobin Bart's hydrops fetalis, homozygous β-thalassemia, and β-thalassemia/Hb E are concerned and programmed for prenatal diagnosis in Thailand [33, 34]. Three important risk alleles (α-thalassemia 1, β-thalassemia, and Hb E) are found in these blood donors and they are at risk of giving birth to babies with severe hemoglobinopathies. Thus, it is very important to characterize the type of hemoglobinopathies and understand the multiple gene-gene interactions in order to provide proper counseling to the blood donors. Furthermore, DNA testing is also necessary to confirm the phenotypes of hemoglobinopathies.

5. Conclusion

This preliminary study demonstrated a significant frequency of α-thalassemia 1 trait, β-thalassemia trait, and Hb E-related disorders in Southern Thai blood donors and revealed similar pattern with lower frequencies in general population because of exclusion criteria of blood donors. To provide the safety of both blood donors and recipients, the screening of thalassemia and Hb E in blood donors was recommended in highly prevalent countries. Both quantitative and qualitative measurements of red blood cells were suggested before transfusing to the patients with red blood cell disorders such as regularly transfused β-thalassemia patients. The data obtained from this study also provide useful information for the prevention and control program of thalassemia in Southern Thai blood donors. Additional samples are required to support the importance of the hemoglobinopathy screening and to validate the prevalence of thalassemia and Hb E in blood donors.

Conflict of Interests

The authors declare that there is no conflict of interests regarding the publication of this paper.

Acknowledgments

The authors are grateful to all blood donors who participated in this study and they thank Miss Chadaporn Jutichob, Miss Amornrat Ruangtong, and Miss Parichart Detpichai and Blood Donation Units of Suratthani Hospital, Trang Hospital, Chumphon Hospital, Phatthalung Hospital, and Krabi Hospital for their kind support in contacting subjects. This work was supported by the National Blood Centre Thai Red Cross Society, Thailand, and the Center for Scientific and Technological Equipment, Walailak University, Thailand.

References

[1] S. Fucharoen and P. Winichagoon, "Thalassemia and abnormal hemoglobin," *International Journal of Hematology*, vol. 76, supplement 2, pp. 83–89, 2002.

[2] S. Fucharoen, P. Winichagoon, N. Siritanaratkul, J. Chowthaworn, and P. Pootrakul, "α- and β-thalassemia in Thailand," *Annals of the New York Academy of Sciences*, vol. 850, pp. 412–414, 1998.

[3] P. Wasi, S. Na-Nakorn, S. Pootrakul et al., "α- and β-thalassemia in Thailand," *Annals of the New York Academy of Sciences*, vol. 165, no. 1, pp. 60–82, 1969.

[4] S. Fucharoen and P. Winichagoon, "Hemoglobinopathies in Southeast Asia," *Hemoglobin*, vol. 11, no. 1, pp. 65–88, 1987.

[5] S. Fucharoen and P. Winichagoon, "Thalassemia in Southeast Asia: problems and strategy for prevention and control," *The Southeast Asian Journal of Tropical Medicine and Public Health*, vol. 23, no. 4, pp. 647–655, 1992.

[6] S. Fucharoen, P. Winichagoon, R. Wisedpanichkij et al., "Prenatal and postnatal diagnoses of thalassemias and hemoglobinopathies by HPLC," *Clinical Chemistry*, vol. 44, no. 4, pp. 740–748, 1998.

[7] A. Chaibunruang, S. Prommetta, S. Yamsri et al., "Molecular and hematological studies in a large cohort of α^0-thalassemia inNortheast Thailand: data from a single referral center," *Blood Cells, Molecules, & Diseases*, vol. 51, no. 2, pp. 89–93, 2013.

[8] V. Viprakasit, C. Limwongse, S. Sukpanichnant et al., "Problems in determining thalassemia carrier status in a program for prevention and control of severe thalassemia syndromes: a lesson from Thailand," *Clinical Chemistry and Laboratory Medicine*, vol. 51, no. 8, pp. 1605–1614, 2013.

[9] M. E. Brecher, *Technical Manual*, American Association of Blood Banks, Bethesda, Md, USA, 15th edition, 2005.

[10] L. P. Meena, K. Kumar, V. K. Singh, A. Bharti, S. K. H. Rahman, and K. Tripathi, "Study of mutations in β-thalassemia trait among blood donors in Eastern Uttar Pradesh," *Journal of Clinical and Diagnostic Research*, vol. 7, no. 7, pp. 1394–1396, 2013.

[11] V. K. Meena, K. Kumar, L. P. Meena et al., "Screening for Hemoglobinopathies in blood donors from Eastern Uttar Pradesh, India," *National Journal of Medical Research*, vol. 2, no. 3, pp. 366–368, 2012.

[12] H. Rosline, S. A. Ahmed, F. S. Al-Joudi, M. Rapiaah, N. N. Naing, and N. A. M. Adam, "Thalassemia among blood donors at the Hospital Universiti Sains Malaysia," *The Southeast Asian Journal of Tropical Medicine and Public Health*, vol. 37, no. 3, pp. 549–552, 2006.

[13] C. L. Lisot and L. M. Silla, "Screening for hemoglobinopathies in blood donors from Caxias do Sul, Rio Grande do Sul, Brazil:

prevalence in an Italian colony," *Cadernos de Saúde Pública*, vol. 20, no. 6, pp. 1595–1601, 2004.

[14] C. T. Acquaye, J. H. Oldham, and F. I. Konotey Ahulu, "Blood donor homozygous for hereditary persistence of fetal haemoglobin," *The Lancet*, vol. 1, no. 8015, pp. 796–797, 1977.

[15] F. Farzana, S. J. Zuberi, and J. A. Hashmi, "Prevalence of abnormal hemoglobins and thalassemia trait in a group of professional blood donors and hospital staff in Karachi," *Journal of the Pakistan Medical Association*, vol. 25, no. 9, pp. 237–239, 1975.

[16] S. S. Chong, C. D. Boehm, G. R. Cutting, and D. R. Higgs, "Simplified multiplex-PCR diagnosis of common Southeast Asian deletional determinants of α-thalassemia," *Clinical Chemistry*, vol. 46, no. 10, pp. 1692–1695, 2000.

[17] M. Lemmens-Zygulska, A. Eigel, B. Helbig, T. Sanguansermsri, J. Horst, and G. Flatz, "Prevalence of α-thalassemias in Northern Thailand," *Human Genetics*, vol. 98, no. 3, pp. 345–347, 1996.

[18] V. Tienthavorn, J. Pattanapongsthorn, S. Charoensak et al., "Prevalence of thalassemia carrier in Thailand," *Thai Journal of Hematology and Transfusion Medicine*, vol. 16, no. 4, pp. 307–312, 2006.

[19] S. Yamsri, K. Sanchaisuriya, G. Fucharoen, N. Sae-ung, and S. Fucharoen, "Genotype and phenotype characterizations in a large cohort of β-thalassemia heterozygote with different forms of α-thalassemia in Northeast Thailand," *Blood Cells, Molecules, & Diseases*, vol. 47, no. 2, pp. 120–124, 2011.

[20] N. Sae-ung, H. Srivorakun, G. Fucharoen, S. Yamsri, K. Sanchaisuriya, and S. Fucharoen, "Phenotypic expression of hemoglobins A_2, E and F in various hemoglobin E related disorders," *Blood Cells, Molecules, & Diseases*, vol. 48, no. 1, pp. 11–16, 2012.

[21] A. Casado, M. C. Casado, M. E. Lopez-Fernandez, and D. Venarucci, "Thalassemia and G6PD deficiency in Spanish blood donors," *Panminerva Medica*, vol. 39, no. 3, pp. 205–207, 1997.

[22] A. K. Tiwari and I. Chandola, "Comparing prevalence of iron deficiency anemia and beta thalassemia trait in microcytic and non-microcytic blood donors: suggested algorithm for donor screening," *Asian Journal of Transfusion Science*, vol. 3, no. 2, pp. 99–102, 2009.

[23] M. K. Alabdulaali, K. M. Alayed, A. F. Alshaikh, and S. A. Almashhadani, "Prevalence of glucose-6-phosphate dehydrogenase deficiency and sickle cell trait among blood donors in Riyadh," *Asian Journal of Transfusion Science*, vol. 4, no. 1, pp. 31–33, 2010.

[24] B. J. Bryant, J. A. Hopkins, S. M. Arceo, and S. F. Leitman, "Evaluation of low red blood cell mean corpuscular volume in an apheresis donor population," *Transfusion*, vol. 49, no. 9, pp. 1971–1976, 2009.

[25] H. D. Alexander, J. P. Sherlock, and C. Bharucha, "Red cell indices as predictors of iron depletion in blood donors," *Clinical and Laboratory Haematology*, vol. 22, no. 5, pp. 253–258, 2000.

[26] D. Maffi, M. T. Pasquino, L. Mandarino et al., "Glucose-6-phosphate dehydrogenase deficiency in Italian blood donors: prevalence and molecular defect characterization," *Vox Sanguinis*, vol. 106, no. 3, pp. 227–233, 2013.

[27] R. O. Francis, J. Jhang, J. E. Hendrickson, J. C. Zimring, E. A. Hod, and S. L. Spitalnik, "Frequency of glucose-6-phosphate dehydrogenase-deficient red blood cell units in a metropolitan transfusion service," *Transfusion*, vol. 53, no. 3, pp. 606–611, 2013.

[28] R. O. Francis, J. S. Jhang, H. P. Pham, E. A. Hod, J. C. Zimring, and S. L. Spitalnik, "Glucose-6-phosphate dehydrogenase deficiency in transfusion medicine: the unknown risks," *Vox Sanguinis*, vol. 105, no. 4, pp. 271–282, 2013.

[29] S. W. Eber, A. Pekrun, A. Neufeldt, and W. Schroter, "Prevalence of increased osmotic fragility of erythrocytes in German blood donors: screening using a modified glycerol lysis test," *Annals of Hematology*, vol. 64, no. 2, pp. 88–92, 1992.

[30] M. Goldman, S. Uzicanin, V. Scalia, and S. F. O'Brien, "Iron deficiency in Canadian blood donors," *Transfusion*, vol. 54, no. 3, part 2, pp. 775–779, 2013.

[31] C. Y. Mantilla-Gutierrez and J. A. Cardona-Arias, "Iron deficiency prevalence in blood donors: a systematic review, 2001–2011," *Revista Española de Salud Pública*, vol. 86, no. 4, pp. 357–369, 2012.

[32] A. Jaovisidha, S. Ajjimarkorn, P. Panburana, O. Somboonsub, Y. Herabutya, and R. Rungsiprakarn, "Prevention and control of thalassemia in Ramathibodi Hospital, Thailand," *The Southeast Asian Journal of Tropical Medicine and Public Health*, vol. 31, no. 3, pp. 561–565, 2000.

[33] S. Fucharoen, P. Winichagoon, V. Thonglairoam et al., "Prenatal diagnosis of thalassemia and hemoglobinopathies in Thailand: experience from 100 pregnancies," *The Southeast Asian Journal of Tropical Medicine and Public Health*, vol. 22, no. 1, pp. 16–29, 1991.

[34] O. Kor-anantakul, C. T. Suwanrath, R. Leetanaporn, T. Suntharasaj, T. Liabsuetrakul, and R. Rattanaprueksachart, "Prenatal diagnosis of thalassemia in Songklanagarind Hospital in Southern Thailand," *The Southeast Asian Journal of Tropical Medicine and Public Health*, vol. 29, no. 4, pp. 795–800, 1998.

Permissions

The contributors of this book come from diverse backgrounds, making this book a truly international effort. This book will bring forth new frontiers with its revolutionizing research information and detailed analysis of the nascent developments around the world.

We would like to thank all the contributing authors for lending their expertise to make the book truly unique. They have played a crucial role in the development of this book. Without their invaluable contributions this book wouldn't have been possible. They have made vital efforts to compile up to date information on the varied aspects of this subject to make this book a valuable addition to the collection of many professionals and students.

This book was conceptualized with the vision of imparting up-to-date information and advanced data in this field. To ensure the same, a matchless editorial board was set up. Every individual on the board went through rigorous rounds of assessment to prove their worth. After which they invested a large part of their time researching and compiling the most relevant data for our readers.

The editorial board has been involved in producing this book since its inception. They have spent rigorous hours researching and exploring the diverse topics which have resulted in the successful publishing of this book. They have passed on their knowledge of decades through this book. To expedite this challenging task, the publisher supported the team at every step. A small team of assistant editors was also appointed to further simplify the editing procedure and attain best results for the readers.

Apart from the editorial board, the designing team has also invested a significant amount of their time in understanding the subject and creating the most relevant covers. They scrutinized every image to scout for the most suitable representation of the subject and create an appropriate cover for the book.

The publishing team has been an ardent support to the editorial, designing and production team. Their endless efforts to recruit the best for this project, has resulted in the accomplishment of this book. They are a veteran in the field of academics and their pool of knowledge is as vast as their experience in printing. Their expertise and guidance has proved useful at every step. Their uncompromising quality standards have made this book an exceptional effort. Their encouragement from time to time has been an inspiration for everyone.

The publisher and the editorial board hope that this book will prove to be a valuable piece of knowledge for researchers, students, practitioners and scholars across the globe.

List of Contributors

Irina Tukan, Irith Hadas-Halpern, Ayala Abrahamov, Deborah Elstein and Ari Zimran
Shaare Zedek Medical Center, Affiliated to the Hadassah-Hebrew University School of Medicine, Ein Karem 91031, Israel University School of Medicine, Ein Karem 91031, Israel

Gheona Altarescu
Gaucher Clinic and Preimplantation Genetics Unit, Shaare Zedek Medical Center, Affiliated to the Hadassah-Hebrew

Arunima Ghosh and Colin A. Kretz
Life Sciences Institute, University of Michigan, Ann Arbor, MI 48109, USA

Andy Vo, Beverly K. Twiss and Jordan A. Shavit
Department of Pediatrics, University of Michigan, Room 8301 Medical Science Research Building III,1150 W. Medical Center Drive, Ann Arbor, MI 48109-5646, USA

Mary A. Jozwiak and Robert R. Montgomery
Blood Research Institute, Medical College of Wisconsin, Milwaukee, WI 53226, USA

Priyanka Saxena and Chhagan Bihari
Department of Hematology, Institute of Liver and Biliary Sciences, D-1, Vasant Kunj, New Delhi 110070, India

Archana Rastogi and Savita Agarwal
Department of Pathology, Institute of Liver and Biliary Sciences, D-1, Vasant Kunj, New Delhi 110070, India

Lovkesh Anand and Shiv Kumar Sarin
Department of Hepatology, Institute of Liver and Biliary Sciences, D-1, Vasant Kunj, New Delhi 110070, India

N. Abdel Karim and C. Siegrist
Department of Internal Medicine, University of Cincinnati College of Medicine, Cincinnati, OH 45267, USA
Division of Hematology and Oncology, University of Cincinnati College of Medicine, 231 Albert Sabin Way, Cincinnati, OH 45267, USA

S. Haider and N. Ahmad
Department of Internal Medicine, University of Cincinnati College of Medicine, Cincinnati, OH 45267, USA

A. Zarzour
Division of Hematology and Oncology, University of Cincinnati College of Medicine, 231 Albert Sabin Way, Cincinnati, OH 45267, USA

J. Ying
Department of Environmental Health, University of Cincinnati College of Medicine, Cincinnati, OH 45267, USA

Z. Yasin
Department of Hematology and Oncology, Baylor College of Medicine, Houston, TX 76706, USA

R. Sacher
Department of Internal Medicine, University of Cincinnati College of Medicine, Cincinnati, OH 45267, USA
Division of Hematology and Oncology, University of Cincinnati College of Medicine, 231 Albert Sabin Way, Cincinnati, OH 45267, USA
Hoxworth Blood Center, University of Cincinnati College of Medicine, Cincinnati, OH 45267, USA

Zeina Al-Mansour and Muthalagu Ramanathan
Division of Hematology/Oncology, School ofMedicine, University ofMassachusetts, 55 Lake Avenue North,Worcester, MA 01655, USA

Diebkilé Aïssata Tolo, Duni Sawadogo, Danho Clotaire Nanho, Boidy Kouakou, N'DogomoMéité, Roméo Ayémou, Paul Kouéhion, Mozart Konan, Yassongui Mamadou Sékongo, Emeraude N'Dhatz, Ismaël Kamara, Alexis Silué, Kouassi Gustave Koffi and Ibrahima Sanogo
Department of Clinical Hematology, Yopougon Teaching Hospital, P.O. Box 632, Abidjan 21, Cote d'Ivoire

Katerina Sarris, DimitriosMaltezas, Efstathios Koulieris, Vassiliki Bartzis,Tatiana Tzenou, Sotirios Sachanas, Eftychia Nikolaou, Anna Efthymiou, Katerina Bitsani, Maria Dimou, Theodoros P. Vassilakopoulos, Marina Siakantaris, Maria K. Angelopoulou, Flora Kontopidou, Panagiotis Tsaftaridis, Gerasimos A. Pangalis, Panayiotis P. Panayiotidis and Marie-Christine Kyrtsonis
Hematology Section of the First Department of Propedeutic Internal Medicine, Laikon University Hospital, Agiou Thoma 17, 11527 Athens, Greece

Nikolitsa Kafasi
Immunology Department, Laikon General Hospital, Agiou Thoma 17, 11527 Athens, Greece

Stephen Harding
The Binding Site Ltd, B15 1QT, Birmingham, UK

Ethan A. Natelson
Professor of Clinical Medicine, Weill-Cornell Medical School and Director, Transitional Residency Program, Houston Methodist Hospital, 6550 Fannin Street, Suite 1001, Houston, TX 77030, USA

David Pyatt
Summit Toxicology, LLP, 1944 Cedaridge Circle, Superior, CO 80026, USA
Schools of Pharmacy and Public Health, The University of Colorado, Denver, CO 80026, USA

Ram Babu Undi, Ravinder Kandi and Ravi Kumar Gutti
Hematologic Oncology, Stem Cells and Blood Disorders Laboratory, Department of Biochemistry, School of Life Sciences, University of Hyderabad, Gachibowli, Hyderabad, Andhra Pradesh 500046, India

Radhika N. Shah, Shila K. Nordone and Jeffrey A. Yoder
Department of Molecular Biomedical Sciences and Center for Comparative Medicine and Translational Research, College of Veterinary Medicine, North Carolina State University, 1060 William Moore Drive, Raleigh, NC 27607, USA
Immunology Program, College of Veterinary Medicine, North Carolina State University, 1060 William Moore Drive, Raleigh, NC 27607, USA

Ivan Rodriguez-Nunez
Department of Molecular Biomedical Sciences and Center for Comparative Medicine and Translational Research, College of Veterinary Medicine, North Carolina State University, 1060 William Moore Drive, Raleigh, NC 27607, USA

Donna D. Eason
Children's Research Institute, Department of Pediatrics, University of South Florida College of Medicine, 140 Seventh Avenue South, St. Petersburg, FL 33701, USA
Immunology Program, H. Lee Moffitt Cancer Center and Research Institute, 12902 Magnolia Avenue, Tampa, FL 33612, USA

Robert N. Haire
Children's Research Institute, Department of Pediatrics, University of South Florida College of Medicine, 140 Seventh Avenue South, St. Petersburg, FL 33701, USA

Julien Y. Bertrand
Department of Pathology and Immunology, University of Geneva School of Medicine, Rue Michel-Servet 1, 1211 Geneva 4, Switzerland

Valērie Wittamer and David Traver
Department of Cellular and Molecular Medicine and Section of Cell and Developmental Biology, University of California at San Diego, 9500 Gilman Drive, La Jolla, CA 92093-0380, USA

Gary W. Litman
Children's Research Institute, Department of Pediatrics, University of South Florida College of Medicine, 140 Seventh Avenue South, St. Petersburg, FL 33701, USA
Immunology Program, H. Lee Moffitt Cancer Center and Research Institute, 12902 Magnolia Avenue, Tampa, FL 33612, USA
Department of Molecular Genetics, All Children's Hospital, 501 Sixth Avenue South, St. Petersburg, FL 33701, USA

Divjot Singh Lamba, Ravneet Kaur and Sabita Basu
Department of Transfusion Medicine, Block D, Level II, Government Medical College & Hospital, Chandigarh 160030, India

Sandra Malak
Hematology Department of the René Huguenin Hospital, Institut Curie, 35 rue Dailly, 92210 Saint-Cloud, France
Ethics Commission of the French Society of Hematology, France

Jean-Jacques Sotto
Ethics Commission of the French Society of Hematology, France
Hematology Department of the University of Grenoble, 38043 Grenoble, France

Joël Ceccaldi
Ethics Commission of the French Society of Hematology, France
Hematology Department of the Robert Boulin Hospital, 33505 Libourne, France

Philippe Colombat
Ethics Commission of the French Society of Hematology, France
Hematology Department of the University of Tours, 37044 Tours, France

Philippe Casassus
Ethics Commission of the French Society of Hematology, France
Hematology Department of the University of Bobigny, 93000 Bobigny, France

Dominique Jaulmes
Ethics Commission of the French Society of Hematology, France
Hematology Department of the University of Saint-Antoine, 75012 Paris, France

Henri Rochant
Ethics Commission of the French Society of Hematology, France
Hematology Department of the University of Créteil, 94010 Créteil, France

Morgane Cheminant
Ethics Commission of the French Society of Hematology, France
Hematology Department of the University of Necker, 75015 Paris, France

Yvan Beaussant
Ethics Commission of the French Society of Hematology, France
Hematology Department of the University of Besanc¸on, 25030 Besanc¸on, France

Robert Zittoun
Ethics Commission of the French Society of Hematology, France
Hematology Department of the Hôtel-Dieu Hospital, 75001 Paris, France

Dominique Bordessoule
Ethics Commission of the French Society of Hematology, France
Hematology Department of the University of Limoges, 87042 Limoges, France

Tariq Helal Ashour
Department of Laboratory Medicine, Faculty of Applied Medical Sciences, Umm Al-Qura University, P.O. Box 7607, Makkah 7152, Saudi Arabia

Abeer Ibrahim
Department of Medical Oncology and Hematological Malignancy, South Egypt Cancer Institute, Assiut University, El Methaq Street, Assiut, Egypt

Amany Ali and Mahmoud M. Mohammed
Department of Pediatrics Oncology and Hematological Malignancy, South Egypt Cancer Institute, Assiut University, Egypt

Annelise Pezzi, Vanessa Valim, Bruna Amorin and Maria Aparecida da Silva
Cellular Therapy Center, Center for Experimental Research, Hospital de Clinicas de Porto Alegre,90035-903 Porto Alegre, RS, Brazil
Postgraduate Course of Medical Sciences, Federal University of Rio Grande do Sul, 90035-903 Porto Alegre, RS, Brazil
Laboratory of Cell Culture and Molecular Analysis of Hematopoietic Cells, Center for Experimental Research, Hospital de Clínicas de Porto Alegre, 2350 Ramiro Barcelos, 90035-903 Porto Alegre, RS, Brazil

Fernanda Oliveira, LauroMoraes and Gabriela Melchiades
Cellular Therapy Center, Center for Experimental Research, Hospital de Clinicas de Porto Alegre,90035-903 Porto Alegre, RS, Brazil

Ursula Matte
Gene Therapy Center, Center for Experimental Research, Hospital de Clinicas de Porto Alegre, 90035-903 Porto Alegre, RS, Brazil

Maria S. Pombo-de-Oliveira
Pediatric Hematology and Oncology Program, Research Center, Instituto Nacional de Câncer, 20230-130 Rio de Janeiro, RJ, Brazil

Rosane Bittencourt and Liane Daudt
Hematology and Bone Marrow Transplantation, Hospital de Clinicas de Porto Alegre, 90035-903 Porto Alegre, RS, Brazil

Lúcia Silla
Cellular Therapy Center, Center for Experimental Research, Hospital de Clinicas de Porto Alegre,90035-903 Porto Alegre, RS, Brazil
Postgraduate Course of Medical Sciences, Federal University of Rio Grande do Sul, 90035-903 Porto Alegre, RS, Brazil
Hematology and Bone Marrow Transplantation, Hospital de Clinicas de Porto Alegre, 90035-903 Porto Alegre, RS, Brazil
Laboratory of Cell Culture and Molecular Analysis of Hematopoietic Cells, Center for Experimental Research, Hospital de Clínicas de Porto Alegre, 2350 Ramiro Barcelos, 90035-903 Porto Alegre, RS, Brazil

Winnie WY Ip
Molecular Immunology Unit, UCL Institute of Child Health, 30 Guildford Street, LondonWC1N 1EH, UK

Waseem Qasim
Molecular Immunology Unit, UCL Institute of Child Health, 30 Guildford Street, LondonWC1N 1EH, UK
Department of Clinical Immunology, Great Ormond Street Hospital, LondonWC1N 3JH, UK

La'Teese Hall, Sarah J. Murrey, and Arthur S. Brecher
Department of Chemistry, Bowling Green State University, Bowling Green, OH 43403, USA

Wai-Yoong Ng and Chin-Pin Yeo
Department of Pathology, Clinical Biochemistry Laboratories, Singapore General Hospital, Outram Road, Singapore 169608

Emmanuelle Dugas-Bourdages and Robert Delage
Centre Universitaire d'Hématologie et d'Oncologie de Québec, CHU de Québec, Hôpital de l'Enfant-Jésus, 1401 18iéme rue, Québec, QC, Canada G1J 1Z4

Sonia Néron
Héma-Québec, Recherche et Développement, 1070 avenue des Sciences-de-la-Vie, Québec, QC, Canada G1V 5C3
Département de Biochimie, de Microbiologie et de Bio-Informatique, Pavillon Alexandre-Vachon, 1045 avenue de la Médecine, Bureau 3428, Université Laval, Québec, QC, Canada G1V 0A6

Annie Roy
Héma-Québec, Recherche et Développement, 1070 avenue des Sciences-de-la-Vie, Québec, QC, Canada G1V 5C3

André Darveau
Département de Biochimie, de Microbiologie et de Bio-Informatique, Pavillon Alexandre-Vachon, 1045 avenue de la Médecine, Bureau 3428, Université Laval, Québec, QC, Canada G1V 0A6

Shamsuz Zaman, Rahul Chaurasia, Kabita Chatterjee, and Rakesh Mohan Thapliyal
Department of Transfusion Medicine, All India Institute of Medical Sciences, New Delhi 110029, India

Carlos Eduardo Coral de Oliveira, Patricia Midori Murobushi Ozawa, Carlos Hiroki, Glauco Akelinghton Freire Vitiello, Roberta Losi Guembarovski and Maria Angelica Ehara Watanabe
Laboratory of Study and Application of DNA Polymorphisms, Department of Pathological Sciences, Biological Sciences Center, State University of Londrina, Rodovia Celso Garcia Cid, (PR 445), Km 380, 86051-970 Londrina, PR, Brazil

Marla Karine Amarante and Aparecida de Lourdes Perim
Laboratory of Hematology, Department of Pathology, Clinical and Toxicological Analysis, Health Sciences Center, State University of Londrina, Londrina, PR, Brazil

Ademola Samson Adewoyin and Jude Chike Obieche
Department of Haematology and Blood Transfusion, University of Benin Teaching Hospital, PMB 1111, Benin City, Edo State, Nigeria

Tolo Diebkilé Aïssata, Clotaire Nanho, Boidy Kouakou, N'dogomoMeité, N'Dhatz Emeuraude, Ayémou Roméo, Sekongo Yassongui Mamadou, Paul Kouéhion, KonanMozart, Gustave Koffi, and Ibrahima Sanogo
Department of Clinical Hematology, Yopougon Teaching Hospital, P.O. Box 632, Abidjan 21, Cote d'Ivoire

Duni Sawadogo
Department of Biological Hematology, Yopougon Teaching Hospital, P.O. Box 632, Abidjan 21, Cote d'Ivoire

Steven M. Prideaux, Emma Conway O'Brien and Timothy J. Chevassut
Brighton and Sussex Medical School, Sussex University, Falmer, Brighton BN1 9PS, UK

Nnamani Nnenna Adaeze and Emmanuel K. Uko
Department of Medical Laboratory Science (Haematology and Blood Group Serology Unit), University of Calabar, PMB 1115, Calabar, Cross River State, Nigeria

Anthony Uchenna Emeribe
Department of Chemical Pathology, University of Abuja Teaching Hospital, PMB 228, Gwagwalada, Abuja, Nigeria

Idris Abdullahi Nasiru
Department of Medical Microbiology, University of Abuja Teaching Hospital, PMB 228, Gwagwalada, Abuja, Nigeria

Adamu Babayo
Department of Medical Laboratory Science, University of Maiduguri, PMB 1069, Maiduguri, Nigeria

Paola Villafuerte-Gutierrez
Hospital Universitario Torrejón de Ardoz, Servicio de Hematología, Calle Mateo Inurria, 28850 Madrid, Spain

Lucia Villalon
Hospital Universitario Fundación Alcorcón, Servicio de Hematología, Calle Budapest 1, 28922 Madrid, Spain

Juan E. Losa and Cesar Henriquez-Camacho
Unidad de Medicina Interna, Sección de Enfermedades Infecciosas, Hospital Universitario Fundación Alcorcón, Calle Budapest 1, 28922 Madrid, Spain

Abuzar Elnager, Wan Zaidah Abdullah and Rosline Hassan
Department of Haematology, School of Medical Sciences, Universiti Sains Malaysia, Health Campus,16150 Kubang Kerian, Kelantan, Malaysia

Zamzuri Idris and Zulkifli Mustafa
Department of Neurosciences, School of Medical Sciences, Universiti Sains Malaysia, Health Campus,16150 Kubang Kerian, Kelantan, Malaysia

Nadiah Wan Arfah
Unit of Biostatistics and Research Methodology, School of Medical Sciences, Universiti Sains Malaysia, Health Campus, 16150 Kubang Kerian, Kelantan, Malaysia

S. A. Sulaiman
Department of Pharmacology, School of Medical Sciences, Universiti Sains Malaysia, Health Campus,16150 Kubang Kerian, Kelantan, Malaysia

Felix Nwajei
Department of Immunology, The University of Texas MD Anderson Cancer Center, 1515 Holcombe Boulevard, Unit 0902, Houston, TX 77030, USA
Graduate School of Biomedical Sciences, The University of Texas Health Science Center at Houston, 6767 Bertner Avenue, 3rd Floor, Houston, TX 77030, USA

Marina Konopleva
Department of Leukemia, The University of Texas MD Anderson Cancer Center, 1515 Holcombe Boulevard, Unit 428, Houston, TX 77030, USA

Amanda J. Moore and Michele K. Anderson
Division of Biological Sciences, Sunnybrook Research Institute, 2075 Bayview Avenue, Toronto, ON, Canada M4N 3M5
Department of Immunology, University of Toronto, Toronto, ON, Canada M5S 1A8

Manit Nuinoon and Warachaya Sengking
School of Allied Health Sciences and Public Health,Walailak University, Nakhon Si Thammarat 80161, Thailand

Kwanta Kruachan and Ubol Sungyuan
Regional Blood Centre XI, National Blood Centre Thai Red Cross Society, Nakhon Si Thammarat 80110, Thailand

Dararat Horpet
Center for Scientific and Technological Equipment, Walailak University, Nakhon Si Thammarat 80161, Thailand